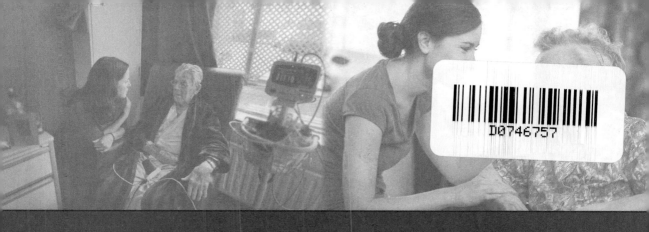

Nursing as Ministry

Kristen L. Mauk, PhD, DNP, RN, CRRN, GCNS-BC, GNP-BC, FAAN

Professor of Nursing
Graduate Program Director
Colorado Christian University
Lakewood, Colorado
President
Senior Care Central/International
　Rehabilitation Consultants, LLC
Ridgway, Colorado

Mary E. Hobus, PhD, MSN, RN

Professor of Nursing
Assistant Director of Nursing,
　Western Colorado
Colorado Christian University
Lakewood, Colorado

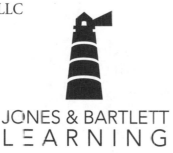

JONES & BARTLETT
LEARNING

World Headquarters
Jones & Bartlett Learning
5 Wall Street
Burlington, MA 01803
978-443-5000
info@jblearning.com
www.jblearning.com

Jones & Bartlett Learning books and products are available through most bookstores and online booksellers. To contact Jones & Bartlett Learning directly, call 800-832-0034, fax 978-443-8000, or visit our website, www.jblearning.com.

Substantial discounts on bulk quantities of Jones & Bartlett Learning publications are available to corporations, professional associations, and other qualified organizations. For details and specific discount information, contact the special sales department at Jones & Bartlett Learning via the above contact information or send an email to specialsales@jblearning.com.

21358-4

Production Credits
VP, Product Management: Amanda Martin
Director of Product Management: Matthew Kane
Product Manager: Tina Chen
Product Specialist: Christina Freitas
Project Specialist: Kelly Sylvester
Project Specialist, Navigate: Kathryn Leeber
Digital Project Specialist: Rachel Reyes
Senior Marketing Manager: Jennifer Scherzay
Product Fulfillment Manager: Wendy Kilborn

Composition: S4Carlisle Publishing Services
Cover Design: Michael O'Donnell
Media Development Editor: Troy Liston
Rights Specialist: John Rusk
Cover Images: © ChameleonsEye/Shutterstock;
 © Alexander Raths/Shutterstock; © Asiseeit/Getty
 Images; © Laflor/Getty Images
Printing and Binding: McNaughton & Gunn
Cover Printing: McNaughton & Gunn

Library of Congress Cataloging-in-Publication Data
Names: Mauk, Kristen L., editor. | Hobus, Mary E., editor.
Title: Nursing as ministry / [edited by] Kristen L. Mauk, Mary Hobus.
Description: Burlington, Massachusetts : Jones & Bartlett Learning, [2021] |
Includes bibliographical references.
Identifiers: LCCN 2019015791 | ISBN 9781284170344 (paperback)
Subjects: | MESH: Parish Nursing | Christianity | Spirituality
Classification: LCC RT51 | NLM WY 86.5 | DDC 610.69--dc23
LC record available at https://lccn.loc.gov/2019015791

6048

Printed in the United States of America
23 22 21 20 19   10 9 8 7 6 5 4 3 2 1

To my husband, Jim, and our many children for their love and support: Rachel and Jim, Kenny and Jen, Dan, Beth and Scott, Jordon, Vika, Daniel, and JJ. To my sweet grandchildren, who give balance and happiness to my life.

To my Mom, Kay Gibson, for being my first example of nursing as ministry in our home and to others.

And finally, to Christian nurses everywhere who are called to nursing as ministry and embrace the work that God has for them.

Kristen L. Mauk

This book is dedicated to my Heavenly Father for graciously answering so many prayers as a registered nurse caring for His children.

To my lovely husband, Steven, and our children and their spouses: Amanda and Bryan, Andrew and Nicole, and Isaiah and Erica, who graciously supported and actively listened through my challenges as a Christian nurse and following God's plan. To my grandchildren, who bring joy and laughter to my life daily.

And finally, to all the colleagues who have been so very faithful, supportive, and courageous to follow God's plan and do His will to bring glory to His name.

Mary E. Hobus

Acknowledgments

The editors give our thanks to colleagues, friends, and family who supported us through this process. We would also like to thank the nursing faculty and leadership at Colorado Christian University for their contributions to this project.

Contents

UNIT I Foundations of Nursing as Ministry   1

UNIT II   The Nursing Process and Ministry   91

UNIT III   Preparing for Nursing as Ministry   143

Chapter 11 Spiritual Gifts in Nursing Ministry 191

UNIT IV Nursing as Ministry at Home and Abroad   211

Chapter 12 Caring for Vulnerable Older Adults Across Settings 213

Chapter 13 Nursing as Ministry for Those in Prison 247

Chapter 14 Poverty and Homelessness 263

UNIT V Developing a Personal Commitment to Nursing as Ministry   343

Preface

*N*ursing as Ministry is targeted at nursing students in faith-based colleges and universities and is intended to serve as a fundamental text to be used in a single course or threaded through the curriculum. It can also be useful to faith-community nurses and to any nurse who wants to practice from a Christian worldview. The purpose of this work is to provide the foundations of Christian nursing as ministry.

This text is distinguished from other books by its pedagogical features, which include Clinical Reasoning Exercises, interviews with nurse leaders, Personal Reflection Exercises, case studies, key points, web-based resources, and suggestions for integrating faith into daily nursing care. Additionally, the work is unique in its edited approach, which incorporates insights from authors from theology, history, nursing, medicine, social work, and pastoral ministry to give a more interprofessional perspective. Collectively, these authors represent academe, research, bedside care, consulting, patient education, church ministry, and mission and global work.

The rationale for developing *Nursing as Ministry* was to fill an identified gap in the market. The editors have worked at faith-based institutions for many years, and they well recognized the need for a contemporary text that was both student friendly and aimed at nursing students in religious universities. Aside from a few classic works, evidence-based textbooks are generally lacking that might provide a foundation for students in Christian or faith-based nursing programs.

This book is divided into logical sections. Unit I discusses the foundation of nursing as ministry, including its historical background, the concept of divine appointments, models for nursing care, and what it means to be a Christian nurse. In Unit II, the nursing process is used to help students and nurses assess, plan, intervene, and evaluate patients from a Biblical worldview. Unit III focuses on understanding the philosophical basis of nursing as ministry, including ways to talk to persons of different worldviews or faiths and how to use one's spiritual gifts. Unit IV presents nursing as ministry at home and abroad, covering unique topics such as working with vulnerable elders, individuals in prison, the poor and homeless, and persons with substance abuse issues; mass disasters; and end-of-life care. Lastly, Unit V focuses on developing a personal commitment to nursing as ministry. This unit includes chapters on caring for one's spiritual self, caring and mentoring others, and Christian-based leadership.

The text has a user-friendly and comprehensive format, with features designed to appeal to today's students. The following pedagogical features enhance students' learning:

- Learning objectives
- Key terms list (with terms highlighted in chapter)
- Tables that summarize key points
- Boxes to highlight interesting information and key practice points
- Pictures, diagrams, and drawings
- Original photographs and figures

- Outstanding Nurse Leader interviews/profiles with photos
- Research Highlights with application to practice
- Evidence-Based Practice features and guidelines
- Clinical Reasoning Exercises
- Personal Reflection Exercises
- Case Studies with questions
- References
- Recommended Readings (including websites)
- Glossary

Students will be delighted to be able to refer to a glossary at the end of the text, as well as to see definitions of key terms immediately on their use within the chapters. Students will also benefit from new online resources and educational materials available from the publisher.

Instructors will find the accompanying online Instructor's Manual to be a time-saving tool. It is designed to provide a complete curriculum for instructors and students, including those who may lack a strong faith-based background. The Instructor's Manual suggests activities for learning and in-class exercises and provides PowerPoint slides for lectures that correspond to student readings in the main text. A Test Bank is also provided. Thus, most of the work of developing a nursing course or integrating portions of it into the curriculum has already been done for instructors.

Foreword

Spiritual care is an essential component of nursing best-practice standards in all settings, but often nurses are not adequately prepared to provide spiritual care, and current educational resources are scarce. For faith community nurses, whose specialty practice focuses on the intentional care of the spirit, finding high-quality educational resources is a struggle internationally. As an educator for both mainstream nursing and faith community nursing practice with a Doctor of Ministry in Global Health and Wholeness, I am excited to find that *Nursing as Ministry* has been compiled to fill the gap between classics, such as Shelly and Miller's 2006 *Called to Care: A Christian Worldview for Nursing*, and the current need for updated nursing spiritual care materials that address the issues and special needs populations of today's nursing practice.

Nursing as Ministry provides perspectives from 29 interprofessional experts focusing on the relationship of nursing and ministry in a user-friendly format with many added beneficial features for both the participant and the instructor. Inclusions such as personal reflections for each chapter and an instructor manual that includes Power Point slides, test questions, and clinical activities makes this text ideal for incorporating into a wide variety of college-level nursing courses.

Sharon T. Hinton, MSN, RN-BC, DMin
Director, Nursing Division, Spiritual Care
    Association
FCN National Project Manager, Westberg
    Institute for Faith Community Nursing
Author, "Nursing in the Church: Insights,"
    Journal of Christian Nursing
Memphis, Tennessee

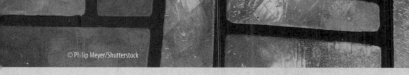

Contributors

Margaret Barnes, DNP, RN, PMHNP-BC
Associate Professor, Post-Licensure Nursing
Indiana Wesleyan University
Marion, Indiana

Anne Biro, MN, RN
ABiro Professional Health Consultancy
Red Deer, Alberta, Canada

Nancy Eckerd, MS, RN
Adjunct Professor
Oklahoma Wesleyan University
Bartlesville, Oklahoma

Alfonso Espinosa, PhD, MDiv, MA
Adjunct Professor of Theology
Saint Paul's Lutheran Church
   of Irvine (LC-MS)
Concordia University
Irvine, California

Kristen J. Goree, DNP, APRN, CNS, FNP-C
Professor of Nursing
Colorado Christian University
Lakewood, Colorado

Kristi Hargrave, MSN, RN
Assistant Professor of Nursing
Colorado Christian University
Lakewood, Colorado

Karen Hessler, PhD, FNP-BC
Professor of Nursing and
   RN-BSN Program Director
Colorado Christian University
Lakewood, Colorado

Mary E. Hobus, PhD, MSN, RN
Professor of Nursing
Assistant Director of Nursing, Western
   Colorado
Colorado Christian University
Grand Junction, Colorado

Steven Hobus, BA, MEd
Principal
Messiah Lutheran Church and School
Grand Junction, Colorado

Tammie L. Huddle, MSN, RN
Assistant Professor of Nursing
Colorado Christian University
Lakewood, Colorado

Cheryl King, MSN, RN, CNS
Assistant Professor of Nursing
Colorado Christian University
Lakewood, Colorado

Luana S. Krieger-Blake, BA, MSW, LCSW
Social Worker (retired)
Hospice of the Visiting Nurse Association
   of Porter County
Valparaiso, Indiana

Becky Le, PhD, RN
Director, Graduate Nursing Program
Oklahoma Wesleyan University
Bartlesville, Oklahoma

Kristen L. Mauk, PhD, DNP, RN, CRRN, GCNS-BC, GNP-BC, FAAN
Professor of Nursing
Graduate Program Director
Colorado Christian University
Lakewood, Colorado
President
Senior Care Central/International
    Rehabilitation Consultants, LLC
Ridgway, Colorado

Jill McElheny, DNP, APRN, CPNP, ENP-BC
Professor of Nursing
Colorado Christian University
Lakewood, Colorado

Eileen Mertens, RN
Registered Nurse (retired)
Delta, Colorado

Rev. Mel Mertens
Minister (retired) and Prison Chaplain
Delta, Colorado

Christina Mulkey, DNP, RN, AGNP-C
Nurse Practitioner
Geriatric and Family Medicine Associates
Wheatridge, Colorado

David Mulkey, DNP, RN, CCRN, CHSE
Nursing Quality Research Specialist
Denver Health
Denver, Colorado

Shirlene Newbanks, DNP, RN
Assistant Dean of Masters in Nursing
    Education and Administration
Associate Faculty
Indiana Wesleyan University
Marion, Indiana

Linda Rieg, PhD, RN, CNE
Professor, Graduate Nursing
Indiana Wesleyan University
Marion, Indiana

Carol Rowley, PhD, RN
Healthcare Educator

John Schreiber, MA, MS, RN
Assistant Professor of Nursing
Colorado Christian University
Lakewood, Colorado

Bob Snyder, MD
President and Founder of IHS Global
Southeastern, Pennsylvania

Tara Stephen, MSN, RN, PHN
Dean of Academic Affairs
Chamberlain University
Downer's Grove, Illinois

Donald W. Sweeting, PhD
President
Colorado Christian University
Lakewood, Colorado

Sam Welbaum, MA, MTS
Adjunct Instructor
Colorado Christian University
Lakewood, Colorado

Barbara White, EdD, RN, CNS
Dean of Nursing and Health Professions
Professor of Nursing
Colorado Christian University
Lakewood, Colorado

Rick Yohn, DMin, ThM
Past Dean of Biblical and Theological Studies
College of Adult and Graduate Studies
Colorado Christian University
Lakewood, Colorado

Reviewers

Betty Leslie Beimel, PhD, RN, CNE
MSN Program Director
Associate Professor
Presentation College
Aberdeen, South Dakota

Elizabeth M. Carson, EdD, RN, CN
Saint Anthony College of Nursing
Rockford, Illinois

Chun Chow, PhD, RN, FNP
Clinical Associate Professor
National University
La Jolla, California

Josie Christian, DNP, RN, PHN
Nursing Department Chair
Assistant Professor
Concordia University
St. Paul, Minnesota

Samantha B. Cussen, MSN, RN
Assistant Professor of Nursing
Indiana Wesleyan University
Marion, Indiana

Celeste Dunnington, PhD
Dean, Associate Professor
Truett McConnell University
Cleveland, Georgia

Shirley Farr, PhD, RN, CNS
Assistant Professor
Director, Entry-Level Masters Program
Azusa Pacific University
Azusa, California

Rosemary Fromer, PhD, RN, CNE
Associate Professor
Indiana Wesleyan University
Marion, Indiana

Ashley Hasselbring, MSN, RN, CCRN
Instructor
University of St. Francis
Joliet, Illinois

Cheryl Lee, PhD, RN, CNE, CWOCN
Associate Professor of Nursing
Assistant Dean for Clinical Education
Carr College of Nursing
Harding University
Searcy, Arkansas

Laura Logan, MSN, RN, CCRN
Clinical Instructor/Faculty
Stephen F. Austin State University
Nacogdoches, Texas

Melinda McLaughlin, MSN, FNP-C
Clinical Assistant Professor
National University
Azusa Pacific University
Azusa, California

Melissa Roberson, MSN, BFA, RN
Assistant Professor
Bon Secours Memorial College of Nursing
Henrico County, Virginia

Diane Smith, DNP, RN, FNP
Assistant Professor
Bon Secours Memorial College of Nursing
Henrico County, Virginia

Michelle Van Wyhe, DNP, ARNP-BC
Associate Professor
Northwestern College
Orange City, Iowa

Margie Washnok, DNP, MS, CNS
Professor of Nursing
Presentation College
Aberdeen, South Dakota

Mark Wilkinson, DNP, MBS, RN
Faith Community Nurse
Assistant Professor
Department of Nursing
Lubbock Christian University
Lubbock, Texas

Dana Collins Windham, MSN, RN
Assistant Professor of Nursing
Louisiana State University at Alexandria
Alexandria, Louisiana

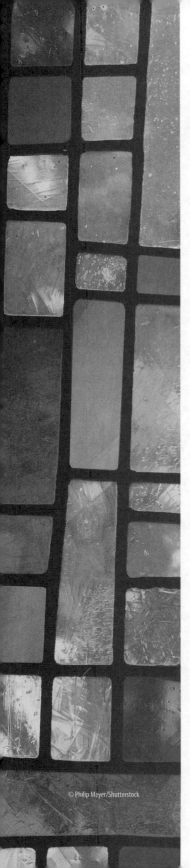

© Philip Meyer/Shutterstock

UNIT I

Foundations of Nursing as Ministry

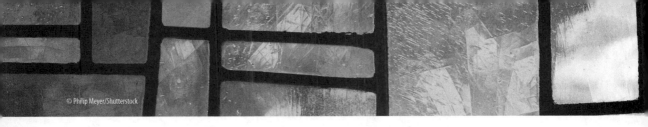

CHAPTER 1

The History of Nursing as Ministry

Donald W. Sweeting, PhD

LEARNING OBJECTIVES

At the end of this chapter, the reader will be able to:

1. Understand the historical roots of nursing as ministry.
2. Begin to develop a personal worldview for nursing.
3. Discuss the concepts of creation, fall, redemption, and consummation.
4. Develop a personal philosophy of nursing as ministry.

KEY TERMS

Creation	History
Florence Nightingale	Worldview

In my adult life, I've been the pastor of two churches, the president of two schools, and a church historian. While teaching church **history** on the seminary level, I have long been fascinated by the extraordinary cultural changes that took place because of the coming of Jesus Christ. One aspect of this is the formative role that Christ's followers have had in health care. In my studies, I've been struck by the fact that there is something very Christian about the hospital and nursing movements.

Today, there is an urgent demand for nurses. The good news is that if you are a halfway decent nurse, you should have job security for the future. In fact, the U.S. Bureau of Labor Statistics (2019) estimates that there will be more than 1 million openings for registered nurses (RNs) in the United States by 2024. In turn, there is a critical shortage of Christian nurses to fill that gap.

There is not simply a shortage of nurses but also a shortage of *good* nurses—that is, nurses who are conscientious, are well trained, and have a deep internal motivation to care for their patients.

▶ The Need for Quality Care

As a layman, there is a great deal I don't know about medicine and nursing. Even so, it feels to me, and to many of my peers, as if the quality of care in the health professions is declining.

I may be wrong, of course. Clearly, our technology is advancing, and we spend more on health care than ever. I recognize that we live in the golden age of knee surgery, of heart care, of biotech marvels, and all that—but it still feels as if the quality of care is declining. My evidence is anecdotal, but I've heard too many others share similar impressions and stories about depersonalized or less-than-competent care to completely dismiss these complaints.

For example, why do even my doctor friends say that if you go to the hospital, don't go alone? That is, you need an advocate to guide you through what feels like an impersonal system (see **CASE STUDY 1-1**).

🔍 *CASE STUDY 1-1*

Just last week my mother-in-law, who is in her 80s, fell and spent a week in the hospital. My wife went with her and was aghast at the oversights of the trauma floor staff. She observed how older people are rushed through the system because of what was described to her as the "pressure from the insurance companies."

On top of this, our nephew, who is eight years old, has been receiving treatment at the local medical center. He's a great little kid, but he had a serious infection. Unfortunately, they kept misdiagnosing it. First it was said to be a stomach problem; then the healthcare personnel called it an appendix problem. Our nephew was an inpatient for three weeks, and the infection got quite serious. For several days, we didn't know if he would make it. In fact, the doctor said that his case involved "a horrible, horrible, horrible, horrible, horrible infection." Now, when a doctor says "horrible" twice, you get freaked out; when he says it five times, then you know it's really bad.

When my sister-in-law and brother-in-law brought my nephew home, he was still vomiting. It was awful to watch him suffer. Eventually, my wife, who is not a doctor, consulted with a physician friend about our nephew's medications. It turns out that the hospital gave this eight-year-old child the wrong medication. They gave him a medication that was for adults and sent him home with that—and for 13 days they kept telling his family it should work. When my wife and sister-in-law approached the dietitian and doctor about this issue, they kept insisting that this was the right medication for the child to take. Finally, one of the nurses looked into the issue and admitted, "You know what? We made a big mistake."

If you had been on the receiving end of this harrowing episode, you would be outraged. We did not sue, nor did we threaten to do so. But we did experience firsthand why a nurse's job is so important. We realized that we need good doctors, assistants, dietitians, and nurses!

Questions

1. Based on this true story from the author, how would you have handled this situation as a Christian nurse?
2. How would you have told the family that a mistake was made?
3. How could this serious situation have been prevented? Where do you think the breakdown in communication occurred?
4. Why is a nurse's job important?

One of my favorite books on medical care is *The Lost Art of Healing*; it was written in 1999 by Bernard Lown. It's a little dated, but nevertheless fascinating. More than 20 years ago, Lown, who worked for four decades as a cardiologist, was writing about how medicine in the United States has lost its way.

According to Lown, there is an unwritten covenant between doctor and patient that is being broken (1999). In his view, healing is being replaced with treating; caring is being supplanted with managing; and listening is being overtaken by technological procedures. Doctors no longer minister: They focus on biological parts that are not functioning right, not on the person.

Lown wrote that a certain pride is instilled into medical students that presents humans as merely biochemical machines. He felt that doctors placed more emphasis on the technical parts of medicine rather than on the more human art of listening (1999). Lown makes the case that doctors must reconnect with their tradition as healers, and that medicine needs a human face.

Here is the view of someone looking at the system from the inside. Lown is not a layman like me, yet he is saying that we're overlooking some very important matters. The challenge to the younger generation, then, is to remake these all-important connections in the very highly specialized and technological environment of contemporary health care.

The business of medicine is huge. Pharmaceutical companies have a major impact on this area, for good and for sometimes not so good. So do insurance companies. But along with this comes the influence of secular worldviews that are now driving the profession.

Other worldviews are now shaping new medical workers coming into the profession. Take, for example, the **worldview** of modernism. Modernism tends to be very scientific and often reductionistic. It might say, "The problem is your organ," and that's all it will look at, rather than the whole person.

Or take the worldview of post-modernism, which tends to be extremely subjective—that is, truth is in the eye of the beholder. It apparently does not have a high view of facts. I cannot image how someone could do science as a thoroughgoing post-modernist.

Or what about the worldview that sometimes describes itself as post-human? Post-humanists (also called transhumanists) talk about redirecting human evolution with new medical techniques and experiments.

Today, we are seeing a drift away from the Christian vision that gave birth to the modern healthcare movement, and toward new secular worldviews that are influencing the field. This is the atmosphere in which you will be practicing nursing. Those of us who are a little older can sense the shift now under way. We have the perspective of another era—one that was admittedly less technically savvy, but one with a more human face. Healthcare practice in this era was driven by a Christian vision of healing and caring for the patient.

This chapter seeks to discuss the Christian foundation for nursing as ministry. I want to acquaint you, or perhaps reacquaint you, with a Biblical basis for nursing, and then bridge from that to see how Christian involvement in the hospital and nursing movements changed history. To do so, we will journey back to the sources (*Ad fontes*) of Christian nursing.

▸ A Biblical Basis for Nursing

Let's begin with Holy Scripture itself and look at some of the key Biblical passages that have shaped the nursing profession. We will start with the Old Testament—specifically, Genesis 1:26–27. At the climax of **creation**, on the sixth day, God created human beings in His own image. Thus, all humans have the dignity that comes from God having stamped His own image on us.

Our dignity is tied to the glory of our Creator, the fountainhead of all dignity. As creatures, our dignity is extrinsic—that is, derived from the God who scoops up dust, molds it into a human being, and breathes into it the breath of life. God assigns to each of us, temporal creatures that we are, eternal significance and worth. As a consequence, every person you meet has God-given dignity.

Look deeper into Genesis 4:9, which provides the fascinating account of Cain and Abel. We sometimes breeze through this passage without paying much attention to its message. It's the story about two siblings who couldn't get along, we tell ourselves. But wait—this is more than just another bad day in paradise!

After Cain takes the life of Abel, God calls Cain to account for what happened. God asks, "Where is Abel your brother?" Cain's reply to God in verse 9: "I do not know; am I my brother's keeper?" That is a profound question. The Lord replies, "What have you done? The voice of your brother's blood is crying to me from the ground." In other words, the dignity of Abel has been violated. Of course you are your brother's keeper, and you have taken his life.

Don't miss the significance of this story. At the beginning of the Bible, God signals that we have a responsibility for the person next to us. All people are created in the image of God, and we are to care for our neighbor. This message is amplified in Leviticus, where God commands, "you shall not stand up against the life of your neighbor" (Leviticus 19:16, English Standard Version [ESV]) and "you shall love your neighbor as yourself. I am the Lord" (Leviticus 19:18, ESV).

Echoing the teaching of Genesis 1, in Exodus we find a fascinating account of the Hebrew midwives. A new Pharaoh noticed that the people of Israel were rapidly multiplying in Egypt. In response, Pharaoh issued a decree to the Hebrew midwives that when a Hebrew boy was born, they were to kill him. The baby girls could live, but not the sons. Exodus 1:17 tells us, "but the midwives feared God and did not do as the king of Egypt commanded them, but let the male children live."

Of course, the main point of this passage is that because of courageous faith of the midwives, Moses was born and he would deliver the children of Israel from Pharaoh's hand. Much later, the Messiah would be a descendant of that line. Even so, it is not insignificant that these midwives had a respect for the lives of these babies and did all that they could to let them live.

Go deeper still in the Old Testament and you come to passages like Psalm 8. In verse 4, the psalmist asks the majestic Lord, "What is man that you are mindful of him, and the son of man that you care for him?" The author then provides the answer: "Yet you have made him a little lower than the heavenly beings and crowned him with glory and honor. You have given him dominion over the works of your hands; you have put all things under his feet" (ESV).

In other words, God has shared His dignity with humankind. He has crowned us with glory and honor. We are created a little lower than the heavenly beings, but higher than the animal world (which also has value and for which we are to care). This psalm is helpful because it lays out an order of being in God's created world and reminds us that we must think rightly about ourselves, according to the Scriptures, not according to the latest trend in political correctness (i.e., speciesism).

Radical animal rights activists no longer recognize the unique dignity of humans, but instead argue that humans have no higher value than animals. Animals and humans are both part of the created order and to be treated humanely. But the Scriptures are clear that humans, though lower than the angels, are given stewardship and dominion over the animals. The peak of creation comes when humans are created and assigned their tasks by God. God was free to give meat to the Israelites in the wilderness (Exodus 16). Jesus was free to eat fish, and he openly proclaimed that humans are of more value than the birds of the air

(Matthew 6:26 and 10:31). Peter's vision in Acts 10 . . . Moreover, erasing the distinction between people and animals leads to *Animal Farm* absurdities—legally, socially, and practically.

In Psalm 139, David says, "O Lord, you have searched me and known me. . . . [You] are acquainted with all my ways." In the middle of this psalm, he says,

> For you formed my inward parts; you knitted me together in my mother's womb. I praise you, for I am fearfully and wonderfully made. . . . My frame was not hidden from you, when I was being made in secret, intricately woven in the depths of the earth. Your eyes saw my unformed substance.

Thus, God was acquainted with this human being before birth. He had great value and worth before he left the womb. David's powerful passage also informs our understanding of how we are to understand ourselves and others, and how we are to treat others.

In the New Testament, early on in the Gospels we see Jesus as he enters his public ministry. What does he do? Matthew 4:23 tells us that Jesus went throughout Galilee teaching in the synagogues, preaching the good news of the kingdom, and healing every disease and sickness among the people. In other words, along with being a preacher of the gospel, he ministered to physical needs. Along with being the Savior, Jesus was a healer.

All four Gospels tell us that Jesus had compassion for the sick. When he trained his 12 disciples, Luke 9:2 tells us Jesus sent them out to do the same thing. They were to preach the kingdom of God and heal the sick. Later in his ministry, Luke 10:9 tells us Jesus sent out an even larger group—72 followers. As before, he charged them to go out, preach the kingdom of God, and heal the sick.

Clearly, Jesus's own ministry, and the disciples' ministry, testify to his work of healing. In addition, Jesus's teaching constantly instructed his followers to care for others. In Mark 12:29–31 after the great commandment to "love the Lord, your God with all your heart, and with all your soul, and with all your mind and with all your strength," Jesus proclaims another commandment like it: "You shall love your neighbor as yourself" (ESV).

In Luke 6:36, Jesus says to his followers, "be merciful, even as your Father is merciful." In Luke 10, we find his parable of the Good Samaritan. Who responds appropriately to the victim who was violently attacked on the Jericho road? Not the priest and not the Levite, "but a Samaritan." This traveler was the one who took pity on the man and bandaged his wounds, put him on a donkey, and took him to an inn to take care of him. Jesus stunned his audience when he said, "You go and do likewise." He said, "do this and you will live." You are to take this Samaritan helper/healer as your model.

In Matthew 25, Jesus says, "I was sick and you visited me" (verse 36). Then he adds, "as you did it to one of the least of these my brothers, you did it to me" (verse 40).

Collectively, these texts testify that Jesus cared about the soul, obviously, because he is Savior. But he also cared about the body and the physical needs of people he met on his path. He commissioned his disciples to do the same.

As we pull all of these texts together, we essentially come up with an outline of a worldview—a Christian worldview that should guide every believer, including those who are called to nursing as ministry.

▶ A Theology of Nursing: A Christian Worldview for Nursing

Creation

A Christian worldview, or what we might call a "theology of nursing," should have four parts. Its foundation is God the creator and the people made in His image. Every person we are asked to care for is created in the image and likeness of God. They are image bearers. For this reason, we are to view them with dignity and respect. We are called to care for them because of who God created them to be.

Fall

The second part of this worldview involves the reality of human sin and what theologians sometimes call "the fall." Through Adam and Eve, humankind rebelled against its maker. Sin entered their hearts; evil twisted everything and there was brokenness and sickness and death. All of us feel this brokenness; we all will experience it. The world is radically out of joint. The messes that we see in the emergency room (ER) or in the hospital room shouldn't surprise us really because we know that things are not the way that they were supposed to be.

Redemption

Now comes the good news: The third part of this worldview involves redemption. God has initiated a rescue operation. He broke into our sin-weary world in the person of His Son. Jesus came to bring salvation—you might say, to put Humpty Dumpty back together again.

Jesus made salvation possible by means of his own intentional, loving, substitutionary atoning death on the cross for sinners. Jesus died so that we might live. He bore our sins in his body and offers us a new standing with God by faith. We can be forgiven, justified (i.e., declared not guilty), because "for our sake he [God] made him [Christ] to be sin who knew no sin, so that in him we might become the righteousness of God" (2 Corinthians 5:21).

Jesus's suffering was redemptive—but that's not where the story ends. He did not stay dead, but rose from the grave. He is alive. The powers of sin and death have been broken. Jesus conquered the grave.

Consummation

In the Bible, then, we have a theology of creation, a theology of the fall, and a theology of redemption. But there is one more piece: consummation. Jesus promised to return and make all things new. When he returns, there will be a new heaven and earth. Meanwhile, as Paul writes in Romans 8, all creation groans and awaits its day of delivery.

As a caregiver, you will hear this groaning more than most people. You will see the realities of human frailness and brokenness more than most. I saw it as a pastor. Pastors, like nurses, are often called into emergencies: We often arrive when people are in the emergency room, and we stand with our flock in the midst of suffering. Like you, we see a lot. And like you, we long for that future day, when "he will wipe every tear from their eyes, and death shall be no more, neither shall there be mourning, nor crying, nor pain any more, for the former things have passed away" (Revelations 21:4).

So What?

Is this worldview familiar to you? I hope it is. But perhaps you are saying to yourself, "Well, so what?" What difference does it make? I believe it makes a world of difference.

It is my conviction that this worldview best describes the human experience, and that it resonates with the deepest questions we have about life. Think about it: Why do we feel as if we have significance and should be treated with dignity? The nihilist's worldview answers that because we came from nothing and will return to nothing, then we have no ultimate significance. No lives really matter. We are a microscopic blip in the cosmos—dust in the wind. The Christian worldview, however, answers that we feel special because we have been created in the image of God.

A second basic question all people have is, "What's wrong with the world, and what's wrong with me?" Do you ever ask that? I do.

We know that things are not the way they ought to be. The older we get, the more we realize that we are all wearing out. We know that someday our hearts will stop beating and our brainwaves will cease. That is not a pleasant thought, but the Christian worldview is not naïve about the world. There is a realism about it.

But then we ask a third basic question: "Given what is wrong, can anyone fix it?" The Bible answers that there is one who came into this world—Jesus Christ—to save us and to rescue us from our ER world.

This prompts a final basic question that we all ask: "Is there any hope for the future?" The Christian worldview answers affirmatively: Christ promised to come again, and when he does there will be a new heaven and earth. This is why we are people of hope.

Many worldviews are naïve about evil, or cannot explain goodness, or have no adequate grounding for human dignity, or offer no hope. In this way, the Christian worldview is different, powerfully different. It not only answers our basic questions but also provides a theology for nursing that gives the whole profession meaning.

Grounded in this worldview, you will not be surprised by the beauty of a person and the intricacy of the way our bodies were designed, nor will you be surprised by the brokenness and the mess that you see. Yet you will not be hopeless, because you know someone has come to help and is there to be called upon. You will be both realistic and hopeful as you enter people's lives and provide compassion, care, and healing.

▶ The Extraordinary Impact of Jesus Christ on the World

For part of my career, I've had the privilege of teaching students about church history. One thing that fascinates me about church history is the extraordinary impact that Jesus had, and the ways in which his coming transformed so many dimensions of human life—education, science, art, music, health care, government, morality, economics, the family, how we think of time, and so on. As discussed in this section, the coming of Christ unleashed a vast humanitarian impulse that continues to resonate today.

Consider the area of language and literacy. Countless people groups all over the world had no written language, until someone brought them the gospel. When they learned about God's love in Jesus Christ, those people suddenly wanted to know more. They wanted to know God's book. So missionaries helped them write down a language, and taught them to read so they could understand the Bible in their own tongue. Yet they still wanted to know more. So missionaries founded schools for their children, and then secondary schools, and later colleges and universities. This pattern played out not only in Western history but all over the world, everywhere that missionaries went. Sadly, this story has been forgotten, or deliberately ignored, in the Western world.

Jesus's effect on education has been extraordinary. The university world of which I'm a part owes a deep debt to the Christian impulses that got it all started. There would be no Christian universities—let alone Oxford, the Sorbonne, Cambridge, or Harvard—if it weren't for Jesus Christ.

There would probably be no nursing profession if it weren't for Jesus. Let me unpack this rather bold statement for you. Think about the Greco-Roman world. As brilliant as they were, Aristotle and Plato argued that most human beings are by nature slavish, and suitable for slavery. According to these philosophers, most people don't have natures worthy of freedom or dignity. Christianity rebukes this message; it says that every single human being is made in God's image and of immense worth and dignity.

Prior to the coming of Christ, in most places, life was very cheap. Jesus and his followers had a revolutionary message: Perhaps we ought to treat our children differently; perhaps we shouldn't sacrifice our children or abandon unwanted infants as many Romans did. Perhaps we should instead save children. Maybe abortion is not a good thing. Maybe we ought to find orphanages to care for unwanted children.

An early Christian writer, Diognetus, put it this way: "Christians marry, as do all. They beget children, but they do not destroy their offspring" (Curtis, 2010, para 2). This idea was later codified into law by Justinian, who outlawed both infanticide and abortion.

And what of the treatment and elevation of women? One major misconception is that Christianity has kept women down. The historical record shows that in the ancient world, a woman's life was very cheap. She was considered to be the property of her husband. Little girls were especially abandoned (exposed to the elements) in culture after culture out of a preference for boys. When missionaries arrived, they pointed out the injustice of this practice. Little girls also have dignity and worth because they are made in the image of God. Husbands are to love their wives sacrificially, just as Christ loved the church.

Something similar happened with slaves. All early empires made extensive use of slave labor, and no one objected to the practice. But then Jesus introduced a revolutionary conception of moral equality in the eyes of God. The idea that slavery was sinful was an idea unique to Christianity and Judaism. It led the church to treat slaves differently and eventually to ban the enslavement of Christians and Jews, which effectively led to the abolition of this practice. Thus, you might say that Christianity helped abolish slavery twice—once in the Middle Ages, and a second time in the 19th century through the efforts of William Wilberforce and others in England. Certainly, some Christians sought to justify this evil enterprise or pushed back on its abolition. Nevertheless, the Bible's teaching on the image of God helped to undermine the legitimacy of slavery.

▶ The Christian Roots of the Hospital/Nursing Movement

The church had much more influence on the history of health care than we realize. In fact, the modern hospital movement can be traced directly back to ancient and medieval Christian institutions.

Of course, it's not that no one else cared for the sick in the ancient world. The Hippocratic Oath, for example, requires physicians to swear by the healing gods to uphold a certain code of medical ethics. The original text is associated with Hippocrates, a Greek physician, who is sometimes called the father of modern medicine.

Some ancient cultures had medical facilities, but they were primarily for royalty, the wealthy, or the military. In ancient Greece, the sick went for healing at the Asclepian temples (associated with the god Asclepios). In the Roman Empire, infirmaries were established for the military. Nevertheless, even this kind of rudimentary care was reserved for the elite, rather than being available to the population at large. Compassion was not a well-developed virtue among the Romans and Greeks; mercy was discouraged.

But with the coming of Christ came a new attitude toward babies, the sick, the disabled, and the dying. The ministry of medical care in early Christianity was church based. Each church established an organized ministry of mercy, usually led by deacons and deaconesses.

A second-century church document called *The Didache* ("The Teaching," circa 96 A.D.) describes early Christian ethics and practices. Notably, it states that Christians are not permitted to procure abortions or commit infanticide.

Rodney Stark (1997), in his book *The Rise of Christianity*, writes about how early Christians in the first and second centuries responded to some of the devastating plagues in the western provinces of the Roman Empire. Quoting early Christian sources, he describes how pagans would push sufferers away, throwing them into the roads before they were even dead. They would often leave town when a major epidemic struck. Christians' response was different: They tended to stay in the cities and nurse the stricken, providing food, water, and basic sanitation. Not all the people they helped were cured, and some of the Christians who helped them died.

Stark quotes Dionysius, the bishop of Alexandria, who described what happened:

> Most of our brother Christians showed unbounded love and loyalty, never sparing themselves in thinking only of one another. Heedless of danger, they took charge of the sick, attending to their every need, ministering to them in Christ, and with them they sometimes departed this life serenely happy for they were infected by others with a disease drawing on themselves the sickness of their neighbors and cheerfully accepting their pains. (Stark, 1997, p. 82)

Stark believed that this outcome left a number of surviving pagans who owed their lives to their Christian nurses in an interesting situation. They began asking: Why were these Christians able to survive in greater numbers than others? Did they enjoy special favor with God? According to Stark, one reason many people were attracted to Christianity in those early centuries is because of the fact that when the plagues broke out, Christians were there to care.

By the fourth century, proto-hospitals had emerged that were founded and funded by religious orders or through the philanthropy of Christian donors. Before the legalization of Christianity, Christian church buildings were forbidden. Consequently, out-in-the-open institutionalized care was rare in that kind of environment. But with the greater toleration of

Christianity and then the Council of Nicaea in 325, suddenly we see a major council issuing decrees not only on doctrinal issues such as the trinity, but also on practical issues—specifically, directing every city with a cathedral to also have a hospital to nurse and heal the sick.

In the eastern Roman Empire, the first Christian hospital was founded by Saint Basil, a monk, in Cappadocia. Subsequently, many hospitals were founded based on the example of Basil's great Basileum and overseen by the Bishop of Constantinople.

In the western Roman Empire, the first hospital was started by a wealthy Christian widow, a disciple of Saint Jerome named Fabiola. Other hospitals eventually began emerging from religious orders tied to monasteries.

For example, Benedict of Nursia founded the monastery at Monte Cassino in 526. Benedict's rule emphasized hospitality to the stranger. Soon, he ordered that every monastery in his order establish an infirmary. At its height, the Benedictine order claimed it oversaw 37,000 monasteries throughout Europe. The Benedictine monastery in Salerno, Italy, founded the oldest and most famous medical school. The first Spanish hospital was founded by Catholics in 580. In 651, the Hôtel-Dieu ("Hotel of God") hospital was founded in Paris by the bishop of Paris, Saint Landry.

In 800, Charlemagne, King of the Franks and Holy Roman Emperor, and considered the Father of Europe, decreed that hospitals that had fallen into disrepair should be restored. He also asserted that every cathedral should have a school, a monastery, and a hospital.

The first hospital in the New World was the Hospital San Nicolas de Bari, founded by the Spanish in Santo Domingo (now the capital of the Dominican Republic). The first hospital in North America, the Jesus of Nazareth Hospital (note the name) in Mexico City, was founded in 1524.

The first hospital in what is now the United States was established in St. Augustine, Florida, in 1598, the hospital of Our Lady of Solitude. In the American colonies, the first hospital was established by Benjamin Franklin and the Quakers—Pennsylvania Hospital. The Red Cross, for its part, was started by an evangelical Christian.

In 1931, American missionaries started a short-wave radio station in Quito, Ecuador, called HCJB, The Voice of the Andes. In the 1950s, they added a hospital to its mission. Today, that hospital is one of the premier hospitals in the whole country. It, too, was inspired by the ongoing influence of Jesus Christ.

Probably the most famous nurse in history was **Florence Nightingale** (**BOX 1-1**). A devoted Christian, she felt called to go to Crimea to nurse British soldiers wounded in the Crimean War. There, she became the first woman to run a field hospital. Later, Nightingale founded a school of nursing in London and lifted the art of nursing to a whole new level. She revolutionized hospital methods in England. She was consulted by kings, queens, and presidents. Despite her fame, she steadfastly maintained that it was God who had called her into this service.

Many of the leading hospitals in cities throughout the world today are products of Christian medical or missionary charity. Besides many Catholic hospitals, many hospitals in North America were founded by Protestant denominations—by Seventh Day Adventists, Baptists, Episcopalians, Lutherans, Methodists, and Presbyterians.

BOX 1-1 Outstanding Nurse Leader: Florence Nightingale

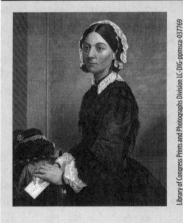

Library of Congress Prints and Photographs Division LC-DIG-ppmsca-037769

Florence Nightingale (1820–1910), known as the mother of nursing, also became known as the "Lady with the Lamp," a name given to her by the soldiers she served in the Crimean War. In her famous book *Notes on Nursing*, Nightingale discussed what she believed nursing was. She considered it to be much like "mothering," focusing on clean air, fresh water, clean bedding, light, a calm environment, and the like (Nightingale, 1859). Through her introduction of hand-washing principles during the Crimean War, infection rates in hospitals were dramatically reduced. The Nightingale Pledge is still recited at nursing graduations throughout the country. Here is the 1935 version:

I solemnly pledge myself before God and in the presence of this assembly, to pass my life in purity and to practice my profession faithfully. I will abstain from whatever is deleterious and mischievous, and will not take or knowingly administer any harmful drug. I will do all in my power to maintain and elevate the standard of my profession, and will hold in confidence all personal matters committed to my keeping, and all family affairs coming to my knowledge in the practice of my calling. With loyalty will I endeavor to aid the physician in his work, and as a "missioner of health" I will dedicate myself to devoted service to human welfare. (Crathern, 1953)

Nightingale stated, "If I could give you information of my life it would be to show how a woman of very ordinary ability has been led by God in strange and unaccustomed paths to do in His service what He has done in her. And if I could tell you all, you would see how God has done all, and I nothing. I have worked hard, very hard, that is all; and I have never refused God anything" (Nightingale, n.d.).

Crathern, A. T. (1953). For the sick. In *In Detroit courage was the fashion: The contribution of women to the development of Detroit from 1701 to 1951* (pp. 80–81). Detroit, MI: Wayne University Press.

▶ Conclusion

Nursing is a strategic discipline that gives students opportunities to serve the Lord and develop a lifetime habit of service. But nursing is also ministry: It prepares people for a noble calling that extends the influence of Jesus Christ.

As a young pastor in northern Illinois, I would often go to the city of Waukegan for hospital visits. At the time, the city had two prominent hospitals: One had no religious affiliation, and the other was Catholic.

One day, I was visiting a young boy from our church who had been run over by a tractor. He was in the ER and was a mess, in horrible condition. In the ER, there was just no sign of hope anywhere—no scripture or anything else to lift the spirits.

Sometime later, I remember going to the other hospital for a similar emergency pastoral visit. It seemed as if every room had a crucifix.

Evangelicals are not big on crucifixes, because we emphasize that Jesus is no longer on the cross, but rather has risen. Even so, I came to really appreciate the presence of a crucifix in a hospital room because it pointed to the one place in history where the pain was extraordinary, but it was not pointless, but rather redemptive. Through the agony of the cross came rescue and hope to a lost and broken world. And to anyone who happens to look to Christ crucified today, there is hope as well. I thought, "Wow, that cross in the hospital makes a difference for people who are in the midst of the valley of suffering and are looking for a shred of hope."

If you are ever on the receiving end of hospital care (as I have been), it makes a big difference if you are surrounded by that kind of hope. It also makes a big difference if you have a doctor or a nurse who will pray for you. It makes a great difference if you have a nurse who will give you excellent care because he or she is working for more than a paycheck. Such a nurse is serving a higher purpose and often sees his or her work as a calling in obedience to Jesus Christ.

You want those kinds of nurses; you don't want the kind who are checking social media and thinking about 100 other things. You want the kind who are devoted and focused.

We often talk about training nurses in the spirit of Florence Nightingale (**BOX 1-2**). At the end of her life, when she was asked how she wanted to be remembered, Nightingale said, "I want to be known as a woman who held nothing back from Jesus." She understood that her role in nursing was as an ambassador of Jesus.

I charge you not only to see nursing as ministry, but also to serve in the name of Jesus, to be motivated by the love of Jesus, to stand in the great Christian tradition of health care that was started by Jesus, and, like Florence

---

BOX 1-2 Evidence-Based Practice Focus

Nightingale was the first nursing theorist, even though she probably would not have considered herself one. She defined 13 canons of environment that included ventilation, light, noise, cleanliness of the room and bed, personal cleanliness, and food. By using the basic concepts of her theory, researchers can manipulate the environment, testing various aspects included in the theory, and examining their effects on health and wellness. For example, researchers have looked at the effects of light on infants in the NICU, the influence of color on mood, and the effect of noise in the ICU on patient recovery (**BOX 1-3**). Nightingale's theory guided the provision of holistic care to persons during her own time, but is still applicable today.

Modified from Pirani, S. A. (2016). Application of Nightingale's theory in nursing practice. *Annals of Nursing and Practice, 3*(1), 1040.

BOX 1-3 Research Highlight

Researchers in this study wanted to examine the difference in auditory function at the neonatal intensive care unit (NICU) discharge, comparing high-risk infant cases that were exposed to the noise of hospital construction and those not exposed. A retrospective descriptive cohort design was used in a sample of 540 infant cases where babies were exposed to hospital construction noise. Newborn hearing screening was done by automated auditory brainstem evoked response (ABER). The difference in auditory function was not statistically significant. The authors concluded that more research is needed to understand whether or not construction noise affects high-risk infants' hearing.

Modified from Willis, V. (2018). The relationship between hospital construction and high-risk infant auditory function at NICU discharge: A retrospective descriptive cohort study. *Health Environments Research & Design Journal, 11*(2), 124–136.

Nightingale, to hold nothing back from Jesus. And if you do, you will make a world of difference.

▶ Clinical Reasoning Exercises

1. What part of the history of nursing as ministry in this chapter most impressed you? Most surprised you?
2. Discuss how believing that all people are made in the image of God would influence your view of even the most challenging of people to care for.
3. Have you thought much about your own worldview? How does it influence your nursing practice?
4. If you had to sum up your worldview in a one-minute speech, what would that sound like? Review the *Understanding Worldview to Minister More Effectively* chapter for help.

▶ Personal Reflection Exercises

As a nurse, you may be involved in a hospital in any of many different cities. But when you get assigned to a particular hospital, look for the cornerstone. Don't look at the new buildings, but rather go to the oldest building and look for the cornerstone that was laid when it was built. Often, though not always, you will find a plaque of some sort to the glory of God, to the care of needy people, or something like that, in the service of God or Christ. In Denver, you might go to Swedish Medical Center. Or go to Littleton Adventist, or Porter Adventist, or Saint Anthony, or Lutheran Medical Center. Why were they originally founded? Nor simply to heal people, but to do so out of a very specific Christian motivation. They are there because of the influence of Jesus Christ.

Try this little experiment. Ask the hospital staff or historian: Do you have a cornerstone? They may think you're crazy. Tell them that you are interested in the history, and then see what you find. Alternatively, ask for a written history of the hospital.

References

Bureau of Labor Statistics, U.S. Department of Labor. (2019). *Occupational outlook handbook: Registered nurses*. Retrieved from https://www.bls.gov/ooh/health care/registered-nurses.htm

Crathern, A. T. (1953). For the sick. In *In Detroit courage was the fashion: The contribution of women to the development of Detroit from 1701 to 1951* Detroit, MI: Wayne University Press.

Curtis, K. (2010). Epistle of Diagnetus quote. Retrieved from https://www.christianity.com/church/church-history/timeline/1-300/epistle-of-diognetus-quote-11629595.html

Florence Nightingale Quotes. (n.d.). *BrainyQuote.com*. Retrieved from https://www.brainyquote.com/quotes/florence_nightingale_752502

Lown, B. (1999). *The lost art of healing.* New York, NY: Ballantine Books.

Nightingale, F. (1859). *Notes on nursing: What it is and what it isn't.* London, UK: Harrison and Sons.

Stark, R. (1997). *The rise of Christianity.* San Francisco, CA: Harper.

Recommended Readings

Fowler, M. D. (1984). *Ethics and nursing, 1893–1984: The ideal of service, the reality of history.* Doctoral thesis, University of Southern California, Los Angeles, CA.

O'Brien, M. E. (2017). *Spirituality in nursing.* Burlington, MA: Jones & Bartlett Learning.

Shelly, J. A., & Miller, A. B. (1999). *Called to care: A Christian theology of nursing.* Downers Grove, IL: InterVarsity Press.

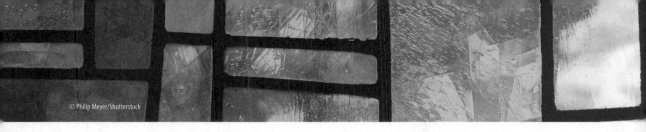

CHAPTER 2

Divine Appointment: Fulfilling Your Call

Barbara White, EdD, RN, CNS

LEARNING OBJECTIVES

At the end of this chapter, the reader will be able to:

1. Describe what "sacred calling" means to the practice of nursing.
2. Analyze your own philosophy of nursing as ministry.
3. Reflect deeply on your "divine appointments" as a professional Christian nurse.
4. Evaluate your nursing practice related to fulfilling God's call for your life.
5. Compare your habits of leadership using the five disciplines of Jesus as discussed in this chapter.

KEY TERMS

Calling
Divine appointments

Prayer
Praying circles

Servant leadership

▶ Introduction

For I know the plans I have for you, declares the LORD, plans to prosper you and not to harm you, plans to give you a hope and a future.

—**Jeremiah 29:11**

In the *History of Nursing as Ministry* chapter, Dr. Donald Sweeting laid the foundation for nursing as ministry as he discussed the history of the profession from a Biblical worldview. This chapter takes a unique path as readers are asked to walk alongside a visionary Christian nurse leader as she shares directly with them her personal story of the sacred **calling** to nursing that is full of **divine appointments** and God-ordained moments. Readers are encouraged to momentarily lay aside the necessity of scholarly note-taking and join this author, Dr. Barbara White, who for many years was the president of Nurses Christian Fellowship International (NCFI), as she writes to you as a friend and a colleague. In a devotional style, Dr. White weaves her story with scripture, wise advice, and reflections for readers about the significance of divine appointments and fulfilling God's call on your life.

▶ The Still Small Voice Is Calling

It was an ordinary Sunday. We had just come home from church and I was standing at the kitchen sink peeling vegetables for dinner. It was a beautiful spring day in Denver—blue sky and fluffy white clouds. In the moment that followed, something amazing, something unforgettable, happened to me. I actually heard God "speak." As I stood there looking out over the backyard, I honestly sensed God's presence and I knew without a doubt that He was speaking to *me*. His voice was not audible, but it was unmistakable. It was as if He had placed His hand on my right shoulder when He said, "Just take what you know and go share it wherever I send you."

Just sharing these words still makes me tingle. The message was vivid, transcendent, and then ended abruptly. "Okay, God," I remember saying. "But where am I supposed to go? And how do I get there? What's next? I'd like the GPS directions, please."

Have you ever felt God's specific call on your life? Do you have a dream? A vision? A passion for what you would really like to do in life? What is your purpose? Why are you here on this earth? Most of us want to make a difference in the world. During my college years, God clearly called me into nursing. I started college as a physical education (PE) major and thought I would be teaching PE to high school students as a career. But then, between my freshman and sophomore years, I needed to find a job to help with college tuition. A friend of my mother from church was the director of

nursing at a small community hospital nearby and offered me a position as a nurse aide. Little did I know how that summer would change my life. As I learned the many tasks of basic care and helping patients with activities of daily living, I discovered the joy of caring for others. When the surgeons asked if I wanted to observe an operation, I was eager to watch and soon learned that our bodies were magnificently made by the Lord in "technicolor."

By the end of the summer, I knew without a doubt that I needed to change majors and become a nurse. I transferred to the university medical center and never looked back. Here is where I was given my first leadership responsibility, as I became class president. I will never forget when the dean had us over to her apartment for dinner and talked with us about professional nursing and our responsibility to move the profession forward. I found my first mentor and knew that someday I wanted to be just like her.

Upon graduation, my heart's desire was clearly set on teaching nursing and becoming dean of a nursing school. But I had no clue how to get there. I stepped out into life confident and expectant.

Many of you are there right now: God has called you and given you a dream, and you want to serve Him with all your heart and soul. But, like me, you may have questions. What specifically do I do? How will I get there? And how will I know I am on the right path? Where do I go from here? It is like a puzzle, Lord. How do I put it all together? When will I finally fulfill your call, Lord?

▶ Moving Toward the Call

I knew God was real. I had a rich Christian heritage. I had been going to church since I was a very young child, made a personal commitment of faith when I was 10, and was baptized at age 12. As a young child, having memorized many Bible verses, I knew that God was trustworthy and that He loved me. As a teenager, I was blessed by going to a church where our entire family was actively involved. On Sunday morning, there was Sunday school and worship service. Sunday evening was youth group and evening service. Wednesday evening was mid-week **prayer** meeting. Once a month, the youth group had a "singspiration" at someone's home after church where we sang hymns and choruses nonstop. All of these experiences are foundational to who I am as a believer in Christ.

During my college years, I became actively involved in Campus Crusade (Cru) and Intervarsity Nurses Christian Fellowship (NCF), where I made lifelong friends. We spent many hours talking, praying together, and seeking the Lord's will for our lives.

In the years that followed, my dream remained like a little flame in the back of my mind and heart. But then, life happened. During my senior year in college, I met the man of my dreams through another divine appointment. A friend had returned home from the Vietnam War and his sister had a "welcome home" party for him. We had all gone to high school together. John, my future husband, was asked to pick me up and bring me to the party. Within three weeks, we were engaged, with a wedding planned for six months later.

My husband and I stayed in the Chicago area for a year as we started our careers. I worked as a staff nurse on a general medical–surgical unit at a large medical center learning the organizational skills, critical thinking, and clinical reasoning needed of any new registered nurse (RN). I learned team nursing as I cared for patients with nurse aides, medication technicians, interns, and residents. We knew from the start that our lives would actually settle in Colorado, a place my husband had grown to love since childhood vacations had taken him to the Rocky Mountains.

When we arrived in Denver, I immediately started seeking a teaching position. A former faculty member from my alma mater was teaching at a diploma school in Denver and arranged an interview for me. I was hired on the spot. I was thrilled, but very naive. Divine

appointment? Absolutely, but not recognized at the time. It was three weeks until fall semester started and I was assigned to teach general medical–surgical nursing. The first topic was renal disease, so I dug into the textbooks and prepared what I thought would be more than sufficient information for this first class. I even prepared a handout. When I was finished "lecturing" only one hour into the three-hour class, I quickly learned that there was much more to effective teaching than I had ever thought about. I had lots to learn—and learn I did. At this point in my life, Colossians 3:23 was my constant prayer: "Whatever you do, work at it with all your heart, as working for the Lord, not for human masters."

By the time I was appointed director of the program in the early 1980s, I had grown in my knowledge and competency in practice and in teaching. To this day, I still hear from former students who confirm that I was able to take complex topics and make them simple enough for new nursing students to understand. I was able to share my faith with patients and students along the way. I loved teaching nursing, and I knew I was in the right place doing the right thing.

And so, life continued. There was graduate school, starting a family and buying a home, and settling into a routine of Bible study groups, church activities, and Sunday school teaching. It took nine years to start our family. Adopting was a time to trust God for His best in our lives and to rejoice as He provided us with just the right children. More divine appointments. Soon the kids grew and we were into soccer and school activities, friends, and family camping and vacations. God was good. Life was great.

In 1986, I was in the process of closing the last diploma school of nursing in the state of Colorado when God again touched my heart with a desire to start a nursing school where we could teach nursing as ministry. It was a rather amazing thought—closing one school of nursing with honor and dignity after having served the area with exceptional new graduate nurses for more than 100 years, and then thinking about starting another school of nursing where scripture could be integrated into every aspect of professional practice. It seemed rather ridiculous and certainly impossible from where I was in life. The nursing profession was changing, and the push for higher education and nursing degrees within the university setting was compounded by the initiation of diagnostic-related groups (DRGs) within hospitals. DRGs "are a patient classification scheme which provides a means of relating the type of patients a hospital treats (i.e., its case mix) to the costs incurred by the hospital" (Centers for Medicare and Medicaid, 2016, p. 1).

The decision to close the school of nursing was a difficult one, but was needed and supported at the time. So, as God once again placed that small desire in my heart, I began to pray and ask God very specifically to show me His plan. A local NCF group of colleagues began to pray with me for just such a program to begin. The Lord began to rekindle my desire to serve Him faithfully for the remaining years of my life, particularly in my professional career. I had been "doing life," and the "stuff of life" happened. But the dream was still there, and a small seed of desire began to grow. As I prayed, it became more focused as God laid on my heart the clear desire to start a nursing school at a local Christian university so that we could teach nursing as ministry. Psalm 34:7 became my new verse to meditate on, claim as a promise, and seek God's perspective: "Take delight in the Lord, and He will give you the desires of your heart."

▶ Heeding the Call

Life continued. As the kids grew up, the days became busier, and the challenges of combining life, parenting, and work became more complex. All of a sudden, I found myself in midlife, now wondering, "Will I ever be able to do something significant for you, Lord?"

I was successful, but was I doing something that God had put me on this earth to do? I really wanted God to use me. Was I doing what God really wanted? Was I living out God's call on my life?

The Holy Scripture records the life stories of heroes of the faith who are really just like us—called by God and learning to live into that call on a daily basis. It started as a typical day but ended unlike any other for David, the shepherd boy. At breakfast, his father and older brothers may have discussed current events and the recent political developments. Israel's neighbors were uneasy and the country's first king was pulling together a national army. None of that mattered much to David. His life was simple (1 Samuel 16).

David had the sheep to worry about. He was responsible, hardy, and brave, and his father had entrusted him with the flock. During the long lazy day under the hot Middle Eastern sun, David spent his time tending the sheep, writing, singing, and dreaming about the world beyond the pasture. The stories he heard were about Noah, Abraham, Moses, and Gideon—stories about faith and honor and destiny. I wonder if David ever thought about his destiny. He probably dreamed the dreams of youth. Will I be a shepherd forever? What if we really do wage war against the Philistines? Could I have a role? Will I ever see faraway lands, meet important people, marry, or have a son of my own?

"David! DAVID!" The shrill call of his father's hired hands brought him back from his daydreams. "Your father needs to see you **now**." As David left the fields and approached the place where the others were gathered, he saw the prophet Samuel. What unfolded next is something I am sure David never could have imagined that morning at breakfast:

> Then the LORD said, Rise and anoint him; this is the one. So Samuel took the horn of oil and anointed him in the presence of his brothers, and from that day on the Spirit

of the LORD came upon David in power. Samuel then went to Ramah. (1 Samuel 16:12–13)

Wow! David woke in the morning as a shepherd boy and went to bed at night as a king. God chose David; He set him apart. God tapped David on the shoulder and called him for a mighty work. But what is amazing is that after he anointed David, Samuel just left. And there was David, left thinking, pondering, and wondering: "I am supposed to be somebody. I am supposed to do something. What now? How do I get from here to there?"

The next morning when David awoke, there was no chariot to take him to the palace. There was no robe or crown or scepter. David's world had turned upside down yesterday, but today it turned right side up again. The next day out in the fields, my guess is that David's question was "What next, Lord? What do I do in the meantime until I become king?"

▶ Waiting for the Fulfillment of the Call

Pastor Rob Brendle, in his book entitled *In the Meantime: The Practice of Proactive Waiting* (2006), states that he sees people do three different things as they wait on the fulfillment of the dreams from God:

- They take control of the plans and get ahead of God.
- They wait a while, forget the plans, and go on to other things.
- They spiritualize the plans and stay stuck, constantly praying but never moving.

In the scripture, a classic example of the first type, a controller, was Saul. Soon after becoming Israel's first king, Saul led the people into battle against the Philistines. As explained in 1 Samuel 13, the overzealous king, eager to bring victory and firmly establish his leadership, took the prophet Samuel's duty into his own hands and ended up botching the whole thing. The one who tries to control the plans tells God in effect: "Thanks for the advice, but I'll take it from here." These people catch the vision, then decide to handle the plans on their own. They run ahead of God and try to make it happen on their own.

Waiting and then forgetting the plan is also a common reaction to the dreams that God entrusts to us. You see, when God whispers in someone's ear, the first response is to become fired up, to pray, and to seek God with passion and determination. Then nothing happens and the waiting begins. These people wake up the next morning and everything is exactly the same as it was before. But instead of responding like David, they figure that maybe the dream really didn't happen and maybe it simply doesn't matter anyway. Whereas controllers disobey God by taking quick action, those who forget disobey God by becoming impatient and going on to other things. When the dreams and plans don't happen according to their timing, or when God doesn't show up like they thought He would, they forget the dream: They simply "walk away," leaving the plans in the dust.

The third choice for waiting on the Lord to act is equally dangerous, as those who spiritualize receive the dream, pray about it, and then pray some more. They talk about the dream and about the "big things" God is doing in the world and how they will be a part of what God is doing someday. They pray and talk, but they are never ready. They have to be more prepared. They want to be involved, but they never take action because fear paralyzes them from pursuing the dream—fear of missing God's will, fear of failing, fear of being viewed as unspiritual. So they wait on the Lord and they watch others doing the "big things" with God. These people are at the opposite end of the controllers. They disobey God by inaction, always waiting for God to do something and never moving forward (Brendle, 2006).

According to Brendle (2006), all three of these decisions are not what God intends. The Bible does not direct us to get ahead of God and take matters into our own hands. Nor are we advised to wait for a little while and then, if it doesn't happen, move on to something else. It also does not encourage us to sit and wait and stay right where we are so that God can eventually find us and move us forward. Look at David. He was anointed king in 1 Samuel 16, but did not actually become king until 2 Samuel 5. David was a youth (probably between 8 and 11 years of age) at his anointing, but was 30 years old when crowned king. In other words, he waited for approximately 20 years to see the fulfilment of that promise from God. Many things happened in David's life between being anointed and putting on the crown: He served in Saul's household and court; he killed Goliath; he developed a great friendship with Jonathan, Saul's son; he spared Saul's life—twice; and he lamented Saul's death. There was a lot of living and a lot of years that passed between David's call and its fulfillment. David lived out the passage of scripture that is my life verse, found in Proverbs 3:5–6: "Trust in the LORD with all your heart and lean not on your own understanding; in all your ways acknowledge him, and he will make your paths straight."

After the diploma school closure, I found a new teaching position at a private university, where I was viewed as an excellent inspirational teacher and had many satisfying experiences with nursing students. I taught theory classes and made clinical site visits throughout the city, encouraging students in their journey toward becoming excellent nurses. I taught interesting nursing courses and was actively involved in NCF both on campus and in the local nurse group. My contacts and collegial relationships grew and flourished. For those things I was eternally grateful and felt humbly privileged. I was happy, and most days were filled with important work. But, deep down inside my soul was a yearning to teach nursing from God's perspective, not just by the textbooks.

In my days of restlessness, the Lord kept drawing me back to His word. 1 Timothy 6:6 says, "but godliness with contentment is great gain." And Paul, one of my favorite New Testament heroes, was so correct in saying in Philippians 4:12, "I have learned the secret of being content in any and every situation." More sin to confess, Lord. Teach me contentment. And He did. He is always faithful to His word. Throughout life, I had rationalized and pleaded with God, all in pursuit of this elusive sense of calling. I waited on the Lord. I believed I was called by God. Forgetting what was behind and straining toward what was ahead, I pressed on and prayed hard, and in those dramatic goose-bump moments at the end of a powerful worship service, I would cry out, "God, please use me!"

This brings me to the very point of this discussion. Suddenly, I realized that those sincerely meant and dramatically expressed petitions in my life were really a little off the mark. Passionately pleading for God to use me was like passionately pleading for fire to be hot or water to be wet. God, by His very nature, uses people. Serving God to advance His kingdom is not something we have to beg Him to do; it is something He has already chosen for us. I've lived most of my life with the notion that God's calling is an event or a position or an achievement, some high rung on the ladder of life that after many years of obligatory climbing, I hope someday to attain. Yet, over the past many years, God has been teaching me that the "calling" is really the "process." God is much more concerned about who we are than about what we do. We never really arrive at our calling: We live into it. In the "meantime" of life, we must trust God. We never really get there, and when we think we do, we invariably learn that what we thought was the end is really just another beginning. God uses everything in our lives to prepare us for what He has in store for us next.

I love Jeremiah 29:11, and I quote this verse often to encourage young people in their calling: "For I know the plans I have for you, declares the Lord, plans to prosper you and not to harm you, plans to give you a future and a hope." What precedes verse 11 is a list of instructions on living, as it were, in the meantime. It is as if God were saying, "Do these things that I am telling you now while you are waiting on the fulfillment of my promise to bring you back from exile and restore your prosperity and joy." In other words, "I have a plan for you. You are called. Therefore, live this way. This is how I want you to live each day, trusting me for the outcome."

Starting in Jeremiah 29:4, notice the "big picture idea": While you are waiting, do life. Be proactive. Don't put life on hold in anticipation of a divine override. Do the work along the way. Take your eyes off yourself and take care of people. Trust, seek, and look to Him for the dream's fulfillment while you grow, stretch, and develop Christ-like character and professional competencies in all the work and circumstances that God allows in your life.

Let's take a closer look at God's instructions to His people. Jeremiah 29:5 states, "Build houses and settle down." While waiting, establish yourself. Don't despise this season of becoming who God wants you to be. Live it and love it! "Plant gardens and eat what they produce." Be productive and create something of worth for the kingdom of God. Do your very best in whatever place God has you. Proactive waiting means doing a great job exactly where you are in the season before the dream becomes reality.

Jeremiah 29:6 says, "Marry and have sons and daughters. Increase in number there, do not decrease." God wants you to grow, stretch, and increase in number while you are here, not once you are there. Opportunities to strengthen our lives abound. Seize them.

Jeremiah 29:7 commands that we "Seek the peace and prosperity of the city to which I have carried you into exile. Pray to the Lord for it, because if it prospers, you too will prosper." Invest your life in others. Serve people and care about their needs, not just your own.

Jeremiah 29:8 states, "Do not let the prophets and diviners among you deceive you." Stay the course of God's call, learn to hear the shepherd's voice, and listen to him. Diligently reject the bad ideas that flood your mind, and cling to God's design alone (Brendle, 2006).

Life is full of special divine appointments orchestrated only by the Lord. We just need to have our Holy Spirit radar open to the opportunities before us. I know that I missed a lot of them simply because I was focused on myself rather than on the Lord and what He had for me. Conviction does not come easy and confession is hard, but they are worth the peace and joy as His forgiveness and grace floods the soul after times of honesty before the Lord.

▶ Questioning the Call

In 2000, I had finally completed my doctoral study. A colleague who was in a responsible position at a local medical center had prayed with me many times about the idea of nursing as ministry and was highly supportive of having nursing students in her facility. The timing seemed so right, at least in my eyes. I was finally ready to do something significant! I walked into the president's office at that local Christian university with a proposal in hand, confident and well prepared.

I walked out totally defeated. The university administration at that time was not able to explore the possibility of such a program. Needless to say, I was devastated. Why, Lord? I thought that this is what I was called to do. Why did I spend all those years preparing? Was all of this doctoral study for nothing? It is only as I look back now that I recognize that this disappointment was truly a God-ordained divine appointment that He had orchestrated for me.

When life gives you a "P" turn instead of a clear left-hand turn, everything seems rather mixed up. Let me explain. In Korea, as we drove throughout Seoul, when we wanted to turn left we were frequently directed to turn right and make a "P" turn: right turn, right turn again at the next block, and finally right turn again at the next block, eventually leading us in the correct direction. I did not know it at the time, but several things had to change, including my direction in life, before God's call, my dream, could become reality. God is continually at work in our lives and in all situations to bring about His divine appointments (Angking, 2012).

It took two years of prayer and wrestling with "What next, Lord?" before I could actually come face to face with who I was and what I was trying to do. I had to "give up the dream." I had to recognize and confess my pride. I needed to be broken of my foolishness and forgiven for my rebellious arrogance. I had to realize that God's timing is always perfect and He is sovereign.

Finally, I surrendered. Finally, I realized that this dream of mine was not about me and what I could do for God. It had to be all about Jesus, and what he could do through us. I needed to get out of the way. Finally, I yielded to the truth that God knows what is best for me. I needed to yield to His will for my life. In John 15:5–11 (New International Version [NIV]), Jesus says:

> I am the true vine, and my Father is the gardener. He cuts off every branch in me that bears no fruit, while every branch that does bear fruit he prunes so that it will be even more fruitful. . . . Remain in me, as I also remain in you. No branch can bear fruit by itself; it must remain in the vine. Neither can you bear fruit unless you remain in me. I am the vine; you are the branches. If you remain in me and I in you, you will bear much fruit; apart from me you can do nothing. . . . I have told you this so that my joy may be in you and that your joy may be complete.

Finally, I came to the realization that I wanted to serve Him no matter what, even if I never got to be a dean of a nursing school where we could teach nursing as ministry. And that's when it happened—the experience that I told you about at the beginning of this chapter. I clearly heard God's still small voice say,

"Just take what you know and go wherever I send you." The door for a nursing school shut, but the dream of teaching nursing as ministry was still alive.

▶ Preparing for the Call

I soon found myself traveling and consulting in China, becoming involved in NCFI, and teaching many places around the world that I had never dreamed of going. Life was good, exciting, and fulfilling. In 2006, I was awarded a Fulbright scholar appointment in Seoul, Korea. But as my husband and I explored the situation and learned we were going to live in a dormitory (of all places, at our age), we became convinced that we could not do it. The financial burden was too great if we tried to rent an apartment. Life in a dormitory would be too hard. I will never forget a phone call from a Korean mentor, who challenged me with a question and a promise from scripture: "Barbara, why are you so worried? Your father knows just what you need, before you ask Him" (Matthew 6:8).

So my husband and I stepped out in faith. Our year in Korea was one of the best years of our life, a time to trust God every day in every way. Our dormitory room turned out to be a five-room apartment, complete with a full kitchen where I cooked American food every weekend for all our new foreign friends. We purchased a car, shopped at Costco, and drove all over that beautiful country. I taught leadership and bioethics, my favorite courses to teach. And I used scripture as the basis of all my teaching, integrating Biblical concepts and promises into each lecture. I was asked to teach and share my expertise with more than 10 university schools of nursing throughout the country. What a privilege! We learned how God "shows up" in so many magnificent ways within uniquely different cultures. Koreans claim 38% of their population as Christian and send out more missionaries per capita than any other country in the world. We worshipped each Sunday at an international church with people from 26 different countries under the teaching and leadership of a pastor from Ghana, who is now one of our closest friends.

My husband and I shared our lives with these special new friends, and God used us in mighty ways. We cooked and served a traditional Thanksgiving dinner to all 60 faculty and staff at the College of Nursing without a single bite of leftover turkey. Turkey is not a food eaten in Korea, so plates of extra meat, stuffing, and cranberry sauce went home to families who had never tasted such a delicious treat. Faculty were surprised at how my husband shared in not only the cooking and serving of the meal but also the decorating of the tables with fall leaves. By contrast, Korean women take full responsibility for all meal preparation and holiday celebrations.

We also had the privilege of sharing parenting principles with obstetric and pediatric nurses from both the education and practice settings. What a joy to bring scriptural principles to bear on topics such as sanctity of life, child care, and discipline. When we shared about adopting our son and daughter, stories of how God provided these special children just for us, there was not a dry eye in the room. Both of our children were clearly divine appointments from the Lord. Later, when our son came to visit us over spring break, he fell in love with an incredible young woman from Kazakhstan, who happened to be an international student at our church. We clearly know now that we had to go to Korea for our son to find his wife.

When I returned from Korea, wonders never ceased, and God's promises never ended. I accepted the new position of dean for nursing at the Christian university where I had hoped and prayed for 20 years about starting a nursing school. Administration now considered nursing a "mission fit." Thankful for God's faithfulness, I stepped into the position in the fall of 2007 clearly knowing that I was called to do this and that God would provide all the resources. His timing, not mine, is always

perfect. Divine appointment? Absolutely. And this time fully recognized. Little did I know, however, how much of a struggle and a challenge it would be.

▶ Confirming the Call

At first, my new role was just a lot of hard work, but then it became more than I could possibly handle. Maybe this was not what I was supposed to be doing. I started telling others that I was there for a reason and a season, and only God knew how long I would stay. In December 2007, just a little more than three months from the excitement of finally being able to live out my dream, I was again discouraged. Maybe I had not heard the Lord correctly. Maybe this was not what God was calling me to do. Maybe I was not in the right place "for such a time as this" after all. "Lord, I need your guidance and wisdom. I need to see all of this from your perspective. Once again, I surrender the entire situation to you. Not my will but your will, Lord," became my prayer.

When my husband and I attended the university Christmas party and the dean of music began singing "How Great Thou Art" in his melodic tenor voice, another touch of God's hand confirmed that this was truly my calling. As he sang, I wept. I knew that I was definitely called to this university at this time to start the nursing program because I knew that being called by God meant that I could not do anything else. Another divine appointment—this one totally confirmed.

For the next three years, after writing more than 4000 pages and 10 reports, it became clear that starting a nursing program at a Christian university was not just about doing the right things; it was about being in the right relationship with the Lord. We were, and continue to be, in a spiritual battle. Ephesians 6:12 tells us "our struggle is not against flesh and blood but against the rulers, against the authorities, against the powers of this dark world and against the spiritual forces of evil in the heavenly realms." But the promise of Ephesians 6:13 has been my prayer: "Therefore, put on the full armor of God, so that when the day of evil comes, you will be able to stand your ground and after you have done everything, to stand." Perseverance and persistence, trusting God for His timing and His sovereignty in every situation, doing my best but leaving the results up to the Lord—these are the scriptural principles on which I firmly stand.

Now as I reflect on the past 12 years, I see God's timing and God's faithfulness in every detail. I sit in awe at what He has accomplished through a highly competent and dedicated faculty and supportive university leadership. Each milestone has a story of God's hand at work. Every accomplishment is filled with divine appointments, situations, or people who have been specifically and unmistakably ordered by God. Each highlight reveals God's goodness and love.

This is His work, not mine. I am just an ordinary person with an extraordinary God, doing the work that God created me to do. Every year is punctuated with another goal completed under exceptional circumstances. So much accomplished in such a short time can only be by the hand of God Himself. When I first walked in the door of the university, the first licensed practical nurse (LPN) students were admitted. They completed the associate degree one year later fully prepared with 100% National Council Licensure Examination— Registered Nurse (NCLEX-RN) exam pass rates. The next year, the first RN to Bachelor of Science in Nursing (BSN) students were admitted, followed by national program accreditation from the Commission on Collegiate Nursing Education (CCNE) shortly thereafter.

In 2011, the first cohort of prelicensure BSN students were admitted and the associate degree nursing students, located in the western part of the state, transitioned to the statewide BSN program by means of a teleconferencing system. By 2013, the BSN program was firmly established and graduating exceptional nurses. In 2015, approval came from the

Higher Learning Commission (HLC) to start a Master of Science in Nursing (MSN) program. This could have happened only as a result of a divine appointment during that year. The curriculum vita (CV) of an exceptional faculty member came to my attention through e-mail. Of course, as only God can provide, she had the exact qualifications needed to lead the MSN program we had proposed. CCNE accreditation followed in 2017.

As our program continued to grow, I once more became convicted of my need for a deeper relationship with God. As God guides, He also provides. And God continued to lay priorities on my heart. More important than program growth and new program development was student and faculty spiritual growth. As a faculty team, we were comfortable praying for and with each other, praying for and with our students, sharing meaningful devotions before each committee meeting and class, and integrating Biblical perspectives into classroom discussions and assignments. But the real challenge for us as a faculty was to grow deeper in our faith and closer to the Lord in the midst of constant change and growth within not just nursing but the university as a whole. Faculty began to prayerfully consider the Biblical themes relevant to each nursing course. They challenged themselves and students to more clearly understand the truth of scripture by developing assignments that required students to dig deep into God's word. The team began to explore their own spiritual giftedness as well as their strengths within the team. Each team member became more vulnerable and grew within the framework of the "body of Christ," as described in 1 Corinthians 12:12–27. As faculty members shared their faith with students and encouraged students to grow in their own faith journeys, the nursing programs became rich with stories of God at work in the lives of students and patients.

One story was so impactful that the student nurse involved was asked to share her story at the county Prayer Breakfast before a room filled with eager listeners. She definitely had a divine appointment the day she cared for a patient on a cardiac step-down unit. Sarah (name changed to protect identity) was a Christian with a strong faith. She prayed for wisdom each day before entering a patient's room. Her patient that day was unstable and frightened. Sarah did her early-morning patient assessments and then reported the findings to her staff nurse. The physician in charge soon came to make rounds and ordered a medication to be given immediately. Being the intelligent and thoughtful student she always was, Sarah quickly looked up the medication and found contraindications based on this specific patient's vital signs and status. Respectfully, she reported her findings to the nurse in charge and refused to give the medication. The physician became quite angry, calling her out for being "only a student" and not following orders. He insisted the medication be given immediately and then left the room. Sarah held her ground and prayed. She rechecked the patient's vital signs and still felt she could not give the medication. The nurse would have to give it instead.

As the nurse was preparing the medication, the patient's monitors began beeping and the room became crowded with staff and doctors. Once the initial crisis was under control, the physician once again asked Sarah if she had given the medication. "No," she replied, "I did not give it." "Good," the physician stated and left the room. Returning to the nurses' station, Sarah found her nurse with tears in her eyes. "How did you know not to give that med?" she asked Sarah. Sarah replied, "Because I took all the steps that I was taught, assessed the patient, and then found contraindications to giving it for this patient. I prayed and I sensed in my heart from the Holy Spirit that I should not give it." The surprised look on the face of the nurse, followed by the words "Good—because if you had, the patient would have gone into cardiac arrest," were confirmation of Sarah's decision.

The nurse then asked Sarah if they might talk about this God to whom Sarah prayed. Sarah met the nurse off shift for dinner and

shared the message of Jesus with her. The nurse's heart was open, and she accepted Christ into her life. In the discussion that followed, the nurse mentioned that she had booked a trip to Israel the next month and was eager to see all these places where Jesus lived and walked. It was a trip she had always wanted to take. As only God could arrange, the tour guide for this specific trip to Israel was Sarah's brother, a local pastor. Texting occurred daily throughout the trip as the nurse was overjoyed with her newfound faith. She was baptized in the Jordan River and came home a new person in Christ. She and Sarah are now friends for eternity.

I look at this situation and praise God that Sarah had the boldness to ask God for wisdom for each patient she cares for and the courage to stand on her convictions. What an example of divine appointments that God arranges for each of us daily, if we are only open to His leading.

▶ Advancing the Call

It was in the fall of 2017 that I first read *Draw the Circle: The 40 Day Prayer Challenge* by Mark Batterson (2012), pastor of National Community Church in Washington, DC. I had received the book at a university women's event during the summer of 2017 but laid it aside. I did not realize that once again, I was at a specific event ordained by God and that He had some special things in store for the year ahead. Thinking it was simply another devotional book, I began a prayer journey with the Lord that would impact my life in profound ways.

I had learned to pray as a child, knowing that prayer was simply talking with God. Whether using a specific format such as adoration, confession, thanksgiving, and supplication (ACTS) or simply having a conversation with my heavenly Father, prayer had always been an integral part of my life. At the school of nursing, we had created a culture of prayer, frequently stopping during the day to pray for specific needs that arose. But this prayer journey was different. Circling 2 Chronicles 7:14 by kneeling before the Lord daily, I found my own prayer life radically changed.

I challenged the faculty with the same encounter as we approached 2018. I knew the school of nursing and its programs in and of themselves were not significant, but our lives were, as we circled this daily promise in prayer. "If my people, who are called by my name, will humble themselves and pray and seek my face and turn from their wicked ways, then I will hear from heaven, and I will forgive their sin and will heal their land."

Based on the legend of Honi the Circle Maker, **praying circles** around our biggest dreams and greatest fears became a powerful new way for me as a leader to experience God's divine appointments and see His hand in our work. I began to realize that I am not accomplishing great things for God, but rather that He is accomplishing great things in me. My job is to pray, trust, and move forward in His power when He opens the doors.

The legend of Honi takes place in the first century B.C., when a devastating drought threatened to destroy a generation. With a six-foot staff in his hand, Honi turned like a math compass, stood inside the circle he had drawn in the sand, and then dropped to his knees and, without a hint of doubt, called on God for rain. His prayer was resolute, humble, confident, and expectant. As the prayer ascended to the heavens, a sprinkle of raindrops descended to the earth. The people rejoiced, but Honi was not satisfied. He prayed again for the rain to fill cisterns and caverns. When it came in a downpour, Honi stayed in the circle and refined his bold request again: "Not for such rain have I prayed, but for rain of your favor, blessing and graciousness." Then by God's grace, when the rain soaked the people's skin, it also soaked their spirit of faith. The circle that Honi drew in the sand became a sacred symbol and testament to the power of God to meet the needs of His people (Batterson, 2011).

My initial circle prayer for 2018 was to settle in, stabilize faculty and staff, and focus on quality within each nursing program. However, God had other plans in mind. By the end of 2017, the university was experiencing exceptional growth. Executive leadership was favorably discussing the need to start the first doctoral program in the university. As deans discussed options and priorities, nursing was selected to lead the way and complete a feasibility study. Never in my wildest dreams or fervent prayers did this possibility ever cross my mind. But with God, all things are possible (Matthew 1:26). God opened the door, the faculty circled it in prayer, and we moved forward to gather data and validate the need. Our two administrative staff had resigned, and with the resignation of a program director, my hopes and prayers for stability were shattered. We knew at some point in time we anticipated expanding the BSN program to campus students. But this dream seemed quite far off, especially knowing that we needed to secure additional laboratory space. Our partnership for lab and simulation with a local hospital had been a wonderful solution for both facilities over the past few years. But now, both institutions were changing and our own lab space was a constant prayer request. I knew we had to wait on God's timing. So my thoughts and prayers turned to the administrative support needs, program leadership, and the doctorate.

At the close of fall semester 2017, during the very last week of school, another divine appointment occurred. We were in the final stages of hiring for a faculty position to teach children and family nursing. As I was heading into the final candidate interview, a new CV from a highly qualified person literally flew into my e-mail box. A phone conversation revealed that she was a perfect fit for the university and felt God's call to Colorado Christian University (CCU). At that point, we already had hired a qualified person for the only available position. However, within the span of 48 hours, there was an unexpected faculty resignation. We then saw that God had orchestrated two new team members, highly energetic, extremely competent, and eager to engage in the work that was before us.

As I think about the past year, I know without a doubt that the God of the universe had His hand on my life and the life of our faculty and school of nursing. He truly cares about every detail of our lives. In a few months, we hired three outstanding new faculty, completed the feasibility study for a doctorate degree, wrote a proposal request to HLC, and became actively involved in state policy issues impacting the nursing profession. The proposal for the first doctorate within the university was submitted in mid-July, with an understanding that the accrediting body would most likely come to make a site visit sometime in the next year.

At the same time, I was clearly nudged by the Lord to talk with the university administration early in the year regarding support for BSN program expansion. This dream, although firmly on the strategic plan for more than 10 years, had never been fully discussed with university leadership. With documented support, we began to circle this issue in prayer, asking God for His perfect timing. In July, through a series of statewide events as well as university growth and support, collaboration began between two very unique and distinct colleges within the university to develop a plan to expand the BSN nursing program to campus-based students as well as adult students. Weekly meetings were attended with great enthusiasm, as faculty in both colleges worked on a specific plan to meet the needs of both student populations without compromising program quality. Key university leaders met with the university president in mid-August.

After a 24-hour prayer vigil, word came back that faculty were to move ahead and submit a request to the nursing board by early September so as to gain a place on the agenda before the end of the year. In Colorado, the Board of Nursing regulates admission numbers for all nursing programs due to limited clinical placement sites. The short time frame between university approval and the need to submit a formal request was next to impossible. We would need to validate our resources to expand.

We needed a lab and we needed additional clinical placement sites—two highly important components of any generic nursing program. It usually takes six months to open a new site, requiring many phone calls, site visits, and clear long-term plans. We had just two weeks. So once again, we drew the circle and prayed.

The request came together more quickly than I had ever seen in all my years of nursing. Within the span of two weeks, we had documented evidence that leased lab space was under renovation and would be ready for occupancy on November 1. The budget for additional university resources and staff had been reviewed and approved. Finally, the additional clinical placement sites in all areas of specialty were secured. In fact, God certainly has a sense of humor, as we were able to submit the request to the Board of Nursing with more than 52 additional confirmed placements instead of the 48 needed. Everyone—faculty, staff, and university leadership—was in awe of what God had done.

Of course, the battle is never over. Even when we know we are doing what we are truly called to do, we do not find God's peace by engaging in excessive planning and attempting to control what happens in the future. I have learned that when my mind spins with plans and success sometimes seems within my grasp, it always eludes me. Just when I think I have prepared for all possibilities, something unexpected happens and throws things into confusion. You see, God did not design us to figure out the future; that is beyond our capability. Instead, God crafted our minds and our hearts for continual communication with Him. We need to trust Him. He wants us to bring Him all of our needs, our hopes, our fears, and our dreams.

▶ Reflecting on the Call to Nursing as Ministry

Nursing has always been viewed as a caring profession. Historically, the profession has roots in the Christian concept of ministry or

---

BOX 2-1 Evidence-Based Practice Focus

An article by Lentz (2018) presents the case for a faith-based palliative care ministry. Faith community nurses (FCNs) are in a unique position to help persons who are in home care prior to hospice (that is, more than six months to live, but with a life-limiting illness). The author suggests that the new role of a palliative care doula (PCD), as a palliative care expert with a faith-based approach, is uniquely qualified to lead a palliative care *ministry* team made up of nurses. Such a care team, coordinated by the PCD, can provide education to patients, families, and parishioners at several key points of care in the dying process prior to hospice.

Modified from Lentz, J. C. (2018). An innovative role for faith community nursing: Palliative care ministry. *Journal of Christian Nursing, 35*(2), 112–119.

BOX 2-2 Research Highlight

Faith community nurses often assume the role of educator in the church or parish, which puts them in a special position to positively influence health behaviors. In this study, clinical nurse specialist students, who were also parish nurses, provided two hours of education each week for six weeks to 11 participants older than the age of 14, with only 4 persons completing all of the sessions. Both older adults and family dyads and triads initially participated, representing teens, adults, and older adults. The educational topics included spiritual growth, stress management, nutrition, physical activity, enhancing self-efficacy, interpersonal relations, and primary and secondary strategies to promote health in adults. The results showed a trend toward healthier behaviors in those who participated, but without statistical significance, which is not surprising due to the small sample size. This study had serious limitations that prohibit generalization of its results, particularly the small sample size, the use of a convenience sample, and a high drop-out rate. However, the topics that formed the education have merit, based on the literature review presented, and the lack of participation in the complete program illustrates a common problem when engaging in community education programs and research.

Modified from Callaghan, D. M. (2016). Implementing faith community nursing interventions to promote healthy behaviors in adults. *International Journal of Faith Community Nursing, 2*(1), 3.

---

service. Although recent changes in healthcare delivery and data measures have focused on the "business" of health and evidence-based practice relying on research, the need to place the whole patient at the center of care remains at the core of nursing practice (see **BOXES 2-1** and **2-2**).

The word *ministry* originated from the Greek word *diakonia*, meaning "service." For years growing up, I heard from missionaries who were in "full-time ministry" either in local or international organizations. In some cultures, such as with my Korean colleagues, after one retires from a professional career, the expectation is to go into "full-time ministry"

serving the Lord throughout the world, meeting the needs of others. But it has always seemed to me that the work of nursing, if truly done from a scriptural perspective, is actually full-time ministry in and of itself. What better way to serve the Lord daily than through nursing? When you think about a 30-year career in the nursing profession, this equates to 62,400 hours of patient care. If all nursing graduates have a 30-year career in nursing, they together will have spent literally millions of hours in caregiving. So why does that matter? That is literally hours and days and years of practicing nursing as ministry, of serving with transformed minds and compassionate hearts.

You never know when or where or how God will invade the routine of your life. In the life of the believer, there are no coincidences. Jeremiah 29:11 assures us that God has a plan for each of us. Right now He is preparing each one of you for the very place that He has for you in nursing. No one else can fill that position. Ephesians 2:10 tells us that "we are God's workmanship, created in Christ Jesus to do good works, which God prepared in advance for us to do." God is always preparing us and positioning us for divine appointments. You will have many of them throughout your career. My prayer for each of you is that you will respectfully and appropriately share the love, compassion, and hope of Jesus with each of your patients during those 62,000 hours of nursing care. Nursing as ministry means serving God and others as Jesus did, as he is our example. The unique calling of the Christian nurse is the realization that one is gifted by God for a specific nursing practice to make a significant difference in the world. Nursing as ministry encompasses evidence-based and compassionate care and is directed by the nurse's faith, which shapes the understanding of roles, privileges, and responsibilities within practice and health care.

Being a Christian nurse does not make one more skilled or competent, nor does it mean that the nurse is more kind, understanding, or compassionate. What we do bring to every clinical situation is our relationship with Jesus, and because of him, we see things differently. Because Jesus transforms us, he works through us to touch others, physically, emotionally, and spiritually. We see brokenness, but we also see the possibility of wholeness. We see suffering, but we also see hope. We see beyond the symptoms and the disease to the person created in the image of God—and that makes a huge difference. Hospitals are filled with holy moments as people come face to face with their mortality and the questions of eternity. The person assigned to the nurse has an eternal soul, a sacred spiritual part of every human being that is immortal. Because of this, I am firmly convinced that nursing is both a scientific discipline and a sacred calling, and that the nurse, no matter the setting, stands on holy ground (O'Brien, 2014).

Faculty have the privilege of teaching and mentoring students through the rigorous process of nursing education. They share their professional knowledge and expertise. But more important, they share their heart and their faith. Nursing instructors of faith know that nursing is a scientific discipline as well as a sacred calling. They are committed to high-quality education based on evidence and the essentials of practice, and they are committed to spiritual formation and growth along the way. We are acutely aware that nurses have the privilege of impacting people's lives physically, emotionally, and spiritually. We know that hospitals, nursing homes, and client's homes are filled with holy moments.

▶ Lessons Learned

As a dean leading a group of dedicated faculty who are committed followers of Christ, God has taught me many lessons in leadership through great authors such as John Maxwell, Robert Greenleaf, Philip Yancey, Os Guinness, and Kevin Leman. My bookshelves are literally filled with great books written by these great men of faith, all containing nuggets of wisdom. One book, however, has been a pillar in my growth as a leader, as the foundational principles it espouses clearly mesh with who God made me to be. *The Servant Leader* by Blanchard and Hodges (2003) challenges the reader to answer two important questions: "Who will you follow?" and "How will you lead?" This text highlights the **servant leadership** principles taught by Jesus. The heart of my leadership, I found, needed to be transformed by examining my motivation, developing Christ-like character, and mastering my pride and fear (Psalm 19:14).

Like any leader, I had to examine my assumptions, set the vision, define and model the values, and create the follower environment—a process that required the renewing of my leadership mind (Romans 12:2). My goal to provide more effective leadership was advanced when my heart and my mind guided my behavior and interactions with others (James 1:22), sometimes called the hands of leadership. Learning about how to effectively manage change and become a performance coach has proved to be an invaluable asset. Finally, forming the habits of effective leadership requires the five disciplines that Jesus practiced during his earthly walk (Psalm 46:10):

- Solitude: spending time alone with God
- Prayer: having a conversation with God and listening to His voice
- Storing up God's Word: meditating on scripture to prepare for the challenges that are yet to come
- Faith in God's unconditional love: proceeding with confidence grounded in trust
- Accountability in relationships: sharing in his vulnerability (Blanchard & Hodges, 2003)

No book, however, is more life changing and has more leadership principles than the Bible itself. The Bible is the Word of God (1 Thessalonians 2:13), truth (2 Timothy 2:15), and alive (Hebrews 4:12); it gives life (1 Peter 1:23) and teaches us how to live (2 Timothy 3:16–17). My best instruction has come from spending time with the Lord, listening to Him, and obeying His precepts. Scripture speaks to my personal development as a wife, mother, friend, colleague, and leader. As I studied heroes of the faith who displayed character, commitment, courage, humility, integrity, and wisdom, I came face to face with my own shortcomings and learned to trust more. Scripture is full of Biblical principles related to accountability, conflict management, decision making, empowerment, stress management, team building, organizational leadership, power, and influence—all skills needed by any leader. As I seek greater understanding of God's love for me through my daily relationships with others,

I am in awe of God's faithfulness, grace, and mercy as He gently draws me closer to Him.

So what are the lessons learned through all of these many years of walking with the Lord in nursing education? Now, nearing the end of my career, I look back with a grateful heart for what God has done in my life. He is truly faithful. And I press on to what is ahead, the next goal or the next challenge that God lays on my heart. I am again reminded that with God, it is not about what we are doing at all, but rather who we are becoming in the process. It is not about doing great things for God, but rather God doing great things in and through us.

Find Your Passion

I often heard my husband say to our kids as they were considering their life work: "Find a job you love. If you do, you will never work a day in your life." Passion is something you love or enjoy doing. Psalm 37:4–5 says, "Take delight in the Lord and he will give you the desires of your heart. Commit your way to the Lord trust in Him and He will do this." To delight in the Lord means that our hearts find joy and fulfillment in Him. When we find satisfaction and worth in God, our hearts long to do His will and our desires begin to match His. As we grow close to Him, get to know Him, and follow him, we recognize that we will never be happy or fulfilled with what this world has to offer. Our hope is in God. He has a specific plan for our lives. God called us first to himself, to follow Jesus and become Christians. But God also has called us to a specific life purpose that is unique to each individual, a particular reason for being. And then God calls us to our immediate responsibilities, those tasks or duties in front of us today. God longs for us to be all that He calls us to be (Smith, 2011). When we listen to God and become a coworker with Him, He directs our steps and uses everything in our life for what He has in mind next. He schedules the divine appointments that result in our assurance that we are doing what He created us to do.

Be Persistent

My husband frequently tells me I have more persistence than anyone he knows.

Determined persistence or perseverance is being tenacious, not giving up, and making the effort to do something and keep doing it until you reach the end. Although surrender and yielding to the Lord was clearly needed for my dream to become a reality, persevering through the trials associated with any position, responsibility, or relationship is what brings maturity of character. As a young woman, someone once asked me what I wanted as my legacy. How did I want to be remembered? I clearly remember saying, "I want to be remembered as a woman of God."

Many times over the past several years, I have found myself quoting James 1:2–4: "Consider it pure joy, my brothers and sisters, whenever you face trials of many kinds, because you know that the testing of your faith produces perseverance. Let perseverance finish its work so that you may be mature and complete, not lacking anything." The scripture does not say "if" you face trials, but "when" you face trials. Everyone faces trials or tribulations in life that test one's patience and endurance. The key is to bring that trial before the Lord, asking what you are to learn and how you are to proceed. The secret is found in Romans 5:3–5: "because we know that suffering produces perseverance; perseverance, character; and character, hope. And hope does not put us to shame, because God's love has been poured out into our hearts through the Holy Spirit, who has been given to us." Only through the power of the Holy Spirit do we mature in character and find hope.

The power of passion and perseverance has been defined as "grit" (Blanchard & Hodges, 2003). Duckworth (2016) sums up her extensive research by saying, "In sum, no matter the domain, the highly successful had a kind of ferocious determination that played out in two ways. First, they are usually resilient and hardworking. Second, they knew in a very, very deep way what it was they wanted. They not only had determination, they had direction" (p. 8). After I took the Grit Assessment Test, the results confirmed that my nature is definitely "gritty." But my prayer is that I will be determined and focused on pursuing only those things that God has called me to do, by the power of the Holy Spirit, by His grace and for His glory.

Draw on God's Power

Anything of eternal value in this life and in eternity is accomplished only by the work of the Holy Spirit in us. I have often heard it said that when God calls us, He also equips us. This was certainly true in my life. Some leadership traits come naturally; many others can be learned. My leadership power is ineffective in every way. It is only in His power that meaningful programs are built and people's lives are impacted. "But you shall receive power when the Holy Spirit has come upon you; and you shall be witnesses to Me in Jerusalem, and all of Judea and Samaria, and to the end of the earth" (Acts 1:8). The Holy Spirit gives us the power to accomplish the work. He is the helper who guides us into all truth, convicts us of sin and transforms us into the image of Christ, and provides wisdom and discernment along the way.

I have often wondered why the dream of teaching nursing as ministry was such a powerful force throughout my life. Why did I want to integrate faith into the profession? The answer is really quite simple. As a Christian, my eternal security is sealed. I know that it is only through the blood shed by Jesus that someday I can enter into heaven. Jesus will stand between me and God Himself because it was His sacrifice on the cross that paid the penalty for my sin. Now that is hope and peace. My life purpose is to inspire hope: That is what I want to do in teaching students, and that is what I believe nurses should do in caring for patients. Nurses should be competent and compassionate, use clinical reasoning, promote health, and inspire hope. Nurses care for the whole person—

🔍 *CASE STUDY 2-1*

Dana is a sophomore nursing student in a public university. She feels that God has been using her family, Christian friends, and life circumstances to point her to change schools to attend a Christian university where she can grow in her faith. Dana has a strong desire to serve on the mission field. As the daughter of missionaries to the Philippines, this has been her heart's passion for many years. However, changing schools would likely result in losing some credits through the transfer and incurring additional costs, setting her back in her goal of getting her BSN in a typical four-year cycle. Dana comes to you, as a fellow Christian nursing student, for advice.

Questions

1. What wise counsel can you give to Dana?
2. How would you pray for her, as a friend and as a fellow nursing student?
3. With whom could Dana talk to find out about faith-based nursing programs in the United States? Is there a list of Christian nursing programs anywhere to which she could refer?
4. Which scriptures could you share with Dana?

body, mind, and spirit. Someday all of us will stand before our maker to give an account of our life. Praise God, I can only stand because of Jesus.

My prayer for you today is that you will seek God with all your heart and that you discover His call for your life. Stop long enough in the hectic chaos of life to listen, really listen, to the still small voice of God (**CASE STUDY 2-1**). Ask Him what plans He has for you. May there be many divine appointments orchestrated by your loving heavenly Father. Once you discover your dream and you know your call, I pray that you will not run ahead of God, do not fall behind God, and certainly do not forget what God has called you to do. Claim God's blessings as you wait and work and live life in the meantime. Seek the face of Jesus and the filling of the Holy Spirit—for it is only in His power that you can accomplish anything of significance.

In the years ahead, my prayer is that many who may read this text will grow in their knowledge of God through recognizing scripture as truth, will experience the joy and peace in life that comes only through knowing Jesus

as Savior and Lord, will mature and be transformed through the power of the Holy Spirit, and will find passion and purpose within the profession so that they can serve Him in nursing—by His grace and for His glory—for such a time as this (Esther 4:14).

▶ Clinical Reasoning Exercises

1. How did you choose nursing as a career? Did you feel the same call from God as Dr. White shared in this chapter? Share your story with at least of one of your peers.
2. Many scripture passages are woven into Dr. White's story. With which of these scriptures do you most identify, and why?
3. This chapter talks about three types of ways to wait after hearing God's call. Discuss these three types, giving examples of characters who illustrate each from the scripture.

▶ Personal Reflection Exercises

1. Have you felt God's call on your life to nursing as ministry? When did this happen? What is your story?
2. What are the major divine appointments in your life that have brought you to where you are now?
3. What part of Dr. White's story resonates most with you?
4. In this chapter, you are encouraged to find your passion. What is your own passion? How does your passion intersect with your God-given gifts and talents?
5. Are you living out God's call in your life? Or have you become sidetracked by the business of life? Which steps do you need to take to accomplish God's calling in your life?
6. Have you ever had a period of waiting to see God's calling fulfilled in your life? What did that look like? How did that feel?

References

Angking, D. (2012). Preparing for nursing ministry. *Journal of Christian Nursing, 21*(1), 59.

Batterson, N. (2011). *The circle maker: Praying circles around your biggest dreams and greatest fears.* Grand Rapids, MI: Zondervan.

Batterson, M. (2012). *Draw the circle: The 40 day prayer challenge.* Grand Rapids, MI: Zondervan.

Blanchard, K., & Hodges, P. (2003). *The servant leader: Transforming your heart, head, hands and habits.* Nashville, TN: Thomas Nelson.

Brendle, R. (2006). *In the meantime: The practice of proactive waiting.* Colorado Springs, CO: WaterBrook.

Centers for Medicare and Medicaid. (2016). Design and development of the diagnosis related group (DRG). Retrieved from https://www.cms.gov/ICD10Manual /version34-fullcode-cms/fullcode_cms/Design_and _development_of_the_Diagnosis_Related_Group _(DRGs)_PBL-038.pdf

Duckworth, A. (2016). *Grit: The power of passion and perseverance.* New York, NY: Simon and Schuster.

O'Brien, M. (2014). *Spirituality in nursing: Standing on holy ground.* Sudbury, MA: Jones & Bartlett Learning.

Smith, G. (2011). *Courage and calling: Embracing your God-given potential.* Downers Grove, IL: InterVarsity Press.

Recommended Readings

MacArthur, J. F. (2017). *Pastoral ministry: How to shepherd biblically.* Nashville, TN: Thomas Nelson.

O'Brien, M. (2017). *Spirituality in nursing: Standing on holy ground.* Sudbury, MA: Jones & Bartlett Learning.

Repo, H., Vahlberg, T., Salminen, L., Papadopoulos, I., & Leino-Kilpi, H. (2017). The cultural competence of graduating nursing students. *Journal of Transcultural Nursing, 28*(1), 98–107.

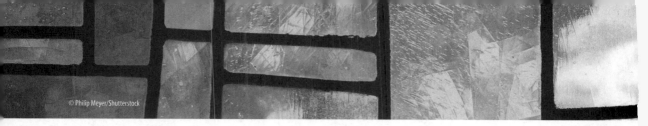

CHAPTER 3

Caring from a Christian Worldview: The Agape Model

Shirlene Newbanks, DNP, RN; **Nancy Eckerd**, MS, RN; **Linda Rieg**, PhD, RN, CNE;
Tara Stephen, MSN, RN, PHN; and **Becky Le**, PhD, RN

LEARNING OBJECTIVES

At the end of this chapter, the reader will be able to:

1. Describe the Christian worldview.
2. Acknowledge the importance of the origin of caring.
3. Discuss how the Fruit of the Spirit may be reflected in nursing care.
4. Explore the personal worldview of the nurse dedicated to the Christian faith.
5. Apply the Agape Model.

KEY TERMS

Agape	Caritas	Imago Dei
Agape Model	Christian worldview	Shalom
Calling	Fruit of the Spirit	
Caring	Holy Spirit	

We Are Mirrors Reflecting Him

He is the Source; we are the "looking" glass.
He is the Light; we are the mirrors.
He sends the message; we mirror it.

We rest in Him—awaiting His call.
And when placed in His hands, we do His work.
It is not about us. It's all about Him.
(Lucado, 2004, p. 32)

Sarah's shoulder leaned wearily against the doorframe of the hospital room; her head too slowly accepted the welcoming support as she waited for her patient to call her for further assistance. It was during this 11th year of her nursing practice, while serving as a weekend charge nurse on an oncology unit, that Sarah experienced a transformation in her personal philosophy of nursing. Learning the mechanics of the functioning human body and the skills necessary to care for the sick and diseased was a major focus as a novice nurse. As she grew professionally from a novice to a competent nurse, there was a strong desire to provide what many perceive to be expert nursing care; however, the increased expectations of hospital administrators and the introduction to new technology resulted in less time at the bedside of the patient, leading to an increased dissatisfaction in her role.

Sarah was weary of the late and long hours of work and the lack of sleep, and she was battling grief from the recent loss of her husband from the dreaded disease of cancer. **Caring** for those who were experiencing the same disease that was her husband's demise only intensified her numbness. Nursing had become a struggle, a duty—merely tasks to perform and a way to provide a living. That night, however, while Sarah was assisting her patient, the patient became more than just an object of duty.

As a Christian, Sarah's personal values and beliefs—specifically, the knowledge that God is the Creator of all things and that He directed her life's path—were never a question in her mind. But that night, they became more than just "head knowledge." As she leaned wearily against the doorframe, Sarah questioned in her mind, "Why am I doing this?" Before the thought had completely slipped away, the **Holy Spirit** strongly impressed upon her heart and mind, saying, "This is one of My created beings and I personally placed this patient under your care." Sarah experienced that night what Nightingale (1992) and others have emphasized as a **calling** from God. Although Sarah's underlying values as a Christian did

not change, her nursing philosophy did. The change did not occur due to her gradual maturity in the profession; instead, nursing became a "calling to serve" as a directive from the Creator Himself.

▶ Nursing as a Spiritual Calling

Historically, many nurses believe that nursing was founded on Biblical principles and that early Christian women felt called to minister and care for the needs of others. In so doing, they demonstrated, or mirrored, the caring characteristics of Jesus Christ (Newbanks, 2015). Throughout history, there have been numerous examples of the link between serving God and health care (**TABLE 3-1**). One of the earliest accounts of nurses demonstrating caring for others is found in Exodus, when midwives would not kill infant boys, because they feared God more than they feared Pharaoh. The relationship between faith and health was foundational with the teachings of Moses and the Levitical laws. At the time, they probably seemed to be just rules to follow, but now we understand that the principles of epidemiology, aseptic technique, isolation, and hand washing were health laws. One of the most well-known Biblical accounts of caring is the parable that Jesus told of the Good Samaritan. In this parable, we discover a man who met the emergent needs of a stranger and recognize the Good Samaritan as reflective of "a neighbor"; understanding the concept of loving your neighbor as yourself. The utmost model of caring is in the form of Jesus Christ himself as he ministered to the needs of many in life, and in death.

Caring was also demonstrated as ministry by early religious orders as they served the sick. St. Benedict founded the Benedictine nursing order. Military, religious, and lay orders of men including the Knights Hospitalers, the Teutonic Knights, the Knights of

TABLE 3-1 A History of Caring

Timeline	Caring: Reflecting	Major Reference	Contribution to Caring from a Biblical/Christian Worldview
Approximately 1450 B.C.	Hebrew midwives	Exodus 1	Example of the call to love God rather than government authorities.
Approximately 1400 B.C.	Moses/Biblical health laws	Leviticus and Deuteronomy	Links between health laws and prevention—even if the cause wasn't understood.
25–30 A.D.	Jesus Christ	Gospel accounts, Luke 10:25–37	Call for compassion, caring, and agape love; serving the poor and helpless; Good Samaritan.
30–100 A.D.	Early church	Matthew 22:36–50; Matthew 25; Acts 6; James 1:27	Deacons and deaconesses caring for the widows, orphans, and sick; loving God and loving others.
1800s	Sisters of Charity, Sisters of Mercy, Deaconesses at Kaiserwerth	Ann Doyle, nursing by religious orders	Provided care to reflect the love of Christ and call to minister to those whom God loves.
1850–1860	Florence Nightingale	*Notes on Nursing*, 1860	Presented nursing as a calling—a means to demonstrate God's love.
1976–present	Sister Callista Roy	Roy, C. (1988). An explication of the philosophical assumptions of the Roy adaptation model. *Nursing Science Quarterly, 1*, 26–34	Roy views human beings as individuals in community with a loving Creator and with others; concept of veritivity. "Persons have mutual relationships with the world and a God-figure" and "God is intimately revealed in the diversity of creation and is the common destiny of creation" (Roy, 1997, p. 45).
1984	Roach	Caring from the heart	Roach's theory of caring brought together aspects of relational ethics, spirituality, and components of caring to inform nursing practice

(continues)

TABLE 3-1 A History of Caring   *(continued)*

Timeline	Caring: Reflecting	Major Reference	Contribution to Caring from a Biblical/Christian Worldview
1994	Ann Bradshaw	*Lighting the Lamp: The Spiritual Dimension of Nursing Care*	An in-depth study of the spiritual dimension of human nature and its place in nursing; presents the Judeo-Christian perspective of a covenant relationship based on love—agape or caritas. Traces the historical development of nursing, with the increasing tensions created by secularization in the profession.
1997	Katie Eriksson	Multiple publications from 1997 onward	Presents the concept of caritas from scripture—agape love—and relates to nursing and caring.
1998, 2008, 2011, 2014	Mary Elizabeth O'Brien	*Spirituality in Nursing: Standing on Holy Ground*	Multiple works that link the love of Christ with nursing care; specifically, that a nursing encounter is a sacred encounter; using the concept of standing on holy ground.
1999, 2006	Shelly and Miller	*Called to Care: A Christian Theology of Nursing* (1st and 2nd editions)	Classical work that compares nursing concepts as seen through a Christian worldview versus post-modern nursing theories.
2004	Cusveller	*Commitment and Responsibility in Nursing: A Faith-Based Approach*	Builds on the scriptural principles of human dignity and the roots of Christian nursing.
2005	Doornbos, Groenhout, and Hotz	*Transforming Care: A Christian Vision of Nursing Practice*	Responds to the question, "How does a commitment to the Christian faith inform the practice of care?"
2013	Campinha-Bacote	*A Biblical Based Model of Cultural Competence in the Delivery of Healthcare Services: Seeing Imago Dei*	Presents a Biblical-based model for the process of becoming culturally competent.

St. Lazarus, and the Hospital Brothers of St. Anthony provided nursing care during the Middle Ages (Rieg, Newbanks, & Sprunger, 2018).

Florence Nightingale witnessed quality care by observing Catholic nuns, who she said made better nurses because they were disciplined and well organized; she also spent time with the Protestant deaconesses at Kaiserwerth, who were well known for caring for the destitute and the training school. Nightingale highly valued education and advocated raising the standard of education for nurses, but she also emphasized nursing as a calling—a vocation: "But more than this, she must be a religious and devoted woman; she must have a respect for her own calling, because God's precious gift of life is often literally placed in her hands" (Nightingale, 1860, p. 71).

The Latin form of the term *vocation* dates back to the 1400s and was defined as "a summons or strong inclination to a particular state or course of action; especially: a divine call to the religious life" ("Vocation," n.d.). As described by Lundmark (2007), the proper title for nursing was heavily debated by the end of the 19th century by nursing organizations and mainstream nursing—namely, whether nursing should be labeled a "vocation" or a "contract." Mainstream medical organizations saw nursing as "particularism, scientism, and more of a contract rather than a vocation" (p. 768). The critical factor for these organizations was that higher education and certification provided competent nurses; therefore, they resisted calling it a vocation, which was perceived as a "virtue of obedience to doctors . . . femininity and motherhood" (p. 768).

Although Nightingale valued education and raising the standard for nursing, it was her perception that, in itself, education should not be the standard by which nurses are measured; instead, nurses should be measured by the standard of their relationship with God (Bradshaw, 1994). Lundmark (2007, p. 767) contends that it is important to use theology-based nursing theories so as to understand the concept

of "vocation" as an intrinsic motivating factor for what motivates a person to choose the profession of nursing and to fully understand nursing itself. Bradshaw perceived the concept of vocation to mean that "Nurses . . . choose to become actualized as a caring person" (Lundmark, 2007, p. 770). In the 1960s and 1970s, nursing turned toward secular values; nevertheless, some Christian nurse leaders advocated a return to the link between faith, calling, and nursing care (see Table 3-1). Viewing nursing as a caring vocation influences how one serves the patient and the community in which the nurse works.

Love and charity, or **caritas**, was originally emphasized as a principal idea in Eriksson's early works (1989, 1997, 2002). Eriksson held that the human being is fundamentally body, soul, and spirit. As such, she asserted that we are religious beings and created in God's image. Therefore, each person deserves dignity, and nurses must accept the responsibility of serving with love and existing for the sake of others. Although other nurse theorists have used this caritas concept, the original scriptures and Biblical understanding of agape love were not preserved in Eriksson's presentation. Instead, in collaboration with several theologians, Eriksson developed a subdiscipline referred to as *caring theology* (Lindstrom, Nystrom, & Zetterlund, 2018).

Shelly and Miller (2006), in their Christian theology of caring, propose that a Christian nurse serves to provide "care for the whole person, in response to God's grace toward a sinful world, which aims to foster optimum health and bring comfort in suffering and death for anyone in need" (p. 250). In accepting this worldview, nursing becomes a "calling" to care for the sick, which cannot be separated from its roots of Biblical teachings (Matthew 25:31–46; Luke 10:33–35; 1 Thessalonians 2:6–8).

In 1905, Weber predicted that the advancement of science and technology would be viewed as progress, and that the epistemology would shift such that the religious principles and "notions of divine authority would fade away and disappear completely" (Fowler, 2012, p. 5). Weber's prediction is supported by contemporary authors who suggest that the Biblical context has been removed from nursing over the years and the perception of what constitutes nursing is changing (Hawke-Eder, 2017; Liaschenko & Peter, 2004; Salladay, 2000).

The concern of some nurses who hold a **Christian worldview** is that nursing is moving toward becoming an occupation rather than a vocation. In addition, the shift of what constitutes a good nurse is moving toward self-sufficiency, professionalism, and academic knowledge (Hawke-Eder, 2017). "Some argue the shift towards academia has left newly qualified nurses ineffective at both performing practical tasks and the interpersonal skills of caring" (Hawke-Eder, 2017, p. 24). This shift has been subtle, and neither obvious nor easy to detect or analyze. Through the years, nursing has been somewhat redefined as a "scientific discipline as well as a profession that requires education and national examination for licensure . . . with a flexible boundary that is responsive to the changing needs of society and expanding knowledge base of its theoretical and scientific domains" (Shelly & Miller, 2006, p. 243; see also Hawke-Eder, 2017). Although education and national examination are essential to the nursing profession, the emphasis on the art of caring has decreased, to the point that nursing has become more of a financial venture and a source of professional career advancement to many practitioners.

For many who hold a Christian worldview, this shift may not be apparent or realized due to either a lack of understanding of nursing theories of other worldviews or a failure to appreciate the danger of embracing theories that include concepts that are contrary to a Christian worldview (Newbanks, Rieg, & Schaefer, 2018). For instance, Shelly and Miller (2006) emphasize that some theories might "open the door to the spirit world Christians are warned against in the Scripture" (p. 51). 1 John 4:1 addresses this point: "Beloved, do not believe every spirit, but test the spirits whether they are of God; because many false prophets have gone out into the world" (New King James Version [NKJV]). In the next section, the Christian worldview is explained further within the description of the nursing metaparadigm.

▶ The Nursing Metaparadigm from a Christian Worldview

Our worldview shapes our responses to life's situations and provides a foundation for our nursing practice. The nursing metaparadigm serves as a framework that nurses infuse with their personal worldview and use to guide their practice. In this chapter, the concepts within this metaparadigm are addressed from the Christian worldview, are based on Biblical truths, and are reflected in the **Agape Model** (**FIGURE 3-1**, **TABLE 3-2**; Eckerd, 2017).

The concept of "caring in nursing moves the term *nurse* to the verb form, *to nurse* or *nursing*"—one of the components of the nursing metaparadigm (Newbanks, 2015, p. 4). Tonges and Ray (2011) contend that the concept of nursing is the act of nurses "demonstrating they care about patients" and propose it "is as important to patient well-being as caring for them through clinical activities such as preventing infection and administering medications" (p. 374). If nursing is grounded only in normative science, known as logical, ethical, and aesthetic ways of thinking, and does not include the concept of caring, it will "likely depict cause-and-effect relationships, depersonalization, detachment, and objectification of person" (Boykin & Schoenhofer, 2013, pp. 96–97). Such a view is too narrow to be considered high-quality care because it ignores the person and family and focuses instead on the disease or the injury, thereby justifying the necessity for Christ-centered patient care.

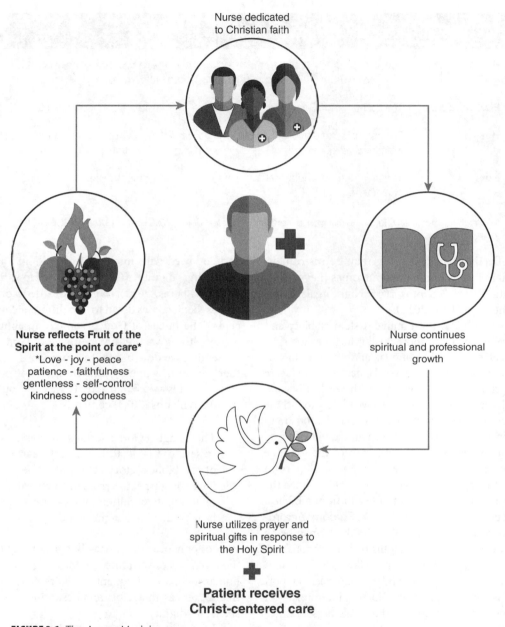

FIGURE 3-1 The Agape Model.

Reproduced from Eckerd, N. (2017). A nursing practice model based on Christ: The Agape model. *Journal of Christian Nursing, 35*(2), 124–130. doi:10.1097/CNJ0000000000000417

Another metaparadigm concept is that of the *environment*. In the Agape Model, this concept is defined as "the spiritual and physical realm where the nurse emulates the agape love of Christ" (Eckerd, 2017, p. 126). Kleffel (2013) maintains that the environment includes all internal and external conditions, circumstances, and influences affecting the person. The nurse may play a major role in assisting the patient in adapting to internal and external environmental stressors that might affect the individual's well-being. The nurse

TABLE 3-2 The Agape Model Metaparadigm Concepts	
Human being	The recipient of Christ-centered care, inclusive of the patient, patient's family, peers, and those with whom the nurse comes in contact, both professionally and personally
Environment	The spiritual and physical realm where the nurse emulates the agape love of Christ
Health	The optimal system stability and well-being of an individual, which includes the spiritual, emotional, relational, and physical dimensions of the recipient of Christ-centered care
Nursing	The practice of providing care to all humankind, revealing the presence and character of Christ

Reproduced from Eckerd, N. (2017). A nursing practice model based on Christ: The Agape model. *Journal of Christian Nursing, 35*(2), 124–130. doi:10.1097 /CNJ0000000000000417

reflecting Christ's caring may be instrumental in improving patient outcomes (Leyva, Peralta, Tejero, & Santos, 2015; Nightingale, Spiby, Sheen, & Slade, 2018).

Health is the optimal system stability and well-being of an individual; it includes the spiritual, emotional, relational, and physical dimensions of the recipient of Christ-centered care (Eckerd, 2017). Holistic health reaches beyond physical, mental, and social well-being to include the spiritual dimension. Research demonstrates a close relationship between an individual's spiritual wellness and the reaction of the immune system function in the healing process (Griffin & Yancey, 2009). Wolterstorff (1994) defined the metaparadigm concept of health from a Biblical standpoint and referred to it as **Shalom**. According to this author, Shalom is "the human being dwelling at peace in all his or her relationships: with God, with self, with fellows, with nature" (p. 251). Shelly and Miller (2006) also support this conceptualization: "Nursing is a ministry of compassionate care for the whole person, in response to God's grace, which aims to foster optimum health (Shalom) and bring comfort in suffering and death" (p. 68).

Unlike other worldviews, the Christian worldview emphasizes that the metaparadigm concept of *person* begins with God as the creator of human beings, created in the image and likeness of God (**Imago Dei**) as physiological, psychological, social, and spiritual beings, and endowed with intellect, free will, and an indwelling dignity (Genesis 1:26; Howard, 2013; Williams, 2013). Williams (2013) concludes that it comes down to two different concepts: "the image of God is something about us, something we are, or the image of God is something we do" (p. 11). In other words, either *person* is a noun, "something about our being," or it is a verb, "an activity we carry out" (p. 40). Williams (2013) contends:

> This imaging God is serious business, so serious that it sits at the very heart of the biblical story. The call to believe the gospel is designed to return us to our first calling, our calling to bear God's image in the world. (p. 44)

We not only bear that image but, according to the teachings of scripture, so does every other human being. Consequently, we are called to treat others as image bearers deserving of respect and dignity.

Ferngren (2009), an early-church historian, proposes that the "teachings on imago Dei were formative in shaping Christian views of humanity, ethics, and ministry" (p. 94). Ferngren also maintains that the doctrine of Imago Dei spurred Christian charity and philanthropy, provided grounds for the belief that human life possesses intrinsic value as a bearer of God's image, gave a new perception on embodiment and human personality, and formed the basis for Christian compassion and care for those in need (Newbanks, 2015). The metaparadigm concept of human being in this text is defined as "the recipient of Christ-centered care, inclusive of the patient, patient's family, peers and those with whom the nurse comes in contact, both professionally and personally" (Eckerd, 2017, p. 126).

When viewed through the lens of a Christian worldview, all of these nursing metaparadigm concepts—nursing, environment, health, and person—are systematically linked and interconnected and reflect the source of caring, caring behaviors, cultural implications, and Biblical scripture (Newbanks, 2015). The origin of caring permeates the framework of the Christian nursing metaparadigm. Just as nursing is considered a central concept in the nursing metaparadigm, so caring is considered a central concept in nursing.

▶ Origin of Caring

One might say that a Christian worldview is born through the transforming power of the Holy Spirit. Until nurses experience a spiritual "awakening" or transformation of the heart, they will not view their practice from a Christian worldview, reflect evidence of practicing the presence of God, see others through His eyes, or reflect His characteristics (Ezekiel 36:26; 2 Corinthians 5:17). According to Grenz and Olson (1996), our spiritual experiences radically affect our worldview. When one considers the Apostle Paul and his experience on the road to Damascus (Acts 9:1–22), we see that his worldview was quickly transformed after his encounter with Jesus. As Johnson (2008) stated, "Perhaps nurses are born, not made" (p. 21). There may be more truth in this statement than Johnson had intended or meant. Jesus told Nicodemus, "You must be born again" (John 3:7, NKJV); in this context, Jesus was referring to a spiritual birth, or reconciliation to God (Newbanks, 2015).

Jesus described the relationship of himself (the vine) and the disciples (the branches). In John 15:5, he said, "I am the vine; you are the branches. The one who remains in me and I in him produces much fruit, because you can do nothing without me" (Christian Standard Bible [CSB]). This metaphor emphasizes the energy and the strength that the branches receive to produce fruit when connected to the vine, with the fruit being the **Fruit of the Spirit** (Parrott, 2018).

As explained by Lundmark (2007), "God's love must be the value system that nursing care is dependent on . . . when God is in me, I am who I should be" (p. 774). This concept is also emphasized in 2 Corinthians 5:17: "Therefore if anyone is in Christ, he is a new creation; old things have passed away; behold, all things have become new" (NKJV). A person who is in Christ (freed from sin and created anew in Christ) no longer serves self, but longs to serve God and others. "We were made to live a life that says, 'Look at God.' People are to look at us and see not US but the image of our Maker" (Lucado, 2018, p. 22).

For a Christian nurse, the virtuous behavior of caring "requires understanding of Agape love" (Campinha-Bacote, 2013, p. 36). This understanding is not innate, nor does it come from a self-image that promotes pride and feeling good about oneself. Instead, Christian nurses see themselves in the light of God's grace and forgiveness, and their dependency upon the renewal of the Holy Spirit allows them to be used to "advance His kingdom and bring joy to others" (Hoekema, 1986, p. 110). As Austgard (2008) shared, "it is only the fruit of Christian belief that can bring about the sincere, self-sacrificing love that can elevate nursing to where it should be . . . without love, nursing is nothing more than a simple craft" (p. 315).

Because of our fallen nature, humans are not able to reflect agape love without having experienced reconciliation with God and an infilling of the Holy Spirit (Romans 5:5; Galatians 5:22). Agape love is "a love that is selfless,

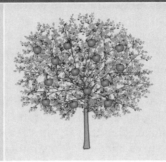

Biblical Practice Points Caring Begins with Christ's Love		
John 3:7 You must be born again. John 15:5 I am the vine; you are the branches. The one who remains in me and I in him produces much fruit, because you can do nothing without me.		2 Corinthians 5:17 Therefore, if anyone is in Christ, he is a new creation. Romans 5:5 This hope will not disappoint us, because God's love has been poured out in our hearts through the Holy Spirit who was given to us. (Christian Standard Bible)

FIGURE 3-2 Biblical practice points.

unconditional, and voluntary loving-kindness" (Campinha-Bacote, 2013, p. 36). We can teach students to care for patients with skills learned through educational strategies. But as the Apostle Paul stressed in Romans 3, compassionate Christian caring, or agape love, comes from the heart as a result of Christ within us; it is not intrinsic to human nature, but rather is a gift from God (Campinha-Bacote, 2013; Shelly & Miller, 2006). Competence without caring often results in robotic, "going through the motions" care. In contrast, bearing the image of God through caring is something that affects our being and is evidenced in the activities we carry out. Selfless caring is reflected as Christian caring. It is who we are, because it is who He is in us (**FIGURE 3-2**).

"It is important the nurse understand the origin of his or her caring and the behaviors that reflect caring, as the capacity to demonstrate caring, or lack thereof, is reflected in his or her nursing practice" (Newbanks et al., 2018, p. 160). Bringing students to the point of reflecting by way of "reexamining, reevaluating [and perhaps even] revising their convictions about God, [themselves], and our world" (Grenz & Olson, 1996, p. 125) may assist them in their practice and help them to answer the question of "why" they do what they do. Providing students with the opportunity to reflect on their worldview for nursing practice—specifically, the presence or lack of caring—is a needed activity that promotes change. Understanding that the source of caring is God and recognizing how caring is demonstrated will provide a foundation for incorporating caring within practice (see **BOXES 3-1** and **3-2**). This reflection may play a major part in this "awakening" or transformation process.

▶ The Agape Model

Every nurse dedicated to Christ has a story to be told regarding the Holy Spirit's influence on his or her practice. This Christian faith-based model is applicable to the clinical nurse, the missionary nurse, the school nurse, the community health practitioner, the nursing educator, the administrator, the advanced practice nurse, and even the new student nurse. When the dedicated nurse commits his or her practice to the Lord, amazing things happen. The purpose of the Agape Model (Figure 3-1) is not only to validate this gold standard of care but also to encourage the novice nursing student to be intentionally bold in his or her practice. The application of this model to the dedicated nurse is limitless, and consists of the highest level of professional, personal, and spiritual standards.

BOX 3-1 Research Highlight

In 2016, Kim and Patterson wanted to see if caring could be taught in a classroom setting. Data were gathered over a four-year period on a total convenience sample of 238 students in a psychiatric–mental health course in a BSN program. Students engaged in a self-awareness, reflective exercise; data were then gathered on an author-developed questionnaire to see if self-awareness actually influenced caring behaviors. The findings support that using self-awareness strategies and quiet time with silence and reflection did have a positive effect on caring behaviors in nursing students.

Modified from Kim, M. S., & Patterson, K. T. (2016). Teaching and practicing caring in the classroom: Students' responses to a self-awareness intervention in psychiatric-mental health nursing. *Journal of Christian Nursing, 33*(2), E23–E26.

BOX 3-2 Evidence-Based Practice Focus

In Dr. Newbanks's (the lead author for this chapter) final project for her doctorate of nursing practice (DNP), she used a critical review of existing literature to develop a middle-range theory on caring from a Christian worldview. Dr. Newbanks discovered that there was a paucity of research on caring from a Biblical worldview. A middle-range theory on Christian caring could guide Christian nurses in their nursing as ministry. Integrative review findings represented by 25 philosophers and nursing theorists showed that "qualitative research was most prevalent (27%) with phenomenological studies (12%) as the second most prevalent type of research study noted" (p. 41), suggesting that caring from a Christian perspective is in its infancy, and that much more research is needed. Characteristics of caring were explored and found to include 15 unique aspects when using a Christian worldview: agape love, accountability, charity, forgiving, faithfulness, generosity, goodness, joy, justness, long-suffering, peacefulness, self-control, self-giving, warmth, and willingness.

The author recommended four areas as ripe for research initiatives: (1) differences in perspectives of characteristics of caring, (2) a 360-degree evaluation of the characteristics of caring, (3) patients' agreement with the study findings, and (4) a Delphi study to confirm the characteristics in this study. Her complete paper on this project is available from ProQuest at the web address listed here.

Modified from Newbanks, R. S. (2015). An integrative critical literature review toward the development of a middle range theory on caring from a biblical Christian worldview (Order No. 10600632). ProQuest Dissertations & Theses Global: Health & Medicine. (1925343218). Retrieved from https://0-search -proquest-com.oak.indwes.edu/docview/1925343218?accountid=6363.

The Agape Model is a tool that describes the development and the character of a nurse who is dedicated to Christ. It is a reflection of the character of Christ manifesting agape love in the nurse's professional and personal life. **Agape** is considered God's self-sacrificial love, love that is charitable, caring for strangers, and love in action versus purely emotional (Eckerd, 2017; MacArthur, 2005). Scripture confirms the critical nature of this sacrificial love: "Truly I tell you, whatever you did for one of the least of these brothers and sisters of mine, you did for me" (Matthew 25:40, New International Version [NIV]).

The Agape Model describes how the nurse, enabled by the Holy Spirit, shows respect regardless of cultural differences or worldviews. Such a nurse is able to achieve excellence in all acts, attitudes, behaviors, thoughts, and deeds. Additionally, the Agape Model defines scriptural guidelines and encourages Christlike qualities that exemplify the excellence of the nurse dedicated to Christ in the delivery of professional standards of care. All core beliefs in this model are found in the Bible, which is considered the ultimate authority, supporting the practice of a nurse dedicated to Christ (Eckerd, 2017).

Statement of Faith

The Agape Model is rooted in a straightforward, Biblically based, nondenominational Statement of Faith:

> God exists in three persons: Father, Son and Holy Spirit. God created the heavens and earth and all things exist by and through Him. The Bible is the inerrant, authoritative Word of God, and together with the indwelling of the Holy Spirit, guides all personal and professional conduct and care provided by the nurse dedicated to Christian Faith. As an offering to God, the dedicated nurse strives for a life reflective of the dedication to a calling from God and belief in the crucifixion and resurrection of Jesus Christ as Lord and Savior, offering salvation and eternal life to all who seek him. (Eckerd, 2017)

The nurse's dedication to Christ is supported by the Statement of Ethos:

> The Agape Model is dedicated to a lifestyle reflecting the character of Christ in both professional and personal life. The reflection is visualized through care, incorporating the Fruit of the Spirit (Galatians 5:22–23) and achieved through committed professional and spiritual growth because of faith, prayer, the use of spiritual gifts and the leading of the Holy Spirit. The nurse dedicated to the Christian Faith is respectful of cultural differences and worldviews and offers

the highest level of excellence in all acts, attitudes, behaviors, thoughts and deeds. This commitment to excellence is viewed as worship and an offering to God. (Eckerd, 2017)

The dedicated Christian nurse's practice and ministry will reflect every aspect of the Agape Model. The Model consists of four intentionally simple constructs (Figure 3-1):

- The nurse is dedicated to Christian faith.
- The nurse continues spiritual and professional growth.
- The nurse utilizes prayer and spiritual gifts in response to the Holy Spirit.
- The nurse reflects the Fruit of the Spirit at the point of care.

The Nurse Is Dedicated to Christian Faith

The Agape Model's main assumption is that the nurse is dedicated to Christ (**FIGURE 3-3**). Becoming a follower of Christ requires that the believer accept Jesus Christ as Lord and Savior. Now a disciple, the believer receives the indwelling of the Holy Spirit. It is the Spirit of God within the believer that sets the dedicated nurse apart by influencing a lifestyle manifestation of the Fruit of the Spirit (Eckerd, 2017).

A	Accept Christ as Savior
G	Grow spiritually and professionally
A	Anticipate Holy Spirit intervention
P	Prayer and spiritual gifts
E	Embrace Fruit of the Spirit

FIGURE 3-3 The Agape Model mnemonic.

Reproduced from Eckerd, N. (2017). A nursing practice model based on Christ: The Agape model. *Journal of Christian Nursing, 35*(2), 124–130. doi:10.1097/CNJ0000000000000417

The nurse dedicated to the Christ also views the nursing practice as a calling or ministry rather than a job. Having been chosen for the profession of nursing, the dedicated nurse views his or her practice as holy ground (Eckerd, 2017; O'Brien, 2011). The dedicated nurse receives Godly instruction from the Holy Spirit, allowing for dedication in service to others, such as is described in 2 Corinthians 5:14–15: "For Christ's love compels us, because we are convinced that one died for all . . . that those who live should no longer live for themselves but for him who died for them and was raised again."

The Nurse Continues Spiritual and Professional Growth

The American Nurses Association's (ANA) *Code of Ethics for Nurses* states, "The nurse owes the same duties to self as to others, including the responsibility to promote health and safety, preserve wholeness of character and integrity, maintain competence and continue personal and professional growth" (ANA, 2015, p. 19). As dedicated nurses committed to our profession, we must fully understand the need for continuing education, which ensures that we apply the highest and best practices in nursing. This practice was encouraged by Florence Nightingale (1860, 1992) in her *Notes on Nursing*, and it continues today through peer-reviewed research and solid, evidence-based practice.

The New Testament of the Bible is rich with instruction for disciples. The nurse dedicated to Christ is encouraged in Colossians 3:10–11 to "put on the new self, which is being renewed in knowledge in the image of its Creator . . . because Christ is all and is in all." Through thoughtful, committed study (2 Timothy 2:15; Romans 12:1–2), the dedicated nurse turns from earthly to Christ-like behavior as an act of worship and under the influence of the Holy Spirit (Eckerd, 2017).

The Nurse Utilizes Prayer and Spiritual Gifts in Response to the Holy Spirit

Communication with God is often accessed through prayer. Dedicated nurses frequently turn to prayer in matters of strength of spirit, guidance, wisdom, knowledge, discernment, boldness, intervention, and any other petition in line with Biblical teaching. Important elements include forgiveness, faith, trust, thanksgiving, praise, and requests for meeting the spiritual, emotional, and physical needs of self and others (Eckerd, 2017). Dedicated nurses consider it an honor to pray for their patients as an integral element of spiritual care. The Apostle James (5:16) tells us that "the prayer of a righteous person is powerful and effective." Nursing research underscores the physical and emotional benefits of prayer in terms of a "positive association between prayer and wellbeing" (Hollywell & Walker, 2008).

Spiritual gifts are imparted by God Himself. Romans 12:68 and 1 Peter 4:10–11 reveal that all Christ-followers are given at least one spiritual gift, handpicked for us, matched to our specific God-given attributes and abilities (Eckerd, 2017). According to Kinghorn (1981), "A spiritual gift is a divine, supernatural ability given by God to enable a Christian to serve and to minister . . . a special tool for ministry" (p. 8). The nurse dedicated to the Christian faith is encouraged to periodically complete a spiritual gifts inventory, such as Kinghorn's (1981) *Discovering Your Spiritual Gifts*. This type of inventory may increase the awareness of one's spiritual gifts, which can then be intentionally practiced. The nurse dedicated to the Christian faith understands that the influence of the Holy Spirit connects the spiritual gift of the dedicated nurse to the needs of the patient at a predetermined spiritual intersection.

The nurse dedicated to Christ is guided by God Himself through the Holy Spirit. He guides us in the spirit of truth, holiness, wisdom, grace, and understanding, and is our

Godly counselor. The Holy Spirit has chosen to work through us to reveal the agape love of Christ to all. It is through the presence of the Holy Spirit in the dedicated nurse's life that our patients experience the love of Christ.

The Nurse Reflects the Fruit of the Spirit at the Point of Care

In Galatians 5:22–23, Paul summarizes the attributes of Christ in nine characteristics: love, joy, peace, patience, kindness, goodness, faithfulness, gentleness, and self-control. Once believers accept Christ as their Lord and Savior, they are enabled, through the Holy Spirit, to reflect the character of Christ in their actions, attitudes, behaviors, thoughts, and deeds (Eckerd, 2017). All nurses dedicated to the Christian faith possess all elements of the Fruit of the Spirit. As we are conformed to the image of Christ, the Fruit of the Spirit is more fully evidenced and demonstrated by the nurse's life, reflecting the agape love of Christ to all persons.

By implementing the Agape Model, the immediate benefit to the nursing profession becomes a Biblically defined view of compassionate care, such as that demonstrated by Jesus in Mathew 14:14: "When Jesus went out He saw a great multitude; and He was moved with compassion for them and healed their sick." Additionally, by offering such Christ-inspired care, the *Code of Ethics for Nurses*, Provision 1, is fulfilled: "The nurse practices with compassion and respect for the inherent dignity,

worth and unique attributes of every person" (ANA, 2015, p. 1). Application of the Fruit of the Spirit, whether in practice or in the dedicated nurse's personal life, is synonymous with excellence in the eyes of God (Eckerd, 2017). The Agape Model offers the highest and best care that a nurse dedicated to the Christian faith can offer.

> Because The Agape Model's focus is on the character of the nurse, it benefits all aspects of patient care. The freshness of approach and delivery will serve to further elevate the nursing profession as a gold standard of care, while setting an example of excellence. Although the primary goal of The Agape Model is for the nurse to emulate the character of Christ, the secondary goal will result in elevated patient satisfaction and outcomes. (Eckerd, 2017)

▸ Application of the Agape Model

The use of the Agape Model in practice is applicable to multigenerational nurses who practice in every healthcare setting. Dedicated nurses should stand out in their personal, professional, and spiritual life by reflecting every aspect of this model within their daily lives, because it represents their life in Christ (**CASE STUDY 3-1**). Just as Christians are recognized

🔍 CASE STUDY 3-1

You arrive on your medical–surgical unit and receive the shift report from the outgoing nurse. The nurse provides a comprehensive report of the patient in room 326, including the patient's physical diagnosis and current assessment data. The patient, Ms. Chase, is a 62-year-old widowed female who lives alone and was admitted yesterday for an exacerbation of chronic obstructive pulmonary disease (COPD). She has a history of bipolar disorder and diabetes mellitus type 2. The patient is a full code, and her oxygen saturation level is stable at 95% on 2 liters of oxygen per nasal cannula.

Her vital signs are as follows: blood pressure, 138/84 mm Hg; heart rate, 76 beats per minute—rate is regular with no abnormal heart sound auscultated; respiratory rate, 18 breaths per minute and unlabored with no abnormal lung sounds auscultated. Oral temperature is 98.8°F. The patient denies pain, with a reported pain level of 0/10. The remainder of the report, including lab values, is unremarkable, except that the night shift nurse adds that the patient has been noncompliant with breathing treatments and the incentive spirometer. The nurse goes on to state, "She is a pretty miserable. If I were you, I would try to stay out of her room as much as possible. She likes to be left alone."

Prior to arriving for each scheduled shift, you undergo a great deal of preparation both mentally and physically. You don the proper attire and equipment; you anticipate the events of the day and mentally prepare to face the challenges. Equally as important as preparing yourself physically and emotionally, as a nurse dedicated to the Christian faith, you prepare for the shift by asking the Holy Spirit to guide you through each and every encounter with patients, family, and coworkers.

Questions

1. As a nurse dedicated to the Christian faith, what steps would you take to prepare yourself prior to arriving for your shift each day?
2. As you prepare to enter the patient's room to meet and assess Ms. Chase, how would you anticipate the Holy Spirit guiding you in demonstrating the Fruit of the Spirit (**TABLE 3-3**) in delivering compassionate care for this patient? Explain your answer.
   Upon assessment, you note that Ms. Chase's oxygen saturation has dropped into the low 90s and her respirations have increased to 22 breaths per minute and are labored. You notice that her nasal cannula is on the bed. While you are reapplying and adjusting her nasal cannula, Ms. Chase suddenly tears it from her face and asks, "Why is this happening to me? Is God punishing me for all of the bad things that I have done in my life?"
3. After addressing the patient's physical needs and ensuring adequate oxygenation and stabilization of her vital signs, how would you approach applying the Agape Model to provide comfort for this patient in light of her previous question about God and His perceived punishment?

Additional resources for case study: NCFI Spiritual Care Materials, https://ncf-jcn.org/resources/spiritual-care-resources

for their fruit, nurses dedicated to the Christian faith will bear fruit in their practice that will be evident to surrounding constituents.

Dedicated nurses (**BOX 3-3**) should integrate Biblical principles, as described in the Agape Model, into every moment of every day, as they interact with their patient as well as with coworkers and others. Furthermore, Christian faculty within faith-based universities should consider integrating the Agape Model into their curriculum. Christian nursing faculty have an obligation to mentor nursing students and to model the likeness of Christ. The Agape Model offers the framework to do just that, while setting the expectation for every nurse to provide Christ-centered, evidence-based care.

▶ Conclusion

This chapter has highlighted the historical journey of caring from a Christian worldview, to enable the nurse to appreciate the roots of Biblical-based caring. The Agape Model was introduced as a framework for providing compassionate care. The challenge for each nurse is to personally reflect on the origin or source of his or her caring.

BOX 3-3 Outstanding Nurse Leader: Jennifer Scott, RN

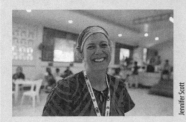

Jennifer Scott

There is no better feeling in my nursing practice than to reflect the heart and character of Christ. I am more than privileged to have been picked by God to represent Him in the field of nursing. The Holy Spirit is the catalyst that took me from a conventional nurse to a kingdom nurse. By allowing the Holy Spirit to lead me in my personal life and nursing practice, I feel so much more love, guidance, calmness, and comfort. I know God's plan for me is to be a Christ-centered nurse, and I rely on the Holy Spirit to guide me. Just looking into someone's eyes or using a simple touch, I will sense the prompting of the Holy Spirit and know in my spirit how God wants me to help people physically, spiritually, or mentally.

Practicing in Canada, I regularly assess the spiritual needs of my patients and their families. My desire is to provide the best care possible for them by showing them the agape love of Christ. By allowing the Holy Spirit to guide me, I can actually feel the difference in the connection I have with my patient.

Every life situation and patient circumstance is different, and I learn from each one of them. By studying the Bible and worshiping God, I'm growing in my faith and desire to become more focused on my profession. I am able to love more, care more, forgive more. By applying my professional instincts, knowledge, and training, and integrating my faith and the guidance of the Holy Spirit, I am sharing the agape love of Christ.

I believe that prayer is so important in everyday life and have come to realize that my nursing practice is a calling. I am doing God's work. I am serving as a conduit to provide excellent care to all, regardless of the circumstances. When you thank God for your blessings and ask God for guidance by embracing the Fruit of Spirit, you are emulating the love of Christ, providing patients with exceptional care focused on their individual needs. This can be demonstrated by a simple touch or look, or the way you perform a nursing intervention.

TABLE 3-3 Fruit of the Spirit Manifested in the Nurse Dedicated to the Christian Faith

Love	The highest expression of dedication and appreciation for the sacrifice of Christ; it requires doing no harm (nonmaleficence), a core element of healthcare oaths and nursing morality (ANA, 2015). The Holy Spirit influences the nurse dedicated to Christian faith in anticipating actions and motives, working to keep the patient free from actual or potential harm. As an act of worship, the nurse dedicated to Christian faith displays caring that goes beyond reasonable, acceptable nursing care, acting as a willing vessel allowing patients to experience God's love and care.	Matthew 7:12; Romans 13:10; 1 Corinthians 13:4–5, 13; Colossians 3:14
Joy	Unlike human happiness, true joy comes from Christ and is present regardless of circumstances. Supernatural joy serves as an insulator and helps provide confident service in the face of undesirable situations. The nurse dedicated to Christian faith has confidence that prayer produces divine results and joy in that God controls all circumstances.	John 16:24; Romans 12:15, 15:13; 1 Corinthians 9:22

Peace	Internal calmness received from God that can be passed to an anxious patient; reflected as confidence in the outcome, regardless of the situation. There are no earthly limits on Godly peace. A peaceful spirit protects the nurse as well as the patient from a sense of chaos. This peace reflects Shalom and secures composure, dissolves fear, and maintains harmony (MacArthur, 2005). Perfect peace comes from God and is often coupled with joy.	John 14:27; Romans 15:13; Philippians 4:4–8; 2 Thessalonians 3:16
Patience	Calm acceptance of people or circumstances results in respect and high regard for others. Combined with prayer, patience allows the dedicated nurse's anxiety to be replaced with focus and confidence and may help diffuse patient anxiety. The nurse dedicated to Christian faith waits on God and the prompting of the Holy Spirit and responds accordingly. The reward is endurance, renewed strength, and divine support, providing the patient with freshness in the delivery of care.	Psalms 75:2; Ephesians 4:2; Philippians 4:6
Kindness	Treating others as God has treated us. The nurse dedicated to Christian faith approaches the patient with knowledgeable, professional confidence and uses tenderness in words and actions. The dedicated nurse's character reveals tenderness generalized to all mankind.	Proverbs 31:26; Ephesians 4:31–32
Goodness	Generosity that springs from kindness. Beneficence, an ethical principle, focuses on the desire to help and advocate for others (ANA, 2015). The nurse dedicated to Christian faith elevates this virtue to a spiritual level by demonstrating the goodness of Christ to others.	Romans 15:14; Galatians 6:10; 1 Timothy 6:18
Faithfulness	The framework required for love and grace flowing from God to the patient. The nurse dedicated to Christian faith remains confident and faithful that the Holy Spirit will direct steps, thoughts, and actions. Daily renewal of the mind and heart is nurtured through scripture and prayer, leaning on God's revelation through the Holy Spirit for understanding.	Luke 16:10–12; Romans 12:2; 2 Corinthians 5:7; 1 John 1:3
Gentleness	Gentleness allows the nurse dedicated to Christian faith to temper aggressiveness in a calm, respectful, and nonthreatening manner. The nurse dedicated to Christian faith invites the Holy Spirit's oversight in striving for gentleness.	Colossians 3:14; 1 Peter 3:15; James 3:17
Self-control	Provides the discipline necessary to be above reproach in character, diligently remaining on task and focusing on the well-being of the patient.	1 Corinthians 9:24–27; 2 Timothy 1:7; Titus 1:8

TABLE 3-4 Applying the Agape Model: Biblical Practice Points		
■ Pray before every interaction with your patient. ■ Be intentional to demonstrate the Fruit of the Spirit in your practice.	■ Identify spiritual distress in your patients. ■ Implement individualized nursing interventions.	■ Identify and develop your God-given spiritual gifts. ■ The results may reflect improved patient outcomes.

▶ Clinical Reasoning Exercises

Explore the Agape Model website and articles at https://agapenursingmodel.com/. Use your Bible as a reference while reading and learning.

1. Discuss the Agape Model with another nursing student in a group setting.
2. Read Exodus 3:4–5. Why is the nurse–patient encounter considered holy ground?
3. From a Christian worldview, discuss what is considered a sacred encounter.
4. How does this apply to you and to your patient?

▶ Personal Reflection Exercises

You have prepared yourself physically, emotionally, and spiritually to care for your clients, including Ms. Chase (Case Study 3-1). You have educated yourself on the Agape Model (**TABLE 3-4**) and understand the importance of displaying the characteristics of the Fruit of the Spirit. You are also familiar with identifying spiritual distress and regularly use evidence-based nursing interventions to assist the patient.

1. What else can you do to ensure that your nursing practice is based on the agape love of Christ?
2. Are you familiar with your own spiritual gifts?
3. Do you believe that your spiritual gifts can lead to change in your approach to patient care and may influence patient outcomes? If so, how?

References

American Nurses Association (ANA). (2015). *Code of ethics for nurses with interpretive statements.* Silver Spring, MD: Author.

Austgard, K. (2008). What characterizes nursing care? A hermeneutical philosophical inquiry. *Scandinavian Journal of Caring Sciences, 22*(2), 314–319.

Boykin, A., & Schoenhofer, S. (2013). Reframing outcomes: Enhancing personhood. In W. Cody (Ed.), *Philosophical and theoretical perspectives for advanced nursing practice* (5th ed., pp. 132–144). Burlington, MA: Jones & Bartlett Learning.

Bradshaw, A. (1994). *Lighting the lamp: The spiritual dimension of nursing care.* Middlesex, UK: Scutari Press.

Campinha-Bacote, J. (2013). *A Biblically based model of cultural competence in the delivery of healthcare services: Seeing Imago Dei.* Cincinnati, OH: Transcultural C.A.R.E. Associates.

Eckerd, N. (2017). A nursing practice model based on Christ: The Agape model. *Journal of Christian Nursing, 35*(2), 124–130. doi:10.1097/CNJ0000000000000417

Eriksson, K. (1989). Caring paradigms: A study of the origins and the development of caring paradigms among nursing students. *Scandinavian Journal of Caring Sciences, 3*(4), 169–176.

Eriksson, K. (1997). Caring, spirituality, and suffering. In M. S. Roach (Ed.), *Caring from the heart: The convergence between caring and spirituality* (pp. 68–84). New York, NY: Paulist Press.

Eriksson, K. (2002). Caring science in a new key. *Nursing Science Quarterly, 15*(1), 61–64.

Ferngren, G. (2009). *Medicine and health care in early Christianity.* Baltimore, MD: The John Hopkins University Press.

Fowler, M. (2012). Religion and nursing. In M. Fowler, S. Reimer-Kirkham, R. Sawatzky, & E. Johnston Taylor, *Religion, religious ethics, and nursing* (pp. 1–26). New York, NY: Springer.

Grenz, S., & Olson, R. (1996). *Who needs theology?* Downers Grove, IL: InterVarsity Press.

Griffin, A. & Yancey, V. (2009). Spiritual dimensions of the perioperative experience. *AORN Journal, 89*(5), 875–882. doi:10.1016/j.aorn.2009.01.024

Hawke-Eder, S. (2017). Can caring be taught? *Kai Tiaki: Nursing New Zealand, 23*(3), 23–25, 46.

Hoekema, A. (1986). *Created in God's image.* Grand Rapids, MI: William B. Eerdmans.

Hollywell, C., & Walker, J. (2008). Private prayer as a suitable intervention for hospitalized patients: A critical review of the literature. *Journal of Clinical Nursing, 18*(1), 637–651.

Howard, T. (2013). *Imago Dei.* Washington, DC: Catholic University of America Press.

Johnson, M. (2008). Can compassion be taught? *Nursing Standard, 23*(11), 19–21.

Kinghorn, K. (1981). *Discovering your spiritual gifts.* Grand Rapids, MI: Zondervan.

Kleffel, D. (2013). Environmental paradigms: Moving toward an ecocentric perspective. In W. Cody, *Philosophical and theoretical perspectives for advanced nursing practice* (5th ed., pp. 168–181). Burlington, MA: Jones & Bartlett Learning.

Leyva, E. A., Peralta, A. B., Tejero, L. S., & Santos, M. A. (2015). Global perspectives of caring: An integrative review. *International Journal for Human Caring, 19*(4), 7–29.

Liaschenko, J., & Peter, E. (2004). Nursing ethics and conceptualizations of nursing: Profession, practice and work. *Journal of Advanced Nursing, 46*(5), 488–495. doi:10.1111/j.1365-2648.2004.03011.x

Lindstrom, U. A., Nystrom, L. L., & Zetterlund, J. E. (2018). Theory of caritative caring. In M. R. Alligood (Ed.), *Nursing theorists and their work* (9th ed., pp. 140–163). St. Louis, MO: Elsevier.

Lucado, M. (2004). *It's not about me.* Nashville, TN: Thomas Nelson.

Lucado, M. (2018). *Unshakeable hope.* Nashville, TN: Thomas Nelson.

Lundmark, M. (2007). Vocation in theology-based nursing theories. *Nursing Ethics, 14*(6). doi:10.1177/0969733007082117

MacArthur, J. (2005). *MacArthur Bible commentary.* Nashville, TN: Thomas Nelson.

Newbanks, R. S. (2015). An integrative critical literature review toward the development of a middle range theory on caring from a biblical Christian worldview (Order No. 10600632). ProQuest Dissertations & Theses Global: Health & Medicine. (1925343218). Retrieved from https://0-search-proquest-com.oak.indwes.edu/docview/1925343218?accountid=6363

Newbanks, R. S., Rieg, L., & Schaefer, B. (2018). What is caring in nursing? Sorting out humanistic and Christian perspectives. *Journal of Christian Nursing, 35*(3), 160–167. doi:10.1097/CNJ.0000000000000441

Nightingale, F. (1860). *Notes on nursing: What it is, and what it is not.* New York, NY: D. Appleton.

Nightingale, F. (1992). *Notes on nursing.* Philadelphia, PA: Lippincott.

Nightingale, S., Spiby, H., Sheen, K., & Slade, P. (2018). The impact of emotional intelligence in health care professionals on caring behavior towards patients in clinical and long-term care settings: Findings from an integrative review. *International Journal of Nursing Studies, 80,* 106–117. doi:10.1016/j.ijnurstu.2018.01.006

O'Brien, M. (2011). *Servant leadership in nursing: Spirituality and practice in contemporary healthcare.* Sudbury, MA: Jones and Bartlett.

Parrott, L. (2018). *Love like that.* Nashville, TN: Thomas Nelson.

Rieg, L. S., Newbanks, R. S., & Sprunger, R. (2018). Caring from a Christian worldview: Exploring nurses' source of caring, faith practices, and view of nursing. *Journal of Christian Nursing, 35*(3), 168–173. doi:10.1097/CNJ.0000000000000474

Roy, C. (1997). Future of the Roy model: Challenge to redefine adaptation. *Nursing Science Quarterly, 10*(1), 42–48.

Salladay, S. (2000). Healing is believing: Postmodernism impacts nursing. *The Scientific Review of Alternative Medicine, 4*(1), 39–46. Retrieved from http://www.sram.org/media/documents/uploads/article_pdfs/4-1-09.Salladay.pdf

Shelly, J., & Miller, A. (2006). *Called to care: A Christian worldview for nursing* (2nd ed.). Downers Grove, IL: InterVarsity Press.

Tonges, M., & Ray, J. (2011). Translating caring theory into practice: The Carolina care model. *Journal of Nursing Administration, 41*(9), 374–381. doi:10.1097/NNA.0b013e31822a732c

Vocation. (n.d.). In *Merriam-Webster*. Retrieved from https://www.merriam-webster.com/dictionary/vocation

Williams, M. (2013). First calling: The Imago Dei and the order of creation: Part I. *Presbyterian, 39*(1), 30–44.

Wolterstorff, N. (1994). For justice in Shalom. In W. G. Boulton, T. D. Kennedy, & A. Verhey (Eds.), *From Christ to the world: Introductory readings in Christian ethics* (p. 251). Grand Rapids, MI: Eerdmans.

Recommended Readings

Bradshaw, A. (1994). *Lighting the lamp: The spiritual dimension of nursing care.* Middlesex, UK: Scutari Press.

Bradshaw, A. (2001). *The nurse apprentice, 1860–1977.* London, UK: Routledge Press.

Campinha-Bacote, J. (2013). *A Biblically based model of cultural competence in the delivery of healthcare services: Seeing Imago Dei.* Cincinnati, OH: Transcultural Associates.

Chapman, E. (2009). *Sacred work: Planting cultures of radical loving care in America.* Nashville, TN: Baptist Healing Trust.

Cusveller, B. (2004). *Commitment and responsibility in nursing: A faith-based approach.* Sioux Center, IA: Dordt College Press.

Deloughery, G. L. (1977). *History and trends of professional nursing.* Saint Louis, MO: C. V. Mosby.

Doornbos, M. M., Groenhout, R. R., & Hotz, K. G. (2005). *Transforming care: A Christian vision of nursing practice.* Grand Rapids, MI: Eerdmans.

Eriksson, K. (1997). Understanding the world of the patient, the suffering human being: The new clinical paradigm from nursing to caring. *Advanced Practice Nursing Quarterly, 3*(1), 8–13.

Eriksson, K. (2006). *The suffering human being.* Chicago, IL: Nordic Studies Press.

Eriksson, K. (2007). The theory of caritative caring: A vision. *Nursing Science Quarterly, 20*(3), 201–202.

O'Brien, M. E. (2008). *A sacred covenant: The spiritual ministry of nursing.* Sudbury, MA: Jones and Bartlett.

O'Brien, M. E. (2011). *Servant leadership in nursing: Spirituality and practice in contemporary health care.* Sudbury, MA: Jones and Bartlett.

O'Brien, M. E. (2014). *Spirituality in nursing: Standing on holy ground* (5th ed.). Burlington, MA: Jones & Bartlett Learning.

Roach, S. (1997). *Caring from the heart: The convergence of caring and spirituality.* Mahwah, NJ: Paulist Press.

Shelly, J. A., & Miller A. B. (2006). *Called to care: A Christian theology of nursing* (2nd ed.). Downers Grove, IL: InterVarsity Press.

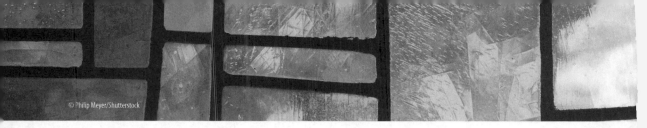

CHAPTER 4

Using Models for Faith-Based Curricula

Kristen L. Mauk, PhD, DNP, RN, CRRN, GCNS-BC, GNP-BC, FAAN

LEARNING OBJECTIVES

At the end of this chapter, the reader will be able to:

1. Examine the relationships among the metaparadigm concepts of person, nurse, health, and environment.
2. Discuss how nurses can work within various curricular frameworks to promote the spiritual health of individuals, families, and communities.
3. Explore the roles of the Christian nurse as scholar, shepherd, steward, and servant.
4. Identify role components of the professional nurse.
5. Define several processes used by the doctorally prepared nurse to impact health outcomes.
6. Appraise two models used in nursing programs/curricula that incorporate spiritual care.

KEY TERMS

Caring	Models	Professional nursing
Environment	Nurse	Theory
Health	Person (personhood)	

Theories or frameworks are useful in guiding nursing practice. While the use of nursing theory has, at times, come under criticism regarding its usefulness in the undergraduate nursing curriculum, models that help nurses understand the metaparadigm concepts of person, health, nurse, and environment can be helpful to both students and practicing clinicians.

A **theory** can be conceptualized as an idea or blueprint that helps explain behaviors, situations, or common problems. **Models** or frameworks are often set forth as part of a theory, but a true theory includes explicit assumptions and propositions that are testable. Examples of grand theories in nursing would include Sister Callista Roy's *Adaptation Model*, Martha Rogers' *Theory of Unitary Human Beings*, Imogene King's *Theory of Goal Attainment*, and Dorothea Orem's *Self-Care Deficit Nursing Theory*. Nursing students and nurses may be familiar with these theories from their study in core courses. In addition to such grand theories, middle-range theories and clinical specialty practice theories may give more detailed guidelines to nursing management of specific disorders or problems. These theories are based on research with unique populations or groups. Thus, nursing students and practicing nurses may use broad theories for general nursing practice or narrow theories to help guide and promote quality health outcomes for certain groups of patients.

Several models have been proposed for various aspects of spiritual care. These include models for spiritual wellness (Christman & Mueller, 2017), transitional care (Ziebarth & Campbell, 2016), and Christian caring in nursing (Rieg, Newbanks, & Sprunger, 2018), among others. Readers are encouraged to look at other chapters in this text for additional theories and models—for example, the *Caring from a Christian Worldview: The Agape Model*, *Spiritual Assessment*, *Role of the Nurse in Disaster Response*, and *Caring for One Another with Christ's Light* chapters. The focus of this chapter is on unique models developed by specific nursing programs to guide curricular development and program planning.

In curricular development, larger, broader theories help to guide educators to develop frameworks or models that can be used to inform curricula and individual courses within a nursing program. When nursing programs are first developed, many factors are considered, including standards of practice, essentials from accrediting bodies, and competencies associated with practice. The philosophy, mission, and vision of the college or university form the foundation for any curriculum of the various programs offered.

The purpose of this chapter is to demonstrate how frameworks and models can be used to guide programs and curricula. Students and nurses should be able to see from a model the focus and emphases of the program. The curricular models for one school and one college of nursing located in different parts of the United States are presented in this chapter. Definitions, concepts, constructs, and processes from these models are explored in relation to their associated mission and vision to demonstrate the use and value of a framework to explain practice, influence research, and inform program learning outcomes. Specific examples within these two curricular frameworks will be given for the baccalaureate, master's, and doctoral levels of practice. The reader may benefit from seeing the connections between major nursing concepts and the development of unique models that support the overarching aims of a college or university.

▶ Colorado Christian University School of Nursing and Health Professions

Every university has mission and vision statements as well as strategic objectives or aims. The vision and mission of individual departments not only reflect those of the parent institution but also incorporate the uniqueness of the specific school or college.

Mission and Vision

The vision of Colorado Christian University (CCU) School of Nursing and Health Professions is *to empower nurses to practice nursing as ministry.* The mission is "to prepare competent, compassionate, moral leaders who excel as servants, shepherds, stewards, and scholars to impact the profession and the world" (CCU, 2019, p. 10).

Major Concepts

As can be seen in the model (**FIGURE 4-1**), the key concepts and terms in the mission statement appear as important components. The CCU model demonstrates Biblical truth as the foundation upon which the curriculum is built, with the liberal arts and sciences coming next, and then nursing as an art and a science. The concepts of the nursing metaparadigm are included in that layer of the foundation. **BOX 4-1** gives definitions of the nursing metaparadigm, adding caring as a key concept.

Several major concepts and constructs influence the program outcomes related to the integration of learning, faith, and practice and form the framework for the curriculum. The major curriculum concepts that are incorporated into course student learning outcomes are the following:

- Integration of learning–faith–practice
- Spiritual formation (forming the beams of the cross)
- Nursing as ministry and competency–character–calling (forming the banner that wraps around the pillars and the cross)
- Interprofessional communication, evidence-based nursing practice, technology management, healthcare delivery, moral leadership, and professionalism (smaller pillars that combine to form a larger column in the model)

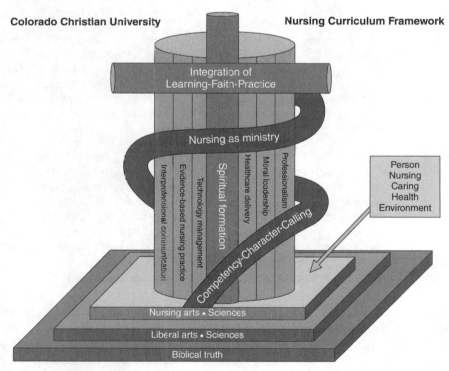

FIGURE 4-1 Curricular model of CCU nursing.

Colorado Christian University (CCU). *Student Handbook 2018–2019.* Used with permission of Colorado Christian University.

BOX 4-1 Definitions of Major Concepts of the CCU Model

Person (personhood) is the result of the creative work of the living, relevant God. The intended purpose of this creative work is to be His image-bearer, reflecting His character and nature to the world around us. We believe in the sanctity of life for all human beings at all stages of existence. We believe that God has designed persons to live independently, interdependently, and dependently. Through cooperation with His purposes, we are empowered to author our purpose in life, our God-inspired life story, and to influence the world around us.

Professional nursing is a scientific practice–based discipline and a sacred calling, oriented toward human good and healing. We believe nursing to be powered by moral good with certain values and standards that support quality of care, professionalism, and moral leadership. Nursing knowledge is the result of scientific inquiry and the integration of physical sciences, social sciences, psychological sciences, and various theoretical propositions. This is the basis for providing the highest-quality, evidence-based nursing practice. Nursing is "the protection, promotion, and optimization of health and abilities, prevention of illness and injury, alleviation of suffering through the diagnosis and treatment of human response, and advocacy in the care of individuals, families, communities, and populations" (American Nurses Association, 2010, p 3).

Caring, as provided by nurses, is always specific and relational: Involvement and caring reside together, resulting in common meanings between nurse and patient (Benner, 1984). Compassionate care is hands-on, patient-centered, physical, and psychosocial; it involves spiritual interventions to meet the needs of patients regardless of how the nurse feels and regardless of the patient's ethnic identity, race, gender, age, status, diagnosis, or ability to pay (Shelly & Miller, 2006). Christian spiritual caring is an act of faith and a response to God's truth and grace through a compassionate presence.

Health is a state of wholeness, well-being, peace (Shalom), and a completeness that permeates all areas of human life. The concept carries with it the idea of universal flourishing and delight or a rich state of existence. We believe health is God's original created goodness, which in its fullest sense is complete physical, mental, and spiritual flourishing that makes possible one's ability to fulfill our created purposes. Such fulfillment brings glory to our Creator. Participation of the nurse in the promotion of health, the prevention of disease, the management of care, and the restoration of Shalom as true health becomes the focus of faith-driven practice.

The **environment** within which the nurse practices nursing comprises the physical conditions and circumstances surrounding the person, and also includes relationships and social structures such as the family, educational system, legal system, and healthcare system. In this environment, interprofessional communication and technology management are essential to deliver high-quality health care. From a Christian perspective, we believe in the Biblical idea of the fallen nature of people and things resulting in evil, suffering, and separation from the Creator, God. Due to this fallen nature, all of the systems in place for intended good are flawed and often ineffective. For the Christian nurse, our concern is for the reconciliation of all things under Christ who is the personification and available fulfillment of Shalom.

Colorado Christian University (CCU). *Student Handbook 2018–2019*. Used with permission of Colorado Christian University.

The CCU doctor of nursing practice (DNP) student handbook explains the relationship between and among concepts within the model this way:

The progressive constructs build from simple to complex and are identified

as competent–caring–calling culminating with nursing as ministry. The program outcome in which faith is integrated into both learning and practice is the cornerstone and capstone of all curriculum development and is depicted by a cross. The cross represents the centrality of Jesus Christ in spiritual formation and integration of faith, learning and practice. The nursing metaparadigm—person, nursing, caring, health, and environment—is embedded in each of the other concepts and constructs. Each course addresses components of the concepts and constructs, with specific content increasing in complexity throughout the curriculum. The concepts and constructs serve as broad categories under which a variety of content can be expressed. (CCU, 2019, p. 14)

Roles of the Professional Nurse as Moral Leader

The roles of the nurse, as seen through a Biblical worldview, encompass moral leadership as a main pillar in the curricular framework. This appears most clearly in CCU's model of the DNP in Visionary Leadership (**FIGURE 4-2**), in which key concepts are emphasized. The cross in the middle of the figure, which was derived from Nurses Christian Fellowship International's model (originally developed by Dr. Barbara White), forms the basis for nursing leadership in conjunction with the general curricular

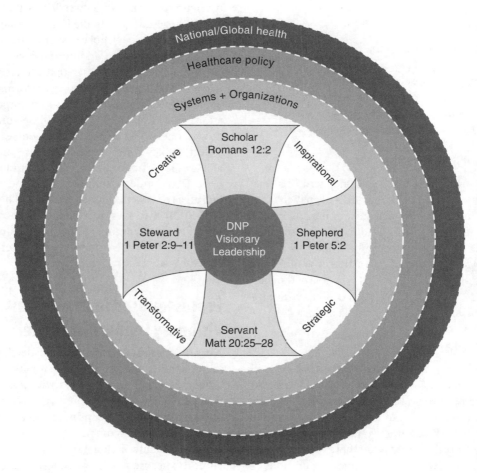

FIGURE 4-2 CCU model of DNP in Visionary Leadership.

model presented earlier. Nursing leadership as portrayed here is central to faith-based nursing. Each role component is discussed next.

Servant

The concept of servant is key to this role component in Christian nursing leadership. The servant leader is first a servant (Coffman, 2017). This type of leadership involves a conscious choice to help others to grow in their personal and professional walks. The nurse leader as servant helps others to pursue health, obtain wisdom, and become more autonomous, thereby encouraging servant leadership in others (CCU, 2019).

Steward

A steward "manages the property, finances, resources and affairs of the organization" (CCU, 2019, p. 15). Stewards are change agents who use the gifts of wisdom and discernment to appropriately manage and allocate resources for the best interests of a facility, group, or organization.

Shepherd

The nurse who leads as a shepherd of a flock nurtures relationships with both patients and the interprofessional team. "In the relationship model of shepherd leadership, the shepherd leader is available, committed and trustworthy, providing direction, correction, mentoring and safety" (CCU, 2019, p. 15). The role of the shepherd is one of humility, protection, encouragement, and care (Lehman & Pentak, 2004).

Scholar

The nurse leader uses transitional research and evidence-based practice to guide care toward positive health outcomes. Critical thinking and wisdom are used to engage in self-reflection and to seek constructive feedback from others. The Christian nurse as a scholar uses best practices to draw the team together in pursuit of the common goal of improving health in persons, families, groups, and populations. Dissemination of research findings through scholarly work is an expectation at the doctoral level of practice in the role of scholar.

Doctor of Nursing Practice Program

In contrast to frameworks or models that may guide an undergraduate curriculum, unique models for various degree levels may be developed. For example, CCU's DNP in Visionary Leadership incorporates the nursing program's leadership model, adding unique processes to the key concepts in the school's mission statement. As illustrated in the model in Figure 4-2, the school envisions that students who graduate with the DNP in Visionary Leadership will be scholars, shepherds, stewards, and servants. In addition, the visionary leader engages in processes that are creative, inspirational, strategic, and transformative, while influencing health systems and organizations, policy, and global health. Based on this model, one would expect to see courses that reflect the key concepts depicted here such as global leadership, healthcare policy, and business. DNP projects may focus on the three foci areas of systems, policy, and global health. **CASE STUDY 4-1** gives an example, with questions for consideration, of how a DNP student might use the CCU model to guide an evidence-based practice project.

Processes Used in the DNP in Visionary Leadership Model

Nurses holding doctorates in leadership or administration are expected to function at a higher level than those nurses with lesser education. Coursework that prepares leaders will encompass a broader scope of practice and will include business acumen, change processes, national and international strategies, advanced clinical expertise, and knowledge of health policy. The processes in the CCU model of DNP in Visionary Leadership are used to influence

🔍 *CASE STUDY 4-1*

Susan is a DNP student in an online program at a large Christian university. She is in her second core course, which covers research and evidence-based practice. The students in this course are asked to use Colorado Christian University's DNP in Visionary Leadership model to formulate a topic and potential setting for their project. In a later assignment, students will develop a clinical question, but for now, the focus is on using this model to guide the project.

Susan has been on several mission trips to Haiti and has a passion for improving the nutritional health of young children living in orphanages. For her assignment topic, she wants to develop a quality improvement project in this area and plans to build on this assignment for her later final DNP project required for graduation. With these factors in mind, answer the following questions.

Questions

1. Which of the three foci of the CCU DNP model would Susan choose in this model? What is the best setting for her project? How do the other foci (in the outer circles) impact the one area Susan would focus on?
2. How would Susan explain the roles of scholar, shepherd, servant, and steward related to her proposed project idea?
3. Which interventions to improve the nutritional health of orphans in Haiti could Susan use to demonstrate creative, inspirational, strategic, and transformative leadership? How would she express these in a future DNP project proposal?

the three focal areas represented by the open systems' circles of systems and organizations, health policy, and national/global health.

Creative

The nurse with a clinical doctorate must be creative in several areas. As an influencer of health systems and organizations, the nurse may need creativity to effect change. Communication with administration and leadership requires creative thinking to engage all stakeholders. Likewise, to introduce changes in health policy, the nurse may need to carefully craft letters, make in-person appointments, or hold key positions on governmental committees and task forces to gain the buy-in of health policy makers. Similarly, to effectively promote health in global populations, the nurse may be called upon to devise interventions beyond the traditional approaches. For example, creative solutions for addressing an issue such as sanitation to ensure clean food and water in an impoverished country must be considered before

introducing traditional medical and nursing care.

Inspirational

Visionary leaders inspire others toward a common goal. The Christian nurse takes inspiration from the teachings of scripture and the example of Jesus Christ. Operating through a Biblical worldview, the doctorally prepared nurse can lead by example, inspiring others to change for positive health outcomes in each of the three focal areas represented in the model. **BOX 4-2** gives an example of an outstanding nurse leader who worked for decades to help develop a theory for Christian nursing.

Strategic

Nurses must be deliberate in their thinking and planning to promote positive health outcomes. Strategic leadership is defined as "the ability to anticipate, envision, maintain flexibility, and empower others to create strategic change as necessary" (Hitt, Ireland, & Hoskisson, 2007,

BOX 4-2 Outstanding Nurse Leader: Linda Rieg, PhD, RN, CNE

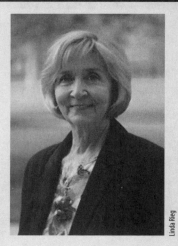

Linda Rieg

Linda Rieg is a professor of nursing at Indiana Wesleyan University and an adjunct faculty member at Colorado Christian University. Dr. Rieg earned a BSN from Edgecliff College, an MBA from St. Xavier University (where she taught for more than 25 years), and an MSN and PhD from University of Cincinnati. She has more than 40 years of experience in a wide variety of nursing clinical, management, and education positions. Dr. Rieg talks about her personal and professional experiences here.

As I reflect on the idea of caring and nursing as ministry, I'm taken back to my early memories of going with my Dad to the hospital as he made pastoral calls. I believe these early experiences—especially watching the nurses as they cared for our parishioners—were key to my lifelong focus on caring from a Christian worldview.

To me, caring was always linked to the characteristics of Christ: compassion, love, and service. As a result, I was moved to become a nurse as a way to serve God through serving those whom He loves. I saw nursing as a natural integration of faith, care, and a committed life to Christ.

Throughout my career as a clinician, administrator, and educator, caring from a Christian worldview was my philosophical/theoretical foundation. Of course, in my early years I wasn't consciously aware of the connection between theory and practice. As a clinician, I simply strived to treat all patients as if I was caring for Christ. Matthew 25:40 was the verse I tried to live: "as you did it to one of the least of these my brothers, you did it to me" (English Standard Version [ESV]). As an administrator, I applied the same principles of caring along with principles of servant leadership with the staff and teams in my area of responsibility.

It was in my role as an educator that I became challenged to intentionally focus on research related to caring and specifically the why—that is, the source of caring. For nurses who embrace a Christian worldview, I felt this source was Christ, but I wanted to validate my thoughts through research.

As a nurse educator, I had a love for nursing history. This was a great fit for my teaching responsibilities, including nursing theory. Most nurses are aware that in the early years, health care was provided as a response to the call on Christians to serve those in need. In the Middle Ages, care was provided by various religious orders that served Christ by caring for the sick and needy. In modern nursing, Nightingale emphasized nursing as a calling—a vocation: "but more than this, she must be a religious and devoted woman; she must have a respect for her own calling, because God's precious gift of life is often literally placed in her hands" (Nightingale, 1860, p. 71). However, as nursing leaders focused on establishing nursing as a profession, the link between service and Christ described by Nightingale seemed to be forgotten.

As a new nurse in the 1960s, I was distressed to see a change in the professional direction. In the late 1960s and 1970s, I saw nursing turning away from our calling and Christian foundations; nursing as ministry was no longer valued. Instead, science was the primary focus, while at the same time migration toward New Age philosophy and secular humanism emerged. What was troubling to me was how many Christian nursing students were drawn to some of these theorists because of the "spiritual" emphasis and caring. However, they did not seem to understand that the spirituality and source of caring for these theories was not congruent with Christianity. When I would discuss these concerns, the students would reply, "But I can't find one that reflects my beliefs as a Christian nurse." This again was a challenge for me to connect with others with similar concerns, do further personal exploration, and conduct qualitative research.

In my search, I found other nurses who had similar concerns about nursing moving away from our foundations. Katie Eriksson was one theorist who linked a theory of caring with Biblical scriptures and principles. Other important nurse leaders who held to the foundations of faith and nursing were Sister Marie Simone-Roach, Sister Mary Elizabeth O'Brien, Judith Shelly, and Arlene Miller. The *Journal of Christian Nursing* was an excellent resource for articles from many other nurses.

As a result, I became more involved in Nurses Christian Fellowship (NCF) and Nurses Christian Fellowship International (NCFI) and developed relationships with some of these authors.

In 2004, I went to the NCFI Congress in Seoul, South Korea, and heard Dr. White discuss the need and opportunities for scholarly collaboration from a Christian perspective. These initial discussions evolved into the International Institute of Christian Nursing (IICN), part of NCFI; eventually I became the director of that organization. A focus of one of the subcommittees was the exploration of caring from a Christian worldview. In addition to findings from the literature, the Lord put many Christian nurses in my "caring" journey. Some of these included Dr. Josepha Campinha-Bacote, Dr. Bart Cusveller, Carrie Dameron, Dr. Shirlene Newbanks, and most recently Nancy Eckerd. Through these relationships, I gained perspectives from many Christian nurses across many countries around the world.

What began as my desire to explain nursing practice and care from a Christian worldview became a collaborative journey with Shirlene Newbanks and Nancy Eckerd. This relationship led to the adoption of the Agape Model described in the *Caring from a Christian Worldview: The Agape Model* chapter of this text.

As I reflect on my path, each step of the journey seems to have led to one more encounter that fueled a passion to develop something that would be congruent for Christian nurses to use in their practice. Corrie ten Boom expressed it best: "This is what the past is for! Every experience God gives us, every person He puts in our lives is the perfect preparation for the future that only He can see" (ten Boom, Sherrill, & Sherrill, 1971, p. 12). I have truly been blessed throughout my life to see how God can orchestrate people, events, and struggles—all for His glory.

Modified from ten Boom, C., Sherrill, E., & Sherrill, J. (1971). *The hiding place.* Lincoln, VA: Chosen Books; Rieg, L. S., Newbanks, R. S., & Sprunger, R. (2018). Caring from a Christian worldview: Exploring nurses' source of caring, faith practices, and view of nursing. *Journal of Christian Nursing, 35*(3), 168–173; Nightingale, F. (1860). *Notes on nursing: What it is and what it isn't.* New York, NY: D. Appleton and Company.

p. 376). CCU has set forth strategic priorities for the university as a whole, and nursing faculty and students are regularly offered opportunities for continuing education in all of these key growth areas.

Transformative

Through the use of strategic leadership in the roles of servant, shepherd, steward, and scholar, the doctorally prepared nurse is able to assist with transformation. As Romans 12:2 says, "Do not be conformed to this world, but be transformed by the renewal of your mind, that by testing you may discern what is the will of God, what is good and acceptable and perfect" (ESV). Not only are faith-based nurses transformed in their own spiritual walk, but they are able to come alongside others in the interprofessional team, as well as patients and families, to facilitate transformative processes that improve their spiritual well-being and overall health. **BOX 4-3** provides an example of how research can be used in the classroom to transform a curriculum in integrating spiritual care education.

▶ Valparaiso University College of Nursing and Health Professions

Mission and Vision

The mission of the Valparaiso University (VU) College of Nursing (CON) is to prepare critically inquiring, competent, and professional nurses who embrace truth and learning and who respect Christian values while promoting health of persons in dynamic healthcare environments. Such environments may be spiritually diverse, although the particular model discussed in this chapter is based on Judeo-Christian values.

Model Concepts

Given its mission, VU CON's Model of Professional Nursing (**FIGURE 4-3**) may be useful in understanding the roles of the nurse in spiritual care. The model incorporates the four metaparadigm concepts considered basic to any nursing

BOX 4-3 Research Highlight

Linda Rieg and colleagues (2018) have studied caring from a Christian perspective. These researchers explored nurses' basis for caring, their faith practices, and views on nursing. A nonexperimental, mixed-methods approach with an international convenience sample of Christian nursing students in two sites yielded 380 surveys. Nursing students reported using Bible reading and prayer most often as frequent faith practices. Seventy-eight percent ($n = 292$) reported believing that nursing is a calling. Additionally, "participants who reported Deity (God, Christ, Holy Spirit) as their source of caring were more likely to view nursing as a calling and report a higher degree of volunteering (serving), giving (financially to a religious community), devotions and prayer (personal walk), and fellowship (meeting with a community of other believers)" (p. 168). Studies such as this one help to shed light on caring from a Biblical worldview and demonstrate the need for more research in this area.

Modified from Rieg, L. S., Newbanks, R. S., & Sprunger, R. (2018). Caring from a Christian worldview: Exploring nurses' source of caring, faith practices, and view of nursing. *Journal of Christian Nursing, 35*(3), 168–173.

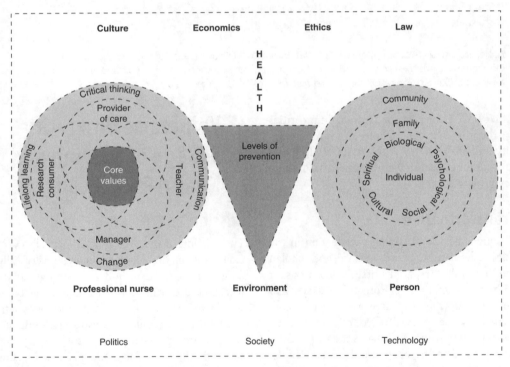

FIGURE 4-3 Valparaiso University College of Nursing's Model for Professional Nursing.
Used with permission from Valparaiso University.

framework: nurse, person, health, and environment (**BOX 4-4**). These four concepts are interconnected in a dynamic, ever-changing milieu influenced by a host of factors, such as socio-economics, politics, and culture.

Four concentric, overlapping circles on the left side of the model depicted in Figure 4-3 represent the professional nurse. Each circle signifies a role component. The common portion of the role components forms the core of

---

BOX 4-4　Definition of Major Concepts in the VU CON Model

Professional nursing is the process by which nurses prepared at the baccalaureate level interact with persons in the dynamic context of the environment to achieve health.

Health is both a dynamic process and a state. As a process, health is movement toward a sense of well-being. As a state, health can be measured by personal and professional standards. The professional nurse interacts with the person using primary, secondary, and tertiary prevention strategies to improve health.

The professional *nurse* uses ethical principles and values to integrate knowledge from the arts and sciences to provide competent care. He or she assumes the role components of provider of care, teacher, manager, and research consumer, using the processes of communication, critical thinking, change, and lifelong learning.

Environment is the dynamic context in which the nurse interacts with the person. Factors influencing the environment include culture, economics, ethics, law, politics, society, and technology.

Persons are individuals, families, or communities. Individuals are holistic beings with biological, psychological, social, cultural, and spiritual dimensions. Families are self-defined groups of individuals who have biological, psychological, social, cultural, or spiritual dimensions. Communities are groups of individuals or families who share common characteristics and work toward a common goal.

---

nursing, which consists of the ethical principles and values that guide nurses. These principles are based on the arts, sciences, and humanities. The core demonstrates that nurses have a scientific and ethical basis for practice.

Surrounding these role components are four essential processes that nurses use daily: critical thinking, communication, change, and lifelong learning. Each process is discussed in more detail later in this chapter.

Health is the entity that brings the nurse and the client together for interaction. Thus, health appears in the middle of the model to represent that connection, which is influenced by the nurse and the person, as well as the environment.

The person appears as three concentric circles and open systems. The person may be an individual, family, or community. Central to the person is a core of values and beliefs that influence the person's practice and sense of self.

Surrounding the entire interaction of person and nursing through health is the environment. Numerous factors influence the environment, as reflected in the model. Examples include sometimes intangible elements such as culture, ethics, law, politics, society, and technology.

This entire milieu of systems is constantly changing and interacting. It forms one picture of professional nursing that may suggest ways to provide spiritually competent care.

Role Components of the Professional Nurse

As identified in the VU model and discussed in this chapter, the four role components of professional nursing include provider of care, teacher, manager, and research consumer. These are further discussed here.

Provider of Care

As a provider of care, the nurse may perform hands-on, direct physical care of patients. Providing spiritual care is just as necessary, but usually less direct than giving a bath or administering medications. The nurse will need to plan spiritual care just as he or she plans physical care. Nurses use the nursing process (assessment, nursing diagnosis, planning, implementation, and evaluation) for this purpose.

Teacher

In the role of teacher, the nurse has many opportunities to assist the person to learn new skills related to spirituality. Perhaps a person wishes to learn to pray or does not know how to study the Bible, but during a crisis or illness feels the need to do so. Other persons may explore different religions if they have not obtained spiritual satisfaction from prior practices. The Christian nurse is often in a position to discuss spiritual questions with patients. Those nurses who have developed a level of expertise and comfort also may teach other nurses to provide spiritually sensitive, competent care in this area. Likewise, hospice nurses frequently address spiritual needs for patients at end-of-life (see the *Nursing Care at End-of-Life* chapter). Nurses are in an ideal place for divine appointments (see the *Divine Appointment: Fulfilling Your Call* chapter) both to give spiritual care and to teach others from the interprofessional team how to do so.

Manager

As a manager, the professional nurse may be called upon to coordinate complex healthcare situations. Overlooking the spiritual needs of the person is common when his or her physical needs are obvious and overwhelming. Some persons may have lost touch with their spiritual selves. Some may no longer be involved in a faith community, although they do remain spiritually connected. Others may not practice a particular faith, yet express a desire to enhance their spirituality. However, during illness, many people wish to reconnect with spiritual support systems, and nurses are in an ideal position to facilitate the rekindling of such relationships.

The nurse as manager may be required to assist families in crisis or to make decisions about whom to involve in the healthcare team. Chaplains are commonly viewed as the key resource for spiritual care, but the family, chaplain, and nurse actually form a spiritual care triad to meet the patient's needs (Sonemanghkara, Rozo, & Stutzman, 2019). Families may have to make difficult decisions about placing

their relatives in long-term care or hospice. These circumstances naturally impose spiritual dilemmas and distress. Spiritual uncertainty is common as people face difficult decisions or death. The astute nurse manager will realize such feelings affect the entire family and make appropriate referrals to the hospital chaplain, sister, priest, or other spiritual leader. Nurse, chaplains, and family members should work together to assure that the spiritual needs of the patient are met.

Research Consumer

As research consumers, nurses must stay aware of current trends and continue to read scholarly publications related to their field of practice. In the area of spirituality, nurses should avail themselves of the many publications (e.g., *Journal of Christian Nursing*) that focus on this important dimension of health care. Nurses can also take advantage of seminars and workshops offered at local, regional, or national levels.

Role Components of the Advanced Practice Nurse

Advanced practice registered nurses (APRNs) have at least a master's-level education, with skills beyond those of the professional nurse. Four types of APRNs are recognized in the United States: clinical nurse specialists (CNSs), nurse practitioners (NPs), nurse–midwives, and nurse anesthetists. The roles of the APRN suggest a higher level of practice, named in the VU CON model as clinician, educator, leader, consultant, and researcher. Each of these components is discussed here briefly as they relate to spiritual care in advanced practice nursing. **FIGURE 4-4** depicts a model for advanced practice nursing.

Clinician

Spiritual assessments are a critical, but often overlooked, part of detailed, holistic examinations (Lewinson, McSherry, & Kevern, 2015; O'Brien, 2017). As a clinician, the APRN has

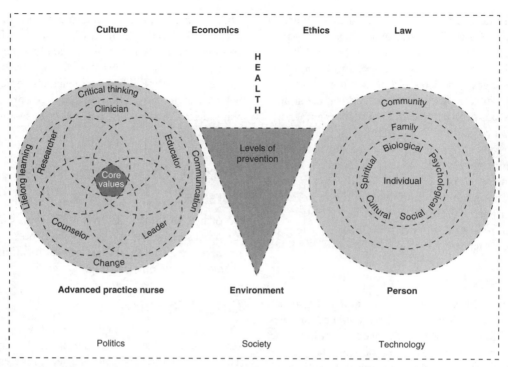

FIGURE 4-4 Valparaiso University College of Nursing's Model for Advanced Practice.
Used with permission from Valparaiso University.

cultivated advanced assessment skills to provide comprehensive care. APRNs have different opportunities than do staff nurses to explore spiritual problems with patients. They may be in unique positions, as primary care providers or educators, to address spiritual concerns. However, the nature of their practice may limit the time available to engage in spiritual discussions. Astute clinicians will look for signs of spiritual distress and use strategies to address the underlying needs.

Educator

The role component of educator is interpreted as an expansion of the role of teacher. A teacher instructs, but an educator uses appropriate theories to skillfully apply the process of teaching and learning. Thus, APRNs are expected to have more teaching expertise than are nurses without graduate education. APRNs addressing spiritual care needs may educate staff, nursing

students, or both in this area. They also may be called upon to speak at conferences or give presentations related to the subject of nursing education. Some APRNs may act as adjunct instructors at universities, serve as clinical scholars, or be certified as nurse educators or in staff development. As an educator, the APRN is in an ideal position not only to incorporate spiritual assessment techniques into practice but also to teach others to do the same.

Leader

As a leader, the APRN takes a proactive approach in providing spiritual care and encourages others to follow this example. Any APRN can assume a leadership role, even if the nurse is not formally employed in a direct management or administrative position. APRNs lead other staff and peers by example. By demonstrating the importance of spiritual care and competence in their own practice, they promote sensitivity to those issues in others. In addition, APRNs often assume leadership positions at various points in their career that provide them with added opportunities to effect changes in policies and procedures.

Nurses with advanced education should be politically active and maintain membership in professional organizations. Some of these organizations have specific goals to address the spiritual needs of patients and families. For example, Nurses Christian Fellowship, an interdenominational group within the InterVarsity parent organization, provides excellent resources and support for nurses focusing on spiritual care.

Consultant

The APRN's role as consultant is important in the spiritual lives of patients and families. APRNs possess the advanced education to act as professional resources for those having spiritual distress during illness or disease. In addition, patients commonly seek from such nurses expert advice on many health-related topics. APRNs should become familiar with the spiritual resources within their communities so that they can more effectively provide information when asked. The role components of consultant and educator may overlap, as seen in the VU model (Figure 4-4). Community leaders may seek the advice of APRNs when planning programs for various groups or ask APRNs to speak in faith-based settings based on their expertise. The APRN who is knowledgeable about spiritual health and well-being is a valuable resource for faith-based communities.

Researcher

The role component of research at the APRN level of practice generally encompasses not only being a savvy consumer, but also actively engaging in research. When they have a master's level of preparation, nurses may serve as members of research teams, provide clinical expertise in research studies, and suggest research ideas and questions. Nurses prepared with the DNP degree are experts in using

evidence-based practice and translating research into practice. Nurses who hold a PhD are prepared to design, conduct, analyze, and evaluate research. APRNs should not only be aware of evidence related to spiritual topics but also formulate hypotheses and researchable questions based on their experience and practice.

Processes Used in Professional Nursing

According to the VU CON model, four major processes help guide professional nursing practice: critical thinking, communication, change, and lifelong learning.

Critical Thinking

Critical thinking is defined as the ability to assess, reason, and arrive at a logical conclusion. The ability to think critically has become an essential expectation for nursing graduates. It is a skill that nurses can improve and hone through study and practice. Critical thinking serves as the foundation for appropriate and planned decision making in nursing. Within the spiritual realm, the ability to reason this way helps nurses to delve into the real problems patients are facing. Ethical decision making—a skill that all nurses must develop—also involves critical thinking and clinical reasoning.

Communication

Communication is probably the most widely discussed process in nursing. Professional nurses must be good communicators to promote health in all dimensions. In the area of spirituality, creating a trusting relationship and being a good listener are essential nursing tasks. Allowing persons to express their feelings of loss, hopelessness, frustration, or anger at God and actively listening help open the doors of communication and facilitate implementation of the caring role of nursing. For many individuals, a time of physical illness is also a time of potential spiritual growth. However, nurses must be aware that spiritual isolation may develop from these same circumstances. Nurses can use strategies to help persons integrate faith and health activities to enhance spiritual wellness, but trust and communication must be present for this outcome to occur.

Change

Facilitating change is a challenging process for nurses, but one in which they engage on a regular basis. Nurses ask patients to change their behaviors, their lifestyles, and their habits. Doing so may require people to give up things that are special to them on many levels. Through change processes, nurses help patients embrace healthier lifestyles. Such change may require examination of a person's core beliefs and values. Although difficult, this process is often necessary to promote health. In some instances, nurses may be called upon to set aside their own beliefs to support the patient's autonomy. In cases in which religious practices are negatively affecting the physical or mental health of one or more people, nurses may use change processes to help people examine the consequences of their decisions and the available options.

Lifelong Learning

Lifelong learning implies that nurses never stop accumulating knowledge. This process affects all the other role components. To remain informed about current research and best practice, nurses must continue to expand their knowledge base. For example, an APRN would not be prepared to act as a consultant without obtaining expertise in the area in question. Many nurses hold certification in a specialty field, and maintenance of such a credential requires continued education through several modalities. These activities may include conference attendance, pursuing higher education, engaging in research, or publishing articles.

Because many nurses report feeling underprepared to meet the spiritual needs of patients (Ali, Wattis, & Snowden, 2015; Giske & Cone, 2015), lifelong learning would include

---

BOX 4-5 Evidence-Based Practice Focus

Loma Linda University School of Nursing (LLUSN) identified strategies for teaching students to provide spiritual care. By purposefully and thoughtfully integrating specific key concepts into the curriculum, the faculty used content and concept mapping techniques to integrate spiritual care into 15 courses. Their model included didactic content identified across these courses, examples of clinical experiences and classroom activities to provide spiritual care in various situations, and specific assignments with readings, personal reflection, and practical applications.

Modified from Taylor, E. J., Testerman, N., & Hart, D. (2014). Teaching spiritual care to nursing students: An integrated model. *Journal of Christian Nursing, 31*(2), 94–99.

---

pursuing knowledge in this subject area. Doing so could take the form of attending a spiritual care conference, readings books or articles on the subject, obtaining a certificate in parish or faith-community nursing, joining a journal club, or having a mentor. Nurses who hold academic positions can promote lifelong learning in spirituality in their students (Taylor, Testerman, & Hart, 2014; White & Hand, 2017) by including content on spiritual care in coursework and encouraging students to continue to pursue expertise in that area (**BOX 4-5**).

▶ Conclusion

This chapter discussed key concepts of the metaparadigm of nursing using two quite distinct models that could be used to guide curricular development. Examples from Colorado Christian University's and Valparaiso University's nursing programs were given. Different levels of education were explored within the models and frameworks. Readers should continue to explore the use of models to help guide curriculum development in faith-based programs. **CASE STUDY 4-2**, as well as the critical

🔍 *CASE STUDY 4-2*

Rose is an 89-year-old widow with three children and eight grandchildren. She has attended the same Presbyterian church for 65 years. Several months ago, Rose found a lump in her breast, but chose to ignore it, fearing it was cancer. She developed increased swelling, hardness, tenderness, redness, and eventually large amounts of purulent discharge from the growing breast mass. Rose did not tell anyone, even her primary care physician, about this condition because she valued her independence and wanted to make her own decisions about having treatment. She did not want to have surgery or chemotherapy, feeling she had lived a good and long life. Rose purposefully hid her discomfort from family members by wearing baggy clothing to disguise the physical changes and withdrew socially to avoid any questions from friends or family members.

When the pain and odor became too great to manage on her own, Rose revealed her condition to her inquiring adult grandson, who insisted that she seek immediate medical attention. Rose was admitted that same day to the acute care hospital with a diagnosis of inoperable metastatic stage IV breast cancer. Refusing any medical treatment, Rose opted for hospice care at home for the remainder of her life. She told the hospice nurse that she is "ready to go home to be with God."

Questions

Using the models presented in this chapter, answer the following questions:

1. Which of the role components of professional nursing would be most important in providing end-of-life care for Rose?
2. What is the role of the family in Rose's care?
3. How would the nurse determine Rose's definition of health?
4. How is the person defined in this situation?
5. Which modifications to the environment can be made to ensure that Rose has a peaceful death?
6. What are some of the major end-of-life tasks that Rose might need to consider? How can the concepts in the models in this chapter help guide the nurse in assisting Rose to prepare for her end of life?
7. How does the nurse provide spiritual support to Rose in this situation?

thinking questions and personal reflections suggested, gives the learner a chance to apply the concepts in this chapter to real-life case scenarios.

▶ **Clinical Reasoning Exercises**

1. Compare and contrast the two models in this chapter. Does one model provide a stronger Biblical worldview to guide the practice of nursing as ministry compared to the other model?

Give examples from the models to support your answer.

2. A BSN nursing student is providing home care to a physician who has a terminal illness. Using the VU CON model for professional nursing, describe how the student would promote health for this dying medical professional. How would the influences of culture, economics, ethics, law, politics, society, and technology impact the practice of nursing as ministry to this particular person?

3. This chapter gives examples of models for nursing practice. In the VU CON

model for advanced practice, how do the role components of the advanced practice nurse (clinician, educator, leader, counselor, and researcher) differ from those of the professional nursing (provider of care, teacher, manager, research consumer) model?

4. The nurse is caring for an elderly patient with dementia whose behaviors include aggression and wandering. Using the CCU model, how would the nurse address the spiritual needs of this person, assuming memory loss is a key factor? How could the nurse show compassion and competence in this situation? How could the nurse act as a shepherd? As a scholar?

5. The CCU DNP in Visionary Leadership model provides guidance in using concepts to enact the roles of servant, steward, shepherd, and scholar. Give two examples of how a family nurse practitioner working in a primary care office, with a heavy caseload of patients, could be creative, inspirational, strategic, and transformative when time is at a premium to complete daily responsibilities. How would an advanced practice nurse in this situation be a visionary leader?

▶ Personal Reflection Exercises

1. Of the models represented in this chapter, with which do you most identify, and why?

2. Have you taken a nursing theory course at any time during your program of study? How did you feel about studying nursing theory?

3. How do you feel in general about nursing theory, frameworks, and models to guide practice? About using models or frameworks to guide your spiritual care of patients, residents, or clients?

4. How could you personally apply concepts from the models in these chapters to your own clinical practice in providing spiritual care?

5. How do you incorporate principles of being a servant, shepherd, steward, or scholar into your nursing practice?

6. Are you comfortable with the processes of communication, critical thinking, change, and lifelong learning? In which of these processes do you feel most proficient? What is one strategy you can use to improve in the area in which you need most improvement?

7. What are some ways that you engage as a clinician, educator, researcher, consultant, and leader in the realm of spiritual care and nursing as ministry? What are your greatest strengths and weaknesses in these roles?

References

Ali, G., Wattis, J., & Snowden, M. (2015). Why are spiritual aspects of care so hard to address in nursing education?: A literature review (1993–2015). *International Journal of Multidisciplinary Comparative Studies*, 2(1), 7–31.

American Nurses Association. (2010). *Nursing: Scope and standards of practice*. Silver Spring, MD: Author.

Benner, P. (1984). *From novice to expert: Excellence and power in clinical nursing practice*. Upper Saddle River, NJ: Prentice-Hall.

Christman, S. K., & Mueller, J. R. (2017). Understanding spiritual care: The faith–hope–love model of spiritual wellness. *Journal of Christian Nursing*, 34(1), E1–E7.

Coffman, T. J. (2017). *Servant leadership: Faculty and student perceptions among Council for Christian Colleges and Universities (CCCU) nursing programs* (Unpublished PhD dissertation). Abilene, TX: Hardin-Simmons University.

Colorado Christian University (CCU). (2019). *DNP student handbook*. Lakewood, CO: Author.

Giske, T., & Cone, P. H. (2015). Discerning the healing path: How nurses assist patient spirituality in diverse health care settings. *Journal of Clinical Nursing*, 24(19–20), 2926–2935.

Hitt, M. A., Ireland, R. D., & Hoskisson, R. E. (2007) *Strategic management: Concepts* (7th ed.). Mason, OH: Thomson Education.

Lehman, K., & Pentak, B. (2004). *The way of the shepherd*. Grand Rapids, MI: Zondervan.

Lewinson, L. P., McSherry, W., & Kevern, P. (2015). Spirituality in pre-registration nurse education and practice: A review of the literature. *Nurse Education Today*, *35*(6), 806–814.

Nightingale, F. (1860). *Notes on nursing: What it is and what it isn't*. New York, NY: D. Appleton and Company.

O'Brien, M. E. (2017). *Spirituality in nursing*. Burlington, MA: Jones & Bartlett Learning.

Rieg, L. S., Newbanks, R. S., & Sprunger, R. (2018). Caring from a Christian worldview: Exploring nurses' source of caring, faith practices, and view of nursing. *Journal of Christian Nursing*, *35*(3), 168–173.

Shelly, J. A., & Miller, A. B. (2006). *Called to care: A Christian worldview for nursing*. Westmont, IL: InterVarsity Press.

Sonemanghkara, R., Rozo, J. A., & Stutzman, S. (2019). The nurse-chaplain-family spiritual care triad: A qualitative study. *Journal of Christian Nursing*, *36*(2), 112–118.

Taylor, E. J., Testerman, N., & Hart, D. (2014). Teaching spiritual care to nursing students: An integrated model. *Journal of Christian Nursing*, *31*(2), 94–99.

ten Boom, C., Sherrill, E., & Sherrill, J. (1971). *The hiding place*. Lincoln, VA: Chosen Books.

White, D. M., & Hand, M. (2017). Spiritual nursing care education: An integrated strategy for teaching students. *Journal of Christian Nursing*, *34*(3), 170–175.

Ziebarth, D., & Campbell, K. P. (2016). A transitional care model using faith community nurses. *Journal of Christian Nursing*, *33*(2), 112–118.

Recommended Readings

Adams, L. Y. (2016). The conundrum of caring in nursing. *International Journal of Caring Sciences*, *9*(1), 1.

Egenes, K. J. (2017). History of nursing. In G. Roux & J. A. Halstead (Eds.), *Issues and trends in nursing: Essential knowledge for today and tomorrow* (pp. 1–26). Burlington, MA: Jones & Bartlett Learning.

Ziebarth, D. (2014). Evolutionary conceptual analysis: Faith community nursing. *Journal of Religion and Health*, *53*(6), 1817–1835.

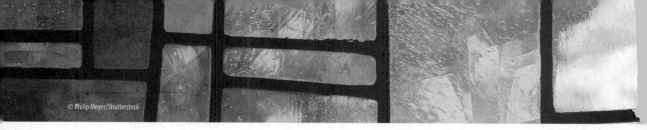

CHAPTER 5

Being a Christian Nurse

Anne Biro, MN, RN; **Carol Rowley**, PhD, RN; and **Bob Snyder**, MD

LEARNING OBJECTIVES

At the end of this chapter, the reader will be able to:

1. Explain the difference between *being a witness* and *witnessing to others*.
2. Differentiate between the faith journey phases of cultivating, sowing, and harvesting.
3. Describe what witnesses can do to help overcome each of the three spiritual barriers.
4. Apply knowledge about the eight Saline Process tools to select ones appropriate for someone you know who is on a faith journey.
5. Formulate options for resolving ethical dilemmas in ways that meet the principles of permission, sensitivity, and respect.
6. Describe how the Saline Process relates to being a Christian nurse.

KEY TERMS

Saline Process	Spiritual history	Spiritual vitality
Spiritual barriers	Spiritual journey	Witness

What does it mean to be a nurse witness? Is that how you would describe yourself? Is that how God would describe you? People's perception of their identities can have a profound impact on how they live their lives and what they expect out of their lives. When considering nursing as ministry, it is important to reflect on the identity of being a witness that God gives His people and how this identity can influence and empower them to participate in His work.

▶ Understanding Identity and Being

Christian nurses who view their profession as ministry are called to embrace their identities as being God's witnesses, God's partners, and God's nurses. The foundation of this call comes from Acts 1:8: "But you will receive power when the Holy Spirit comes on you; and you will be my witnesses in Jerusalem, and in all Judea and Samaria, and to the ends of the earth" (New International Version [NIV]). In this verse, **witness** is used as a noun, not a verb. This distinction emphasizes that Jesus primarily called His disciples to live life embracing their true identity as opposed to performing religious activities. True identity is not subject to significant variability: It should be consistent through variable conditions. In contrast to the consistency of identity, actions are frequently initiated and paused or stopped. Being a witness, therefore, is an identity to be maintained throughout one's life regardless of circumstances.

When considering what it means to be God's witness, it is helpful to distinguish between the contributions of an eyewitness and an expert witness. Eyewitnesses are asked to describe something from personal experience. In contrast, expert witnesses are enlisted to provide precise and accurate information on a topic in which they have achieved a higher level of mastery than would be expected in the general population. In Acts 4:13, Luke recounts how certain authorities responded to testimony given by Peter and John: "When they saw the courage of Peter and John and realized that they were unschooled, ordinary men, they were astonished and they took note that these men had been with Jesus." The impact of Peter's and John's witness did not come from theological expertise, but rather from having spent significant personal time with Jesus. All nurses should be able to provide detailed knowledge in the art and science of nursing that is developed over time through continual study and practice. Nurses who have an ongoing relationship with Jesus should be able to communicate through words and actions how encountering Jesus impacts their lives.

Being in relationship with Jesus is fundamental to being God's partner. Partnership involves the idea of a shared goal or vision. If partners are heading opposite directions, relationship problems are predictable, and accomplishment of any objectives may be hindered. In Matthew 10:25, Jesus indicates that the goal of disciples is to become like their teacher. Being in partnership with God challenges His disciples to deliberately choose to seek His presence and understand and embrace His priorities. Although those who partner with God may not see, hear, or feel Him in physical ways, they are never left alone or isolated. In every circumstance, God is available to teach, strengthen, and encourage those who partner with Him.

Being God's nurse is a special partnership available to Christians who are called not only to live as identifiable reflections of Jesus but also to engage in the healing ministry. They recognize that people are created body, soul, and spirit, and that the ramifications of this creation are eternally significant for each person. Beyond delivering a specified scope of professional skills, nurses are called to have and reflect God's love and compassion for those with whom they interact. Ultimately, Christian nurses are called to deliver nursing care on earth while living out the culture of heaven.

This chapter expounds on how to live and work in such a way that others are given an opportunity to encounter their living and loving Creator. Christian nurses have the opportunity to be Jesus's witnesses not only to patients but also to everyone with whom they interact. In this chapter, terms such as *patients, clients, colleagues,* and *others* can be used interchangeably. This chapter describes a framework for living as a witness: the **Saline Process**. The Saline Process has been implemented in numerous countries throughout the world. As is indicated by the name, witnesses are encouraged to be like saline—a specific solution of salt and water that sustains life. This analogy emphasizes how it is important for witnesses to balance God's love and truth in their interactions with others. As this chapter unfolds, the reader will be introduced to key principles and tools in the Saline Process that help healthcare providers ethically and effectively share God's love and truth with people in ways that can help them draw closer to Jesus. As this chapter is only a condensation of some of the key concepts in the Saline Process course, it is recommended that readers interested in learning more participate in a full Saline Process Witness Training.

▶ Being God's Witness

Being created in the image of God (Genesis 1:27) gives people an opportunity to display a degree of His attributes. While Eve and Adam's choice to rebel against God's plan marred that ability, Jesus's declaration that his Holy Spirit–empowered disciples would become his witnesses brings renewed hope for participating in this high calling. Many nurses find it challenging to know how to accurately and effectively accomplish this task in their work environment or in a multicultural setting. Indeed, styles that may be appropriate in one setting may be viewed as offensive in another. God's witnesses desire to reflect Jesus in a way that builds bridges instead of barriers.

In this regard, it is important for God's witnesses to consider 1 Peter 3:15: "But in your hearts revere Christ as Lord. Always be prepared to give an answer to everyone who asks you to give the reason for the hope that you have. But do this with gentleness and respect." A witness's interactions with others should be marked with permission, sensitivity, and respect. This, of course, is expected of any healthcare worker's interactions with a patient, family member, or colleague. Nurses do this when they take vital signs, administer medications, delegate activities to an aide, or consult with other healthcare professionals. God's witnesses need to remember that not only are they created in God's image but they are also called to treat others with the honor due to those who have been created in His image.

Being Motivated by God's Love

Love for God and others is the core motivation for being God's witness. John reveals that the first step to loving was receiving God's love: "We love because he first loved us" (1 John 4:19). Thus, it is essential that God's witnesses experience His lavish and steadfast love. When nurses are filled with God's love, this love can then overflow to people for whom they care. Loving others includes caring for a person's body, soul, and spirit. While much of nursing care involves addressing a person's physical needs, God's nurses must remember that the body for which they are caring is associated with a spirit and a soul. A person's spiritual health has consequences not only in life on earth but also after passing from this life into eternity. Being motivated by God's love prompts God's witnesses to care not just for people's temporary physical and emotional needs, but for their eternal spiritual needs as well. Answering God's call to be His witnesses demonstrates sincere love for God as well as for others.

Being Identified as Salt and Light

In further exploring the identity of God's witnesses, it is instructive to consider Jesus's words to his disciples about salt and light:

> You are the salt of the earth. But if the salt loses its saltiness, how can it be made salty again? It is no longer good for anything, except to be thrown out and trampled underfoot. You are the light of the world. A town built on a hill cannot be hidden. Neither do people light a lamp and put it under a bowl. Instead they put it on its stand, and it gives light to everyone in the house. (Matthew 5:13–14)

Jesus told his disciples that they were salt. In life and in health care, salt is both common

• You can be gentle & respectful but still offend.

and essential. In cooking, it is used to season and preserve food; in health care, isotonic saline is commonly used for hydration, irrigation, and cleansing. It's easy to see salt when many crystals are together in a salt shaker. In contrast, when it is mixed in a liter of intravenous fluid or a container of food, it is not visible. Nevertheless, its presence can change hypotonic water into an isotonic solution or give bland food a delicious taste. Salt does these things reliably and predictably because it maintains unique chemical properties.

After Jesus told his disciples that they were salt, he also gave them the identity of light. Like salt, light is both common and essential. Without light, people cannot visually perceive their surroundings. The purpose of light is to illuminate the environment; indeed, as Jesus pointed out, a hidden light is pointless. Without light, people remain in darkness. Light also has specific properties, such as the ability to be reflected. A source of light can be extinguished, but while present, light remains light—whether it is bright or dim, its identity does not change.

What does it mean for God's witnesses to be salt and light? Both salt and light have an effect on their environments. Salt impacts on contact. It can improve the taste of food. It is also essential for maintaining healthy fluid and electrolyte levels in the body. It has cleansing properties. Salt makes things taste better and function efficiently. Likewise, God's witnesses can have contact with people in ways that make the environment more pleasant or comfortable. In a healthcare setting, being salt might look like giving a patient or colleague a word of encouragement or helping a coworker at a stressful time. Keeping one's spoken and body language clean and not engaging in gossip are other examples of being salt. By acting in these and similar ways, God's witnesses can make a positive and noticeable impact on their environment.

While salt works to improve things on contact, light makes things visible. In terms of being God's witness, being light makes God more visible to those present. One example of this would be offering, with sensitivity, permission, and respect, to pray for someone who is confronting an overwhelming situation. Because the act of being light makes Jesus visible through the witness, it takes more courage than being salt, which is appealing but often invisible. Both salt and light, however, are part of a witness's identity.

In conjunction with maintaining our identity as salt and light, it is important to recognize the effect that a witness's attitudes, words, and actions can have on others. For all God's witnesses, balancing truth and love is important. Continuing the analogy of saline, it is essential that therapies involving sodium be strategically regulated. While an infusion of 0.9% saline can provide life-saving rehydration, a solution of 3.0% saline can precipitate a serious adverse reaction because of its hypertonicity. Conversely, infusing a solution of 5.0% dextrose may be insufficient for restoring health to a hypovolemic or hyponatremic patient. When acting as a witness, only truth without love could provoke a very negative reaction, perhaps similar to an allergic reaction. Only love without truth could abandon a person to an eternity apart from God. An effective witness balances truth with love to provide the spiritual equivalent of 0.9% saline—the exact solution that reflects God's love and truth so as to promote spiritual life and health.

Of course, administering ever-increasing amounts of sodium is generally not therapeutic in patient care. Instead, the goal is to provide the correct dose of the needed element. Both the appropriate amount and the chemical identity of sodium are important. Similarly, one's impact as a witness does not necessarily increase by saying more, speaking more loudly, or working harder. Effectiveness starts with living out one's identity as a witness of Jesus. When one's life is filled with Jesus and his love, that love will overflow from one's heart and mind to one's actions and interpersonal relationships. Thus, being an effective witness comes from overflow, not overwork; it's not about doing more, it's about truly being who one is called to be.

▶ Being God's Partner

Jesus told his disciples, "You did not choose me, but I chose you and appointed you so that you might go and bear fruit—fruit that will last" (John 15:16). Jesus called his followers to live lives of eternal impact. While much in this physical world will not pass into eternity, a person's soul will. What happens to each soul is important. Peter wrote about God's desire for people to be saved, explaining that God is "not wanting anyone to perish, but everyone to come to repentance" (2 Peter 3:9). Because of Jesus's great love for people, He willingly paid the price of his earthly life to offer reconciliation to all. Recognizing that God wants and offers the opportunity for imperfect people, made acceptable because of Jesus, to partner with Him in bringing others to salvation should give God's partners a sense of humility and sobriety as they live out this calling.

Recognizing Barriers to Living Our Identity

An understanding and acceptance of our identity as being salt and light is important to embracing God's identification of us as His witnesses, but how we express this identity is also important. Taylor, Park, and Pfeiffer (2014) conducted qualitative research to better understand how Christian nurses' religiosity impacted their practice, specifically with regard to providing spiritual care. Nurses in the study were motivated to reflect God's love and were open to praying with and for patients, as well as praying for guidance for themselves as they cared for their patients. They also felt building relationships and sensitively following patient responses regarding spiritual care were important, as it was possible for offense to occur if care was provided in a manner unwelcomed by the patient.

should we let offense deter us?

Yet, many Christian healthcare workers struggle with knowing how best to provide spiritual care. McSherry and Jamieson's (2011) study of more than 4000 nurses in the United Kingdom (74.3% of whom self-identified as Christian) revealed that 95.5% of them had interacted with one or more patients with spiritual needs. Nevertheless, only 5.3% of the nurses reported feeling that they could always meet the spiritual needs of their patients, and 92.2% stated that they could meet these needs only sometimes. A total of 79.3% either agreed or strongly agreed that spiritual care education for nurses was inadequate.

This theme of inadequate education for addressing patients' spiritual needs was also recognized when Dutch Christian healthcare professionals were surveyed regarding faith and their healthcare practice. Cusveller, van Leeuwen, and Schep-Akkerman (2015) concluded that "Christian professionals do not ask for lectures on the way things are or how things should be in healthcare. They have a need for training, tools, role models, and best practices of transparent participation by Christians in healthcare" (p. 30). Equipping healthcare workers with practical skills and tools to live as witnesses is one of the core purposes of the Saline Process.

Journeying with Others

When one reads through the Gospels, it becomes clear that Jesus did not have only one strategy for ministering to people. As Jesus joined with what the Father was doing (John 5:19), his interactions with people could look quite different, depending on each person's situation. In John 4, Jesus compared the agricultural process with reconciling people back into a restored relationship with God. This is a useful analogy even today (**FIGURE 5-1**). The goal is a big harvest, but before harvest time, the soil must be cultivated and prepared before seeds can be sown. The soil needs to be cleared of things that would hinder growth, such as rocks, roots, or weeds. Once the ground

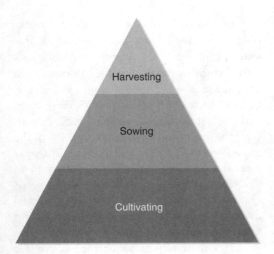

FIGURE 5-1 Cultivating, sowing, harvesting.

Reproduced from International Health Services (IHS). (2015). *The Saline Process trainer's manual.* Southeastern, PA: Author.

has been prepared, seeds need to be planted. While everyone works with a view toward the harvest, if no one participated in the laborious activities of cultivating and sowing, the harvest would be limited or nonexistent. Harvest, then, is not an isolated event, but rather the culmination of a process that unfolds over time. In the same way, a person's moment of reconciliation with God may be preceded by many small steps leading to the confession of Jesus Christ as Lord and Savior.

This concept of people being on a journey toward God can be visualized with the Engel Scale, as modified by IHS Global (International Health Services [IHS], 2015). This process-related model of spiritual decision making was initially conceptualized by Viggo Søgaard while he was studying at Wheaton Graduate School. James Engel subsequently revised this concept and published the model, which depicts the process of someone moving from having no knowledge of the gospel to becoming a reproducing believer (Engel & Norton, 1975). Many modifications of the Engel Scale exist, and the Modified Engel Scale shown in **TABLE 5-1** is derived from the work of Walt Larimore and Bill Peel, in conjunction with Christian Medical and Dental Association (CMDA) USA. The Modified Engel Scale

as used in the Saline Process is a tool to help us understand that the journey to becoming a believer in God can be a process that may occur in stages (IHS, 2015).

The Modified Engel Scale gives God's partners an overview of different stages that may be experienced in someone's **spiritual journey**. Some people may be at a stage in their spiritual journey in which the soil of their hearts needs to be cultivated with love and mercy to prepare their hearts for a future time of sowing. As Paul reminded Christians, God's kindness is a catalyst in bringing people to repentance (Romans 2:4). Other people may be actively engaged in trying to learn who Jesus is or what it would be like to follow him. God's partners need to meet people where they are. Trying to jump ahead into a different season is likely to be frustrating, unfruitful, and potentially harmful. God's partners can trust God to be working at the right pace in someone's life and need to focus on fitting into God's plan by loving and caring for people where they are. In this way, our nursing care becomes patient centered.

For nurses, it is particularly important to trust God's love and plan for the people whom they encounter. Nurses might meet some patients only for a moment, after which they will never care for them again. Nurses might see other patients once but have a longer time to interact. In different situations such as physical rehabilitation or chronic disease, they may experience ongoing encounters with a person. In each situation, nurses need to focus on that moment—connecting and participating by being salt and light. When the interaction is over, they can trust that God will still be working in the person's life, drawing that person to Himself. Progress may seem slow and sometimes may even seem to go backward. The witness's job is not to judge the person, but rather to listen to God's direction of how to give that person a touch from God.

As people encounter God's message of reconciliation, they may have different responses. Luke recounts an example of this

TABLE 5-1 Modified Engel Scale

Disciple	Chooses to live by faith	**+5**	**Multiplying**	**Speaks to:** The whole person **Addresses:** Social barriers **Overcomes:** Isolation **By:** Participation in body **Goal:** Growth **Answers:** Will I live for Christ? **Example:** Jerusalem church (Acts 2:41–47) and Samaritan awakening (Acts 8:4–8) **Tools:** Prayer, questions, gospel presentation, spiritual referral team
	Chooses to share faith with others	**+4**		
	Makes Christ-like choices	**+3**		
	Joins in community life	**+2**		
	Assimilates God's Word	**+1**		
Believer	Trusts in Christ	**0**	**Harvesting**	**Speaks to:** The will **Addresses:** Volitional barriers **Overcomes:** Indecision, unwillingness to change **By:** Prayer and persuasion **Goal:** Trust Christ **Answers:** Will I trust Christ? **Example:** Paul before Agrippa (Acts 26:1–29) **Tools:** Prayer, questions, gospel presentation, spiritual referral team
	Turns from self-trust	**−1**		
Seeker	Sees Christ as the answer	**−2**		
	Recognizes own need	**−3**		
Spectator	Considers the truth of the gospel	**−4**	**Sowing**	**Speaks to:** The mind **Addresses:** Intellectual barriers **Overcomes:** Ignorance, misconceptions, error **By:** Presentation **Goal:** Understanding **Answers:** Who is Jesus? What does he want from me? **Example:** Ethiopian eunuch (Acts 8) **Tools:** Prayer, faith flags and faith stories, truth prescriptions, gospel presentation, spiritual referral team
	Understands the implications	**−5**		
	Aware of the gospel	**−6**		
Skeptic	Recognizes relevance of the Bible	**−7**		
	Looks positively at the Bible	**−8**	**Cultivating**	**Speaks to:** The emotions **Addresses:** Emotional barriers **Overcomes:** Indifference, fear, and antagonism **By:** Your presence **Goal:** Trust you **Answers:** What's in it for me? **Example:** Nicodemus (John 3) **Tools:** Prayer, questions, spiritual history, faith flags and faith stories
	Recognizes difference in the messenger	**−9**		
Cynic	Aware of the messenger	**−10**		
	Going own way	**−11**		
	Avoids the truth	**−12**		

Modified with permission from Dr. James Engel © IHS Global, Inc. (2015).

phenomenon in Acts 17:16–34. After Paul arrived in Athens, he began to share the gospel with Jews and philosophers. Eventually, he was invited to expound on this message in front of an assembly. After Paul concluded his presentation, the response of the listeners was recorded: "When they heard about the resurrection of the dead, some of them sneered, but others said, 'We want to hear you again on this subject.' After that, Paul left the Council. Some of the people became followers of Paul and believed" (Acts 17:32–34a). This passage includes three types of responses to the gospel. The first response mentioned was not simply voicing disagreement with the message, but also expressing negative emotions. The next response was wanting to hear more, a more thoughtful reaction that engaged the intellect. Finally, the passage describes people who expressed belief in Jesus's resurrection and made a commitment to follow Paul's teaching. Other passages of scripture describe times when people decided not to follow Jesus. One example is the rich ruler who walked away from Jesus after being told to sell his possessions and give to the poor (Luke 19:16–22). This type of response involves volition—making a choice to do or not do something. These three types of responses (emotional, intellectual, and volitional) can still be encountered today.

Overcoming Spiritual Barriers

The three types of responses reflect different types of barriers that prevent people from putting their faith in Jesus, which can be viewed as **spiritual barriers** (**FIGURE 5-2**). While only God can remove spiritual barriers, witnesses can help lower barriers through understanding each of these barriers and responding appropriately.

Emotional barriers are frequently the result of bad experiences with religion. Sadly, too many people have experienced rejection or abuse from the church or religious people. Some people may blame God for difficult situations in their lives. If they are confronted with a religious message, they may react angrily. In this situation, God's witness should remember that "A gentle answer turns away wrath, but a harsh word stirs up anger" (Proverbs 15:1). It is God's kindness that leads people to repentance

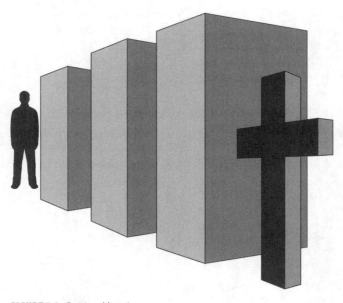

FIGURE 5-2 Spiritual barriers.
Reproduced from International Health Services (IHS). (2015). *The Saline Process trainer's manual*. Southeastern, PA: Author.

(Romans 2:4). Through their presence, witnesses build trust and consistently reflect God's gentleness and kindness while depending on God to lower emotional barriers.

Other people may simply not be aware of God's plan for reconciliation. They may be open to learning more if this plan is communicated with permission, sensitivity, and respect. Paul wrote in 2 Timothy 2:24–25 that a witness must be able to teach in a manner that is humble and avoids arguing. Witnesses should communicate truth with patience and gentleness, trusting God to bring others to a knowledge of Himself.

When people understand God's invitation to follow Him, they are confronted with making a choice that will change their life. Depending on their culture, the cost of following Jesus may include rejection by family members, loss of employment, or even possible death. For everyone, it includes recognizing Jesus as Lord and Savior and coming into alignment with God's authority. As witnesses interact with people encountering volitional barriers, God is calling for His people to stand in the gap (Ezekiel 22:30) and be steadfast in prayer (James 5:16). God's witnesses can be assured that their prayers have great effect as God works in lives to lower volitional barriers.

As indicated in the Modified Engel Scale (Table 5-1), different people may face different barriers at different times in their lives. Some people may progress in a linear manner through the different barriers, while others may go back and forth, and some may experience only one or two barriers. A witness's loving presence to overcome emotional barriers, the presentation of Biblical truth to overcome intellectual barriers, and prayer and persuasion to overcome volitional barriers are reflected in Paul's exhortation to the Colossians:

> Devote yourselves to prayer, being watchful and thankful. And pray for us, too, that God may open a door for our message, so that we may proclaim the mystery of Christ, for which I am in chains. Pray that I may proclaim it clearly, as I should. Be wise in the way you act toward outsiders; make the most of every opportunity. Let your conversation be always full of grace, seasoned with salt, so that you may know how to answer everyone. (Colossians 4:2–6)

▶ Being God's Nurse

Those who embrace the call to be one of God's nurses have the opportunity to bring a heavenly perspective and understanding to the ministry they offer through nursing (**BOX 5-1**). Doing this successfully requires that Christian nurses maintain **spiritual vitality** and influence while being diligent to always interact with others using permission, sensitivity, and respect. Through recognizing the spiritual barriers of those they encounter, they can make wise choices in how to best offer others a touch from God and a glimpse of who He is.

Maintaining Spiritual Vitality and Influence

Nurses who seek to live as God's witnesses need to maintain spiritual vitality. Spiritual vitality refers to the condition of one's spiritual health, which is maintained and increased by drawing life from Jesus. As recorded in John 15:5, Jesus testified: "I am the vine; you are the branches. If you remain in me and I in you, you will bear much fruit; apart from me you can do nothing." Spiritual vitality is achieved by staying connected to Jesus. This can be experienced in several ways, such as by participating in personal and corporate worship, reading the Bible, praying by oneself or with partners, confessing one's failures, and receiving forgiveness. Being in an accountability or mentoring relationship can facilitate growth and provide encouragement. Even if people have drifted away from God for a season, God is ready to welcome them back. Maintaining

BOX 5-1 Outstanding Nurse Leader: Dr. Barbara Ihrke

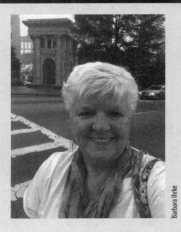

Barbara Ihrke

Dr. Barbara Ihrke has been a nurse for more than 40 years and is currently the leader of the nursing program at Indiana Wesley University. She describes being a witness of Jesus as her identity—a normal, everyday part of who she is. She credits the Saline Process Witness Training (SPWT) with freeing her to be a witness and releasing her from expectations that some Christians have in regard to outcomes. As a nurse, Ihrke says that focusing on harvesting in the healthcare setting might be appropriate about 1% of the time, but that one can always cultivate and sow. She has found faith flags and faith stories to be the tools she uses the most.

As head of the nursing program, Ihrke often works with visiting scholars and professors from other countries. On one occasion, when arranging a meeting with a visiting professor who had previously identified herself as being from a different religious background, Ihrke mentioned that she would be available after her morning routine of reading and exercise. The professor asked what Ihrke read each morning, and Barbara replied that she read the Bible. The professor verbalized interest in beginning to read the Bible, and eventually made a decision to trust in and follow Jesus.

This is one story of Ihrke's use of faith flags in everyday life. In this situation, the faith flag led to a conversation, and eventually a commitment to Christ. At other times, when there isn't any interest in further conversation, Ihrke isn't discouraged, as she trusts God for the outcome. Faith flags and stories have become an everyday part of her life as a witness to Jesus.

a connection with Jesus is essential for God's witnesses to have positive spiritual influence.

While witnesses endeavor to stay connected to Jesus, as part of humility it is important to recognize that the goal is not pretending to be perfect or denying weaknesses. Even with one's best intentions and efforts in being a witness, there may be times when mistakes are made or events take an unexpected turn. Scripture is filled with followers of God who didn't always get it right, including Abraham, Moses, Miriam, David, Martha, and Peter. One's failures and mistakes will never surprise God. When honestly evaluated, failures may even provide opportunities for growth and maturity. The Holy Scripture promises that those who humble themselves before God will be uplifted (1 Peter 5:6). God makes it clear that His desire for those who have fallen short of the desired standard is restoration, and He wants those who follow Him to be sensitively involved in this restoration process (Galatians

6:1). The whole body of Christ will benefit if witnesses stay connected to Jesus, stay connected to each other, don't give up on each other, and keep each other accountable in a spirit of love and humility.

Along with encouraging spiritual vitality, the Saline Process identifies five specific characteristics that contribute to a person's spiritual influence, referred to as the Five C's:

- Christ-like **C**haracter
- Professional **C**ompetence
- **C**ompassion
- Wise **C**ommunication
- **C**ourage

God's nurses should reflect Christ-like character in their words and actions. Thankfully, they do not have to do this in their own power. In Galatians 2:20, Paul explains: "I have been crucified with Christ and I no longer live, but Christ lives in me. The life I now live in the body, I live by faith in the Son of God, who loved me and gave himself for me." Witnesses have the opportunity to show the Jesus in them to those they encounter. They can show Jesus to others as they respond to both ordinary and stressful situations with love, humility, integrity, and wisdom.

In addition to demonstrating Christ's character, God's nurses should strive to deliver professionally competent care to their patients. Christian nurses must avoid relegating the provision of physical care to a subordinate level, while prioritizing spiritual care. The Bible teaches us that human beings are made in God's image (Genesis 1:27) and that we are to treat the body with respect (1 Corinthians 6:12). Therefore, instead of providing only cursory or outdated physical care, God's nurses should be delivering the best possible evidence-based care to their patients.

In maintaining spiritual influence, showing compassion is also important. While compassion comes easily to some nurses, others may feel awkward giving emotional or spiritual comfort to people in distress. Even those to whom compassion comes easily may find times when they have nothing left to give. Yet, all of God's nurses need to be faithful in reflecting God's character of compassion. In 2 Corinthians 1:3–4, Paul explains that as Christians receive comfort from a compassionate God, they can extend this comfort to those who are suffering. If patients face the fear or loneliness of being ill or the loss of being able to care for themselves, nurses can use their compassionate presence, gentle words, and appropriate touch to bring comfort.

Another characteristic of spiritual influence is wise communication. Proverbs 18:21 reminds us that "The tongue has the power of life and death," and Colossians 4:6 instructs that our conversation should be "seasoned with salt." Undoubtedly, communication entails much more than words. People communicate by the tone of their voice, the volume of their voice, the expression of their face, and in many other nonverbal ways. Just as technical skills can be honed with practice, so nurses can seek to improve their effectiveness in communicating therapeutically. Along with the way, striving for cultural competence in caring for patients from diverse backgrounds should not be neglected, as different cultures may express needs differently, and appropriate strategies for meeting these needs may vary by culture. God's nurses can make a habit of praying for guidance to make each patient encounter therapeutic. Sometimes even a brief comment or gentle touch can make a big difference to distressed or lonely people.

The last of the Five C's is courage. For the gospel to be clearly understood to the degree that someone can choose to put their faith in Christ, more than kindness is required—the message of Jesus must be communicated. In some places, spiritual care or nurse-initiated conversations related to spirituality are discouraged or restricted. Receiving training in how to ethically and appropriately provide spiritual care can help witnesses take steps forward in sensitively communicating about Jesus. Besides becoming equipped, partnering with others in prayer and accountability is another way to help build courage. While challenges may occur, it is important to never give up the pursuit of Christ-like character, professional competence, compassion, wise communication, and courage.

Creating a Safe Environment

A safe environment helps people feel accepted and at ease. If a patient wants to discuss something of a personal nature, nurses should help create spaces that protect patient confidentiality consistent with ethical nursing practice. If spiritual topics are addressed, it is important for witnesses to avoid using words that contribute to misunderstanding or negative emotional responses. Some people have spiritual barriers that make them uncomfortable discussing spiritual issues. Pursuing spiritual conversations or topics in these situations can create feelings of unease and add further barriers.

BOX 5-2 Research Highlight

Taylor et al. conducted descriptive and correlational research investigating nurses' opinions related to (1) having religious or spiritual conversations with patients, (2) sharing their personal religious or spiritual beliefs with patients, and (3) praying with patients. Participants were also asked questions regarding their personal religiosity, prayer, tendency to share personal religious beliefs, and tentativeness of their convictions. The majority of the 445 participants were Christian (92.9%), female (92.1%), from the United States (90.8%), and not employed by a religious organization (65.4%). The vast majority of respondents held the opinion that these activities were appropriate either in certain circumstances or in any situation. Notably, only 1.6% believed that nurses should never discuss religious or spiritual matters with patients except during screening, and 11.8% believed that nurses should discuss them only after patient initiation. Similarly, a minority of respondents believed that disclosing one's personal spiritual or religious beliefs and praying with patients should be done only at patient request (28.8% and 24.8%, respectively) or never (6.7% and 6%, respectively). With respect to a nurse's personal spiritual life, higher intrinsic spirituality scores were associated with belief in the appropriateness of disclosing beliefs and initiating prayer, while higher scores related to the tendency to share personal beliefs were associated with agreement about the appropriateness of all three activities. Spirituality of nurses was associated with belief in the appropriateness of self-disclosure and prayer in nursing.

Modified from Taylor, E. J., Park, C. G., Schoonover-Shoffner, K., Mamier, I., Somaiya, C. K., & Bahjri, K. (2018). Nurse opinions about initiating spiritual conversation and prayer in patient care. *Journal of Advanced Nursing, 74*(10), 2381–2392. doi:10.1111/jan.13777

Nurses should avoid consciously or unconsciously manipulating people to make religious commitments based on some indication that they might receive better care, less expensive care, or some other benefit. Judgmental attitudes or harsh words also create spiritual barriers. Nurses need to remember that it is God's kindness that encourages people to turn to Him (Romans 2:4), not their sermons, conditions, or condemning attitudes. Nurses need to discern where patients are on their faith journey and respond appropriately (**BOXES 5-2** and **5-3**). Creating a safe environment requires the nurse to focus on helping overcome patient barriers in an effective manner.

Using Eight Practical Tools to Help People on Their Faith Journey

The Saline Process describes eight tools that can be used at different stages of a patient's journey. These tools, when applied with permission, sensitivity, and respect, can help remove

BOX 5-3 Evidence-Based Practice Focus

Although spiritual care is always part of holistic care, many nurses do not receive formal education about how to actually provide it. Wittenberg et al.'s 2017 study surveyed oncology nurses about their experiences with spiritual care. Nurses reported that patients most often were the ones who initiated conversations about spiritual care, and this occurred mainly when they faced end-of-life or were experiencing spiritual distress. Approximately one-third of the nurses in this sample shared their own personal stories of faith with patients when appropriate and used similar strategies discussed in this chapter; they reported that this intervention also strengthened their own faith. The findings from this survey demonstrate the need to include in the curriculum ways for nurses to address spirituality with patients.

Modified from Wittenberg, E., Ragan, S. L., & Ferrell, B. (2017). Exploring nurse communication about spirituality. *American Journal of Hospice and Palliative Medicine, 34*(6), 566–571.

emotional, intellectual, and volitional barriers. The eight tools are prayer, questions, spiritual history, faith flags, faith stories, truth prescriptions, gospel presentation, and the spiritual referral team.

The first tool, prayer, is used throughout the entire process. In everything that is done, prayer is useful for guiding and empowering the life of a witness. Nurse witnesses commit to pray for their workplaces and to continue to seek God's leading in their lives. When possible, it is helpful for nurses and other Christian healthcare workers to pray together. Discernment should be used when considering praying for patients or praying with patients. Nurses are also obligated to adhere to the policies and procedures of the facility regarding spiritual support to patients.

The second tool in the Saline Process is questions. Questions, when used effectively, communicate care and interest in a person's life. The right questions help people express their physical, psychosocial, and spiritual needs. A skilled nurse will use a variety of question types, such as open and closed, probing, and reflective questions. As competent and genuinely compassionate care is delivered, trusting relationships can be built that open doors for deeper conversations. Gently asking wise questions may uncover deeper needs that only Jesus can meet. In the midst of asking questions, listen carefully to what the patient is sharing; also listen carefully to the Holy Spirit, who can direct each conversation. Many times, patients have spiritual needs, but they may be hidden behind physical, emotional, and social problems. Guided by the Holy Spirit, nurses' questions can show interest in each patient's life and help uncover possible barriers between that patient and Jesus.

As nurses perform health assessments on their patients, they need to remember to ask questions not only about their patients' physical, emotional, and social health, but also about their spiritual conditions. It is important to recognize that people's spiritual beliefs can impact their healthcare decisions (Silvestri,

Sommer, Zoller, & Nietert, 2003). **Spiritual history,** the third tool, is a specific set of questions about a person's spirituality. A variety of standardized spiritual histories have been developed, including FICA (Pulchalski & Romer, 2000) and HOPE (Anandarajah & Hight, 2001) (see the *Spiritual Assessment* chapter). Among the standardized spiritual histories, different terminology is used. When conducting a spiritual history, it is helpful to phrase questions using words familiar to the patient. Depending on the situation, the nurse can discern if it is most appropriate to ask the entire set of questions or if only one or two questions are warranted.

Faith flags and faith stories are two tools that identify the nurse as a follower of Jesus and give an idea of what this means. A faith flag consists of two key elements: (1) expressing common ground related to the patient's situation and (2) making a statement that identifies the nurse as a follower of Jesus. For example, if the patient expresses sorrow about a loss, the nurse might compassionately say, "I also had a time of grieving, but God gave me peace in the midst of it." If the patient asks the nurse to explain, a faith story related to the situation could be shared. The nurse should receive permission prior to sharing a personal experience with the patient. Because the faith story is about a personal experience, the nurse must be careful not to insert opinions or suggestions about what the patient should do. The faith story takes only one or two minutes to relate. Both faith flags and faith stories need to be communicated using words that are common in everyday language that someone without Bible knowledge can understand. Referencing specific churches or denominations should be avoided, as the goal is pointing people toward Jesus. In sharing faith flags and stories, the nurse needs to be careful not to create barriers or an unsafe environment.

The sixth tool is the truth prescription. A truth prescription gives the patient something to do, read, or watch that helps the person experience Biblical truth in a personal way. For example, when caring for a patient who is fearful, if the patient is open to it, the nurse might recommend reading Isaiah 41:10 three times a day: "So do not fear, for I am with you; do not be dismayed, for I am your God. I will strengthen you and help you; I will uphold you with my righteous right hand." Another truth prescription could be watching a Christian inspirational movie or taking action to restore a relationship. Truth can have a powerful impact on a person; thus, as with the principle of a saline solution, it is important to regulate the strength and frequency to promote a therapeutic effect.

As emotional and intellectual barriers are removed, the time may come when people want to hear an explanation of God's plan for salvation. In 1 Peter 3:15, witnesses are instructed to always be ready to give an answer when asked about their hope in Christ. Giving a gospel presentation usually works best if the witness has practiced and become comfortable with explaining the message. Several different methods may be used to help explain how to be reconciled to God. Similar to faith flags and stories, a witness should be able to explain the gospel message clearly and concisely in common, everyday language.

Paul encouraged Christians to "make the most of every opportunity" (Colossians 4:5). As God's witnesses, nurses should be alert for ways to partner with God in being salt and light. At some points in the patient's spiritual journey, it may be best to make a referral to someone better equipped to help the patient. This may be due to time constraints faced by the nurse, lack of expertise, the need of the person to connect with someone who has been in a similar situation, or the patient leaving the healthcare setting. A useful tool at this time is the spiritual referral team. It is helpful for a nurse witness to develop a list of people who have the potential and are willing to follow up on a variety of spiritual needs. These people should exhibit Christ-like character, professional competence, compassion, wise communication,

and courage and should always maintain confidentiality. Examples of people on a spiritual referral team may include a person who has gone through a similar experience, a colleague, a hospital chaplain, or a pastor. Before referring the individual, be sure to obtain the consent of the person being referred.

▶ Conclusion

Effective spiritual care is patient and moves according to God's timing. Because of the eternal ramifications related to people being reconciled to God, witnesses might feel a sense of urgency for getting others to make a statement of faith in Jesus. However, God's witnesses can have confidence that God, "who wants all people to be saved" (1 Timothy 2:4), is already at work in each person's life. As Christian nurses care for others, they need to trust God's love and sovereignty. While God works in people's lives, God's partners need to stay connected to Him, listen to Him, and join Him in what He is doing.

Nurses can provide excellent holistic care to their patients each day in a way that positively impacts their physical, emotional, social, and spiritual health (**CASE STUDY 5-1**). To accomplish this, God's nurses need to be filled with God's love. They need to maintain professional competence as well as their own spiritual vitality, viewing themselves as God's partners as they encounter people at various phases on their journey to Jesus. Empowered by the Holy Spirit, nurse witnesses are salt and light when they give patients a touch of God's compassion and communicate God's truth with courage. Ensuring permission, sensitivity, and respect, they can use the eight Saline Process tools to help lower spiritual barriers in those persons with whom they interact. In this ministry, nurses can focus on being witnesses who view each patient interaction as a divine appointment, reflecting God's love to the patient and trusting God for the results.

🔍 *CASE STUDY 5-1*

Nurse Sarah works in the orthopedics department in a large hospital. Two weeks ago, a 25-year-old female, Jessica, was brought to the emergency department via ambulance for severe trauma after a motor vehicle accident. She had an elevated blood alcohol level on arrival. She required emergency surgery for her multiple injuries. Jessica was transferred yesterday from the intensive care unit to the orthopedics department, where she is continuing her recovery and will soon begin physical therapy.

As Sarah was checking Jessica's peripheral IV, she noticed scarring on Jessica's wrists. When reviewing Jessica's past medical history, she noted there had been a prior suicide attempt. Jessica's emergency contact is listed as her aunt. Sarah suspects that Jessica's current health problems are more than just physical and wants to follow up with her before she is discharged.

Questions

1. If you were Sarah, how would you start this conversation?
2. What are some questions that Sarah can ask Jessica to learn more about her emotional and social problems?
3. Based on this scenario, which spiritual barriers do you suspect may be present in Jessica's life? What are some ways Sarah could be salt and light without creating any new spiritual barriers in Jessica?

▶ Clinical Reasoning Exercises

1. Interview a Christian who decided to follow Christ after becoming an adult. Ask the person to describe reasons for not choosing Christ before this time. Identify which types of spiritual barriers were experienced and how the barriers were overcome.

2. Read the article by Saguil and Phelps (2012). Practice taking a spiritual history with one friend or colleague using one of the methods described in the article. Describe in your journal how healthcare decisions might be impacted by the person's spiritual worldview. Based on what the person told you, what are appropriate ways for you to be a witness to Christ for this person? Evaluate how well you think the interview process went. Are there things that you would do differently the next time you take a spiritual history?

3. Identify a challenging time in your life in which you experienced God's help. Construct a faith story by writing a three- to four-sentence description of this event and the way in which Jesus helped you. Identify how you could find common ground with a patient through this situation (e.g., dealing with anxiety, disappointment, or loneliness). Using the area of common ground, write a single-sentence faith flag.

▶ Personal Reflection Exercises

1. Think of a situation at school or work when you were the only Christian in the midst of others who did not have a relationship with Jesus. Did they know

you were a believer? How did you let them know this? If they did not know you were a believer, why do you think this was? How did being a Christian affect your relationship with this group? Do you think that you were able to be salt and light in this situation? Why or why not?

2. Was there ever a time when you saw or heard about a Christian talking about Jesus or religion to someone who was not yet a follower of Christ in a manner that you felt was inappropriate or unhelpful? Why did you think the Christian's actions were not helpful? How did the listener respond? How did you respond to the situation? Can you think of a better way that the Christian may have communicated in that situation?

3. Have you ever had the opportunity to work with a team of other Christians in a school or healthcare setting? What were the benefits to you personally with respect to working as a team with other Christians? What were the benefits to the work/setting/patients because there was a team of Christians collaborating? What were the challenges of working on this team?

References

Anandarajah, G., & Hight, E. (2001). Spirituality and medical practice: Using the HOPE questions as a practical tool for spiritual assessment. *American Family Physician, 63*, 81–89.

Cusveller, B, van Leeuwen, R., & Schep-Akkerman, A. (2015). Being the minority: Christian healthcare providers in the Netherlands. *Journal of Christian Nursing, 32*(1), 26–30.

Engel, J. F., & Norton, W. (1975). *What's gone wrong with the harvest: A communication strategy for the church and world evangelism.* Grand Rapids, MI: Zondervan.

International Health Services (IHS). (2015). *The Saline Process trainer's manual.* Southeastern, PA: Author.

McSherry, W., & Jamieson, S. (2011). An online survey of nurses' perceptions of spirituality and spiritual care. *Journal of Clinical Care, 12*(11–12), 1757–1767.

Pulchalski, C., & Romer, A. L. (2000). Taking a spiritual history allows clinicians to understand patients more fully. *Journal of Palliative Medicine, 3*(1), 129–137.

Saguil, A., & Phelps, K. (2012). The spiritual assessment. *American Family Physician, 86*(6), 546–550.

Silvestri, G. A., Sommer, K., Zoller, J. S., & Nietert, P. J. (2003). Importance of faith on medical decisions regarding cancer care. *Journal of Clinical Oncology, 21*(7), 1379–1382.

Taylor, E. J., Park, C. G., & Pfeiffer, J. B. (2014). Nurse religiosity and spiritual care. *Journal of Advanced Nursing, 11*(70), 2612–2621.

Recommended Readings
Spiritual Care

Fawcett, T. N., & Noble, A. (2004). The challenge of spiritual care in a multi-faith society experienced as a Christian nurse. *Journal of Clinical Nursing 13,* 136–142.

Minton, M. E., Isaacson, M., & Banik, D. (2016). Prayer and the registered nurse (PRN): Nurses' reports of ease and dis-ease with patient-initiated prayer request. *Journal of Advanced Nursing, 72*(9), 2185–2195. doi:10.111/jan.12990

Ronaldson, S., Hayes, L., Aggar, C., Green, J., & Carey, M. (2012). Spirituality and spiritual caring: Nurses' perspectives and practice in palliative and acute care environments. *Journal of Clinical Nursing, 21*(15–16), 2126–2135.

Vance, D. L. (2001). Nurses' attitudes towards spirituality and patient care. *Medsurg Nursing, 10*(5), 264–268.

van Loon, A. M. (2005). Commentary on Fawcett and Noble (2004), The challenge of spiritual care in a multi-faith society experienced as a Christian nurse. *Journal of Clinical Nursing, 14,* 266–268.

Wittenberg, E., Ragan, S. L., & Ferrell, B. (2017). Exploring nurse communication about spirituality. *American Journal of Hospice and Palliative Medicine, 34*(6), 566–571.

Spiritual History

Borneman, T., Ferrell, B., & Puchalski, C. (2010). Evaluation of the FICA tool for spiritual assessment. *Journal of Pain and Symptom Management, 40*(2), 163–173.

Saguil, A., & Phelps, K. (2012). The spiritual assessment. *American Family Physician, 86*(6), 546–550.

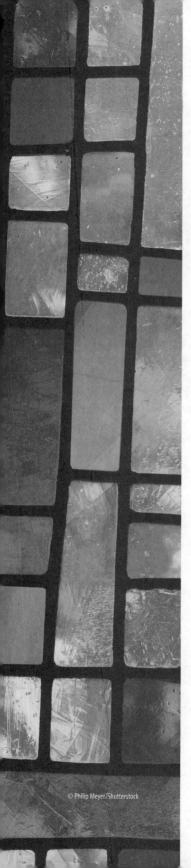

© Philip Meyer/Shutterstock

UNIT II

The Nursing Process and Ministry

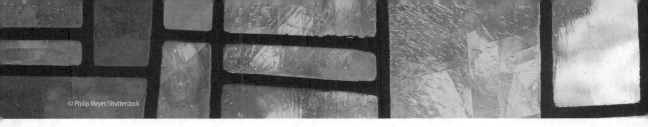

CHAPTER 6

Spiritual Assessment

Kristen J. Goree, DNP, APRN, CNS, FNP-C

LEARNING OBJECTIVES

At the end of this chapter, the reader will be able to:

1. Describe the spiritual assessment process in accordance with the Spiritual Care Implementation Model.
2. Identify key questions found in a spiritual screen and the role of the nurse in screening for spiritual distress.
3. Differentiate the types of information gathered by the various spiritual history tools and by whom such tools should be administered.
4. Recognize the role of the chaplain or other spiritual care provider in obtaining a professional spiritual assessment.
5. Examine the health implications and Joint Commission regulations associated with the assessment of spiritual needs.

KEY TERMS

Nursing process
Professional spiritual
  assessment
Spiritual assessment

Spiritual Care Implementation
  Model
Spiritual care methods of
  inquiry

Spiritual care provider
Spiritual distress
Spiritual history
Spiritual screen

For many Americans, the term *spirituality* is linked to the values and beliefs that surround the Christian faith. According to a Gallup poll, 73% of Americans identify themselves as Christian, with Protestants making up the largest religious group (Newport, 2017). Despite the continued prevalence of Christianity in the United States, 6% of Americans subscribe to another faith, while 21% report no faith at all (Newport, 2017). Due to this variance, several definitions of spirituality have emerged in the literature over the last decade (Hughes et al., 2017; Steinhauser et al., 2017). According to Steinhauser et al. (2017), these definitions are typically represented by one of the following overarching concepts: "diverse spiritual or religious beliefs, rituals and practices, coping, distress, relationship with the transcendent, sense of meaning, or life purpose" (p. 429).

Of all the concepts presented, the most frequently utilized are those that define spirituality in connection to ultimate meaning, purpose, and relationship. For Christians, meaning and purpose are discovered within the context of a higher power, the one true God. Here, meaning is found in loving God, loving others, and living out the purpose by which one has been equipped and called (Ephesians 2:10; Matthew 22:36–40; Romans 8:28). Furthermore, made in the very image of God (Genesis 1:27, 5:1; John 4:24), the human spirit longs to be connected in relationship to its maker and through such relationship finds love, joy, and peace (Galatians 5:22–23; John 15:5). According to the Barna Group (2017), prayer and the reading of scripture are the tools most commonly used to foster this type of relationship. In contrast, individuals who believe themselves to be spiritual, but not Christian or religious, are more likely to be polytheistic and/or believe God to be represented by "a state of higher consciousness that a person may reach" (Barna Group, 2017, para. 7). For these individuals, meaning and purpose are found within the relationships to self, nature, and others. Such relationships are strengthened through the preferred spiritual practices of nature immersion, solitude, reflection, or personal meditation (Barna Group, 2017).

Despite the vast differences in how the concepts of meaning, purpose, and relationship play out in the lives of the religious and the non-religious, both groups have the potential to identify with these terms in their own way. Given this level of inclusivity, such terms have been incorporated into the definition of spirituality put forth by the National Consensus Project for Quality Palliative Care Guidelines (NCP Guidelines). The NCP definition, which was developed by a community of hospice and palliative care leaders from across the country, is one of the most widely agreed-upon and utilized definitions within the palliative care and hospice community (Steinhauser et al., 2017). As presented at the International Consensus Conference of 2012, the NCP defines spirituality as "a dynamic and intrinsic aspect of humanity through which individuals seek meaning, purpose, and transcendence, and experience relationship to self, family, others, community, society, and the significant or sacred. Spirituality is expressed through beliefs, values, traditions, and practices" (National Coalition for Hospice and Palliative Care [NCHPC], 2018, p. 32).

▶ The Nursing Process

Assessing spiritual well-being in patients is not new to nursing, but rather has been foundational to nursing practice as part of a holistic model of care. Seeing the patient as more than just a physical entity, nurses care for the mind, body, and spirit. According to the American Nurses Association's *Nursing 2015 Code of Ethics*, "optimal nursing care enables the patient to live with as much physical, emotional, social, and religious or spiritual well-being as possible" (Fowler, 2015, p. 179). Furthermore, the spiritual beliefs of the patient are to be respected and taken into consideration when formulating a patient's plan of care (Fowler, 2015).

Traditionally plans of care are created by moving through the **nursing process**, a critical-thinking framework that includes the stages of assessment, diagnosis, planning, implementation, and evaluation (American Nurses Association [ANA], n.d.; Fowler, 2015). Because needs must be identified before such a plan of care can be developed, however, the first step in the spiritual care planning process is the administration of a spiritual assessment.

▶ The Spiritual Assessment

In the most basic sense, a **spiritual assessment** can be viewed as the collection and analysis of data to evaluate the spiritual needs and resources of a patient within the healthcare setting (Cadge & Bandini, 2015). While such a definition outlines which data are to be collected and for what purpose, it fails to clarify the process by which such information should be obtained. According to the NCP Guidelines, the collection of spiritual data should not be conducted by the nurse in isolation, but rather as part of a collaborative effort. When the nurse is working as part of an interprofessional team, data should be gathered using one of the three potential **spiritual care methods of inquiry**: spiritual screening, spiritual history, or the professional spiritual assessment. Each method requires a different level of time and expertise for its application, so not all providers should utilize each method (Balboni et al., 2017; NCHPC, 2018).

While nurses may gather spiritual data utilizing either spiritual screening or spiritual history tools, a professional spiritual assessment should be completed by a **spiritual care provider** such as a chaplain, religious leader, spiritual counselor or director, pastor, or faith community nurse or provider (Balboni et al., 2017; NCHPC, 2018). This process has been depicted within the **Spiritual Care Implementation Model**, which was originally delineated by Puchalski et al. (2009) and can be applied to both the inpatient and outpatient clinical environment.

Spiritual Screen

Of the three spiritual care methods of inquiry, the spiritual screen is the most simplistic and is the method most commonly used by nurses (**CASE STUDY 6-1**). According to the definition presented at the "State of the Science in Spirituality and Palliative Care" conference, a **spiritual screen** "evaluates the presence or absence of spiritual needs and/or distress with the goal of identifying those in need of further spiritual

🔍 CASE STUDY 6-1

A 37-year-old male with a 15-year history of chronic back pain is admitted to the hospital for his second back surgery in three months. When conducting the admission health history, you learned that the patient's religious affiliation is Christian. Upon reassessment, the patient appears depressed, staring out the window when you try to make conversation and answering in a monotone voice with only one- or two-word responses.

Think about nursing care as it relates to this patient:

1. What is an appropriate response by you as the nurse?
2. Which question(s) might you ask?
3. Which spiritual care method of inquiry would this line of questioning fall under?

The nurse completes a spiritual screen and offers to pray with the patient. The patient responds by stating, "I don't think that it will do much good. I don't think God is interested in helping me right now."

Based on the patient's response, the nurse asks the patient if he would like to speak to a chaplain. Somewhat reluctantly he agrees.

4. What nursing diagnosis might be appropriate for this patient?
5. What spiritual care method of inquiry do you anticipate the chaplain will utilize to further assess the spiritual needs of this patient?
6. How can improving the spiritual well-being of this patient impact his health outcomes?

assessment and care" (Balboni et al., 2017, p. 442). Typically administered as part of a nursing admission health history, a spiritual screen should include questions that address more than just the religious affiliation of the patient; that is, it should include one or two questions aimed at uncovering the presence of spiritual distress (NCHPC, 2018).

The nursing diagnosis of spiritual distress is one of five diagnoses approved by NANDA International (NANDA-I) that relates to the topic of spiritualty or religion (**TABLE 6-1**). According to NANDA-I, **spiritual distress** is "[a] state of suffering related to the impaired ability to experience meaning in life through connections with self, others, the world, or a superior being" (Herdman & Kamitsuru, 2014, p. 372). Experienced by 40.8% of patients with cancer undergoing chemotherapy treatment, spiritual distress can manifest itself in the form of alienation, anxiety, body image disorders, burden to family, crying, feeling disconnected, fatalism, fear, need for forgiveness, desire to die, guilt/punishment, hopelessness, impaired role performance, insomnia, lack of dignity, feeling abandoned by relatives and friends,

loneliness, questioning identity, refusing to interact with significant others, issues surrounding relationship with God, social isolation, uncertain future, worthlessness, and physical symptoms (Martins & Caldeira, 2018).

One example of a spiritual screening tool is the Religious Struggle Spiritual Screen developed by Fitchett and Risk (2009). Composed of three main questions, this screen is intended to quickly identify patients experiencing spiritual struggles so that an appropriate chaplain referral can be made (**FIGURE 6-1**). For individuals who do not immediately claim spirituality, two separate questions can be used.

Although often utilized at the beginning of care, spiritual screens should not be conducted at only one point in time. As the trajectory of a patient's illness changes, so, too, can the individual's ability to cope or find strength/comfort (NCHPC, 2018). While reassessment does not always need to involve the application of a specific tool, the nurse should continuously screen for spiritual distress or the desire for chaplain visitation.

One way to rescreen patients for the potential of spiritual distress is by assessing for the presence of spiritual pain. In a study by Mako, Galek, and Poppito (2006), spiritual pain was described to patients as "a pain deep in your being that is not physical" (p. 1108). In this same study, 96% of patients with cancer reported experiencing such pain, which was further expressed as feelings of abandonment by God, regret, depression, anxiety, or disconnectedness from God, family, or spiritual community. Another important finding in this study was the discovery of a significant correlation between the depression scores of patients and the presence of spiritual pain, with more depressed patients experiencing greater spiritual pain (Mako et al., 2006). Given this correlation, it would be prudent for the nurse as part of ongoing patient assessments to explore patient cues that suggest depression or spiritual distress. Verbal cues that could suggest spiritual pain might include a depressed affect or comments made by the patient about never getting better or inquiry as to why God would allow such an illness or injury to happen to him or her.

TABLE 6-1 NANDA-I Spiritual Nursing Diagnoses, 2015–2017
Nursing Diagnosis
Impaired religiosity
Risk for impaired religiosity
Readiness for enhanced religiosity
Spiritual distress
Risk for spiritual distress
Readiness for enhanced spiritual well-being

Data from NANDA International (NANDA-I). (2018). *NANDA International Nursing Diagnoses: Definitions and Classification 2018–2020* (11th ed.). New York, NY: Thieme.

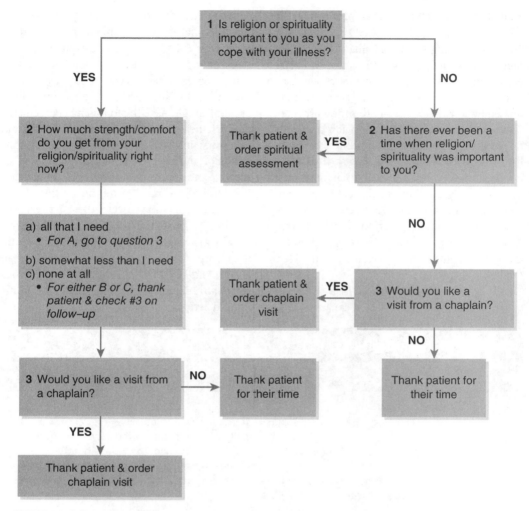

FIGURE 6-1 Religious struggle spiritual screen.

Reproduced from Fitchett, G., & Risk, J. L. (2009). Screening for spiritual struggle. *Journal of Pastoral Care and Counseling, 63*(1–2), 1–12. Copyright © 2009 SAGE Publications. Reprinted by permission of SAGE Publications, Ltd.

Given the frequency with which spiritual pain and depression appear in patients, it seems logical to heed previous recommendations in the literature and treat spirituality distress as a vital sign (Bultz et al., 2011; Puchalski et al., 2009). A potential question that could easily be incorporated into routine nursing assessments might then be, "Are you experiencing any depression or spiritual pain related to your illness?" Positive answers could be briefly explored by the nurse, if comfortable, or could be immediately followed by a question about the patient's desire to talk with a chaplain.

Spiritual History

The **spiritual history** is more inclusive than the spiritual screen and comprises questions that uncover values, preferences, and needs that influence the patient's plan of care or ability to effectively cope with the present health crisis (LaRocca-Pitts, 2012; NCHPC, 2018). Spiritual histories are typically completed during the initial contact with the patient as part of a comprehensive hospital history and physical examination, or in the outpatient setting as part of a complete health history during an annual physical examination or new clinic visit (Balboni et al., 2017; NCHPC, 2018; Puchalski, 2014). According to the Spiritual Care Implementation Model, the bedside nurse or social worker may conduct a history; nevertheless, an initial spiritual history is more typically conducted by a primary care or admitting provider (advanced practice nurse, physician assistant, or physician). This reality should not preclude the bedside nurse from reviewing spiritual history tools, however, as spiritual discussions may spontaneously arise in which such tools may be useful in guiding the conversation. If a spiritual need is identified, then a referral to a spiritual care provider should be triggered and a more thorough spiritual assessment completed (NCHPC, 2018).

To assist with the spiritual history-taking process, more than 40 different spiritual tools have been developed by practicing nurses, physicians, social workers, chaplains, and researchers (Cadge & Bandini, 2015). Despite this wide array of tools, not all are well suited for the clinical environment. Based on the frequently cited work by Koenig (2007), a spiritual history tool should have the following characteristics: brief; easy to recall; effective in obtaining necessary information; patient-centered, focusing on the patient's beliefs; and validated as credible and appropriate by experts in the field.

One of the most commonly utilized assessment tools that meets these criteria is the FICA Spiritual History, which was created by a physician, Dr. C. M. Puchalski, from the George Washington Institute for Spiritual Health (**TABLE 6-2**). The FICA tool focuses on spiritual/religious faith, influence, community, and actions of care.

TABLE 6-2 FICA Spiritual History Tool	
Acronym	**Questions**
F	Faith and Belief ■ "Do you consider yourself spiritual or religious?" or "Is spirituality something important to you?" or "Do you have spiritual beliefs that help you cope with stress/difficult times?" (Contextualize to reason for visit if it is not the routine history). ■ If the patient responds "No," the health care provider might ask, "What gives your life meaning?" Sometimes patients respond with answers such as family, career, or nature. ■ (The question of meaning should also be asked even if people answer yes to spirituality).
I	Importance "What importance does your spirituality have in your life?" "Has your spirituality influenced how you take care of yourself, your health?" "Does your spirituality influence you in your healthcare decision making?" (e.g., advance directives, treatment, etc.)
C	Community "Are you part of a spiritual community?" Communities such as churches, temples, and mosques, or a group of like-minded friends, family, or yoga can serve as strong support systems for some patients. Can explore further: "Is this of support to you and how?" "Is there a group of people you really love or who are important to you?"
A	Address in Care "How would you like me, your healthcare provider, to address these issues in your healthcare?" (With the newer models including diagnosis of spiritual distress A also refers to the "Assessment and Plan" of patient spiritual distress or issues within a treatment or care plan).

© Christina M. Puchalski, MD, 1996. Puchalski, C., & Romer, A. L. (2000). Taking a spiritual history allows clinicians to understand patients more fully. *Journal of Palliative Medicine, 3*(1), 129–137.

Another commonly cited spiritual history tool created by a physician is the HOPE model (**TABLE 6-3**). In this model, the first question does not center on spiritual beliefs, but rather the patient's source of hope and strength. According to Anandarajah and Hight (2001), leading the patient in this way helps to create an open conversation, as the language of

TABLE 6-3 HOPE Spiritual History Tool	
Acronym	**Questions**
H	Sources of Hope, meaning, comfort, strength, peace, love, and connection ■ What in your life gives you internal support? ■ What are your sources of hope, strength, comfort, and peace? ■ What do you hold on to during difficult times? ■ What sustains you and keeps you going? ■ For some people, their religious or spiritual beliefs act as a source of comfort and strength in dealing with life's ups and downs—is this true for you? If no, was it ever? If yes, what changed?
O	Organized religion ■ Do you consider yourself to be part of an organized religion? ■ How important is this to you? ■ Which aspects of your religion are helpful and not so helpful to you? ■ Are you part of a religious or spiritual community? ■ Does it help you? How?
P	Personal spirituality and Practices ■ Do you have personal spiritual beliefs that are independent of organized religion? What are they? ■ Do you believe in God? ■ What kind of relationship do you have with God? ■ Which aspects of your spirituality or spiritual practices do you find most helpful to you personally? (e.g., prayer, meditation, reading scripture, attending religious services, listening to music, hiking, communing with nature)
E	Effects on medical care and End-of-life issues ■ Has being sick (or your current situation) affected your ability to do the things that usually help you spiritually? (Or affected your relationship with God?) ■ Is there anything that I can do to help you access the resources that usually help you? ■ Are you worried about any conflicts between your beliefs and your medical situation/care/decisions? ■ Would it be helpful for you to speak to a clinical chaplain/community spiritual leader? ■ Are there any specific practices or restrictions I should know about in providing your medical care? (e.g., dietary restrictions, use of blood products) ■ If the patient is dying: How do your beliefs affect the kind of medical care you would like me to provide over the next few days/weeks/months?

religion and spirituality can sometimes be a barrier to sharing beliefs. As the history unfolds, the focus moves from the more generalized questions of hope to more specific questions surrounding organized religion, practices, and their impact on care.

Although less publicized in the literature, another tool that incorporates hope was created by Dr. Judith Allen Shelly (2017), a nurse and minister. As a Christian and publications director for Nurses Christian Fellowship, Shelly based her tool on the writings of the Apostle Paul (**TABLE 6-4**). In 1 Corinthians 13:13, Paul states, "And now these three remain: faith, hope and love. But the greatest of these is love" (New International Version [NIV]).

In 2015, Dr. W. Larimore, a Christian physician, expanded upon the typical components found in a spiritual history tool to assess for "spiritual struggles" that had been identified in the literature and linked to increased mortality rates. According to Larimore (2015), patients who admitted to questioning God's love for them, or wondered whether God had abandoned them, or felt punished by God for a lack of devotion, were at a 16% to 22% higher risk of mortality than those who answered no to these types of questions. Based on these findings, Larimore developed the LORD's LAP tool (**TABLE 6-5**).

TABLE 6-4 Faith, Hope, and Love Spiritual History Tool	
Categories	**Questions**
Faith	■ Are you connected with a faith community? Do they know you are here? ■ Would you like me to notify your pastor or hospital chaplain that you are here? ■ What spiritual practices are meaningful to you? How can I help you to continue those practices while you are here? ■ How has your illness affected your relationship with God? ■ Is prayer helpful to you? ■ How can I pray for you? ■ Would you like me to pray for you? ■ Which Bible verses have been most meaningful to you?
Hope	■ How are you coping with your illness? ■ How does your faith help you cope with suffering? ■ What do you hope for beyond this life? ■ What do you fear the most? ■ What gives you the most joy and satisfaction in life?
Love	■ Who provides you with the most love and support? Are they able to be present with you now? ■ Do you believe that God loves you? If not, what seems to stand in the way? ■ Are there people you need to forgive? ■ Do you want to ask anyone to forgive you?

Data from Shelly, J. A. (2017). Spiritual assessment. In *CSB Nurse's Bible* (pp. 1097–1098). Nashville, TN: Holman Bible Publishing.

TABLE 6-5 LORD's LAP Spiritual History Tool	

Acronym	Questions
L	Lord ■ May I ask your faith background? Do you have a spiritual or faith preference? Is God, spirituality, religion, or spiritual faith important to you now, or has it been in the past?
O	Others ■ Do you now meet with others in religious or spiritual community, or have you in the past? If so, how often? How do you integrate in your faith community?
R	Religious struggles or Relationship ■ If the L and O questions have indicated that the person is religious, then assess LAP questions. f not, share a brief faith flag.
D's	Do ■ What can I do to assist you in incorporating your spiritual or religious faith into your medical care? Or, is there anything I can do to encourage your faith? May I pray with or for you?
L	Love ■ How has this illness caused you to question God's love for you?
A	Abandon ■ How has this illness led you to believe God has abandoned you? Have you asked God to heal you and He hasn't?
P	Punish ■ Do you believe God or the devil is punishing you for something?

From Larimore, W. (2015, Fall). Spiritual assessment in clinical care part 2: The Lord's LAP. *Today's Christian Doctor*, p. 29. Retrieved from https://x362 .blob.core.windows.net /downloads/5bf87413431f4b17bfe833e491ad26e5 -461f62f3-8e49-402a-9ae3-e3d9add2f26b.pdf. Used with permission from Christian Medical & Dental Associations.

Embedded within this tool is the opportunity to share a faith flag with those who do not currently identify with Christianity. Larimore (2015) provides an example of the delivery of a faith flag in the following statement:

Even though religion and spirituality are not important to you now, I often see patients who, when facing a health crisis or decision, will begin to have spiritual thoughts or questions. When I was younger, I had similar questions that resulted in my coming into a personal relationship with God. I just want you to know that if you ever want to discuss these things, just let me know. (p. 27)

Faith flags are discussed in more detail in the *Being a Christian Nurse* chapter.

Professional Spiritual Assessment

Although spiritual history tools can uncover a great deal of information, it is believed that a more comprehensive assessment is required to develop a plan of care that best meets the spiritual needs of the patient (LaRocca-Pitts, 2015). A **professional spiritual assessment** is "an in-depth ongoing process of evaluating a patient's spiritual needs and resources completed by chaplains or other individuals possessing advanced training in spiritual care" (Balboni et al., 2017, p. 444; see also Puchalski et al., 2009). Given the spiritual expertise and time that are required to conduct such an assessment, according to Hughes et al. (2017), this task should ideally be completed by a board-certified chaplain. When such a professional is unavailable, another spiritual care provider can be utilized (Balboni et al., 2017).

Historically, professional spiritual assessments have been conducted by chaplains using individualized narrative-based assessment approaches. While such methods are still practiced today, there has been a push in the field of palliative care to use more standardized tools that are quantifiable and tested for reliability and validity (Balboni et al., 2017). According to Balboni et al. (2017), the use of such tools has the advantage of more easily communicating assessment findings and the proposed plan of care to patients, family, and the healthcare team.

One example of a standardized tool that has demonstrated reliability in the literature is the Spiritual Distress Assessment Tool (SDAT; Balboni et al., 2017; Monod et al., 2010). Based on the Spiritual Needs Model, which defines the four dimensions of spirituality and five corresponding needs, the SDAT includes a set of standardized questions for interview and analysis purposes (**TABLE 6-6**). After patient consent is obtained, these interview questions should be asked by the chaplain over a 20- to 30-minute time period. At the completion of the interview, analysis of information related to the five spiritual needs is conducted and a score awarded that reflects the severity of unmet needs or the presence or absence of spiritual distress (Monod et al., 2010).

▸ Nursing Implications of the Spiritual Assessment

The nursing assessment process is a wonderful example of interprofessional care. Through such collaborative efforts, the team has the ability to effectively assess the spiritual needs of the patient and ultimately formulate a plan of care to improve the patient's spiritual health. Benefits to improving spiritual health are many, but some of the outcomes recorded in the literature include reductions in pain, depression, and risk of suicide (Hui et al., 2011; Kopacz, Hoffmire, Morley, & Vance, 2015; Mako et al., 2006).

Despite the positive health outcomes associated with spiritual assessment, nurses sometimes perceive the issue of spirituality as a private one for patients and, therefore, are hesitant to engage in conversations of a spiritual nature (Gallison, Xu, Jurgens, & Boyle, 2013). It is important for the nurse to realize that research has demonstrated that patients desire the opportunity to discuss spirituality in connection with their medical care (Williams, Meltzer, Arora, Chung, & Curlin, 2011). According to Williams et al. (2011), when such conversations are allowed to unfold, patients are more likely to rate their hospital experience as having provided the highest level of care.

Given patients' desire for spiritual openness and the positive impact of spirituality on health and hospital ratings, it should be no surprise that The Joint Commission

TABLE 6-6 Spiritual Distress Assessment Tool (SDAT)

Spiritual Needs Model	Patient Interview	Interview Analysis	
Spiritual dimension and need associated with the spiritual dimension	**Set of questions for patient interview**	**Questions for analyzing the interview and identifying unmet spiritual need**	**Scoring of unmet spiritual need (range from 0 to 3*)**
Meaning ■ Overall life balance **Need for Life Balance** ■ Need to maintain and/or rebuild an overall life balance ■ Need to learn to "live with" an illness or disability	Does your hospitalization have any repercussions on the way you live usually? Is your overall life balance disturbed by what is happening to you now (hospitalization, illness)? Are you having difficulties coping with what is happening to you now (hospitalization, illness)?	How does the patient speak about his or her need for life balance? Is the overall life balance of this patient disturbed?	To what degree does the *Need for Life Balance* remain unmet? ■ 0 ■ 1 ■ 2 ■ 3
Transcendence ■ Anchor point exterior to the person **Need for Connection** ■ Need for beauty ■ Need to be connected with the personal existential anchor	Do you have a religion, a particular faith, or spirituality? Does what is happening to you now change your relationship to God or to your spirituality? (closer to God, more distant, no change) Is your religion/spirituality/faith challenged by what is happening to you now? Does what is happening to you now change or disturb the way you live or express your faith/spirituality/religion?	How does the patient speak about his or her need for connection? Is his or her need for connection disturbed?	To what degree does the *Need for Connection* remain unmet? ■ 0 ■ 1 ■ 2 ■ 3

(continues)

TABLE 6-6 Spiritual Distress Assessment Tool (SDAT) *(continued)*

Spiritual Needs Model	Patient Interview	Interview Analysis	
Values ■ System of values that determine goodness and trueness for the person; the system is made apparent in the person's actions and life choices **Need for Values Acknowledgment** ■ Need that caregivers understand what has value and significance in his or her life **Need to Maintain Control** ■ Need to understand and be involved in caregivers' decisions and actions	Do you think that the health professionals caring for you know you well enough? Do you have enough information about your health problem and the goals of your hospitalization and treatment? Do you feel that you are participating in the decisions made about your care? How would you describe your relationship with the doctors and other health professionals?	How does the patient speak of his or her need that caregivers understand what has value and significance in his or her life? How does the patient speak of his or her need to understand and be involved in caregivers' decisions and actions?	To what degree does the *Need for Values Acknowledgment* remain unmet? ■ 0 ■ 1 ■ 2 ■ 3 To what degree does the *Need to Maintain Control* remain unmet? ■ 0 ■ 1 ■ 2 ■ 3
Psychosocial Identity ■ The environment (society, caregivers, family, close relations) that maintain the person's particular identity **Need to Maintain Identity** ■ Need to be loved, to be recognized ■ Need to be listened to ■ Need to be in contact (in particular with the person's faith community and other people) ■ Need to have a positive self-image ■ Need to feel forgiven, to be reconciled	Do you have any worries or difficulties regarding your family or other persons close to you? How do people close to you behave with you now? Does it correspond with what you expected from them? Do you feel lonely? Could you tell me about the image you have of yourself in your current situation (illness, hospitalization)? Do you have any links with your faith community?	How does the patient speak of his or her need to maintain identity?	To what degree does the *Need to Maintain Identity* remain unmet? ■ 0 ■ 1 ■ 2 ■ 3

* 0 = no evidence of unmet spiritual need; 1 = some evidence of unmet spiritual need; 2 = substantial evidence of unmet spiritual need; 3 = evidence of severe unmet spiritual need.

Reproduced from Monod, S. M., Rochat, E., Büla, C. J., Jobin, G., Martin, E., & Spencer, B. (2010). The Spiritual Distress Assessment Tool: An instrument to assess spiritual distress in hospitalised elderly persons. *BMC Geriatrics*, *10*(88), 1–9.

(an organization that accredits hospitals and healthcare organizations to qualify for Medicare and Medicaid reimbursement) mandates that a spiritual assessment be conducted on every patient that is admitted to an acute care or nursing home facility (Joint Commission, 2010, 2018). Not only do medical facilities need to identify spiritual issues that impact spiritual well-being, but according to The Joint Commission (2010), they must also accommodate identified religious/spiritual beliefs and practices. To ensure that such regulations are upheld, the nurse plays an important role in the spiritual assessment process and the delivery of spiritual care.

▶ Conclusion

As the first stage in the nursing process, the assessment of spiritual needs is foundational to holistic nursing care. The assessment process is completed through the utilization of several spiritual care methods of inquiry (spiritual screening, spiritual history, or the professional spiritual assessment) and through the collaborative efforts of many different members of the healthcare team. The nurse plays a vital role in ensuring that spiritual distress is identified during the screening process (see **BOXES 6-1**, **6-2**, and **6-3**), that referrals are appropriately made to spiritual care providers,

---

BOX 6-1 Outstanding Nurse Leader: Kara Palfy, MSN, APRN, AGNP-C

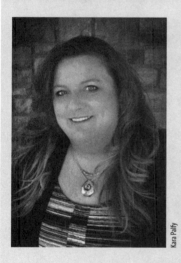
Kara Palfy

My journey as a nurse began in 1992. I had been trained in the U.S. Army, but after coming home, I never felt satisfied with my work. I did private pediatric nursing, then worked on a memory care unit in a skilled nursing facility. I remember feeling really helpless when watching as people died with their symptoms terribly undertreated. When I witnessed the difference in experience with a hospice team in place, I knew that hospice nursing was what I wanted to do.

I have been a hospice nurse since 2001 and am able to provide comfort and knowledge to people dying at home. For me, hospice provides a unique opportunity to step into the middle of a person's chaos and provide care that makes a difficult situation a little better. I heard someone liken the dying process to the birthing process and have found it to be so true. We have the opportunity to "birth" someone out of this life; it takes patience and sometimes even pacing. A person's spirituality, or lack thereof, can provide as much comfort as it can fear.

Eventually, I learned of the devastating impact of spiritual distress on the well-being of patients at the end-of-life. When distress does occur, I am thankful to be part of a hospice care team.

For the majority of my time as a hospice nurse, I was not a believer. As I look back over the years, it is easy to see a string of missed opportunities when it comes to assessing the spiritual needs of my patients. I admit that because I didn't have a faith of my own, I didn't prioritize spiritual needs and place them on an equal footing with those of a physical nature. I recall feeling that I often had "more pressing issues," including medications, equipment, and acute symptom management, and instead relied on the spiritual care coordinator to ask questions of a spiritual nature. After I came into relationship with Christ in 2013, however, I discovered a whole new appreciation for spirituality and its impact on health and well-being. I was on fire for the Lord and was eager to talk to everyone about how Jesus Christ had

(continues)

BOX 6-1 Outstanding Nurse Leader: Kara Palfy, MSN, APRN, AGNP-C   *(continued)*

changed my life. Even now, I look for openings in conversations to talk about faith when I visit with patients, such as a Bible in the patient's home or a beautiful cross necklace that I can comment on. If given an open invitation by the patient, I am prepared to share my story.

In 2015, I earned my MSN as an adult–gerontology nurse practitioner. Although I am still in hospice on a part-time basis, I am now able to assess the spiritual well-being of patients within my own practice. I now understand the important role that spirituality plays and strive to assist my patients by caring for the whole person. Although it is easy to want to go back in time and change things in my past, I have chosen to appreciate the journey and to use what I have learned in the past to benefit my patients of today.

BOX 6-2 Research Highlight

A study by Gallison et al. (2013) assessed the practices and barriers to spiritual care experiences by nurses in an acute care medical center in New York. A total of 227 nurses working on oncology, critical care, step-down, geriatrics, research, or general medical units received a Spiritual Care Practice (SCP) questionnaire via e-mail. Of those invited to participate, only 113 completed the SCP in its entirety and were ultimately included in the study.

Results from this study indicated that although 96% of nurses agreed that spiritual care is within the role of a nurse, only 39% of them were providing the spiritual support at the ideal level predetermined by the researchers. Most commonly, nurses agreed with survey statements that indicated that barriers to spiritual care included time (68%) and the view that a patient's spirituality is private and, therefore, should not be assessed by the nurse (50%). Additional theme analysis on open-ended responses suggested the following barriers: time (39%), system barriers (30%), patient resistance (17%), and lack of appropriate education (17%).

Nursing students in educational institutions and nurses in clinical practice should discuss potential barriers openly so that strategies can be discovered to improve the spiritual care of patients. Nurses must remember that spirituality is a component of holistic nursing care and has the potential to impact health outcomes.

Modified from Gallison, B. S., Xu, Y., Jurgens, C. Y., & Boyle, S. M. (2013). Acute care nurses' spiritual care practices. *Journal of Holistic Nursing, 21*(2), 95–103. doi:10.1177/0898010112464121

BOX 6-3 Evidence-Based Practice Focus

Fifty healthcare providers (29 nurses, 11 physicians, 4 social workers, and 6 others) participated in a pilot study that aimed to increase the level of spiritual care provided to patients. To increase spiritual and religious care, healthcare providers were enrolled in a five-month fellowship program known as Clinical Pastoral Education for Healthcare Providers (CPE-HP). The CPE-HP program, which is accredited by the Association for Clinical Pastoral Education, was delivered through the chaplaincy department. Following the completion of 100 theory hours, 300 clinical hours, and weekly assignments such as reflective logs and case study presentations, participants reported a 61% increase ($p < 0.001$) in the number of religious/spiritual conversations with patients, a 95% increase in the frequency by which they engaged in prayer ($p < 0.001$), and a 33% increase overall in their perceived ability to provide spiritual care. The ability to provide spiritual care included criteria such as conversing with patients or families to identify spiritual needs, participation in spiritual assessments, and spiritual care plan formulation and implementation.

Offering the CPE-HP program in hospitals and palliative care/hospice facilities throughout the United States could significantly improve the quality, frequency, and ease with which nurses engage in the spiritual assessment process and facilitate the planning and implementation of spiritual care.

Modified from Zollfrank, A. A., Trevino, K. M., Cadge, W., Balboni, M. J., Thiel, M. M., Fitchett, G., ... Balboni, T. A. (2015). Teaching healthcare providers to provide spiritual care: A pilot study. *Journal of Palliative Medicine, 18*(5), 408–414. doi: 10.1089/jpm.2014.0306

and that all elements of well-being (mind, body, and spirit) are incorporated into the patient's plan of care.

▶ Clinical Reasoning Exercises

Explore the spiritual history videos created by the George Washington Center for Spirituality and Health (https://www.gwumc.edu/gwish/ficacourse/out/main.html). Using the FICA tool in Table 6-2, obtain a spiritual history on a peer, friend, or family member and record your findings as a narrative under each corresponding letter:

- F:
- I:
- C:
- A:

Analyze and synthesize your findings. If this person was your patient, how would this information shape your nursing care?

▶ Personal Reflection Exercises

Although this tool is typically completed by a spiritual care provider, perform a professional spiritual assessment on yourself utilizing the Spiritual Distress Assessment Tool (SDAT) in Table 6-6. Record your answers

to the interview questions for each identified need, and then analyze and score your findings. To complete this exercise you will need to reflect on a current or past illness experience for which you received medical care.

Following the completion of this exercise, answer the following reflection questions:

- What have you learned about your own need for connection to God or the transcendent?
- What spiritual needs were identified?
- What is your risk level for the presence of spiritual distress?

Develop a plan of care for yourself as to how you will either improve your spiritual well-being in the areas of need identified or seek help for the spiritual distress you are experiencing.

References

American Nurses Association (ANA). (n.d.). The nursing process. Retrieved from https://www.nursingworld .org/practice-policy/workforce/what-is-nursing/the -nursing-process/

Anandarajah, G., & Hight, E. (2001). Spirituality and medical practice: Using the HOPE questions as a practical tool for spiritual assessment. *American Family Physician, 63*(1), 81–88.

Balboni, T. A., Fitchett, G., Handzo, G. F., Johnson, K. S., Koenig, H. G., Pargament, K. I.,... Steinhauser, K. E. (2017). State of the science of spirituality and palliative care research part II: Screening, assessment, and interventions. *Journal of Pain and Symptom Management, 54*(3), 441–452.

Barna Group. (2017, April 6). Meet the "spiritual, but not religious." *Releases in Faith & Christianity.* Retrieved from https://www.barna.com/research/meet-spiritual-not-religious/

Bultz, B. D., Groff, S. L., Fitch, M., Blais, M. C., Howes, J., Levy, K., & Mayer, C. (2011). Implementing screening for distress, the 6th vital sign: A Canadian strategy for changing practice. *Psycho-Oncology, 20,* 463–469. doi:10.1002/pon.1932

Cadge, W., & Bandini, J. (2015). The evolution of spiritual assessment tools in healthcare. *Society, 52,* 430–437. doi.org/10.1007/s12115-015-9926-y

Fitchett, G., & Risk, J. L. (2009). Screening for spiritual struggle. *Journal of Pastoral Care and Counseling, 63*(1–2), 1–12.

Fowler, M. D. M. (2015). *Guide to the code of ethics for nurses with interpretive statements: Development, interpretation, and application (*2nd ed.). Silver Spring, MD: American Nurses Association.

Gallison, B. S., Xu, Y., Jurgens, C. Y., & Boyle, S. M. (2013). Acute care nurses' spiritual care practices. *Journal of Holistic Nursing, 21*(2), 95–103. doi: 10.1177/0898010112464121

Herdman, T. H., & Kamitsuru, S. (Eds.). (2014). *Nursing diagnoses 2015–2017: Definitions and classifications* (10th ed.). Chichester, UK: Wiley Blackwell.

Hughes, B., DeGregory, C., Elk, R., Graham, D., Hall, E. J., & Ressallat, J. (2017, March). Spiritual care and nursing: A nurse's contribution and practice [White paper]. Retrieved from https://healthcarechaplaincy.org/docs/about/nurses_spiritual_care_white_paper_3_3_2017.pdf

Hui, D., de la Cruz, M., Thorney, S., Parsons, H. A., Delgado-Guay, M., & Bruera, E. (2011). The frequency and correlates of spiritual distress among patients with advanced cancer admitted to an acute palliative care unit. *American Journal of Hospice and Palliative Medicine, 28*(4), 264–270.

Joint Commission. (2010). Advancing effective communication, cultural competence, and patient- and family-centered care: Roadmap for hospitals. Retrieved from https://www.jointcommission.org/roadmap_for_hospitals/

Joint Commission. (2018). Standards interpretation frequently asked questions (FAQs). Retrieved from https://www.jointcommission.org/standards_information/jcfaq.aspx?ProgramId=0&ChapterId=0&IsFeatured=False&IsNw=False&Keyword=spiritual%20assessment&print=y

Koenig, H. G. (2007). *Spirituality in patient care: Why, how, when, and what* (2nd ed.). West Conshohocken, PA: Templeton Foundation Press.

Kopacz, M. S., Hoffmire, C. A., Morley, S. W., & Vance, C. G. (2015). Using a spiritual distress scale to assess suicide risk in veterans: An exploratory study. *Pastoral Psychology, 64,* 381–390. doi:10.1007/s11089-014-0633-1

Larimore, W. (2015, Fall). Spiritual assessment in clinical care part 2: The Lord's LAP. *Today's Christian Doctor.* Retrieved from https://x362.blob.core.windows.net/downloads/5bf87413431f4b17bfe833e491ad26e5-461f62f3-8e49-402a-9ae3-e3d9add2f26b.pdf

LaRocca-Pitts, M. (2012). FACT, a chaplain's tool for assessing spiritual needs in an acute care setting. *Chaplaincy Today, 28*(1), 25–32.

LaRocca-Pitts, M. (2015). Four FACTs spiritual assessment tool. *Journal of Health Care Chaplaincy, 21,* 51–59. doi: 10.1080/08854726.2015.1015303

Mako, C., Galek, K., & Poppito, S. R. (2006). Spiritual pain among patients with advanced cancer in palliative care. *Journal of Palliative Medicine, 9*(5), 1106–1113.

Martins, H., & Caldeira, S. (2018). Spiritual distress in cancer patients: A synthesis of qualitative studies. *Religions, 9*(10), 1–17. doi:10.3390/rel9100285.

Monod, S. M., Rochat, E., Büla, C. J., Jobin, G., Martin, E., & Spencer, B. (2010). The Spiritual Distress Assessment Tool: An instrument to assess spiritual distress in hospitalized elderly persons. *BMC Geriatrics, 10*(88), 1–9.

National Coalition for Hospice and Palliative Care (NCHPC). (2018). *Clinical practice guidelines for quality palliative care* (4th ed.). Richmond, VA: Author. Retrieved from https://www.nationalcoalitionhpc.org/ncp/

Newport, F. (2017, December 22). 2017 update on Americans and religion. *Gallup.* Retrieved from https://news.gallup.com/poll/224642/2017-update-americans-religion.aspx

Puchalski, C. M. (2014). The FICA spiritual history tool. *Journal of Palliative Medicine, 17*(1), 105–106. doi:10.1089/jpm.2013.9458

Puchalski, C., Ferrell, B., Virana, R., Otis-Green, S., Baird, P., Bull, J.,... Sulmasy, D. (2009). Improving the quality of spiritual care as a dimension of palliative care: The report of the Consensus Conference. *Journal of Palliative Medicine, 12,* 885–909. doi: 10.1089=jpm.2009.0142

Shelly, J. A. (2017). Spiritual assessment. In *CSB nurse's Bible* (pp. 1097–1098). Nashville, TN: Holman Bible Publishing.

Steinhauser, K. E., Fitchett, G., Handzo, G. F., Johnson, K. S., Koenig, H. G., Pargament, K. I.,... Balboni, T.A. (2017). State of the science of spirituality and palliative care research part 1: Definitions, measurements, and outcomes. *Journal of Pain and Symptom Management, 54*(3), 428–440.

Williams, J. A., Meltzer, D., Arora, V., Chung, G., & Curlin, F. A. (2011). Attention to inpatients' religious and spiritual concerns: Predictors and association with patient satisfaction. *Journal of General Internal Medicine, 26*(11), 1265–1271. doi:10.1007/s11606-011-1781-y

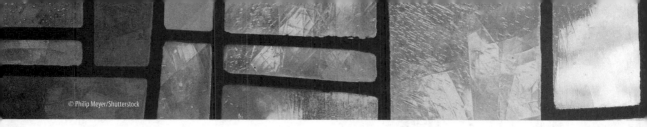

CHAPTER 7

Planning, Goals, and Interventions Related to Spiritual Care of the Patient

Kristi Hargrave, MSN, RN

LEARNING OBJECTIVES

At the end of this chapter, the reader will be able to:

1. Recognize that spiritual care is complex and that a traditional approach of ADPIE may not always fit the situation.
2. Distinguish when and how to plan for spiritual needs of patients, implement goals, and carry out interventions that foster holistic care.
3. Assess which interventions are most appropriate for a specific patient.
4. Synthesize the patient's spiritual needs with the care that can be offered by the interprofessional team.
5. Create an individualized, patient-focused response to spiritual needs that is guided by the Holy Spirit.
6. Execute a care plan for a patient that involves a spiritual component.

KEY TERMS

ADPIE	Guided imagery	Therapeutic communication
Bibliotherapy	SMART	

▶ Planning, Goals, and Interventions

This chapter addresses how to approach spiritual care using the nursing process, while acknowledging its limitations within this multifarious issue. It is important to recognize that nurses are humans first, and nurses second. They must, at times, rely on their innate inclinations and intuition to address patients' spiritual needs as they become evident. Discussions may turn spiritual when it is least expected. Interactions with patients cannot always be planned out. Nurses can try to utilize a systematic approach, but they must also remain flexible, take advantage of opportunities to address spiritual needs as they arise, and count on their communication skills, training, preparation, and most importantly, the Holy Spirit to guide them.

▶ Background

The human body is complex, yet nurses learn how to approach it using the nursing process and critical thinking to address physical needs. From the beginning of nursing school, students study how to systematically approach a patient using the **ADPIE** model: Assess, Diagnose, Plan, Implement, and Evaluate. While this approach can be used when caring for patients' physical needs, often nurses are challenged in finding the best ways to approach spiritual needs using this model. In some situations, it simply doesn't fit. This possibility of mismatch can be challenging for concrete thinkers and detailed planners, as flexibility is often needed due to the complexities of human emotions and spirituality. Often, there is not a single correct approach to complex spiritual issues. Nonetheless, the nursing process can often be adapted to help patients with spiritual needs, just as it can be tailored to patients' physical needs.

Nurses may encounter numerous obstacles to spiritual care, such as personal intimidation and lack of comfort in dealing with spiritual interventions. Although nurses often cite spiritual care as an important component in holistic care, they frequently feel unprepared to meet the spiritual needs of their patients (Murphy, Begley, Timmins, Neill, & Sheaf, 2015). Nurses may feel as if they lack the training or Biblical knowledge needed to address these types of issues. They may also fear saying the wrong thing or being uncomfortable with sensitive dialogue of a spiritual nature.

Thus, part of strengthening this aspect of care is to first acknowledge that nurses may not have the same confidence in their ability to care for patients' spiritual needs as they do in their ability to care for patients' physical needs. This comes as no surprise, as many nursing programs, and even nursing textbooks, do not adequately address this topic or prepare nurses to implement spiritual care (Murphy et al., 2015). McEwen (2004) analyzed more than 50 books recommended for hospitals and found that while some of them contained a passing mention of religion or patients' psychosocial needs, rarely did nursing textbooks devote an entire chapter to spirituality. Another study examined spiritual content in undergraduate pediatric nursing textbooks and found that in many cases an *entire textbook* would not mention even once the spiritual needs of a child and his or her family (Murphy et al., 2015). How could this critical element be omitted from a book that is supposed to be used to train nurses in holistic care? It is no wonder that nurses may feel abandoned and left to figure out how to provide spiritual holistic care for their patients on their own.

▶ Planning and Goals

Spirituality is a shared characteristic of all human beings, despite their culture or individual religious beliefs. This concept allows the nurse, as a co-spiritual being, to interact with people on deep and personal issues. Despite a lack of training to address specific cultural or religious practices, nurses can show support, love, and care for another being, and thereby make an impact on that person's life.

Unfortunately, not all interactions with patients are positive, and sometimes the best intentions can still cause frustration. Consider the story of Job in the Old Testament. His friends came to comfort him in a time of intense suffering and despair, and they did not support his spiritual well-being. In fact, they did just the opposite: Job's friends made things worse. They accused Job of doing something wrong to bring about his suffering and assumed that it was God's punishment. Although they meant well, their words to Job were neither true nor uplifting.

As this story suggests, good intentions do not always produce a positive outcome. Nurses must be sensitive to the patient and ensure that spiritual care does not come across in a condemning or blaming manner. Not all patients will be receptive to a nurse's plan for how to help them spiritually. Nonetheless, this does not mean there is no value in attempting to help. Seeking to understand a patient's cultural background and religious preferences is a means to connect to the patient and provide valuable interactions based on the patient's unique needs.

Part of a nurse's job is to meet the patient and family where they are spiritually. During a nurse's career, he or she may find inspiration within a family. For example, a family may have such amazing kindness, perspective, and strength that they actually encourage the nurse spiritually, rather than vice versa. Other families may respond to illness or tragedy with anger or emotional isolation from those around them. It is not the nurse's job to judge their response to adversity, but rather to meet them where they are and investigate how to best support them emotionally and spiritually.

Not every interaction will fit into a care plan. How can one plan for interactions that spontaneously arise? Nurses must embrace those moments of divine appointment as they come and find time to connect with patients as more than just physical beings. On the whole, some interventions can be planned as part of the nursing process, but extemporaneous interactions often provide unexpected opportunities for quality spiritual care.

It is widely accepted that spiritual care is a key component in a person's health and can provide great value to patients and families during trying times. Studies conducted on patients with advanced cancer have found that when spiritual needs are addressed, quality of life is improved, medical costs are reduced, and patients become more receptive to hospice care (Balboni et al., 2011; Balboni et al., 2013). Other studies have shown that patients report greater satisfaction in their healthcare experience if spirituality is addressed (Astrow, Wexler, Texeria, He, & Sulmasy, 2007; Williams, Meltzer, Arora, Chung, & Curling, 2011). Patients deserve to have their spiritual needs heard and addressed, especially amidst the stress of a critical illness. In fact, The Joint Commission requires spiritual assessment (see the *Spiritual Assessment* chapter) as a component of spiritual care (Taylor, 2002). This organization does not, however, detail how the nursing process can be specifically applied to best accomplish this task. Each nurse must determine how to tend to a particular patient's spiritual needs most effectively. Healthcare systems, as a whole, should collectively examine how to improve training and equip nurses to meet the spiritual needs of their patients.

Once a spiritual issue or concern has been identified, the next step is to plan how to approach the issue in a way that is both sensitive and supportive to the patient. Planning, or purposefully thinking in advance, for spiritual care must be individualized and should include appropriate nursing interventions and the desired outcomes (Taylor, 2002). If the assessment has already been completed, the nurse has engaged in sufficient dialogue with the patient and can begin to personalize a plan for approaching the individual's spiritual needs. The nurse should take into consideration the patient's willingness to discuss spirituality based on previous interactions. It is also important to remember that relationships between nurses and patients often grow with time. As trust develops, patients may be more willing to discuss personal or spiritual concerns with their nurse if given the opportunity. With this in mind, the nurse should intentionally keep the subject of spirituality open to discussion throughout the patient's stay.

There are several practical ways in which this plan can be executed. As the relationship between nurse and patient grows, the nurse could periodically ask questions that open the door for spiritual dialogue or offer personal testimonies that share how the Lord has met the nurse's own spiritual needs. Questions such as the following may be asked:

- How are you feeling about your relationship with God during this time of stress?
- How are you dealing with your diagnosis from a spiritual perspective?
- How are you processing your thoughts about dying in relationship to your spiritual beliefs?

These questions could be helpful in keeping the conversation open and continuing to touch base with the patient on spiritual matters.

Nursing education teaches that a plan should be specific to each patient, and that goals should be **SMART**: Specific, Measurable, Achievable, Relevant, and Timely. For example, a specific plan could be to request a referral for a priest, pastor, or other professional religious specialist to talk with the patient, with a goal that the patient will meet with the chaplain for 30 minutes to process emotions related to his or her diagnosis or loss. In other cases, a general or broader plan may be more appropriate if the nurse isn't quite sure about the best path for the patient. A more general plan may be to continue to seek opportunities to discuss how the patient is processing emotions and spiritual concerns related to a cancer diagnosis, with a goal that the patient is able to communicate his or her needs related to spiritual

distress. Neither of these approaches is wrong, in that people have different needs at different times. Part of the planning phase should include reassessments of patients to see if they are still in the same place spiritually, or if their needs may have changed. Patients, especially those who are anticipating death, may transition through the stages of grief. During this time, the initial plan may need to be adapted to meet the ever-changing needs of the patient.

Unbound Medicine (2018) describes some specific priorities for addressing spiritual distress or potential for spiritual distress. One nursing priority should be to assess causative or contributing risk factors. Another priority for this condition is to assist patients in dealing with their feelings or the situation they are in. Additionally, the nurse should work collaboratively with patients and interdisciplinary teams to set goals that help patients to move forward. Thus, the plan of care should include who is involved in the planning and what, if any, teaching will be involved. Desired outcomes or goals could include that the client will be able to do the following:

- "Identify meaning and purpose in own life that reinforces hope, peace, and contentment.
- Verbalize increased sense of connectedness and hope for future.
- Demonstrate ability to help self and participate in care.
- Participate in activities with others [and] actively seek relationships.
- Discuss beliefs and values about spiritual issues.
- Verbalize acceptance of self as being worthy, not deserving of illness or situation, and so forth." (Unbound Medicine, 2018, para. 7)

Setting goals for spiritual care often focuses on helping the patient process spiritual concepts or thoughts. Accomplishing a spiritual goal can be challenging, as many such goals are not as concrete and measurable as other more physical objectives. Nonetheless, the overarching goal is to assist the patient through means that foster enhanced spiritual well-being. Ideally, goals should be action oriented, time specific, and measurable. The nurse should always seek to set goals in collaboration with the patient. In turn, the nurse's role is to advocate for what the patient desires or the family desires, if appropriate. Thus, the goals may come from things the patient or family have verbalized that they would like to achieve. Some examples include these identified by Weiss (2011):

- Mr. S. stated, "I want to keep Bessie at home until she dies."
- Mrs. T. stated, "I want to live to see my daughter married in three weeks. After that, I will be at peace and ready to die."
- Mr. W. wants to reconnect with his faith congregation by attending church when able and/or have the church elders visit him at home.
- The patient wants to reconcile with his brother who lives out of state.
- The patient hopes she won't die alone—she fears her family won't be with her at that time.

Nurses do not have to hide that they are trying to help the patient spiritually. If the initial assessment did not illicit enough information to develop a patient-centered goal, then it may be helpful to ask the patient directly what the goals should be. A nurse could be quite straightforward with a patient about this point: "Mr. Smith, part of providing care for your entire being while you are in our facility includes spiritual care. Do you have any spiritual needs or goals that I can assist you with?" Other questions may be more indirect, such that the nurse could work them into a conversation to gain more information. For example, a nurse could ask, "What brings you comfort and strength?", "Is there anything I could do to help with this?", or "What do you need to have spiritual peace with your disease process?" (Weiss, 2011). Options for patient goals may include ideas such as that the patient will do the following:

- "Find fulfillment in self, others, work, leisure, and/or higher power

- Accept the limitations of humanity/themselves
- Take time to meditate or communicate with God
- Investigate and interpret illness within the context of meaning
- Balance the spiritual with physical and emotional needs" (Seidl, 1993, p. 49)

It can be challenging to obtain all of this information in a way that the nurse can plan and document, but here are some suggestions. First, the nurse can communicate with the patient and assess the patient's spirituality per guidelines at the facility and various assessment techniques, documenting the patient's response. Then a diagnosis can be made:

- Spiritual distress
- Potential for spiritual distress
- Potential for enhanced spiritual well-being

Next, describe what the diagnosis is related to:

- Anxiety about or fear of something
- Disconnection or conflict with family or friends
- Expressed concern with meaning of suffering or death
- Need for hope, peace, or joy
- Inability to participate in religious practices due to physical disability (Taylor, 2002, p. 153)

In charting this information, the nurse should include how this diagnosis is manifested and how the nurse came to this conclusion. For example, the documentation may include the statement "as evidenced by": "The patient may have potential for enhanced spiritual well-being related to a disconnection with family as evidenced by the patient stating that he hasn't talk to his father in the last five years and he wishes he could make things right."

The next step is planning for what outcomes the nurse would like to see in regard to the specific patient need. These could include the criteria previously discussed or other options such as that the patient will do the following (Taylor, 2002):

- Express movement toward satisfactory answers or meanings
- Verbalize less anxiety or fear
- Report an increased sense of harmony with self, friends/family, or deity
- Participate in religious practice or with religious community members
- Identify meaningful ways to express self, experience joy, or increase creativity outlets related to spiritual needs

Lastly, the nurse would plan for which interventions would best fit the patient and accomplish the desired outcome. Interventions, like those discussed in the next section, turn good intentions into actions that nurses can take to assist a patient. The effectiveness of the interventions implemented should be evaluated, and then a determination made of whether a change in the plan is needed or whether the objective has been met. This is how the traditional nursing process typically works for spiritual care.

▶ Interventions

To be the hands and feet of Jesus, nurses must take action. The idea of a prescriptive process by which healthcare workers address and plan for spiritual interventions or actions that intercede for a spiritual purpose may seem challenging, or even inappropriate to some (Pesut & Sawatzky, 2006). However, nurses may already do this to a great extent and not give themselves credit for their interventions. Nurses, by nature, are often helpers. Nurses may see a need and address it without writing up an official care plan for it. How often have nurses put a hand on a person's shoulder when she is crying or sat down with a patient just to listen? Nurses innately know that these interventions are appropriate, yet they may never be documented; despite its informal nature, such care provides spiritual and emotional support, nonetheless.

The interventions that a nurse completes should be specific to each patient and to the issues at hand. Patients experience spiritual challenges in their own unique way, and not everyone will respond to the same intervention. Intervening isn't about pushing a plan onto a patient or forcing the nurse's religion onto a person with a different religion. Instead, intervening is about meeting patients where they are and offering options that may help them work through spiritual issues. The patient may be ready to receive helpful interventions, or not. Some people, due to their stage of grief, respond by pushing people away and closing off emotionally. The nurse should keep in mind that even if a person is not ready to discuss spiritual needs when the nurse first approaches the individual, the patient may be in a completely different emotional place on another day. People change as they move through the stages of grief and acceptance. A person may also experience grief over a lost limb, a child with a disability, news of impending death, or a new diagnosis of a chronic health issue. For many patients, the diagnosis of acute illness, especially a cancer diagnosis, carries an emotional burden that may cause them to either lean on their spirituality for strength or question their spirituality within the context of disappointment about their health. Throughout the process of grief and suffering, there are opportunities to help patients through various interventions.

Therapeutic Communication

Therapeutic communication is a purposeful verbal interaction between a healthcare provider and a patient with a goal of having a meaningful dialogue that fosters understanding. Nurses must realize that patients are not looking for clichéd answers, or even advice in most cases. Responding with such a prescriptive or rote answer is a mistake that nurses with good intentions can sometimes make. Rather than give answers, nurses should strive to reflect and offer choices to the patient.

An example situation could be that a patient expresses anger at God for a diagnosis of cancer. He may say, "I don't know how God could allow this to happen to me. He can't possibly be a loving God." The nurse has many options for how to respond. Most importantly, the nurse should be genuine and try not to give canned responses such as "God has a reason for everything" or "God will not give you more than you can handle." This type of cliché shuts the patient down in the communication pattern and may cause the patient to feel the nurse is minimizing his emotions. A reflective statement may be appropriate to continue the conversation: "It sounds as if you are questioning why God would allow this to happen to you and if He really loves you? Those are honest questions."

As a follow-up, the nurse could offer a couple of options to allow the patient to choose what to do next: "Would you like for me to ask a pastor or counselor to come talk to you, or do you need time to pray and reflect on this more?" If the patient says he would be open to talking with a pastor, then the nurse can find out if the patient already has someone whom he would want you to contact, or if the nurse should request that a hospital chaplain come by. If the patient says he just wants more time, the nurse could simply say, "I am glad you felt comfortable sharing that with me. Do you mind if I follow up with you in a few days to see if you have processed that question any more or if there is anything I could do to offer you support?"

Additionally, patients could be involved in formulating a plan of action. The nurse could ask, "If you feel upset or angry, what do you think would be a healthy way to process those emotions?" Also, validation may be a technique of comfort. An example would be to relate to the patient: "Struggling with spiritual issues related to your diagnosis can be quite common for cancer patients as they process all that they are going through physically, spiritually, and emotionally." Also, open-ended questions can be offered that demonstrate empathy:

"If you think of any way that I can help you, or even if you just need a hand to hold and a listening ear, please let me know." Therapeutic communication utilizes a variety of methods that help nurses establish a rapport with patients and helps them process their thoughts and emotions.

Keep in mind that nonverbal communication is also important to demonstrate engagement with the patient in the conversation. For example, nurses should engage in appropriate eye contact with patients. Try not to look away in an uncomfortable manner if the patient is discussing challenging topics. Nurses should also make sure to not have prolonged and awkward eye contact that may create undue stress for the patient. Also, be aware that some cultural norms exist and should be respected in regard to eye contact. If the nurse comes across as uncomfortable, then the patient is less likely to openly discuss his or her needs. Nurses should demonstrate compassion through their words and their nonverbal cues.

Options for structured frameworks exist that can help guide healthcare providers in their communication with patients regarding spiritual issues. Sinclair and Chochinov (2012) discuss how the mnemonic SACR-D can be used to help patients with existential and spiritual needs, especially in comprehensive palliative care. **BOX 7-1** provides details on this framework and an option for spiritual care.

Being Present

Even when all the right therapeutic techniques are used, patients may not know what they need or how to be supported. In this case, the best intervention may be to simply have a compassionate presence. Being present may be achieved through active listening, or simply spending time with a patient to bring joy and a smile. In other instances, a moment of sitting silently while the patient cries or placing a hand on the patient's shoulder demonstrates a compassionate presence.

BOX 7-1 Research Highlight

Communicating with Patients About Existential and Spiritual Issues: SACR-D Work

According to Sinclair and Chochinov (2012), communicating with patients regarding spiritual and existential needs is a core element, especially for comprehensive palliative care. They use the mnemonic SACR-D to summarize this communication process.

S: Self-awareness and spiritual sensitivity are the first step in this framework. Clinicians who embrace their spirituality have been reported to have "lower incidence of professional burnout, significant and sustained changes in levels of compassion, attitude, and work satisfaction, and increased meaning of life" (Sinclair & Chochinov, 2012, p. 73).

A: Assess patients' spirituality through extrinsic and intrinsic means, including asking about spiritual history. The FICA spiritual assessment tool is one means of examining a patient's spiritual background and needs.

- F: Faith and Belief
  - Do you consider yourself spiritual or religious?
  - What gives you meaning in life?
  - Do you have spiritual beliefs that help you cope with stress/difficult times?
- I: Importance
  - What importance does your spirituality have in your life?
  - Has your spirituality influenced how you take care of yourself in this illness?
- C: Community
  - Are you part of a spiritual or religious community?
  - Is this a support to you and if so, how?
- A: Address in Care
  - How would you like your healthcare providers to use this information about your spirituality as they care for you?

C: Compassionate presence is a more intrinsic means of connecting with a patient in a positive and caring way. One study found that practitioners who had a friendly, warm, or reassuring relationship were considered by patients to be more effective communicators than practitioners who kept consultations formal and didn't offer reassurance (Stewart, 1995).

R: Refer a patient to the most-suitable professional resource as needed.

D: Dialogue with patients in a manner to communicate effectively and exquisitely by paying attention to the patient's language and perspective. Strive to choose words that help to connect with the patient and that the patient will understand while striving sensitively to explore the patient's spiritual orientation.

Data from Sinclair, S., & Chochinov, H. M. (2012). Communicating with patients about existential and spiritual issues: SACR-D work. *Progress in Palliative Care*, 20(2), 72–78. doi.org/10.1179/1743291X12Y.0000000015

This may seem simple, but nurses are often challenged to find the time to carry out all of the little things due to time restraints. Nurses often care for multiple patients, are stretched thin for time, and rely on multitasking to make the most of their time due to high staffing ratios. It is important to realize that there is value in slowing down if at all possible. Scripture reminds us that "There is a time for everything" (Ecclesiastes 3:1) and that we should "Be still and know that I am God" (Psalm 46:10). Jesus inferred that there are appropriate times to slow down and not be busy in the story of his visit with Mary and Martha (Luke 10:38–42). It may take only 5 to 10 minutes out of a 12-hour shift to make patients feel as if the nurse cares and supports them holistically. A few minutes in prayer can make a difference in a patient's life. The nurse must establish a priority that spiritual needs are of utmost importance and just as valuable as the physical interactions.

Despite the value to the patient of the nurse being present, some nurses may find that they want to minimize time spent with patients that is not for a specific physical intervention, as a form of avoidance and out of a fear of getting too personal with patients. They may feel uncomfortable with a patient asking difficult questions and not feel equipped to respond to such queries. Nurses do not have to be perfect communicators, counselors, or pastors to respond effectively. In fact, sometimes the response could be as simple as "I wish I had the right words to say to help you feel better. I can sit with you, though." This implies empathy and care even though there is no answer. Truthfully, we may not ever have an answer to challenging questions that patients ask, especially to the tried-and-true question of "Why?" A nurse does not have to know the answers or how to respond, but just acknowledge the patient and be a sounding board of compassion and love.

It can be helpful for nurses to find their own inner calm and peace so that they will be able to be receptive to others (Taylor, 2002). Some nurses may not feel comfortable with spiritual interventions of praying, reading scriptures, listening, or counseling a patient about spiritual concerns (O'Brien, 2014). If this is the case, nurses should find a way to still meet their patients' holistic needs through referrals or other means while evaluating their own spirituality and challenging themselves to grow in this area.

Prayer

Prayer is another tool that is available to nurses both personally and professionally. Prayer has been documented in the literature to be helpful in many contexts (O'Brien, 2014). It can be difficult to define prayer, however, and it may mean different things to different people. In fact, Carretto (1978) went as far as to say that "we can never define what prayer is," as it involves "communicating with a mystery" (p. 75). It is challenging to put spiritual concepts into earthly words; however, a clear, concise, or even educated understanding of prayer is not necessary for the power of prayer to be effective. Eloquent prayers are not heard any better than simple words. In fact, God even understands the language of a sigh, groan, or moan (Giordano, 2009). Scripture details how the Holy Spirit can even intercede for Christians when the person cannot express in words what his or her spirit needs to convey to the Lord (Romans 89:26). God hears the pleas and the hurts, just as He hears the praises. Prayers do not have to be long, either. Indeed, Matthew 6:7 guides believers to not babble on with many words. Shelly and Fish (1995) declare that a short and simple statement to God on the patient's behalf is often best, expressing the patient's hopes, fears, or needs and acknowledging God's capacity to help and meet the patient in his or her situation. This concept goes back to the value of being genuine.

Nurses can offer to pray with a patient either out loud or silently. The patient must be accepting of this intervention for it to be appropriate. The nurse must always ask permission to pray with a patient or family members out of respect for their beliefs and values. Additionally, nurses should be cautious when they pray to not force their own agenda (Taylor, 2002). For example, praying "Lord, please help Mrs. Smith to accept that she is dying and be at peace spiritually" may reflect the nurse's position—but the patient may still be praying for healing and want to continue to fight the disease (Taylor, 2002). Sometimes paraphrasing what the patient has expressed is a way to pray for the patient without making personal assumptions—for example, "Father God: Mrs. Smith says she is tired, but wants to keep fighting. Please help strengthen her and show her your love." Prayer is one way to demonstrate support for the patient, but it is also an intimate act and should be approached respectfully (Taylor, 2002).

Spiritual Referrals

Nurses should acknowledge their own limitations and realistic time restraints within the context of spiritual care. Many times the nurse may have great intentions of wanting to help a patient spiritually or emotionally, but that is beyond the scope of what can realistically be accomplished during the nurse's shift or within the boundaries of the nurse's training. When it comes to providing spiritual care, most nurses are generalists and may need to coordinate the services of a specialist (Taylor, 2002). Sometimes patients need more spiritual guidance, counseling, or discussion than the nurse can accommodate. It is important that nurses do not consider this reality to be a failure on their part, but rather recognize it as a responsible move to advocate for the patient. Just as there are times when a nurse must call a physician to address a patient's physical need, so there are times when the nurse must reach out to a pastor, priest, rabbi, or spiritual leader for support as an intercollaborative team member.

The Joint Commission requires that institutions have formal arrangements to provide chaplain services to patients (Taylor, 2002). However, because patients will have various religious preferences, it is important to find out if they wish for the nurse to contact a specific type of clergy member on their behalf. Even if the nurse does not subscribe to the same religious tenets as the patients, he or she should try to make the best referral to an appropriate match for that patient (O'Brien, 2014). Distinctions should be recognized among the various religions when making such referrals. For instance, not all Western religions would be addressed by the same pastor, just as the Eastern religion of Buddhism would not be a best match with a Hindu referral.

Get to know your patients and ask questions to identify the best referrals. For example, many patients may identify as Christian, but some may differ in their preference to talk with a Catholic priest or a Protestant pastor. Some may even have a preference that is more specific than just stating a certain denomination preference. If possible, try to make the most specific referral for clergy to aid the patient. If an exact match for the referral is not available, let the patient know that you realize that such a referral may not be a perfect fit with the patient's belief system, but a hospital chaplain is available to be a resource and is trained to help people of various religions and cultures. Nurses can explain that professional chaplains merge theology and psychology and are often trained to specifically assist in health-related transitions or spiritual challenges (Taylor, 2002).

The Little Things

Nurses see patients in their most vulnerable and challenging times. The nurse has a role of honor and privilege to listen to very personal stories and emotions that the patient wouldn't normally share with a stranger. Sometimes being an active listener for a few minutes is the intervention, sometimes it is a smile, and sometimes it is holding a hand to show support. As Brault (1986) wrote, "Enjoy the little things, because someday you may look back and realize they were the big things" (p. 139). This point is important for nurses to remember, in that the little things are often the things that make people feel cared for. In fact, one study by Taylor and Mamier (2005) found that patients with cancer may appreciate a variety of interventions that encourage independent personal spiritual development, such as informing patients of spiritual resource options available to them. Even humor has been found to have a role that is important to patients (Taylor & Mamier, 2005). Thus, not every conversation has to be a serious discussion of heavy, spiritual issues to be effective and helpful to the patient. All patients must process their own emotions, in their own time. Nurses have the opportunity to reassure patients that searching for meaning or insight from an illness or tragedy is a normal response and that the human spirit is resilient (Taylor, 2002). To be able to provide any kind of love, support, or guidance is a gift that the nurse can offer out of service to the Lord. This is truly nursing as ministry in everyday practice.

Sometimes, nurses use their own God-given discernment skills to know when and how to respond appropriately. These are not skills that a classroom or a book can teach a nurse. Nurses who may be uncertain of how to best intervene can pray for wisdom and discernment regarding how to handle a situation or seek guidance from other more experienced or respected nurses. New nurses will continue to grow throughout their careers as they learn how to respond in difficult situations. With that caveat in mind, nurses must recognize that every situation is unique. What worked with one family or patient may not be effective with another. Caregivers must be sensitive to nuances and not try to apply a "one size fits all" approach to spiritual care when planning for interventions; instead, they should appreciate that trying something with love is often better than trying nothing out of fear of failure or rejection.

The actual role of a nurse may transcend what many people may initially think of as the traditional nurse role as seen in the media—that is, giving shots, starting IV lines, and taking patients to surgery. Nurses have opportunities to make an impact by serving people in God's love every day. Serving patients in a variety of ways is often most effective. Nurses can offer hope to patients by sharing stories of patients who have made it through similar circumstances. A simple act of therapeutic touch, such as putting a hand on a crying patient's shoulder or holding a patient's hand as he or she prays, can help patients feel that they are not alone.

Implementing a meaningful ritual could also be therapeutic to facilitate spiritual healing. Nurses can teach patients about simple relaxation techniques, such as counting backward from 10, that could help when they are feeling overwhelmed or have high levels of anxiety. Likewise, nurses can introduce breathing techniques or other calming meditations such as **guided imagery**, which can help to relax patients and bring spiritual peace. What may seem like a small change can demonstrate that a nurse cares and is going the extra mile. Loving actions, gestures, or words of support done in a genuine fashion, often mean just as much to families as the quality physical care (**CASE STUDY 7-1**).

🔍 *CASE STUDY 7-1*

Family-Centered Care

Meghann and Ziggy Guentensberger went through what no parent would ever want to endure when they lost their child Rylie, when she was only 12 years old. Rylie was hit by a car and spent 28 days in the pediatric intensive care unit (PICU) before she died. The family shared their experience and perspective on those 28 days with nursing students to help them gain insights from this tragedy. Even though nurses may often see tragedy, the family encouraged the students to not become callous as practicing nurses.

The Guentensbergers stressed that nurses should not be afraid to make a human connection with families. Moreover, they challenged nursing students to not just go through the motions of caring physically for a patient without taking time to get to know the patient and their family. During their ordeal, nurses helped the Guentensbergers feel known and supported by asking questions, by discussing their daughter by her name (Rylie) instead of avoiding using her name, and by talking to

(continues)

Rylie even when everyone knew she was so heavily sedated that she probably couldn't understand what they were saying. They also noted that nurses would sometimes seem to read them or pick up on their body language and would intercede. Meghann explained how one nurse took her for a walk outside the unit to help her get away for a few much-needed minutes one day when she felt a high level of stress. The family felt spiritually and emotionally supported by healthcare workers through a variety of actions that some might consider to be just "the details."

During their child's 28-day stay, the Guentensbergers had only one nurse whom they asked to not care for their daughter again. The issue wasn't that the nurse wasn't qualified or trained appropriately, but rather that she was rigid and didn't show compassion in her interactions with the family. As evidenced by this example, the role of a nurse is expected to be much different than that of many other caregivers. Families don't always expect to connect to and be supported by every person whom they encounter in the hospital, but they do often have that expectation of their relationship with their nurse. It is an honored role. Nurses are privileged to participate in the most delicate and treasured intimate moments with families, from bringing a child into the world, to being in the room when their loved one takes a last breath. The impact that nurses make may well depend on their ability to take their nursing practice out of just the physical realm and concurrently offer spiritual and emotional support as well.

Questions

1. What advice would you give to a new nurse or nursing student based on an experience you have had with a family in crisis?
2. How could you positively impact a family with a loved one who is nonresponsive?
3. Have you had any personal experience with a friend's or family member's care in a hospital setting that you learned from? Describe your take-away messages, good and bad, and explain how this experience would frame your care as a healthcare provider.

Music Therapy/Music Listening

There is something special about music that touches the spirit and transcends religious preferences. Listening to prerecorded music, or having someone play live music for a patient, can be considered an adjunct therapy offered for patients to reduce stress or a spiritual aid. According to music therapist Raymond Leone (2018), singing music in a hospital room can help people connect to each other and to their thoughts and feelings. Religious or worship music can provide a means for the patient to detach from the worries of the present and focus on the worship of a higher power. Many studies in music have found that music can positively influence self-reported scores of anxiety and lower an elevated heart rate

related to stress or worry (Bae, Lim, Hur, & Lee, 2014; Jimenez, Escalona, Lopez, Vera, & DeHaro, 2013; Li & Dong, 2012).

Of course, people find different types of music enjoyable and relaxing. Patients should be given options for which kind of music they would enjoy listening to the most: gospel, folk, country and western, traditional religious hymns, classical, or praise and worship. If patients cannot speak, check with family members to ask which kind of genre they embraced before their illness so they can enjoy music.

Sutherland (2005) points out that the Bible tells of how King Saul called young David to play his music to help with his emotional and spiritual distress. O'Brien (2006) shares a story of how a respiratory therapist started playing a guitar for one of his patients who had trouble breathing and found that her breathing calmed and eased after the intervention. Leone (2018) found that music can arouse a patient who may suffer from dementia to recall and enjoy lyrics that had been memorized in the past, bringing the patient to a temporary alert state. Sacred music can aid in increasing spiritual awareness in a patient, having a powerful impact (Taylor, 2002). Music affects people in ways that nurses may not completely understand, but they can certainly see the responses and smiles of a patient.

Scripture Reading and Bibliotherapy

For many people of faith, reading God's word is a daily ritual of great meaning. For others, it is something they turn to for strength, wisdom, or support. For still others, it may be a foreign idea to read or turn to scripture. Nurses can learn where patients stand on this issue and how they feel through engaging in open dialogue with the patient or their family. No matter the category into which a patient falls,

bibliotherapy or reading spiritually uplifting materials and sacred writings could be offered as a spiritual intervention (Taylor, 2002).

If a patient already has a practice of reading the Word of God, then the nurse's role could be to facilitate this ritual by making sure the patient has the Bible or book of choice. If patients are limited physically due to illness or disability and unable to read on their own, the nurse can read or have a family member or volunteer read scriptures or a favorite book to the patient as an intervention.

If a patient does not normally read the scriptures but would be open to this practice as an aspect of spiritual care, then the nurse could help find a verse or passage that might bring hope, comfort, or peace. It may even be a good idea to have a few favorite "go-to" passages written down to share as opportunities arise and if appropriate within the context of spiritual care. Note that practice should not involve forcing a patient to listen to a nurse reading long chapters of scripture or unwanted mini-sermons: Nurses should be sensitive and not overbearing. Sharing just a verse or two is often enough to bring spiritual encouragement (**BOX 7-2**).

BOX 7-2 Author's Personal Story

My beloved grandmother, who was a believer in Christ, died from cancer. There came a time in her disease process where she could no longer read or even communicate with me. I felt somewhat helpless as a family member. I found a little book containing scriptures that were separated out by categories such as hope, trust, and love. The week preceding her death, I brought that book with me on my visits and took turns reading scriptures from each category out loud to her at various times. It was a little odd at first, as it was a one-way conversation, but I held out hope that she could hear me. This was something that I could do as a family member to try to bring her comfort.

Family and friends often want something of importance to do so that they can feel needed and helpful. Scripture reading can be delegated to loved ones or friends. You can reassure them that they are making a difference, as there are many documented cases of patients who have come out of a coma or heavy sedation and remembered what people said to them during this period (Sheehan, 2010). It is important to share this message with families, so that they don't feel as if reading to a loved one who is unresponsive is a wasted effort. Quite the opposite—it is most respectful to assume that the patient can hear everything that is said in the room. Encourage the family to find an intervention of value, whether it is scripture reading or some other act of compassion.

Another option is to offer this intervention to family members or close friends of the patient. Scripture reading can bring hope, comfort, and peace through meaningful words of divine inspiration.

Facilitating Relationships and Forgiveness

Many people desire to come to the end of life in a peaceful and harmonic state with close relationships intact. However, it is quite possible that patients may be in spiritual distress due to an unresolved issue with a family member or friend. A patient may be holding onto resentment, hurt, or anger that weighs heavy on the heart. These issues, if left unresolved, can be quite impactful not only to the patient, but also to the other person involved.

The scriptures guide Christians to "get rid of all bitterness, rage, anger, brawling and slander, along with every form of malice. Be kind and compassionate to one another, forgiving each other, just as in Christ God forgave you" (Ephesians 4:31–32, New International Version [NIV]). Yet, forgiveness can be one of the most difficult things for people to achieve, as pain and resentment can run deep. When people go through serious illness, suffering, or approaching death, they sometimes will become more reflective on their life, considering forgiveness as a form of closure. Forgiveness allows people to move on from the past and release negative emotions. Enright (2018) describes how forgiveness may start with an inner quality of motivation to rid oneself of resentment. Many complex psychological reasons explain why people are challenged with forgiving, but they are beyond the scope of this chapter. Thus, it may be necessary to get a referral for some patients to talk with a licensed professional counselor to aid in the process of forgiveness.

The paradigm of spirituality entails examination of connectedness interpersonally, intrapersonally, and transpersonally as related to human health and well-being (Reed, 1992). It can be quite challenging to go from a place of anger or bitterness to a place of genuine compassion. Relationships make people vulnerable, but often so do disease and the dying process. Patients may open up to caring and trustworthy individuals around them during critical illnesses, such as nurses. If a patient expresses to the nurse that he or she has a relationship issue that is unresolved, the nurse can probe what the patient is ultimately seeking or needing. For example, if the nurse senses bitterness or resentment from the patient, a therapeutic response could be "It sounds as if you still feel some resentment toward that person. How do you think that resentment impacts you?" Nurses can express that their goal is for the patient to have a sense of peace and fulfillment that could be gained by forgiveness. They can facilitate forgiveness by asking, "Are you ready to forgive that person?" or "What is stopping you from forgiving that person?"

To understand forgiveness, a person should also understand what forgiveness is not. As Wilhoit (2008) explains, "Forgiving is not forgetting.... Forgiving is not excusing.... Forgiving is not ignoring.... Forgiving is not necessarily to offer unconditional trust" (p. 201). It may be important for the patient to view the offender as separate from the offense (Wilhoit, 2008). In other words, people are more than their mistakes or sins. A question that can be helpful to consider is "Could there have ever been a time in my life when I did something to offend or hurt another person?" We would want forgiveness and not to be judged based on that one offense, no matter how severe it might be.

Jesus is the ultimate example for forgiveness. As followers of Christ, we are commanded to also forgive as He forgave us (Colossians 3:13; Matthew 6:14–15; Luke 17:3–4; Ephesians 4:32).

Another aspect important to hurting patients is to see themselves as more than their wound (Wilhoit, 2008). The Bible guides us to live in harmony and turn the other cheek, letting go and forgiving rather than taking things into our own hands. The God of all the universe wants us to forgive.

For some patients, forgiveness may be a single decision that is made with finality; for others, it may be more of a process. Wilhoit (2008, p. 201) explains one possible progression:

1. Consider how you were forgiven.
2. Be realistic. Name the sin against you for what it truly is. Limit your expectation of what will result from forgiveness.
3. Share the pain.
4. Accept the time forgiving may take.
5. Understand what it means to "forgive and forget." God cannot forget our sins in the sense that He loses them from His memory. Instead, by forgetting those sins, He sets aside the punishment we deserve. So when we "forget" the offense done to us, it means we will not in the future "use" the offense as a reason to punish the offender.
6. Learn ways to break the chain of self-enslavement to bitter thoughts.

Patients do not have to have reconciliation so as to have forgiveness in their heart. Enright (2018) describes the difference between forgiveness and reconciliation by stating that "forgiveness is a moral virtue in which the offended person tries, over time, to get rid of toxic anger or resentment and to offer goodness of some kind to the offending person" (para. 3), whereas reconciliation can be seen as more of a "negotiation strategy in which two or more people come together again in mutual trust" (para. 3). Patients can reconcile by extending an olive branch that shows they are willing to try, willing to forgive, willing to move on. Prayer should be a part of this process as Christians seek to have God's character. A prayer could be for "God to restore the trust

in a relationship" or for "God to help the person surrender resentment every time it creeps back in." Satan does not want patients to have healthy, restored relationships where there is forgiveness and reconciliation.

As nurses and as Christians, we can work collaboratively with counselors, pastors, and social workers. Collectively, the team can offer aid to facilitate forgiveness. Forgiveness can have huge impacts on the peaceful passing of a person and help to decrease spiritual distress that a patient may have from unresolved issues.

▶ Holistic Care

When nurses plan and intervene with patients to help them not only physically but also spiritually, they care for the patient holistically. Holistic care looks at many aspects of a person and his or her environment. It has a long and rich history in nursing: Florence Nightingale even examined this connection and engaged in nursing by practicing holistic care. Holistic nurses are often described by patients as nurses who "truly care" (Practical Nursing.org, 2018). Some interventions related to holistic care could include the following (PracticalNursing .org, 2018, para. 5):

- Learn the patient's name and use it.
- Make good, strong eye contact.
- Ask how a patient is feeling and sincerely care.
- Smile and laugh when appropriate.
- Use therapeutic touch.
- Assist patients to see themselves as people who deserve dignity.
- Preserve the patient's dignity.
- Educate the patient on the importance of self-care.
- Ask the patient how you can reduce his or her anxiety or pain.
- Use nonpharmacologic methods of pain control such as imagery, relaxation techniques, and more.
- Encourage the patient and assist as needed with alternative treatment

modalities; never underestimate the benefit of a massage, aromatherapy, or music.

■ Ask if the patient has certain religious, cultural, or spiritual beliefs; be sensitive and accepting if the patient does.

Synthesis and Practical Application

Nurses want to be more than competent—they want to be exceptional. An exceptional nurse finds a way to give care that is holistic yet balanced. Being an excellent nurse may mean being vulnerable and making human connections. It may mean that the nurse cries with a patient, feels pain with a family, or struggles with his or her own emotions and spirituality. The challenges that patients go through are hard and real, and nurses are on those front lines with them. They may be there only for a season, but their interaction during that time is crucial in shaping the long-term takeaway message for the patient or family member. Maya Angelo famously said, "I've learned that people will forget what you said, people will forget what you did, but people will never forget the way you made them feel" (McLeod, 2018, para. 19). Nurses have an impact on how patients feel during every day of their service.

Nursing is a ministry and an opportunity to impact others with God's love and compassion.

The mission of a Christian, as described in Matthew 22:36–40, is to love God and love one's neighbor. Christian nurses can serve the Lord with their work as ministry by thinking of their patients as their neighbors. Colossians 3:23–24 encourages all people to work as if they are working for the Lord, not for human masters. With this point in mind, nurses are able to serve even the most difficult patients as they work toward their highest calling, to honor God by their work. The interventions that nurses carry out are often messy; in fact, some people could never fathom the work that nurses do. The spiritual component of dealing with patients is often messy as well, as a person may be broken in spirit and need the love of a forgiving God. It is from a place of love that nurses can respond in service to the Lord, carrying the sometimes-heavy load of healing and providing hope.

Nurses should approach each patient with humility and with a servant's heart (**BOX 7-3**). Approaching the patient with humility and offering options demonstrate that each person ultimately gets to make his or her own decisions on the individual's spiritual journey. Be respectful of each person and his or her spiritual or religious preferences. The patient's spiritual and religious preferences may not be

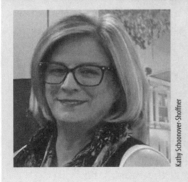

According to Schoonover-Shoffner, her vision for NCF is "that we encourage you in the ministry of nursing, helping you think Christianly about what you do. Colossians 2:6–10 summarizes how I pray NCF helps you grow and be strengthened spiritually, discerning Biblical truth from worldly wisdom, and realizing the authority you have in Christ as a Christian nurse:

> So then, just as you received Christ Jesus as Lord, continue to live in him, rooted and built up in him, strengthened in the faith as you were taught, and overflowing with thankfulness. See to it that no one takes you captive through hollow and deceptive philosophy, which depends on human tradition and the basic principles of this world, rather than on Christ. For in Christ all the fullness of the Deity lives in bodily form, and you have been given fullness in Christ, who is the head over every power and authority.

Schoonover-Shoffner and her physician husband, Richard, have three adult children. Her home is in Kansas, where she lives with her husband and many beloved pets. She participates in weekly Bible study, and also plays the piano for worship at her church.

Schoonover-Shoffner provides an excellent example of a unique way that a nurse leader can influence nursing as ministry through her own professional "interventions." As a Christian nursing journal editor, she assures that only the best evidence-based practice articles are published, and she helps to advance faith-community nursing. As the NCF director, she is a leader/mentor for nurses throughout the United States and the world.

what the nurse personally believes, but that is between the person and God. It is not the place of the nurse to judge a person; that is Jesus's role, and nurses are simply the hands and feet of our Lord in service. Christians would love to see everyone come to know the Lord Jesus as their own personal Savior, but the nurse may or may not be able to be a part of this decision. Nevertheless, the nurse may be planting seeds that will in time reap a harvest. Nurses must not think of interactions with patients as a burden to save the world, but rather should be available as doors open for communication to discuss the gospel's message. There can certainly be an aspect of witnessing for the Lord that nurses do either through their caring actions or through sharing the gospel with a receptive patient (**BOX 7-4**).

▶ Conclusion

This chapter has discussed planning, goals, and interventions available to help a patient with spiritual issues. By no means did it provide a complete list of interventions. Nurses must follow their instincts when working with patients, especially when guided by the Holy Spirit to interact with patients in the most meaningful ways. They should attempt to utilize the nursing process when possible to help with spiritual issues, but also remain flexible so they can make changes and initiate impromptu interventions when necessary to help the patient spiritually and emotionally.

Addressing this task may influence nurses' spirituality as well, prompting them to work through their own spiritual questions or battles. There may even be times when nurses need spiritual support as well and should seek resources for themselves (see the *Caring for One's Spiritual Self* chapter). Some days, the job may be emotionally taxing and cause nurses to question their role. On other days, working with patients may inspire nurses and bring utmost satisfaction for a job well done.

Nurses have new patients each day and new challenges; no day is the same on the job. We have a unique opportunity to care for people in an intimate and personal way, touching people physically, emotionally, and yes, even spiritually.

BOX 7-4 Evidence-Based Practice Focus

Creating a Culture for Evidence-Based Practice in the Faith Community

The author describes how she feels it is an ethical responsibility to use the best knowledge available to inform practice and express Christian love, care, and respect for the people whom she serves.

Faith community nursing is a specialty that falls under community health. The standards for the professional faith community nurse (FCN) state that the nurses in this specialty also integrate evidence and research into practice. An interdisciplinary research committee was established at a nondenominational Christian nonprofit organization focused on finding solutions for homelessness and addictions. A doctoral-level-prepared parish nurse took the lead on this new research committee, which had a goal of enhancing program effectiveness through scientific evidence and a best-practice model.

First, a long-term addiction recovery program was identified as a priority need. The community-based participatory research (CBPR) model was adapted to create evidence-based practice (EBP). The starting point of the committee was to discuss the question "How does a long-term addict get well?" and establish goals. A literature review was conducted on how to measure success in recovery. Additionally, residents, staff, and board members were surveyed to define their own definition of recovery success. Three elements emerged as common measures of success:

- Sustained sobriety
- Spiritual growth
- Employment

Ultimately, the strategies used to incorporate research/EBP into faith-based ministry for this organization included strategies for success such as the following:

- Identify the most immediate need(s) in the community.
- Create structures to integrate research and EBP on key priorities into the community.
- Educate community members on the meaning and value of research as well as planning/decision-making.
- Involve as many members as possible in various aspects of research or EBP.
- Use appropriate resources from outside the community.
- Set up systems/plans to ensure adherence to rigorous ethical standards for research.
- Ensure that the process of research/EBP is transparent.

Lashley, M. (2013). Creating a culture for evidence-based practice in the faith community. *Journal of Christian Nursing, 30*(3), 158–163.

▶ Clinical Reasoning Exercises

Stories of Music

A worship pastor, Steve, went to visit a long-time friend in the hospital, bringing his guitar. He ministered to his friend through song, singing and playing at his bedside. He played some spiritually uplifting songs and some secular songs that he knew his friend loved, such as songs by Johnny Cash. The experience was a time of joy and uplifted the patient's spirits. It enabled the friends to bond as they reminisced over music and memories.

Questions

1. How did music impact the patient's hospital stay?
2. Do you think this intervention altered the patient's self-report of pain during the visit?

Jacob's grandmother has Alzheimer's disease. His mother is a choir director, and Jake grew up with music in his home. Most of the time Jacob's grandmother cannot have meaningful dialogue and interaction due to memory loss. When Jacob and his mother visit his grandmother, they sing to her and she is able to recall lyrics and sing along. It is a time of joy for the family, as the music seems to bring his grandmother temporarily back to them as she claps and sings along. This can be spiritually uplifting for all of them as they sing praise songs to the Lord together.

Questions

1. Why is this response meaningful to the family?
2. Why do you think the grandmother had a temporarily increased state of alertness and comprehension when the music was played?

▶ Personal Reflection Exercises

1. How comfortable do you feel discussing spirituality with your patients?
2. What experiences have brought you to a place of comfort talking about spiritual things with patients? Alternatively, what experiences have become barriers to doing this in practice?
3. How do you balance your personal faith and sharing this faith at work with the constraints of your health system? If you work in a faith-based organization, does this make it easier to implement spiritual interventions?
4. Which of the nursing interventions to address a patient's spiritual needs have you used so far? Are

there any that you use more frequently? What ideas has this chapter given you related to how you can better meet the spiritual needs of your patients?

References

Astrow, A., Wexler, A., Texeira, K., He, M., & Sulmasy, D. (2007). Is failure to meet spiritual needs associated with cancer patients' perception of quality of care and their satisfaction with care? *Journal of Clinical Oncology*, *25*(36), 5753–5757. dx.doi.org/10.1200/jco.2007.12.4362

Bae, I., Lim, H., Hur, M., & Lee, M. (2014). Intra-operative music listening for anxiety, the BIS index, and the vital signs of patients undergoing regional anesthesia. *Complementary Therapies in Medicine, 22*, 251–257.

Balboni, T., Balboni, M., Enzinger, A., Gallivan, K., Paulk, M, Wright, A.,... Prigerson, H. (2013). Provision of spiritual support to patients with advanced cancer by religious communities and associations with medical care at the end of life. *JAMA Internal Medicine, 173*(12), 1109–1117. doi.org/10.1001/jamainternmed.2013.903

Balboni, T., Balboni, M., Paulk, M. E., Phelps, A., Wright, A., Peteet, J.,... Prigerson, H. (2011). Support of cancer patients' spiritual needs and associations with medical care costs at the end of life. *Cancer, 117*(23), 5383–5391. doi.org/10.1002/cncr.26221

Brault, R. (1986, September). Quotable quotes. *Reader's Digest*, 139. Retrieved from http://rbrault.blogspot.com/p/who-wrote-enjoy-little-things.html

Carretto, C. (1978). *Summoned by love*. Maryknoll, NY: Orvis Books.

Enright, R. (2018) Why forgiving does not require an apology. *Psychology Today*. Retrieved from https://www.psychologytoday.com/us/blog/the-forgiving-life/201804/why-forgiving-does-not-require-apology

Giordano, C. (2009). With groaning which cannot be uttered. Retrieved from http://www.allaboutgod.net/profiles/blogs/with-groanings-which-cannot-be

Jimenez, M., Escalona, A., Lopez, A., Vera, R., & DeHaro, J. (2013). Intraoperative stress and anxiety reduction with music therapy: A controlled randomized clinical trial of efficacy and safety. *Journal of Vascular Nursing, 31*(3), 101–106.

Leone, R. (2018). Music is connection... music is beauty... even in a hospital room. Retrieved from https://www.linkedin.com/pulse/music-connectionmusic-beautyeven-hospital-room-leone-mmt-mt-bc-?articleId=6448604783250014208#comments-6448604783250014208&trk=prof-post

Li, Y., & Dong, Y. (2012). Preoperative music intervention for patients undergoing cesarean delivery.

International Journal of Gynecology and Obstetrics, 119, 81–83.

McEwen, M. (2004). Analysis of spirituality content in nursing textbooks. *Journal of Nursing Education, 43*(1), 20–30.

McLeod, L. (2018). Be the leader they want. *First Impressions Magazine.* Retrieved from http://www.firstimpressionsmag.com/be-the-leader-they-want.html

Murphy, M., Begley, T., Timmins, F., Neill, F., & Sheaf, G. (2015). Spirituality and spiritual care: Missing concepts from core undergraduate children's nursing textbooks. *International Journal of Children's Spirituality, 20*(2), 114–128. doi.org/10.1080/1364436X.2015.1055458

O'Brien, M. E. (2006). *The nurse with the alabaster jar: A Biblical approach to nursing.* Madison, WI: NCF Press.

O'Brien, M. E. (2014). *Spirituality in nursing: Standing on holy ground.* Burlington, MA: Jones & Bartlett Learning.

Pesut, B., & Sawatzky, R. (2006). To describe or prescribe: Assumptions underlying a prescriptive nursing process approach to spiritual care. *Nursing Inquiry, 13*(2), 127–134.

PracticalNursing.org. (2018). The importance of holistic nursing care: How to completely care for your patients. Retrieved from https://www.practicalnursing.org/importance-holistic-nursing-care-how-completely-care-patients

Reed, P. G. (1992). An emerging paradigm for the investigation of spirituality in nursing. *Research in Nursing & Health, 15*, 349–357. doi:10.1002/nur.4770150505

Seidl, L. G. (1993). The value of spiritual health. *Health Progress, 74*(7), 48–50.

Sheehan, M. (2010). *Healing prayer on holy ground: A cardiologist discovers God's presence in the lives of his patients.* Lake Mary, FL: Creation House

Shelly, J. A., & Fish, S. (1995). Praying with patients. *Journal of Christian Nursing, 12*(1), 9–13.

Sinclair, S., & Chochinov, H. M. (2012). Communicating with patients about existential and spiritual issues: SACR-D work. *Progress in Palliative Care, 20*(2), 72–78. doi.org/10.1179/1743291X12Y.0000000015

Stewart, M. A. (1995). Effective physician–patient communication and health outcomes: A review. *Canadian Medical Association Journal, 152*(9), 1423.

Sutherland, K. (2005). Can music help heal us? The first recorded use of music as an instrument of healing in the Bible. *Journal of Christian Nursing, 22*(3), 29–31.

Taylor, E. J. (2002). *Spiritual care: Nursing theory, research, and practice.* Upper Saddle River, NJ: Prentice Hall.

Taylor, E. J., & Mamier, I. (2005). Spiritual care nursing: What cancer patients and family caregivers want. *Journal of Advanced Nursing, 49*(3), 260–267. doi: 10.1111/j.1365-2648.2004.03285.x

Unbound Medicine. (2018). Nurse's pocket guide: Spiritual distress and risk for spiritual distress. Retrieved from https://nursing.unboundmedicine.com/nursingcentral/view/nurses-pocket-guide/308560/all/Spiritual%20Distress%20and%20Risk%20for%20Spiritual%20Distress

Weiss, S. (2011, April 19). Spiritual care assessment: Measurable goals and outcomes. Retrieved from www.nacc.org/docs/resources/Suzanne%20Weiss%20spiritual%20assessment%20measureable%20goals-outcomes.pdf

Wilhoit, J. (2008) *Spiritual formation as if the church mattered: Growing in Christ through community.* Grand Rapids, MI: Baker Academic.

Williams, J., Meltzer, D., Arora, V., Chung, G., & Curling, F. (2011). Attention to inpatients' religious and spiritual concerns: Predictors and association with patient satisfaction. *Journal of General Internal Medicine, 26*(11), 1265–1271. dx.doi.org/10.1007/s11606-011-1781-y

Recommended Readings

Del Valle, S. (1980). Spiritual care and the nursing process. *Australasian Nurses Journal, 9*(7), 12–13.

Taylor, E. J., Mamier, I., Ricci-Allegra, P., & Foith, J. (2017). Original article: Self-reported frequency of nurse-provided spiritual care. *Applied Nursing Research, 35*, 30–35. doi.org/10.1016/j.apnr.2017.02.019

Westera, D. (2017). *Spirituality in nursing practice: The basics and beyond.* New York, NY: Springer.

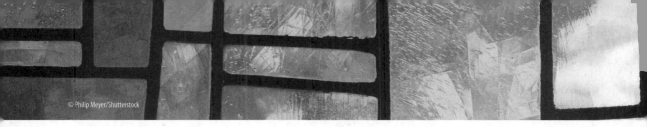

CHAPTER 8

Spiritual Evaluation

Tammie L. Huddle, MSN, RN, and **Mary E. Hobus**, PhD, MSN, RN

LEARNING OBJECTIVES

At the end of this chapter, the reader will be able to:

1. Understand the importance of evaluating the effectiveness of spiritual interventions.
2. Discover the importance of nursing as ministry through spiritual evaluation.
3. Determine the registered nurse's (RN's) role in spiritual evaluation as a RN, an instructor, and a student.
4. Value nursing as ministry and the patient's spirituality.
5. Assess the effectiveness of the patient's response to prayer.

KEY TERMS

Evaluation
Nursing process/care plan

Patient/client
Spiritual care plan

▶ Spiritual Evaluation

The nursing process consists of five components: assessment, nursing diagnosis, planning (including goals and outcomes), interventions, and evaluation (*Nurse's Pocket Guide*, 2018). All of these components work collectively to assist the healthcare team to provide the best care for the **patient or client**. This chapter discusses the evaluation stage of the nursing process as well as the process of putting all

of the components together as a spiritual care plan is developed for the patient or client.

Provision 4 of the *Code of Ethics for Nurses* speaks directly to this issue, outlining the accountability and responsibility for nursing practice: "The nurse has authority, accountability, and responsibility for nursing practice; makes decisions; and takes action consistent with the obligation to promote health and to provide optimal care" (Fowler, 2015, p. 59). Each step of the nursing process is essential

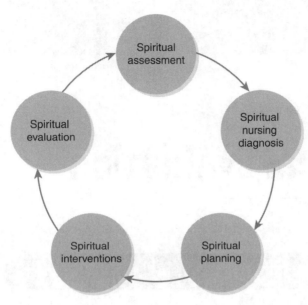

FIGURE 8-1 Nursing process circle.
T. Huddle (2019). Used with permission.

in providing high-quality care. During evaluation, we ask questions such as "Why did this happen?" or "What can I learn from this occurrence on the medical–surgical floor?" As registered nurses (RNs), we recognize the significance of continuous monitoring of the patient's status and evaluating the effectiveness of the nursing care provided. The RN knows this is a continuous process and that the plan of care must be changed if needed based on the clinical decision making of the RN.

Nurse's Pocket Guide (2018) defines the **evaluation** component of the nursing process as "determining the client's progress toward attaining the identified outcomes and monitoring the client's response to and effectiveness of the selected nursing interventions." Although the evaluation stage is the "last" in the nursing process, all components are continually reviewed and modified as the care team "evaluates" the patient/client's response. The RN is vital in the reassessment of this process specific to how the patient/client is responding to the spiritual care plan, whether the goals and

outcomes are still relevant, and whether the interventions are still appropriate. **FIGURE 8-1** illustrates how the **nursing process/care plan** is a continuous circle; thus, by providing spiritual care, the RN is not just caring for the patient/client's body but also his or her mind, soul, and spirit.

▶ Nursing as Ministry

The connection of caring for the whole person—body, soul, mind, and spirit—allows the RN to minister and connect holistically with the patient/client, thereby providing nursing as ministry. The Bible reminds us that the Lord desires to refresh souls. Psalm 23:2 states, "He makes me lie down in green pastures, He leads me beside quiet waters, He refreshes my soul" (New International Version [NIV]). Although the patient/client might not be lying down in "green pastures," his or her soul still needs to be refreshed. Nursing as ministry allows the RN to provide comfort, strength, compassion, kindness, encouragement, hope, and spiritual support to the patient/client. Through understanding how to complete a **spiritual care plan**, the RN is able to provide for the specific needs of the patient/client rather than assuming what the patient/client desires. During this time, the RN must be sensitive to the patient/client.

Sensitivity on the part of the RN is important when the RN is completing a spiritual assessment for the patient/client (see the *Spiritual Assessment* chapter). Being ill or needing treatment can be very intimidating. In turn, the patient/client may feel vulnerable and not desire to share more than necessary. Nurses who acknowledge this vulnerability can help to alleviate the patient's/client's fears. This occurs when the RN chooses to fully listen, chooses to have a willing heart to hear and not judge, and chooses to see the patient/client as a person, rather than as just a number, a disease, or a task to complete.

The following true story describes an event that happened to a patient when the patient was getting checked into a doctor's appointment. For this purpose, the patient's name will be Sonja and the RN's name will be Louise. Louise had Sonja sit on the exam table and then started to ask Sonja the typical questions of why she was seeing the doctor, which allergies she had, and so on. During this time, Louise was focused on the computer and did not recognize that Sonja was worried about the visit. As Louise was finishing the tasks that needed to be completed, she then asked Sonja how her day was going. Sonja started to share about her fears regarding this doctor's visit, but quickly recognized that Louise was not truly paying any attention to anything that she was saying. So Sonja started to say, "blah, blah, blah, blah, blah." It took a moment for the nurse to realize that Sonja was literally saying, "blah, blah, blah"; when she did, both nurse and patient started to laugh. Louise recognized that she was choosing to complete the task and not choosing to fully focus and

hear what the patient was saying. Louise apologized to Sonja and said that the reminder to focus on her as the patient was a valuable lesson learned that day. Because of the honesty and integrity of this nurse, Sonja did end up sharing her fears with Louise. The nurse was then able to offer spiritual and emotional support to Sonja.

Through humbling herself and choosing to refocus on the patient, this nurse showed vulnerability with the patient. This vulnerability took bravery on the nurse's part and earned trust with her patient. By being brave, the RN can enter into the patient's/client's life and show willingness to care for and provide for patients/clients regardless of differing opinions, thoughts, and ideas (**BOX 8-1**). Entering into someone's vulnerability requires trust from both the patient/client and the RN.

Now is the time to put all the information from the spiritual assessment and the planning stage to form a spiritual care plan. **CASE STUDY 8-1** allows the student nurse to practice developing such a plan. To facilitate the development of this care plan, the author has presented the patient history as well as the answers that the patient shared when the FICA spiritual assessment was performed. The student is asked to use this information to develop the remainder of the care plan. Through putting the spiritual care plan into practice, the reader will be able to solidify and understand how to utilize the information that went into the development of this plan.

🔍 *CASE STUDY 8-1*

Spiritual Care Plan
General Patient Information
Scenario:

Patient initials: JD   Age: 37-year-old male   Room #: 12

Chief complaint: Chronic back pain

Admitting diagnosis: Patient to have spinal fusion revision this hospitalization

Past medical history: 15-year history of back pain; depression

Past surgical history: Spinal fusion 3 months prior to this admission

Allergies: Sulfa

Current medications: Vancomycin (prophylactic prior to surgery); oxycodone

Current vital signs and pain level: Blood pressure, 128/66 mm Hg; pulse, 76; respirations, 18 breaths/min; temperature, 98.2°F; oxygen saturation, 92% on room air; pain level, 8/10 and increasing with movement

In Case Study 8-1, information is gathered from the patient/client's chart that is important as the RN starts to formulate a plan for the patient and to understand which types of questions, assessments, and other tools the RN will be completing with the patient/client. According to *Taber's Medical Dictionary* (which is available via Nursing Central), this process is part of "an orderly approach to administering nursing care so that the patient's needs are met comprehensively and effectively" ("Nursing Process," 2017).

Spiritual Assessment

A spiritual assessment of the patient in this case study was performed. Here were the results:

SPIRITUAL ASSESSMENT

Note: *The "patient's" comments are italicized.*

FICA Spiritual History Tool
1. Faith and Belief
   - Do you consider yourself spiritual or religious?
     - *Yes, I am spiritual. I grew up in the church and have relied on God throughout my life.*
   - Do you have spiritual beliefs, values, or practices that help you cope with stress/difficult times?
     - *Yes, I pray and read the Bible. I value time with others, respect, and privacy.*
   - If no, what gives your life meaning?
2. Importance
   - What importance does your spirituality have in your life?
     - *My spirituality has strong importance to me, but I have been questioning why God is punishing me and why would He put me through all of this pain. I just don't understand why He would do this when I was following Him. I mean, I'm a good person and try to treat people with respect. I'm a good worker but haven't been able to work, which has caused strain on my family.*

- Has your spirituality influenced you in how you handle stress?
    - *Yes and no. I pray and ask God to take away the pain, but then I get discouraged and withdraw from my family and from God. I don't think God is interested in helping me.*
- Does your spirituality influence you in your healthcare decisions? If so, are you willing to share those with your healthcare team?
    - *No.*

3. Community
- Are you part of a spiritual or religious community?
    - *Yes, I belong to the local church on the corner.*
- Is this of support to you and if so, how?
    - *Sometimes, but I've been dealing with this pain for so long and now I'm more depressed and withdrawn that I don't think they know how to help me anymore. They help my children and my wife but I'm hopeless.*
- Is there a group of people you really love or who are important to you?
    - *My wife, my children, my parents, my siblings.*

4. Address in Care
- How should I address these issues in your health care?
    - *Stop my pain.*

Data from Puchalski, C. M. (2014). The FICA spiritual history tool. *Journal of Palliative Medicine, 17*(1), 105–106.

Taber's Medical Dictionary describes assessment as "the systemic collection of all data relevant to the patients, their problems, and needs" ("Nursing Process," 2017). The spiritual assessment that the RN completes is very relevant to the needs of the patient (see Case Study 8-1). The RN must remember to assess the patient/client's body, soul, mind, and spirit.

Spiritual Nursing Diagnosis

Nursing diagnosis is defined by NANDA International (n.d.) as a "clinical judgment concerning a human response" that "provides the basis for selection of nursing interventions to achieve outcomes for which the nurse has accountability." Because the RN is accountable for the care provided to the patient, the RN must take care in the selection of the appropriate nursing diagnosis that matches what was found through review of the patient/client's general information and the spiritual assessment. If the RN is engaged and focuses on the patient/client, then the nursing diagnosis will be more appropriate for the patient/client.

NURSING DIAGNOSIS

Based on the spiritual assessment, which nursing diagnosis would best fit this scenario?

Spiritual distress related to chronic illness, loss of independence, and reliance on others as evidenced by the patient stating that he is wondering why God is punishing him and his inability to work at this time.

Reproduced from *Nurse's Pocket Guide*. (2018). Spiritual distress and risk for spiritual distress. Retrieved from https://nursing.unboundmedicine.com/nursingcentral/view/nurses-pocket-guide/308560/all/Spiritual_Distress_and_risk_for_Spiritual_Distress

Spiritual Goals and Outcomes

Two important factors when developing an appropriate goal and outcome for a patient/client are that the goal/outcome must be patient specific and that the goal is written as a SMART goal.

PATIENT GOALS AND OUTCOMES

Based on the spiritual assessment, which goals would best fit the nursing assessment and nursing diagnosis of the patient in our case study?

Goals:
- The patient will discuss spiritual beliefs and values specific to the current pain.
- The patient will identify meaning and purpose in his own life that reinforces hope in the current situation.
- The patient will meet with his pastor or hospital chaplain for 30 minutes prior to patient discharge to discuss spiritual interventions (such as praying or reading his Bible) to help provide distraction, refocusing, and/or relief from pain.

Questions

1. Per the *Planning, Goals, and Interventions Related to the Spiritual Care of the Patient* chapter, are the above goals SMART goals?
2. If not, how could you revise them to be SMART goals (specific, measurable, attainable, relevant and timely)?

What outcomes would best fit the nursing assessment, nursing diagnosis, and goals?

Outcomes:
- The patient will report an increased sense of harmony with the deity.
- The patient will identify ways to increase meaning and hope in his current situation.

Reproduced from *Nurse's Pocket Guide*. (2018). Spiritual distress and risk for spiritual distress. Retrieved from https://nursing.unboundmedicine .com/nursingcentral/view/nurses-pocket-guide/308560/all/Spiritual_Distress_and_risk_for_Spiritual_Distress

---

Spiritual Interventions

Taber's Medical Dictionary describes intervention as the "determination of expected patient-centered outcomes, objective methods of evaluating patient progress toward the contributory goals, and optimum courses of action to resolve the problems identified and achieve the desired results" ("Nursing Process," 2017). Interventions are identified here that would be the best fit for this patient.

Spiritual Evaluation

Once the interventions have been implemented, the RN should review whether the goals and outcomes were met, not met, or partially met. The RN will then need to reassess the patient and update the spiritual care plan accordingly.

Evaluation entails returning to the patient/client to determine whether the goals and outcomes have been met and if the interventions have been effective in the care of the patient. At this time, the RN reevaluates the full spiritual care plan and makes adjustments accordingly. The previous portions of the nursing process include "doing," but the evaluation phase allows for "being" with the patient and making sure that the care plan is patient/client focused.

INTERVENTIONS BASED ON GOALS/OUTCOME

Which interventions would best fit for this patient?

Examples:

- Provide compassionate presence through the use of active listening, sitting silently when the patient is struggling with pain, and offering to hold the patient's hand during painful procedures to promote trust and comfort for the patient.
- Offer to pray and/or read the Bible for/to the patient.
- Offer the patient a visit from the hospital clergy or clergy of the patient's choice.
- Provide music to help lower anxiety when pain level is high.
- Offer journaling as a way for the patient to share thoughts, ideas, prayers, and so on during this time.
- Request a visit from the patient's pastor and/or the hospital chaplain.

Reproduced from *Nurse's Pocket Guide*. (2018). Spiritual distress and risk for spiritual distress. Retrieved from https://nursing.unboundmedicine.com/nursingcentral/view/nurses-pocket-guide/308560/all/Spiritual_Distress_and_risk_for_Spiritual_Distress

EVALUATION BASED ON GOALS/OUTCOMES

One of the goals was to have the patient's pastor or the hospital chaplain visit the patient for 30 minutes prior to discharge to discuss what spiritual tools the patient can use when in pain. The suggestions were prayer and reading the Bible.

One intervention included the RN requesting a visit by the pastor or hospital chaplain. A second intervention was the RN offering to pray with and/or read the Bible with the patient.

As the RN was evaluating whether this goal was met, not met, or partially met, the RN recognized that while the pastor and hospital chaplain were called to visit the patient, they were not available prior to the patient's discharge. The patient was in severe pain and asked the RN to pray with him and to read Psalm 23 to him. The RN recognized that this goal was partially met. The RN was able to help the patient through prayer and reading the Bible while he was in pain. Per the patient, the prayer and the reading of Psalm 23 calmed him and allowed him to "relax so my back wasn't so tense."

The goal was then revised to state "Patient to meet with pastor after discharge for 30 minutes per week for 2 to 4 weeks to pray with him and seek out Bible passages that will help him with distraction, refocusing, and/or relief of pain.

Questions

1. Do you agree that the goal was partially met? Why or why not?
2. How would you change the goal or interventions?

▶ Evaluating the Effectiveness of Spiritual Evaluation

The RN who is evaluating the spiritual care plan developed in Case Study 8-1 may recognize that offering prayer to the patient as a way to help promote hope could cause either reassurance for the patient or discomfort. Sensitivity comes back into play here, as the RN must realize and receive cues from the patient and not promote or force the RN's own agenda or cause added burden for the patient. In one investigation of praying for patients, the authors noted that RNs should "offer prayer if they have received consent, provided local policies and protocols are in place to support prayer as a therapeutic intervention" (French & Narayanasamy, 2011, p. 1203).

The Tale of Two Student Nurses

As a Christian student nurse or Christian RN, there may be times when praying for a patient and/or family member is an important intervention. The intent behind the request to pray for the patient or family member is very important when offering prayer as an intervention.

For example, during clinicals, a nursing student, whom we will name Joann, prayed for all patients regardless of whether the patient requested prayer. Joann felt it was her "duty" to pray because she was a Christian and that was what was going to "help" the patients. Because the intent was for Joann to "complete a Christian task," the patients felt coerced, as if the prayer was forced upon them, and unable to refuse the prayer. The nursing school was contacted after multiple patients complained to the hospital staff regarding how "forceful the student was" specific to prayer.

Another nursing student, whom we will name Jim, recognized that his patient was in spiritual distress and that prayer could be an effective intervention. Jim spoke with the patient, offered prayer as an intervention, and was told by the patient that the patient did not want prayer. Jim then reevaluated the plan of care and made revisions accordingly. The student nurse was sad that the patient did not want prayer, but he recognized that this was about the patient and honored the patient's request. Jim kept the focus on the patient.

Facilitating Prayer

If the nurse's evaluation reveals that the patient does not wish to participate in prayer, the nurse can still offer prayers in private for this patient. Following are examples of prayers that can be said aloud or silently. Prayer is simply talking to God. He lends His ear to

hear and desires to provide for those who call upon Him. He is faithful. If unsure as to what to say, then praying the scripture is powerful.

- Dear Lord Jesus, I ask that you would intervene and support my patients/clients as they walk through this journey. Please give them faith, hope, healing, and guidance. Thank you. In Jesus's name, Amen.
- Psalm 86:1: "Hear me, Lord, and answer me, for I (my patient/client) is poor and needy."
- Psalm 143:1: "Lord, hear my prayer, listen to my cry for mercy; in your faithfulness and righteousness come to my (patient/client's) relief."

▶ Conclusion

Nursing as ministry keeps the patient at the center. By focusing on the patient, the RN is able to provide care that is specific and directed toward the patient (**CASE STUDY 8-2**). Knowing how the patient responds through the evaluation process is vital to supporting, guiding, and providing for the patient's spiritual needs. **BOX 8-2** contains an example of a RN who exemplifies nursing as ministry. **BOXES 8-3** and **8-4** provide additional information on students' understanding of spiritual care.

▶ Clinical Reasoning Exercises

1. A BSN nursing student is providing care to a RN who has breast cancer, and has just returned to her room after a mastectomy. The student knows it is important to evaluate the patient's level of pain and her dressing. Why is evaluation an important ongoing process for this patient? Why might

🔍 *CASE STUDY 8-2*

As a RN, you are providing care in the neonatal intensive care unit (NICU) to three premature infants. One of the "preemies" has been diagnosed with several birth anomalies that are incompatible with life. The RN is providing comfort measures for this infant. The family has been informed by the neonatologist that their baby will not survive due to the birth anomalies. Sister Rebecca, who is also an RN, is helping you during this time. The parents have requested that their child be baptized. Sister Rebecca asks the priest who is on call to baptize the baby, but the priest refuses to come to the bedside in the NICU. As the RN, you are angry and can't understand why the priest will not grant the parent's request of baptism for this child of God. Sister Rebecca and you as the RN baptize the baby; within the hour, the baby dies as the parents hold their little one. In your heart, you know you did the right nursing procedure by baptizing this child.

Questions

1. As a RN, you work in a faith-based acute care health setting. You have a close relationship with God and have learned about spiritual care. How did you develop your spiritual beliefs and values in God?
2. How do you maintain your spiritual beliefs and values? Do you read the scriptures, pray, attend church, or have time for reflection?
3. How do you deal with your feelings of anger toward the priest who refused to baptize a child of God?
4. From actively listening to these parents, do you think baptizing their child was important to them? What should the RN do if he or she does not believe in infant baptism?
5. Would you be comfortable in baptizing this preemie?
6. As an RN, how do you evaluate the decisions that you made and the response of anger that you had?

BOX 8-2   Outstanding Nurse Leader: Windie Her, RNBC, BSN, MA, CPXP

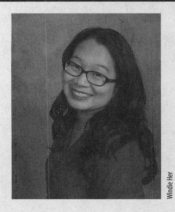

Windie Her is a passionate servant leader who aspires to believe, encourage, and empower all those whom she encounters. She believes that no matter what capacity you are in, you are a leader and can make a positive change for others. Her has more than a decade of experience in the healthcare field in a variety of roles and specialties and has worn many different hats. She's been a Nightingale nominee, float pool nurse, nurse educator, and nurse manager, and she currently works as a patient experience manager. Her has excelled as a nurse leader through her relationships with others. She is genuine and honest, and she chooses daily to be fully present. She has a gift for making others feel important and encouraged. Her was chosen as a nurse leader because of the huge difference she makes in the lives of all those people whom she touches. Her love for the Lord shines forth even if she doesn't say anything about the Lord. She exudes a welcome spirit and truly lives out nursing as ministry.

(continues)

BOX 8-2   Outstanding Nurse Leader: Windie Her, RNBC, BSN, MA, CPXP   *(continued)*

Her believes that her mission field is her "everyday, ordinary life" (Romans 12:1–2, Message King James Bible [MSG]). Because of this, she enjoys going to work every day, trusting that God will lead her in all that He is calling her to do. She knows that she is right where God wants her to be and prays each day to be used by God.

Her originally received her bachelor's in science in nursing from Walla Walla College, School of Nursing in Oregon. She went on to receive her master's in arts in leadership from the Denver Seminary in Denver, Colorado. Her nursing degree as well as her leadership degree have allowed Her to excel as a nurse educator, as a nurse manager, and currently as a patient experience manager.

Her has been married for 15 years and has four children, ages 11, 9, 7, and 5. Outside of her work, her great source of pride and joy is being a full-time mother of four and a wife. She enjoys devoting time to her family, traveling, and spending time outdoors hiking, biking, or going to the beach.

Her's family legacy is amazing, as her family (parents and grandparents) were refugees from Vietnam. Her family has deep roots in the relationships they build with others, in serving the Lord, and in giving thanks to the Lord for His provision for their family. Her parents instilled the belief in her that God brought their family to live in the "land of opportunity" and encouraged her to continue to live out her faith in thanksgiving to the Lord. Her grew up knowing that God truly blessed her family. She continues to be active in her church through women's and children's ministries as well as leading a young couples group with her husband.

When discussing the content of this chapter (spiritual evaluation), Her's eyes lit up, she sat a little straighter, and her excitement for this topic bubbled up (her excitement and joy in life is very contagious). She shared the following:

- Spiritual evaluation is a time when you review all that has been done for the patient while ensuring that the patient remains at the center. Another key piece is to make sure that all team members have been included in the spiritual care of the patient.
- The spiritual evaluation process is where we connect with our heart, our head, and our hands. The Bible reminds us in Mark 12:30 to "Love the Lord your God with all your heart and with all your soul and with all your mind and with all your strength" (NIV). The evaluation stage of the nursing process allows for this vulnerability and provides an opportunity to share Jesus's message with the patient through fully relying on and loving the Lord with all of the body, soul, mind, and spirit.
- Jesus reevaluated as he healed. He is our example of evaluating the care we provide to our patients/clients. For example, when Jesus healed a blind man in Mark 8, he reevaluated him, asking the man:

    "Can you see anything now?" Jesus asked him. The man looked around. "Yes!" he said,
    "I see men! But I can't see them very clearly; they look like tree trunks walking around!"
    Then Jesus placed his hands over the man's eyes again and as the man stared intently,
    his sight was completely restored, and he saw everything clearly, drinking in the sights
    around him. (Mark 8:23–25, The Living Bible)

- When she worked with a patient with end-stage disease, she was able to make a spiritual connection with the patient. This patient confided that when he was younger, he tried to commit suicide but saw Jesus. The patient said that he heard Jesus say, "It's not your time yet." At the time of this interaction with Her, the patient was older and was in the process of dying. Her was able to pray with and for this patient. A little while later, this patient started to code (heart stopped beating)—the team was there and a vent was placed. The family was really struggling because they didn't understand what was happening spiritually as well as physically. The patient's wife and family did not want to let go of the patient. Her was praying silently, asking the Lord how to help. She felt led to approach the wife and shared with her: "I know I haven't met you yet; however, I was able to talk with your husband. Your husband knows God and trusts God. Let's allow God and the patient to decide when he should go home to heaven." Her knew that this interaction was from the Lord because it was not something she would ever share with a family member. The wife was very receptive to Her's message. Because of this intervention, the focus returned back to what was best for the patient and a peace came into the room that was not there originally.

- Be willing to be a part of God's process and calling—it's not about us, but about what God wants to do in and through us. Patients expect good care when they come into the hospital. Let's surprise the patient through being authentically present and by building relationships with our patients.

Her shared, "I encourage you to pray every morning or evening on your way to work. Pray for your patients, your peers, your leaders, and your organization. Pray that God will lead you to where He wants you to go, doing what He is calling you to do. Pray for guidance, especially in the tough moments of your calling as a nurse. God will guide you as you are faithful to Him." Her exemplifies this devotion over and over.

BOX 8-3 Research Highlight

Brown, Humphreys, Whorley, and Bridge researched the significance of senior BSN student nurses' perceptions of spiritual care education and whether the graduate students were ready to provide spiritual care to others. The researchers state, "Research is limited regarding self-perceived competence of nursing students to provide spiritual care" (p. E5). Data were collected by using a mixed methods design incorporating both qualitative and quantitative approaches. The qualitative approach gathered data from 45 students during their senior exit interviews in a face-to-face group. The quantitative approach gathered data from 30 students who completed the Spirituality and Spiritual Care Rating Scale (SSCRS). The survey results demonstrated a strong perception that the BSN students were ready to provide spiritual care upon graduation.

Modified from Brown, K., Humphreys, H., Whorley, E., & Bridge, D. (2019). Ready to care? Student nurse perceptions of spiritual care education. *Journal of Christian Nursing, 36*(1), E5–E10. doi:10.97/CNJ0000000000000579

BOX 8-4 Evidence-Based Practice Focus

Pittroff and Hendricks-Ferguson (2018) have studied "the importance of academic nurse researchers partnering with clinical nurses for clinical research." A four-hour training session was planned to assist clinical nurses in participating in evidence-based practice as part of a palliative care end-of-life communication-focused research study. The purpose of the study was to evaluate the effectiveness of the research training techniques. The authors used the analogy from Matthew 28:19–20 in their writing, noting that academic nurse researchers should collaborate with clinical nurses to utilize evidence-based practice to inform nursing practice for high-quality care. The results indicated that the training was acceptable.

Modified from Pittroff, G. E., & Hendricks-Ferguson, V. L. (2018). Preparing clinical nurses for nursing research: Evaluation of training procedures in a palliative care pilot study. *Journal of Christian Nursing, 35*(1), 38–43. doi:10.1097/CNJ0000000000000462

the RN need to make clinical decisions when providing care to her patient and what decisions might they be? As an RN, which other components of the nursing process might you use with this patient and why?

2. This chapter discusses the importance of spiritual evaluation, which can occur across the life span. You are the RN in an outpatient department caring for a 6-year-old female scheduled for surgery within the hour. As you finish your assessment, you ask your patient if there is anything else that she needs before going to surgery. She replies, "I would like to see a pastor before surgery." As an RN, you have three other patients waiting to be checked in for surgery. Describe your responsibility in providing spiritual support for this child. Why are you accountable for this request of spiritual support?

▶ **Personal Reflection Exercises**

1. How does implementing a spiritual care plan for a patient help that patient?

2. How does evaluating the goals, outcomes, and interventions help support the patient?

3. Is prayer always appropriate as a nursing intervention? Why or why not?

4. As a student nurse or RN, how do you see yourself interacting with patients on a spiritual level?

5. Are there any boundaries that the RN must be aware of when working with patients and families specific to a spiritual plan of care?

6. How would you answer the FICA spiritual assessment questions? Did you learn anything new about yourself?

7. Can you think of a time when prayer would have been an appropriate intervention for a patient?

8. Has there been a time when you wanted to pray with a patient or family member but held back because of fear?

9. Do you have a prayer that you say for your patients/clients?

10. What scripture might you use to pray for/with your patient/client?

11. Write out a prayer you might say for a patient/client.

References

Fowler, M. D. M. (2015). *Guide to the code of ethics for nurses with interpretive statements: Development, interpretation, and application* (2nd ed.). Silver Spring, MD: American Nurses Association.

French, C., & Narayanasamy, A. (2011). To pray or not to pray: A question of ethics. *British Journal of Nursing, 20*(18), 1198–1204.

NANDA International. (n.d.). Nursing diagnosis. Retrieved from http://www.nanda.org/nanda-i-resources/glossary-of-terms/

Nurse's Pocket Guide. (2018). The nursing process and planning client care. Retrieved from https://nursing.unboundmedicine.com/nursingcentral/view/nurses-pocket-guide/308575/all/The_Nursing_Process_and_Planning_Client_Care

Nursing process. (2017). In D. Venes (Ed.), *Taber's medical dictionary.* Philadelphia, PA: F. A. Davis.

Recommended Readings

Adkins, C. S. (2015). Evaluating theory from a Christian perspective: Transformative learning theory. *Journal of Christian Nursing, 32*(2), 112–115. doi:10,1097/CNJ.000000000000154

Henderson, D. L., & Powers, C. F. (2016). Are faith community nurses using the *Scope and Standards of Practice? Journal of Christian Nursing, 33*(1), E1–E6. doi:10.12097/CNJ.0000000000000245

Schoonover-Shoffner, K. (2013). Praying with patients. *Journal of Christian Nursing, 30*(4), 197. doi:10.1097 /CNJ.0b013e3182a6eaba

Stryker, R. (2010). Spiritual care: An unexpected lesson. *Journal of Christian Nursing, 27*(1), 28–31. doi:10 .1097/01.CNJ 0000365988.79894.be

Taylor, E. J., Testerman, N., & Hart, D. (2014). Teaching spiritual care to nursing students: An integrated model. *Journal of Christian Nursing, 31*(2), 93–99. doi:10 .1097/CNJ.000000000000058.

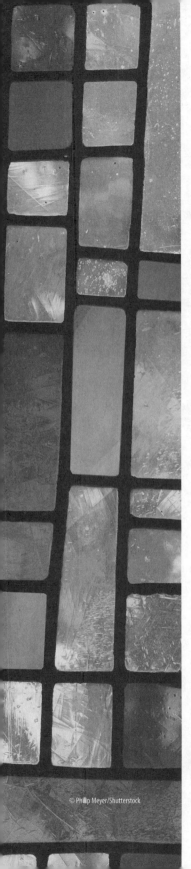
© Philip Meyer/Shutterstock

UNIT III

Preparing for Nursing as Ministry

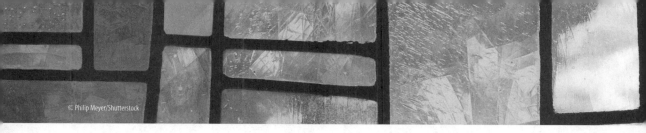

CHAPTER 9

Understanding Worldview to Minister More Effectively

Samuel Welbaum, MA, MTS

LEARNING OBJECTIVES

At the end of this chapter, the reader will be able to:

1. Understand the concept of worldview in relationship to nursing as ministry.
2. Discuss the philosophical underpinnings of a worldview.
3. Discover one's own worldview.
4. Describe strategies for demonstrating the love of God within nursing for those of different worldviews.

KEY TERMS

Meaning	Subjective
Objective	Worldview

Have you ever tried to have a conversation with someone who does not speak your language? Perhaps your native tongue is English, and you're trying to have a conversation with someone who speaks only Spanish. In this situation, there might be some overlap in some of the words, but rather quickly it will become apparent that communication will be rather difficult. Perhaps you turn initially to the illogical, but oddly popular, technique of speaking more loudly and more slowly. Of course, if someone doesn't speak your language, being louder really won't help matters. A more effective approach would entail pointing at objects and gesturing in ways that you hope transcend language. That might net some positive results, but they will still be rather limited. Your best bet if you desire to talk with someone who speaks only another language is to either hire an interpreter who knows both languages or learn the other language yourself, so you can communicate with the person in question.

This scenario of two people speaking two different languages is one that we've seen often enough that it's easy to wrap the mind around. We can understand the confusion, the frustration, the bewilderment. One person says "table"; the other says "mesa." So how can they ever communicate clearly? However, another version of this scenario plays out far more often and leads to even greater confusion, yet is much less widely recognized.

Suppose that instead of two people speaking different languages, we now have two people who are speaking the same language. Let's say that both have English as their native tongue. Does the fact that two people are speaking English guarantee that both are speaking the same language? In one way, yes—but in another way, not at all. Language allows people to communicate what is inside their heads to someone else; however, that person understands it based on what is in the message recipient's head and translates it accordingly. I have no control over what someone else hears me say. I can control the words that I say, but not how the other person takes them. This is the heart of the issue of **worldview**.

This chapter discusses how to engage in conversation with someone who, even though she might speak the same language on the surface that you do, does not *speak the same language underneath* that you do, if that distinction makes sense. To put it another way, this chapter seeks to help readers learn how to serve in the ministry of nursing, when those persons to whom you are ministering are of another religious tradition, or reject belief in God, or deny the importance of thinking about the meaning of life or the topic of the divine in general. It is not meant to be a step-by-step guide on how to address these families

of belief (many other excellent books exist that do so), but instead suggests a way of thinking through how to communicate with those persons with whom we disagree. This chapter engages the reader in a philosophical look at some deep questions that, when answered according to the scriptures, allow nurses to be more effective in their caring ministry.

To address this topic, the term *worldview* will be defined, and readers are encouraged to identify the facets of their own worldviews. Then, we will consider how to identify another person's worldview, and how the nurse can "put on" that worldview to think about or see the world in the same manner that the other does. The chapters concludes by thinking through the issue of how to disagree well, and considering when that disagreement perhaps does more harm than good. All ministry is based on relationships, and disagreement can either deepen or fracture a relationship, so wisdom and timing are key. First, however, we consider the topic of worldview itself.

▶ What Is a Worldview?

The term *worldview* originated in the late 18th century and was first used by the Prussian philosopher Immanuel Kant. Kant's epistemology predicated that humans participate in the creation of knowledge by taking sense data from the world as it is and putting those data into mental categories that create the phenomena that we experience. For example, when I look at a car, I never view the car as it is in the world, but only as it appears to me. Thus, in Kant's usage, worldview means how I sense the world, or how the physical world is constructed in my head.

Over time, the concept of worldview began to evolve and move beyond mere physical representation, asking larger questions. The term *worldview* was not used by the 19th-century Danish philosopher Søren Kierkegaard, but the concept of "lifeview" was. Kierkegaard developed a system in which a person lives in a sphere, or stage, of existence; this sphere, in turn, determines how life is perceived. If someone is in the aesthetic sphere, then life is about pleasure; in the ethical sphere, it's about morality; and in the religious sphere, it's about faith. People in the three spheres of existence will look at the same event and respond very differently because of their differing vantage points. While the aesthete might look at an extravagantly wealthy person with great envy, the religious person—the "Knight of Faith," as Kierkegaard called the archetype of this sphere—might look at the aesthete with pity because of all the distractions that fill his life.

In the 20th century, thinkers such as Ludwig Wittgenstein and Thomas Kuhn expanded the concept of worldview even further. Wittgenstein emphasized the use of language games, noting that the very words we use have meaning only in particular contexts when addressing particular people. Consider the word *who*. When pronounced, the word *who* in English is an interpersonal interrogative, but in Hebrew *who* (written "hu") is the third person masculine singular pronoun, the equivalent of the English word *he*. Or consider another example: What does the word *bad* mean? In most settings, it means either "morally wrong" or "of a poor quality"; however, as typified by Michael Jackson's song, in the 1980s *bad* meant the exact opposite of its usual meaning, denoting something of a rather high quality. Thus, when we communicate, even the words that we use are particular to our own usage, and those who understand us most are the people who use words in a similar way or play a similar language game.

Kuhn emphasized the concept of a "paradigm shift." Such a shift occurs when either a discovery or a realization affects the consciousness of an individual, or the collective consciousness of a society, in such a way that it completely changes the way in which topics are approached or questions are asked. Consider the shift one goes through as a child when she realizes that Santa Claus's arrival on Christmas Eve is just a game her parents have been playing

with her, and all those gifts are from them, and her parents have been eating the cookies all along. Suddenly, it seems as if the child lives in a different world than the slightly more magical one that she inhabited a few minutes prior. Suddenly getting to bed early on December 24 is not as important, nor does the fear of a stocking full of coal burn as brightly. This is a minor example, but Kuhn suggests that science, and every sphere of life, operates within these paradigms, and our paradigm fully colors how we approach the world.

This brief history of the concept of worldview could (and should) be expanded, but it brings us to a place where we can consider how the word is used now, and how it might be applied to your interactions with coworkers or those who are in your care. Today, there are any number of suggestions about how one might define worldview and various tests to understand what a worldview is. Ravi Zacharias (2018) notes that a worldview must provide existentially satisfying answers to questions of origin, meaning, morality, and destiny. J. P. Moreland (2017) couches worldview as a set of habits that form our background beliefs about the world. James Sire (2009), one of the foremost scholars in the area of worldview studies, offers this expanded definition:

> A worldview is a commitment, a fundamental orientation of the heart, that can be expressed as a story or in a set of presuppositions (assumptions which may be true, partially true or entirely false) that we hold (consciously or subconsciously, consistently or inconsistently) about the basic constitution of reality, and that provides the foundation on which we live and move and have our being. (p. 20)

Sire's definition emphasizes that worldviews form the foundation of a person's entire way of being. Every action, every thought, every word, and everything that a person does is guided by, understood in light of, or done because of that person's worldview.

A person's worldview is fundamental to his or her way of being, but we must recognize that it consists of "givens," or ideas that are assumed, or presumed, by the individual without argument. Perhaps another way of saying this is that these are ideas that are argued *from*, not argued *to*. Given your trust in your senses' ability to convey knowledge about the world, I could make an argument that it is going to rain (it looks overcast, it feels cold or humid, and so on), or that my dinner is burnt (looks black, smells charred, tastes dry, and so on). Both "it's going to rain" and "my dinner is burnt" are ideas that I argue *to*—but to argue *to* something, I have to be arguing *from* something. In this case, it's the idea that your senses convey accurate information about the world. I do not need to convince you that your senses convey accurate information about the world; in fact, I would need to make a valiant effort to convince you that they don't convey accurate knowledge about the world. Everyone presumes that his or her senses convey accurate knowledge about the world; it is not until supplied with a reason to the contrary that someone believes she might not be able to trust her senses. A colorblind person does not come to the conclusion that he is colorblind without evidence that the world is not as his senses perceive it.

It is perhaps best to understand a worldview as an interpretive matrix through which a person "reads" the world. We interpret, understand, and react to every event that happens based on our own presuppositions. These presuppositions—or givens, to use my earlier term—form in a multitude of ways. Sire's definition indicates that these worldview concepts can be unconscious. Your worldview is shaped by your culture, your religion, your family of origin, the media you ingest, and any other myriad of things. It is likely that two people with similar upbringings and life experiences will have very similar worldviews; however, personality traits also help shape our worldview.

In a very real way, every person on the planet lives in his or her own little world, in that we all interpret the world from our own vantage point. A 62-year-old introverted optimistic Asian American Buddhist male who grew up in a politically liberal family living in San Francisco will read the world very differently than does a 28-year-old extroverted pessimistic Hispanic American Evangelical Christian female who grew up in a politically conservative family living in Dallas. Each of those factors listed to describe the people in question affect and shape his or her worldview.

The task, then, is to figure out how to communicate effectively across worldviews. It is certainly a difficult task, but before we start attempting to communicate across worldviews, we need to first establish what our own worldview is.

▶ How Do I Determine My Own Worldview?

If a worldview is a set of givens, or presuppositions, that one reasons or operates from, and an interpretive matrix through which one reads the world, then what views or beliefs make up a worldview? As noted earlier, Zacharias (2018) has said that a worldview answers questions related to origin, meaning, morality, and destiny. Within this framework, a person's worldview answers some major questions: How did we get here? Why are we here? How should we act? Where are we going? Immediately upon reading those questions, you likely had at least a vague answer of some sort to each one. Those answers, when pushed far enough, reveal your worldview.

A Framework for Worldview

Have you ever had a conversation with a 5-year-old? Children of this age love to ask "Why?" about things that seem very clear to us. However, after a series of "whys" it becomes apparent that we lack some answers. Say that you tell the 5-year-old that you need to go to work. He asks, "Why?" You say, "To make money." He asks, "Why do you need money?" You respond, "So we have a place to live." He asks, "Why do we need a place to live?" You say, "So we have a place to sleep at night, and a place to put all our stuff." He asks, "Why do we need all this stuff?" You exasperatedly say, "Because we like our stuff and we would be sad without it." This goes on and on until finally you say, "That's just the way it is." When you hit that bedrock, you've discovered your worldview.

It may be helpful here to expand the list of questions that we are addressing by again turning to Sire's work *The Universe Next Door* (2009). In this book, Sire lists eight questions, the answers to which form the bedrock of your worldview.[1]

1. What Is Prime Reality?

What is ultimately the most real? Phrased another way, what thing exists in such a way that if he/she/it didn't exist, nothing else would? Perhaps that answer is God, or a plurality of gods, or a spirited cosmos, or merely material reality. At the core, if we follow the train of "why" back far enough, we discover something that we see everything else resting upon. The answer to this question sets the stage for the answers to the remaining seven questions.

2. What Is the Nature of External Reality?

This question seeks to explore what type of place we understand the universe to be. Is it created? Is it ordered, or is it chaotic? Was it designed, or does it hinge upon chance? Is matter simply physical, or is it spirited? As an example, if someone says that she is trying to determine what the universe wants for her, what does this statement indicate that she

believes about the universe? It appears that because she believes the universe has a want or a desire for her to do a certain thing, that the universe must be alive in some manner.

Or consider another example: If someone in your care asks you to pray for him, he is communicating that he believes that the material world that we live in is such that a spiritual entity can act and affect that matter. How different is that belief than the one signaled if the same patient were to ask you to send positive vibes his way? In the former, the presumption is that material reality is affected by physical individuals supplicating a divine or spiritual agent; in the latter, material reality seems to be affected by physical individuals directly. The latter belief seems to presume a greater power for the human person than the former, though the person asking for "good vibes" is not aware of it.

3. What Is a Human Being?

Are humans merely highly advanced animals? Perhaps something like a computer with meat and skin on us? Entities made in God's image? Or perhaps gods in waiting? The answer to this question is incredibly important in the medical field, particularly in areas of medical ethics. When does a human start being a human person? Peter Singer (n.d.), a noted ethicist at Princeton University, has asserted in various settings that a human person is an entity who can anticipate the future, and has wants and desires about the future. As a newborn baby has no concept of her existence over time, Singer asserts that she is not a person; therefore, if her parents and doctor agree that due to severe disability, it is better to end this infant's life than to allow her to live, it is not the same as killing a person. In fact, if parents decided to kill their newborn who is not severely disabled, Singer believes that action is wrong,

---

1 These questions are taken from Chapter 1 of the fifth edition of Sire's *The Universe Next Door*, with my commentary/explanations included.

but not as wrong as if a person were to have been killed; moreover, it is wrong only because other families would have been happy to love and raise the child.

While this is an extreme example, it demonstrates the ramifications of how one answers this question. In many spheres of existence, it is assumed that there is a particular dignity to humanity; however, this question calls you to ask yourself, "Where does that dignity come from?" It also challenges us to think about the way we talk about ourselves. The human body was not described in mechanical terms until the Industrial Revolution, and the human brain was not discussed in computer or digital terms until the 1970s. It isn't surprising that people did not describe the human as a computer before computers were invented. However, it does indicate that we are very comfortable using things that humanity has created as a metaphor for understanding humanity—a metaphor that can become more than a metaphor, and perhaps cognitively normative.

4. What Happens to a Person at Death?

This question addresses a person's absolute destiny. When this life ends, what comes next? Clearly, the answers to the three preceding questions inform this one. It would make no sense for a person to believe that humans are merely material, yet also believe that after death our souls face judgment. If humans are not souls, or if we do not have any nonmaterial part to our existence, then nothing of our identity continues on after death. That is not to say that nothing of "us" carries on, merely that our identities do not. I once spoke with an atheist who took great comfort in the fact that once she died, her particles would float out into the world. Her line of thinking was similar to that of noted atheist Carl Sagan (1980): "The cosmos is within us. We are made of starstuff. We are a way for the universe to know itself." While his statement almost sounds

pantheistic, Sagan wasn't claiming that the universe is conscious, but rather that humans are nothing more than a clump of particles that have gained consciousness.

There are plenty of implications for how one lives based on the answer to this question. Do our actions have eternal significance? Or is death the end? Think of it this way: Within 300 years, you and everyone who will ever meet you will be dead. Unless you do something of vast historical significance, such as found a country or cure a disease, within 400 years your name will be forgotten and listed only on a few family trees somewhere. This outlook admittedly sounds bleak—but is it the full story? If you believe in reincarnation, you will agree with the atheist that the particles that made up your body will move on, but your soul (or a rough equivalent) will still exist here on Earth, just in another body. If you hold to Christian theism, you believe that our souls will never cease to be; thus, in 400 years' time, while forgotten on Earth, you will be awaiting the judgment.

To push this point even further, if someone holds to a works-based understanding of the afterlife, perhaps something like that depicted in the TV show *The Good Place*, then you'll analyze each action to consider the eternal consequences of what is currently being done. The question of "Have I done enough good?" will never leave. This uncertainty is why the prophet Muhammad said that even he didn't know what his fate would be when he stood before Allah (Sura 46).

5. Why Is It Possible to Know Anything at All?

Compared to the last few questions, this one is a bit more esoteric, albeit rather telling. People believe that they have accurate knowledge about the world, and that they can think through and apply that knowledge. But why is that the case? Right now, as you're reading this page, why are you able to do so? One answer might be that humans have evolved sensory abilities over time, and due to natural selection, sensory faculties that favor the emergence of consciousness developed. This stance raises another question: What makes us think that our knowledge is accurate? An implication of holding to mere survival of the fittest as the cause of knowledge acquisition is that this process does not tend to develop accurate systems, but rather useful ones.

Put another way, when I see a ball coming at my face, I move because I trust my sense of sight and believe that it is aimed at revealing the world as it is. However, I also have stopped my car in the middle of the night waiting for a mailbox to cross the road because I mistakenly thought it was a person. In both cases, I believed that my senses were revealing the world as it is. In the second instance, though, my senses were mistaken. What if they were always mistaken this way because that bent has some evolutionary advantage? What if I don't even exist and my consciousness is merely an illusion? Descartes rejected this idea famously by attempting to doubt himself, but concluded, "I think, therefore I am." His contemporary, philosopher Daniel Dennett (1991), among others, has called even this point into question, saying that perhaps we don't exist.

Another possible answer is that humans are made in the likeness of a God or are designed by a God in such a way that we are able to understand the created order. According to this view, our ability to understand the world is connected to our creation. Humans are able to understand the world because we've been crafted this way. This idea is found not just in Christian theism, but even in the unique theism of Aristotle, who believed that "By nature, all men desire to know."

6. How Do We Know Right and Wrong?

Morality is a universal human phenomenon, but what does a person mean when she says that something is "morally right"? Some have said that morality is based on the character of God, and humans know moral truths because they were made by a moral God. This understanding of morality means that we know right and wrong because they are **objective** facts that exist in the outside world. Another possible response is that morality is not absolute, but rather subjectively useful; that is, humans have evolved into moral creatures because certain acts are better for the survival of our species. Or perhaps morality is completely relative to times and cultures. In this answer, what is morally right or wrong changes over time not due to new information, but rather due to new societal inclinations. The philosopher David Hume went so far as to say that morality is actually nothing more than emotions. When a person says, "This is wrong," what that individual actually means is "I have negative feelings about this." That might be true for the person saying it, but it is necessarily applicable to anyone other than the person speaking.

The thing to notice about these answers is that they all fall into one of two types: Either morality is an objective fact of the cosmos and applies to everyone at all times, or morality is changeable and applies to different people and cultures in different ways. The key to this worldview question is trying to decipher which a person believes. When people make statements such as "Murder is wrong," they almost always mean it in an objective way that applies to all people at all times. Indeed, if they didn't, they would say something more akin to "Murder is often wrong" or "Murder is currently wrong." The difficulty for many systems that lack a divine being (and some that have one) is in trying to determine which criteria constitute right and wrong. In his book *The Moral Landscape*, self-proclaimed theist and religious critic Sam Harris (2010) presents a naturalistic system of objective morality dependent on positive brain states, but does not present an argument as to why we should care that others are experiencing positive experiences beyond "That's the right thing to do," which itself asserts the question without addressing it.

7. What Is the Meaning of History?

Where is everything headed? We've already addressed what happens when we die, but this question wants to know the **meaning** of everything that happens prior to that point. Is history building toward anything? Perhaps not. A consistent atheist could say that history is completely chaotic and random. In contrast, following the work of Hegel, many atheists have suggested that history is progressing toward utopia—a time when there is no religion and no elite class, and everyone is satisfied and in harmony. Hegel himself believed that history was the story of God coming to self-realization. Others have posited that history is the battleground for good and evil, and eventually one will emerge as victorious. Many theistic religions understand history as the arena in which God accomplishes His purposes, in which people encounter the divine.

The point of interest here has to do with purpose. If a person says, "I'm just waiting for the universe to show me a sign," then it is clear that he believes that the universe has a will or a desire of some sort. Statements that indicate something either was, or was not, meant to be indicate an intentionality or a design in our lives. No one who believes that the world is random can consistently believe that she was meant to get a certain job. That's inconsistent.

8. What Personal, Life-Orienting Core Commitments Are Consistent with This Worldview?

This final question asks you to look back over your answers to the first seven questions. These answers form the bedrock, the foundation of your worldview, but they are not the totality of it. Everyone has a different experience of the world, so even within the naturalist or the Christian worldview, everyone will have a slightly (to incredibly) different understanding of the world. This fact is vital to understand when you begin to have conversations with others. Using Sire's first seven questions as a framework can help you understand the general trajectory of an individual's thought, and perhaps make some very educated guesses; however, each person is an individual and needs to be addressed as such.

Now that we've taken the time to analyze our own beliefs and have begun to come to terms with the way we see the world, we can begin to think through how to have conversations with people who don't share our worldview. At the beginning of this chapter, I used the analogy of trying to communicate to someone who speaks another language. That is the very task that cross-worldview communication seeks to perform. You will find that you communicate much more easily with people who share your core convictions. So many conversations today fail to bear any fruit because people assume that everyone thinks in exactly the same way they do. But this is like being at the Olympic Village and assuming that everyone speaks German. Certainly the Germans do, and people from many other countries may have some overlap between their own languages and German, but a large contingent of the athletes won't understand a word of German. Your goal in communicating—not only as a nurse, but in life in general—is not merely to be able to talk with people who share your views, but also to learn to communicate well across worldviews. The way one does so is by learning how to think in other people's worldviews.

Thinking in Other Worldviews

To continue the language analogy, it is easy enough to walk up to someone and ask, "Spreken Sie Deutch?" or "Habla Español?" to determine if he or she speaks either German or Spanish; however, you won't have the same success approaching someone and asking, "Spreken Sie New Age pantheism?" or "Habla naturalistic materialism?" It would be nice if communication was that simple, but sadly it is not. Thus, in our desire to minister effectively, we need to be able to determine people's worldviews, and learn how to think from their point of view. This is not an easy task for many reasons. Perhaps the most obvious is that if the other person's worldview is not yours, you are merely pretending to be in that worldview, so the thinking won't come as naturally. In fact, it may draw you to conclusions that make you uncomfortable.

That said, if we cannot walk up to someone and ask which worldview that person speaks, we need to be able to determine it in other ways. The key to this is, quite obviously, communication. When you enter a patient's room, you are going in blind. You probably have a name, a medical history, and a very safe assumption that the individual would like to get better—but that tells you very little about the beliefs of the person with whom you are speaking. In most situations, the general ideas floating around a culture will have, in some way, influenced the person you're speaking with. Making this assumption becomes a launching pad from which you can begin to trace the patient's worldview framework.

In many cases, your interactions may be minimal: The patient might be gone in a few hours and never seen again, so your communication will be mostly mechanical. However, for those patients with whom you will be interacting for days or perhaps longer, or in your interactions with people in the everyday world, the first key to understanding what they think is to listen to what they say. This sounds like common sense, but listening is a lost art. Often people are distracted in communication, or they are waiting their chance to talk rather than actively listening. This phenomenon is so pervasive that people often are longing for a chance to speak and to be heard.

Think of it this way: If you visit the hair salon or the barbershop, do you expect the stylist/barber to talk more than you? Of course not. And the good stylist knows that and will do whatever is necessary to keep you talking. The same is true with a bartender, or a waiter, or a member of any other service profession. These professionals are well aware that part of their

job is to allow their clients to feel heard. As a nurse, you have a unique opportunity to allow people who are often sad, lonely, bored, and perhaps depressed to talk and build some sort of a community in what can feel like isolation. But that means you need to talk less than the patient does. Certainly, you will need to talk, interact, and build a relationship. Be aware, though, that while you have coworkers, family, friends, and others to talk to, sometimes the patient has only you. Many people pay counselors a large amount of money just to have someone to talk to; as a nurse, you get to be that person for so many people in the hospital setting.

As a person talks, note what he or she says and start to ask the worldview questions to yourself. If a patient says that people are praying for him, that remark doesn't tell you anything about his worldview necessarily. In contrast, if the patient says that he has asked people to pray for him, now we know something about what he believes. A person does not ask for prayer unless he believes in a higher being (or he's doing it as a means of appeasing someone). In the same vein, if someone says, "In a past life I'm sure...," that might be an indication she holds to reincarnation. However, you also have to note how she said it. Was she laughing? Did it sound like a joking statement? Did she sound serious? Often when listening, we need to hear not only the words, but also the way the words are said.

Clearly, it can be difficult to fully grasp what a person believes because communication involves so many nuances. Does a certain intonation mean sarcasm for this patient, as it does in another? Does that sigh mean sadness, or does it signal contentment? These types of communication barriers can be overcome only by the intentional work of caring about a person and getting to know that individual not merely as a patient, and not merely as a problem you need to resolve before taking your break, but as a person made in God's image. As you determine to care for your patients in this way, you will begin to understand their beliefs more, and you will find it easier to think the way that they think. Doing this will help you communicate more readily with them on all topics, but in particular on issues of spiritual depth.

Possibly the largest chasm to cross in understanding someone's worldview is the same chasm that we face in understanding our own worldview. Oftentimes, we do not believe what we say we believe. However, we know it about ourselves. Because we cannot read our patients' minds, we cannot determine if what they are saying indicates what they actually believe, or what they want to believe, or what they think they believe. It might seem odd to suggest that people don't believe what they say they believe; however, it happens often. Consider a person who smokes cigarettes. At this stage, it is very unlikely that she doesn't know that smoking is harmful for her; in fact, she will probably affirm that she believes smoking is harmful for her—and yet she still smokes. This disparity leaves us with two possible conclusions: (1) While the person intellectually affirms that smoking is harmful, she doesn't actually believe that it will harm her; or (2) she does believe that smoking can or will harm her, but she doesn't care. The first conclusion is frequently correct, as people often know that something is harmful, yet still do the action. Michel Foucault (1990), a philosopher and founder of the Burning Man festival, died of AIDS because, while he knew going to San Francisco bathhouses of the early 1980s was risky, he still pursued this behavior. He even went so far as to claim that "sex is worth dying for" (p. 156).

In many cases, for both yourself and your patients, what you do might be a better indication of your real worldview, or what you truly believe, than what you say you believe. The person who absolutely does not believe in ghosts has no need to be scared of a haunted house, and an atheist has absolutely no reason to pray. In fact, if an atheist/materialist in your care asks for prayer, it may be a crack in the armor that has been built up to suppress the fact that, according to Romans 1, at their core, everyone believes in God.

Because you will be constantly gaining new information about your patients' beliefs, you need to be constantly restructuring where you place them in a worldview structure. Mind you, you also need to be doing the same thing to yourself. If you have a deeply held belief and then realize that all of your actions contradict it, you need to ask yourself if you actually believe it. All relationships are dynamic, and as they deepen, you will see that beliefs are constantly changing, strengthening, and weakening—and it takes time and effort to keep up with all the ebbs and flows. However, doing so helps make you a more compassionate person and, in turn, a more compassionate nurse.

Thinking in Another Person's Worldview

Before we discuss how to think in other worldviews, it is important to stress that thinking like someone else does not mean agreeing with someone else. A large communication gulf exists in our society because too often people have equated trying to understand how someone else thinks with agreeing with that person's conclusions. This association isn't completely unmerited. In many cases, when we begin to think like another person, two things happen.

First, we begin to understand how the other person makes certain connections that our own mind wouldn't naturally put together. This experience of seeing connections in other worldviews can begin to make those worldviews make sense in such a way that you might call your own views into question, particularly if you begin to find this other worldview's connections to be more intellectually satisfying.

Second, thinking in someone else's worldview begins to humanize the person and builds empathy for that individual. When you put on someone else's world for an hour or so, and then you return to your own, you become less callous and stoic toward the other person's worldview. Even if you still adamantly disagree with those beliefs, you are often a bit softer toward the person, and if you care for the person, you become somewhat more likely to alter your views. These two phenomena are the great fear in our present culture: If we begin to think like someone else, and that person does not return the favor, then we might begin to soften, and it will be harder to disagree and shun those outside our religious, political, racial, gendered, or other tribe. However, learning this skill is vital to communication, and to every form of ministry.

Another point to consider when trying to think like another person is to realize that, while that person's conclusions might make sense in his or her worldview, that **subjective** experience does not change objective reality. Conversely, because every person is a subject, when we think about the objective, we always think about it subjectively. For example, when it is 77°F in a room, it is objectively 77°F in a room. However, my friend and I can have different subjective experiences of that objective reality. When the temperature is 77°F outside, my friend might put on a sweater because she's a little chilly. In contrast, I will have a fan on, if not the air conditioner, because my subjective experience of 77°F is different than hers, even though the temperature is objectively the same. When we approach matters of creation, meaning, purpose, and other big issues, it is possible for a person to have a coherent worldview, or draw a coherent subjective conclusion, that is not objectively true.

This last point is key for understanding how to think like other people. It is very easy for us to dismiss other people's arguments or conclusions as being wrong, but we have to ask how they came to that conclusion. Perhaps they reached this conclusion in a goodhearted or noble manner, but their starting place was wrong. Just as in algebra class back in high school, it helps here to show your work to determine where things went wrong, or perhaps went in a different direction. If someone believes life has no purpose, but he also believes that there is no God and everything is a product of chance, energy, and time, then he has a fairly consistent belief. You can see how he came to that conclusion. That does not mean that the person is right that objectively life has no meaning, but it does mean that subjectively the way he reads the world leads to

that conclusion. Understanding that the starting point of his belief lies in a universe created by random chance, you can now try to think the way he does, try to inhabit that world, and then start to ask questions (to yourself, not necessarily to the patient) that you, as a visitor to this world, wouldn't understand. If life has no purpose, can we say that anything is actually getting better? How can we say things are morally better than other things?

Perhaps a good example of this phenomenon is the abortion debate. The conversations that happen around the topic of abortion are heated, entrenched, and almost never helpful. This lack of progress reflects that in almost every conversation one has on the matter, and in almost every debate that one sees on the matter, the people involved are having two different conversations. This shouldn't surprise us: They are coming from two different worlds, and if both sides could put on the other person's worldview just for an hour, the conversation would look very different. The fact that both parties are having different conversations can even be seen in the names used for the two sides, for example, pro-choice and pro-life. Although these labels are presented as opposites, the opposite of "choice" is not "life," and the opposite of "life" is not "choice." If you were to ask a pro-choice person if she is pro-death, she would almost certainly say no. Conversely, if you were to ask a pro-life person if she is pro-totalitarianism, she also would most assuredly say no. These labels tell us nothing about the objective reality of abortion, but they tell us a great deal about the subjective reality of those involved in the conversation.

The person who claims to be pro-choice is starting from a place in which her position is arguing about the rights of the woman carrying the baby. The person who is pro-life is starting from a place in which she is arguing about the rights of the baby in the womb. Almost universally, what is revealed in these conversations is that both sides affirm women's rights, and both sides cherish the lives of babies; the tension between them arises from the worldview starting place as to whether the entity in the womb is a human person or a potential human person. For this reason, the labels "pro-choice" and "pro-life" should really be replaced with the more accurate "pro-abortion on demand" and "anti-abortion on demand," respectively, in that the latter labels are less rhetorical and focus more particularly on the actual debate. These labels also reveal that the heated debates over the conclusions that people have drawn are actually based on initial presuppositions.

Of course, the debate does not automatically evaporate if both sides think like the other—but it does allow for better conversation. Statements like "Pro-life people don't respect women" and "Pro-choice people don't care about babies" disappear when we understand that fundamentally while we subjectively believe that the other's view indicates an objective dismissal of women's rights/baby's rights, the other person subjectively doesn't believe so. Understanding this fact allows us to try to inhabit the other's view and to show disparities within it. For the pro-life person, for example, the goal then becomes not to win a debate about a baby's right to life, but rather to help the pro-choice person see that the entity in the womb is a human person. That becomes a constructive discussion.

This example may have seemed like a long rabbit trail, but it is a key example of the importance of trying to think in another person's worldview. When someone says something that you find shocking, and perhaps unbelievable, it is helpful to stop and ask, "How did he get there?" Realizing that he is relying on a different framework than you have adopted can be a great tool to understanding how this shocking conclusion makes sense to him. Further, by being able to put on his worldview assumptions, you can see more fully how he drew these conclusions (**CASE STUDY 9-1**). One way to practice this is to watch your favorite

🔍 CASE STUDY 9-1

Sally and Sherman are expecting their first child. At a routine physician's visit, they are told that the baby has a chromosomal abnormality and will have Down syndrome. The parents are devastated. After hearing the news from the Christian physician, the couple is still sitting in the exam room: Sally is weeping, and Sherman is visibly angry. Sally was raised in a strict Catholic home and would never consider an abortion. Sherman claims to be an atheist and wants Sally to abort the baby. Sally has already refused to have this conversation, but she is not sure that she can care for a baby with serious physical problems. If you were the nurse entering the room in this situation, immediately after the news was given, what would you do?

Questions

1. What is the first thing you would say to this couple?
2. What worldview does Sherman probably hold? What worldview does Sally hold? How can you better relate to them in this situation if you understand their worldview?
3. What options do you think the physician presented to them? How do you give information to this couple without violating your own personal beliefs about the sanctity of life? About when life begins?
4. Where can you refer Sally for comfort and support?
5. Can you use therapeutic listening in this situation? What about prayer? What are some appropriate strategies in this case, given the difference in Sally's and Sherman's worldviews?
6. How would you deal with Sherman if he asks you about abortion clinics or physicians who perform abortions?
7. How do you feel about a situation in which it is known that a child will be born with a disability or abnormality?

movie or TV show and ask yourself, "How did the villain come to those conclusions?" Think through the villain's position and see if you can come to an understanding of why the villain is doing what he or she does—but perhaps stop before you see the villain as the hero.

As we conclude this section, it is important to again emphasize that things in the world are objectively one way or the other. Things are objectively morally right or morally wrong; however, from our standpoints we interact with these objective realities in a subjective manner. The hope, the goal, is to understand the objective world accurately, and to assist others in augmenting their subjective understanding of the world to mirror the objective reality of the world. This task requires prayer, patience, boldness, intentionality, and a constant stream of nourishment from the one who created objective reality in the form of His word and His people.

▸ Communicating Your Worldview Indirectly

One last point to consider as we think through the matter of worldview and communication is that very often, owing to the nature of your workplace, you won't be able to initiate explicitly Christian conversations. If a patient starts the conversation, there may be ways to guide it there, or if you have a visible tattoo or an accessory of a Christian nature, that might spark a question. Nevertheless, more often than not, your ministry will have to be one that is not expressly verbally Christian, though that does not mean it is not deeply rooted in the gospel or in your Christian conviction.

The phrase "Preach the gospel always, use words when necessary" has become a Christian cliché that is either deeply loved or adamantly despised. This quote is often attributed to St. Francis of Assisi, even though it has never been found in any of his writings and does not appear anywhere until the late 1980s (almost 1000 years after Francis's death). Nevertheless,

whoever made up the phrase understood St. Francis rather well, because it does sound like something he would say. Those who dislike this phrase do so because they see it as an excuse to never share the gospel verbally. They look at Paul's statements such as Roman 10:14—"How then will they call on him in whom they have not believed? And how are they to believe in him of whom they have never heard? And how are they to hear without someone preaching?"—and properly conclude that saving faith in Christ only comes from the explicit communication of the gospel.

Still, there is merit to what this cliché says. St. Francis emphasized the dynamic relation between God and His creation, in which His love is constantly changing the created world, and His creation is constantly pouring forth praise (hence the hymn "All Creatures of Our God and King"). Seen in this light, the quote may be alluding to what Paul chastises the Corinthian church for in 1 Corinthians 13:1: "If I speak in the tongues of men and of angels, but have not love, I am a noisy gong or a clanging cymbal." Salvation comes by hearing, but if what is heard is not loving, then it often does more harm than good.

In your position as a nurse, you will very rarely be able to explicitly share the gospel (though you should pray often for the opportunity to do so). Instead, you should seek to display the transforming power of the gospel in how you care for your patients, in how you talk to and about your coworkers, in how you treat staff in other departments, and so on. The great commandment tells us that we are to love God and love our neighbor as ourselves. The love of neighbor comes from our love of God. In the same way that when we love a person, we start to care for the music, movies, and shows that that person loves, so the more that we love God, the more that we will love what God loves. Because God loves all people, deeply loving God will transform you into a nurse who sees the patient not as a problem to fix, but as a person loved by God, and who sees your annoying coworker not as a person to tolerate, but rather as an image bearer of God whose eternal soul God deeply cares about—and therefore you ought to as well.

In light of the command to love so deeply, we can see that while communicating the gospel always requires words, embodying and living out the transforming truth of the gospel is something that we do implicitly every hour of the day. In fact, if we don't, our shortcomings call us to return to our own worldview and question what we hold at the center of our belief system. You may not be able to expressly communicate initially that God loves a coworker, or a patient in your care, but you can communicate that you deeply care for them, because if you are following Christ fully, you do. From there, you can wait for opportunities to explicitly express your worldview in ways that make sense in light of their worldview, so as to cross the "language divide" that we introduced at the beginning of this chapter. Maybe you'll have the opportunity, or maybe you won't. In any case, you do have the opportunity to be the manifestation of God's compassion for this patient, for this coworker, and for this person. To do nursing as ministry, you seize upon that opportunity and praise God for the chance to love the neighbor in this way.

▶ Clinical Reasoning Exercises

Read the Taylor et al. (2018) article summarized in **BOX 9-1**. Explain your agreement or disagreement with the researchers' general conclusion based on their data: "Nurses working in a faith-based organization were 276% more likely to believe they could initiate such conversation and 153% more likely to think they could initiate an offer of prayer" (p. 2381).

1. Do you think that this result can be generalized to most faith-based nurses?
2. Have you ever worked with a faith-community nurse? Do you

have one in your place of worship? What is the role of that nurse within the church? Explain how he or she could use an understanding of others' worldviews (**BOX 9-2**) to provide culturally sensitive care in the community environment or within the church.

▶ Personal Reflection Exercises

Answer the eight questions posed in the first part of this chapter. What does this tell you about your own worldview? On what do you

BOX 9-1 Research Highlight

The researchers in this study used a cross-sectional quantitative design to explore nurses' opinions about starting religious or spiritual conversations during patient care. An online survey was used to collect data from 445 nurses in a convenience volunteer sample. The survey measured various aspects of religiosity and nurses' opinions about introducing spiritual care with patients. The findings showed that the vast majority of nurses (90%) believed it was appropriate to start a conversation about spiritual things, and 75% of nurses responding would use self-disclosure or offer prayer with patients. The more religious a nurse rated himself or herself, the more likely he or she was to initiate such a conversation. "Nurses working in a faith-based organization were 276% more likely to believe they could initiate such conversation and 153% more likely to think they could initiate an offer of prayer" (p. 2381). Thus, a nurse's personal faith and working environment were found to influence whether the patient's spirituality was discussed.

Modified from Taylor, E. J., Gober-Park, C., Schoonover-Shoffner, K., Mamier, I., Somaiya, C. K., & Bahjri, K. (2018). Nurse opinions about initiating spiritual conversation and prayer in patient care. *Journal of Advanced Nursing, 74*(10), 2381–2392.

BOX 9-2 Evidence-Based Practice Focus

In this edited medical book with many contributors, the authors discuss spirituality in nearly every medical specialty. Within the 22 chapters, there is content on religion and spirituality in obstetrics/gynecology, pediatrics, family practice, psychiatry, family medicine, surgery, gerontology, oncology, palliative care, the intensive care unit, medical ethics, education, and nursing. Perspectives from many different disciplines, including sociology, law, theology, and psychology, are provided. The authors state that the book's purpose is to explore questions that arise about religion and spirituality in real-life patient cases provided by each of the chapter authors. This work represents an interprofessional look at the topic but emphasizes the physician as the leader of the team.

Modified from Balboni, M., & Peteet, J. (Eds.). (2017). *Spirituality and religion within the culture of medicine: From evidence to practice*. Oxford, UK: Oxford University Press.

base your assumptions? How would you describe your worldview?

1. Have you worked with patients whose worldview was radically different than your own?
2. How did you feel about this? Were you able to approach the subject of spiritual care?
3. What is your own personal style for integrating spiritual care with your daily nursing?
4. How comfortable do you feel initiating a discussion about spiritual things with your patients or residents? Why do you think you feel comfortable or uncomfortable?

References

Dennett, D. C. (1991). *Consciousness explained*. New York, NY: Back Bay Books.

Foucault, M. (1990). *The history of sexuality* (reissue ed., Vol. 1). *Vol. 1. An introduction*. New York, NY: Vintage.

Harris, S. (2010). *The moral landscape: How science can determine human values*. New York, NY: Free Press.

Moreland, J. P. (2017). *Kingdom triangle: Recover the Christian mind, renovate the soul, restore the spirit's power*. Grand Rapids, MI: Zondervan.

Sagain, C., & Malone, A. (Director). (1980). The shores of the cosmic ocean. In *Cosmos*. Arlington, VA: PBS.

Singer, P. (n.d.). Frequently asked questions. Retrieved from https://petersinger.info/faq/

Sire, J. W. (2009). *The universe next door: A basic worldview catalog* (5th ed.). Downers Grove, IL: IVP Academic.

Zacharias, R. (2018). Think again: Deep questions. Retrieved from https://www.rzim.org/read/just-thinking-magazine/think-again-deep-questions

Recommended Readings

Barnum, B. S. (2011). *Spirituality in nursing: The challenges of complexity*. New York, NY: Springer.

Duckham, B. C., & Schreiber, J. C. (2016). Bridging worldviews through phenomenology. *Social Work & Christianity*, *43*(4), 55–67.

Galloway, S., & Hand, M. W. (2017). Spiritual immersion: Developing and evaluating a simulation exercise to teach spiritual care to undergraduate nursing students. *Nurse Educator*, *42*(4), 199–203.

O'Brien, M. E. (2003). *Parish nursing: Healthcare ministry within the church*. Sudbury, MA: Jones and Bartlett.

O'Brien, M. E. (2017). *Spirituality in nursing*. Burlington, MA: Jones & Bartlett Learning.

Shelly, J. A., & Miller, A. B. (2006). *Called to care: A Christian worldview for nursing*. Downers Grove, IL: InterVarsity Press.

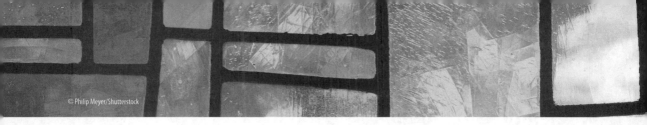
© Philip Meyer/Shutterstock

CHAPTER 10

Nursing as Ministry for Diverse Populations and Faiths

Alfonso Espinosa, PhD, MDiv, MA.

LEARNING OBJECTIVES

At the end of this chapter, the reader will be able to:

1. Describe the role of the Christian nurse.
2. Understand that the one who nourishes must be nourished.
3. Apply the universal articles of the faith to everyone served.
4. Analyze those being served to find common ground and build bridges for the gospel.
5. Evaluate responses to find new ways for expressing love, mercy, and compassion through other avenues if necessary.
6. Create a personalized approach for living out God's bearing and carrying toward diverse populations and faiths.

KEY TERMS

Divine monergism
God-man
Image of Christ
Objective gospel

Original (hereditary) sin
Subjective faith
Universal atonement
Universal truths

Vicarious satisfaction
Vocations

▶ Nursing and Its Relationship to the Ministry of Jesus Christ

Nursing is a God-given vocation, a calling that innately reflects the very nature of God. By understanding the basis for this assertion, we become able to demonstrate why nursing is ideally suited for serving people from diverse populations and faiths. First, however, we need to consider the Biblical foundations as to *why* nursing represents the nature of God. Once this is established, the universal application of God's love and mercy—regardless of culture or creed—will be evident.

Biblical Foundations

Deuteronomy 1:31: "God carried you"

In Exodus 34:6, God reveals Himself to Moses as "merciful and gracious" (English Standard Version [ESV]), and St. John states in the New Testament, "God is love" (1 John 4:19). Streaming from His love and mercy is the concrete evidence of His nature—namely, the *doing* of love and mercy. When someone is thirsty, love and mercy give drink. Any other "love" or "mercy" that is unwilling to *act* is merely theoretical and non-authentic. Nursing from a Christian perspective to diverse populations and faiths is helped by this insight on the nature of God: "God is merciful. God shows favor—*khesed* [the Old Testament Hebrew word for lovingkindness, steadfast love]—to man in spite of the unworthiness of man caused by his miserable condition of sin" (Espinosa, 2016, p. 211). This crucial insight informs us that God *is* in this way—merciful, loving, and compassionate—regardless of the condition of the object of His mercy and love. That is, the inherent impartiality of the Hippocratic Oath is consistent with God's very nature of love and mercy.

There is nothing within the one for whom He is loving and merciful toward that negates God's compassion. Likewise, there is nothing within the one whom the nurse serves that disqualifies this person from God's love and mercy for him or her, regardless of any prejudice within the society that would discriminate against the one served. It is really that simple: Those who represent God (such as the Christian nurse) represent these attributes of His nature to all they serve. The Christian nurse, therefore, is an ambassador of God's universal love and mercy.

Such service *must* act—concretely—and be received by the one being served. Intentionality translates into actual helping. It is easy to talk about love and mercy, but the goal in Christian nursing is for these properties to be *incarnational*. St. James warns against the delusion of words (or mere intention) without action: "If a brother or sister is poorly clothed and lacking in daily food, and one of you says to them, 'Go in peace, be warmed and filled,' without giving them the things needed for the body, what good is that?'" (James 2:15–16). Nursing happens to be a natural launching pad for genuine mercy and lovingkindness, the very manifestation of God's presence in the world.

Nursing comes from the Latin word *nutrire*, which means "to nourish." *Nurse* in Latin is *nutrix*. This concept "to nourish" is fascinating as expressed in the Holy Scripture. The New Testament includes a Greek word—*tropophoreo*—that means "bring one nourishment." This same Greek word was used in the Greek translation of the Old Testament (known as the *Septuagint* or *LXX*) demonstrating that this idea is included in *both* testaments.

The Greek word *tropophoreo* appears within Deuteronomy 1:31. The one who engages in this action exemplifies the concept of to "bring one nourishment" (Liddell & Scott, 1968, p. 1828). It is helpful, however, to consider the actual Old Testament Hebrew word—and therefore the older word—translated as *tropophoreo* in the Greek.

The original Hebrew word in Deuteronomy 1:31 is *nasa*. *Nasa* means—specifically—"bearing or carrying" (Harris, Archer, & Waltke, 1980, p. 601). The translators of the *LXX* believed that the best way to describe the Lord helping His people in Israel was via nourishing them (or, if we may be so bold, nursing them). The actual Hebrew word may refer to bearing physical loads, but it is also the same word used to describe what Christ did for us when he bore the sins of many (Harris et al., 1980, p. 601). Isaiah 53:4 states in reference to the Christ, "Surely he has borne our griefs and carried our sorrows." That is, *nasa* has a range of meaning, and it is enlightening to see how bearing/nourishing relates to the saving work of Jesus Christ.

Let us consider Deuteronomy 1:31 more closely. This verse describes a more practical kind of bearing: "[The Lord your God was with you] in the wilderness, where you have seen how the Lord your God carried you, as a man carries his son." *Nasa* is here depicted as God *carrying* his people. Nurses help the languished person; they sustain the one in need. Nurses enter the lives of sufferers and help bear their load. Certainly, such bearing by the Lord must have been multifaceted, and nursing reflects this sense of bearing and carrying those whom nurses serve.

It is easy to see the mercy–love connection—living as an expression of the very nature of God—in this bearing/nourishing. Galatians 6:2 says, "Bear one another's burdens, and so fulfill the law of Christ." And what is the law of Christ? It is love (see the "new command" of Christ as recorded in John 13). What does love do? It bears the burdens of others. What do nurses do? They bear the burdens of others. Nurses demonstrate the love and mercy of God in concrete ways that help and nourish those whom they serve. They epitomize and make incarnational the love of Christ by bearing and carrying the one in need; in turn, the one in need is nourished and helped.

This is an inspirational way of seeing Christ in the nursing ministry vocation. Christ bears us up as he helps, heals, and saves. Furthermore, concepts such as bearing and carrying elicit the idea of physical contact. This is not an incidental point: Jesus made physical contact a regular part of his public ministry. The Gospels record numerous accounts of Christ healing as he touched. As the incarnate God, Christ did not *need* to touch to heal (as if his power depended on it), but his bearing/nourishing ministry was made manifest through physical contact nonetheless, and the receiver of his love was powerfully affirmed in his love *through* his touch.

Mark 1:40–41 is an example of Christ having physical contact with those he served. In this text, a leper implored Christ and knelt before him. He said to the Lord, "If you will, you can make me clean." The next verse (41) records: "Moved with pity, [Jesus] stretched out his hand and touched him and said to him, 'I will; be clean.'" Jesus had love and mercy toward the leper, and his touching him signified the Lord's bearing/nourishing ministry to a man who was otherwise considered an outcast in his society. In such scenes, we are led to the result of Christ's ministry as echoed in Psalm 103:2–3, "Bless the Lord, O my soul, and forget not all his benefits, who forgives all your iniquity, who heals all your diseases." And again—concretely—when did the Lord especially do this? He did so as Isaiah described Christ bearing our griefs and carrying our sorrows (see Isaiah 53:4), which, of course, applies to the Lord's cross at Calvary.

Acts 13:18: "[God] put up with them"

The Greek word *tropophoreo* ("to bring one nourishment") is also used in the New Testament itself (Liddell & Scott, 1968). Acts 13:18 provides further insight: "And for about forty years he put up with them in the wilderness." This translation "put up with them" inherently signals patience and long-suffering (extended and genuine love through sacrificial service). Bauer (1979), in *A Greek–English Lexicon of the New Testament*, define the word in Acts 13:18 specifically as "[to] carry in one's arms, i.e., care for . . . someone (tenderly)" (p. 828). Furthermore, the root word, *trophos*, means "nurse" (p. 827). The word is recorded in 1 Thessalonians 2:7: "But we were gentle among you, like a nursing mother taking care of her own children." Indeed, this biblical nursing is characterized by tenderness.

This insight from Acts 13:18 (and its complement from 1 Thessalonians 2:7) adds tremendous reason to view the nursing vocation as holy and as an occasion for expressing God's peculiar care for people. Christian nurses are not simply going through the motions. The one they are bearing up and nourishing is the one they "carry" in a tender way. That is, nurses in Christ not only bring with them the love and mercy of Christ in their actions, but they do so tenderly, which is the heart of Christ. God's love and mercy reside in the spirit of Christian nurses as they serve. This is not "putting up with [those served]" begrudgingly, but willingly, with the goal of expressing the tender care residing in the nurse whose life is in Christ. In this way, the Christian nurse becomes the epitome of what a Christian is. This is how Martin Luther described it in *The Freedom of a Christian* written in 1520:

> Hence, as our heavenly Father has in Christ freely come to our aid, we also ought freely help our neighbor through our body and its works, and each one should become as it were a Christ to the other that we may be Christs to one another and Christ may be the same in all, that is, that we may be truly Christians. (Luther, 1957, pp. 367–368)

The Church, the Body of Christ, Has Always Served This Way

Around the time of Cyprian (A.D. third century), the Christian church had been—and continued to be—the center of caring for those in need. Uhlhorn (2007) records this important history: "As yet institutions did not exist. There was no need of houses of hospitality, houses for foreigners, orphanages, hospitals, so long as every Christian house was an asylum" (p. 123). This was the tradition of the church. Christians' heartbeat and impulse were to live out faith in Christ by serving those in need. It is important to be aware that when Christ teaches examples of piety (holy living) in the Sermon on the Mount at Matthew 6, he begins with almsgiving (giving to the needy). The church was quite simply concerned for the well-being of others; it was following Jesus's teaching.

Acts 2 provides immediate insight into the life of the earliest Christian church. After St. Luke gives a lucid description of the public worship services at verse 42, we encounter this description of the daily life of Christians in the church at verses 44–45: "And all who believed were together and had all things in common. And they were selling their possessions and belongings and distributing the proceeds to all, as any had need."

Evidence shows that for the first 300 years of its existence, the church's strong practice was to bear and nourish those who were sick, especially if they were fellow Christians. Eusebius, the ancient Christian historian, preserved a letter from Bishop Dionysius of Alexandria that describes the nursing activity of the early church within the Body of Christ. It is remarkable:

> Most of our brethren, in the fullness of their brotherly love, did not spare themselves. They mutually took care of each other, and as instead of preserving themselves they attended on the sick, and willingly did them service for Christ's sake, they joyfully laid down their lives with them. Many died after having been by their exertions the means of restoring others. The best among the brethren, many presbyters, deacons, and distinguished

laymen ended their lives in this manner, so that their deaths, which were the result of piety and strong faith, seem not inferior to martyrdom. Many who took into their hands and laid upon their bosoms the bodies of Christian brothers, closed their mouths and eyes, and reverently interred them, soon followed them in death. (Uhlhorn, 2007, pp. 188–189)

Advancing into the fourth century, as Uhlhorn (2007) puts it, "the whole period had a strong propensity to institutions" (p. 324). Matching these institutions were the corresponding servants. These Christians were doing the Biblical verb *diakonein* ("to minister, to provide for, or to help someone"); those who served in this ministry were *diakonos* ("deacons") and took part in the general service called *diakonia*, which means "ministry" or "service" (Olson, 1992, pp. 22–23). In the Holy Scripture, these words are also applied to Jesus himself (Matthew 20:28; Mark 10:45; Luke 22:27), his followers, and their work (Olson, 1992, p. 23).

To bear the title *diakonos* is to be known for giving—to an extraordinary degree—basic help. It might even be rendered as "busboy" (Keller, 1997, p. 56). Keller writes, "This is the Christian pattern of greatness and the pattern of Christ's work. He came to render the most humble, basic kind of service" (p. 56). While the disciples debated about which of them was the greatest, the Lord Jesus Christ described Christian distinction this way as recorded at Luke 22:26b: "Rather, let the greatest among you become as the youngest, and the leader as one who serves." Such service emulates the service of Christ.

Olson (1992) points out that the "diaconal care of the sick and dying developed in the fourth and fifth centuries into an order of men called *parabolani* [or "sick-nurse" in the Christian Church (Liddell & Scott, 1968, Supplement p. 114)] who attended the sick in some larger eastern churches such as that of Alexandria" (p. 61). Uhlhorn (2007) describes their duties as including the seeking out of the sick and suffering so as to lead them into the hospitals, and then attend on them while there.

By the reign of Emperor Justinian in the sixth century, the emperor's legislation had established a wide gamut of institutions, which included *nosocomia* ("houses for the sick") (Uhlhorn, 2007, pp. 329–330). Both the formation of hospitals and those who served in them were well on their way. What is humbling (and exciting) to consider, however, was that such servants were and are in the image of Jesus Christ, who, according to Matthew 20:28, "came not to be served but to serve, and to give his life as a ransom for many."

▶ The Service Ministry of the Christian Nurse

As the prior discussion suggests, today's nurse who follows Jesus is conducting a continuation of the service rendered by the diaconate, those who serve in the **image of Christ**. The very origins of nursing are steeped in showing Jesus's love and mercy through the care of the sick and the suffering. Christian nurses bring Christ to those whom they serve and imitate Jesus, who came not to be served, but to serve. The early Christians demonstrated this so powerfully that it was easy to see their bearing, nourishing, and carrying. They did so sometimes—as has been noted—even to the extent of giving up their own lives to serve others. It is hard to think of other **vocations** that so innately show the love of Christ to the world.

Given the clear correspondence between nursing and the ministry of Jesus Christ, it is beneficial to consider Jesus's own ministry. By considering the Lord's way firsthand, the nurse becomes better informed about the ministry of those who seek to be his ambassadors to the world. Much may be gleaned from the Lord's ministry that may powerfully equip the Christian nurse.

At the same time—and here we enter the most important part—we cannot reduce nursing to the task of simply replicating and imitating the Lord Jesus Christ. There is only one Savior. There is only one Lord. What is crucial to grasp in the consideration of his ministry is that he is the nurse of nurses. He is the helper of those who help. He is the healer of those who heal. He is the one who bears those called to bear. We must understand that the Christian nurse is as much an object of Christ's love and mercy as anyone whom the nurse will serve. We continue by considering the Lord's one-of-a-kind ministry, which is not so much about a call for emulation as it is a call for personal reception. In this way, Christ is formed in the servant of God. In this way, Jesus works through nurses, who in themselves can do nothing (John 15).

The Unique Ministry of the Lord Jesus Christ Empowers the Christian Nurse

Luke 10:25–37: The Parable of the Good Samaritan

The terminology "Good Samaritan" is well known in the world of medicine. Indeed, many hospitals and medical centers use this name. In addition, the label "Good Samaritan" is often applied to any person who comes to the aid of another, especially if the one helped faces dire circumstances. It is not uncommon for national news stories to highlight the "Good Samaritan" who saves the life of another. Indeed, this terminology has popular, cultural usage. The true significance of the symbol-metaphor, however, can be properly known only in its original context—namely, the Holy Scriptures, and specifically in St. Luke's Gospel, the tenth chapter, verses 25–37:

> [25]And behold, a lawyer stood up to put him to the test, saying, "Teacher, what shall I do to inherit eternal life?"

> [26]He said to him, "What is written in the Law? How do you read it?" [27]And he answered, "You shall love the Lord your God with all your heart and with all your soul and with all your strength and with all your mind, and your neighbor as yourself." [28]And he said to him, "You have answered correctly; do this, and you will live." [29]But he, desiring to justify himself, said to Jesus, "And who is my neighbor?" [30]Jesus replied, "A man was going down from Jerusalem to Jericho, and he fell among robbers, who stripped him and beat him and departed, leaving him half dead. [31]Now by chance a priest was going down the road, and when he saw him he passed by on the other side. [32]So likewise a Levite, when he came to the place and saw him, passed by on the other side. [33]But a Samaritan, as he journeyed, came to where he was, and when he saw him, he had compassion. [34]He went to him and bound up his wounds, pouring on oil and wine. Then he set him on his own animal and brought him to an inn and took care of him. [35]And the next day he took out two denarii and gave them to the innkeeper, saying, 'Take care of him, and whatever more you spend, I will repay you when I come back.' [36]Which of these three, do you think, proved to be a neighbor to the man who fell among the robbers?" [37]He said, "The one who showed him mercy." And Jesus said to him, "You go, and do likewise."

As Arthur A. Just Jr. (1997) points out, it is typically assumed that this story is a lesson in morality. Such a view contends that the Good Samaritan teaches us how to treat our neighbor. This interpretation, however, misses the crucial point: *Jesus* is the Good Samaritan. All the other characters in this account are reflections of sinful humanity.

At first glance, this seems overstated. Doesn't Jesus direct his listener in the simplest terms: "go, and do likewise"? Isn't this as clear as moral imperatives come? The answer is, "It depends." If one approaches this story as a command for us to do something in an effort to be righteous and justified in ourselves (as the lawyer approached it), then the moral imperative will set us up for utter and complete failure. In our sin, we are unable to serve to this extent. We are just too instinctual about self-preservation. More will be said in a moment when we consider the conduct of the priest and Levite.

In contrast, if it is believed upon (trusted in the heart) and confessed (with our sincere words) that Jesus Christ is the only true Good Samaritan, then Christian nurses may then go forth by learning how Christ might work *through* them as the true Good Samaritan. That is, the moral imperative can be fulfilled only by Christ, whether in terms of his public ministry conducted 2000 years ago or through his current ministry lived in and through his servants. Either way, Christians never pat themselves on the back, thinking they have—in themselves—the strength or the wherewithal to live such a life of selfless sacrificial bearing. Such a life is Jesus's life alone.

In the Biblical era, the way to Jericho included navigating a perilous canyon, the perfect location for robbers and thieves to hide and wait for their victims. Keller (1997) paints the comparison of walking through a dangerous dark alley at night in modern times and being fully aware of the danger, then seeing a total stranger lying on the ground dying (or at least appearing as though dying). Is it a trap? Are those who did this to the dying man still close by? Does it appear that this man on the ground is about to die anyway? Should a person risk his or her own life in this case, or take the smarter route and find assistance to bring back? It is easy to imagine many reasons one might hesitate to do anything at all.

The excuses for inaction, however, are punctuated in the parable's introduction of the priest and Levite. This argument would assuredly appeal to the lawyer listening to Christ's answer to his question, "And who is my neighbor?" The desire of the sinful ear, mind, and heart is to stick to legalities. Pastors, nurses, and other servants all want to know—for their own justification for action or inaction—about the law. What is right? What is wrong? This is a stumbling block for every servant of the Living God.

Dietrich Bonhoeffer (1955) is profound in describing our legalistic tendencies in his book *Ethics:* "For man in the state of disunion good consists in passing judgment and the ultimate criterion is man himself. Knowing good and evil, man is essentially judge" (p. 30). Here, universal service and compassion are limited because the person who claims to know God will easily justify why he or she might serve some, but not others. Sinful humanity wants to take God's place and become a judge: "Some deserve my service; others do not." In the Good Samaritan story, the lawyer was this way, and so was the priest and Levite.

Jesus intends for all who have sin to be able to relate. If one were to simply reason, "Well, I have no choice but to serve anyone I am assigned to serve, so of course I will serve anyone," then such reason focuses only on the external action to the exclusion of the internal impulse. Are *all* served with the same love and mercy despite their status, their legal innocence or guilt, their goodness, their evil, and/ or their resemblance to obvious stereotypes? If we are honest, then Jesus's story of the Good Samaritan will convict us.

If anyone might be the exception to judgmental legalism, then one might expect the priest and Levite to meet that criterion. Unfortunately, they merely punctuate the problem. They were associated with the temple in Jerusalem. As Joel B. Green (1997) points out, their inclusion highlighted what every Jew was aware of: There were "boundaries between clean and unclean, including clean and unclean people . . . their association with the temple commends them as persons of exemplary piety whose actions would be regarded as self-evidently righteous" (p. 431). Their walking past the man lying for dead was proof that they believed their status exempted them from helping the man left for dead. Because they loved their self-righteousness, they cut themselves off from having love and mercy for the dying man.

Bonhoeffer (1955), however, does not restrict love to a quality generated by human affection, conviction, or action. It is even more than the *action* discussed in the first section of this chapter. Bonhoeffer explains: "Love, then, is the revelation of God. And the revelation of God is Jesus Christ. . . . Love is not an attitude of men but an attitude of God" (pp. 50–51). The only way *any* person can be recognized as *neighbor* is through the absolute and unconditional Savior of *all*, who is in his very nature love and mercy. In Christ, there is never differentiation between people served. The lawyer needed teaching on this point because his question implied that—in his mind—some people were *not* his neighbor (Just, 1997, p. 452).

To help the hard-hearted lawyer, Jesus continued to tell the story by introducing someone who would surely be among those excluded from the lawyer's version of *neighbor*. The Lord Christ introduced—from a Jewish/true Israelites' perspective—a scandalous figure: a Samaritan. Samaritans were people from the northern kingdom who embraced open idolatry; they were half-breeds and sworn enemies. Indeed, when Jesus himself had offended the Jews, they called *him* a Samaritan while rejecting him (John 8:48). That is, Jews rejected Samaritans, holding them without any esteem and only contempt.

This sworn and hated enemy, however, is the one who did not act in the same way as the priest and Levite. This traveler—this Samaritan despised by Jews—was the one who helped the dying Jewish man (our clue that the dying man was Jewish is the fact that he was traveling from Jerusalem). In other words, the Samaritan was the person with so much love and mercy that he freely saved the life of his sworn enemy.

Who does this? Who loves this way? There is only one answer: the Lord God. The lawyer's definition of *neighbor* was too limited. Jesus's definition includes all people with compassion overflowing. Keller (1997) describes this compassion:

> This compassion was full-bodied, leading him to meet a variety of needs. This compassion provided friendship and advocacy, emergency medical treatment, transportation, a hefty financial subsidy, and even a follow-up visit. (p. 11)

Christ presents himself as the Good Samaritan with love and mercy for every single human being who has ever lived, is living, or will live. And—as Just (1997) describes—Christ makes God our neighbor so that we are healed and forgiven of our sinful limitations, so that Jesus says to us, "As I live in you, you will have life and will do mercy—not motivated by laws and definitions, but animated by my love" (p. 454).

Matthew 11:28–30: "Come to me . . . and I will give you rest"

What is perhaps even more compelling for helping us see Jesus's universal compassion and his willingness to help and nourish anyone in need is his direct call and invitation as recorded in Matthew 11:28–30. These words are both powerful in their inclusivity and comforting in their merciful expression; they are sheer gospel that draws the sufferer to Jesus:

> Come to me, all who labor and are heavy laden, and I will give you rest. Take my yoke upon you, and learn from me, for I am gentle and lowly in heart, and you will find rest for your souls. For my yoke is easy, and my burden is light.

Here again, the proper application for the Christian nurse seems counterintuitive. It is easy to imagine that the moral of this text is that we should emulate Jesus while learning from him to be gentle, lowly at heart, and so on. The truth, however, is not only more realistic, but infinitely more empowering and encouraging. Instead of taking his words as a call to *imitate* Christ, we must know our proper place in the Lord's teaching. If we are to be the beneficiaries of Jesus's gracious invitation, then we must be—de facto—those who "labor and are heavy laden." If the Christian nurse cannot confess as much, then burnout is just around the corner.

It is easy to read this chapter or any other on the service of Christian nursing, especially as it pertains to God's way in Christ, and get excited to the extreme. Nurses might imagine themselves to be so equipped by the Holy Spirit that they take on the contours of super-servants, so strong and so spiritual that they might expect to move mountains daily with unlimited energy and enthusiasm. After all, they have Jesus. After all, they are born again by water and the Spirit. While not denying that the Christian is certainly in Christ and born-again, such misguided enthusiasm misses the insight of Matthew 11:28–30.

In this passage, Jesus reveals that those whom he blesses and those joining him by coming to him (or being drawn to him) are "laboring" and "loaded down" (heavy laden). These individuals are the ones described earlier who receive "bearing and carrying." These are the people whom nurses serve. But before nurses serve anyone else, *they* must be served. They must see and confess how they themselves are laboring and are heavy laden; they must recognize just how much they need rest.

Notice that this call and invitation of Christ is described as *being drawn*. This terminology reflects the original language used in the scripture. The call from Jesus is a gospel-call. It is a call of love and mercy so powerful that it enables the weak and helpless sinner to rise up and go to Jesus. The picture is not radically different from the **divine monergism** described in John 11, where Jesus called Lazarus to come out of the tomb. This call "draws and moves and at the same time holds out to us all that Jesus has" (Lenski, 1943, p. 456). It is not dissimilar from the gracious and kind host inviting the hungry, "Come and eat!" The invitation itself fills the hungry with strength to come and partake with great relief and joy. Such a call would never receive a begrudging or resentful response.

This insight in and of itself should cause the nurse to step back and reevaluate. The Christian nurse does not approach those who are weak as if he or she—the nurse—is strong. Instead, the Christian nurse serves the weak as one who is also weak. We have all heard about the importance of empathy in demonstrating true compassion. In interpreting Matthew 11:28–30, we realize that there is never a need to pretend that we do not relate to weakness. It is true: The servants of God are also weak. They, too, have experienced the mercy and nourishing they offer to those whom they serve. They, too, are weary and heavy laden with their "suffering, unrest, trouble, fear, grief, pain, an evil conscience, against which [people] rebel so vainly, [and these add] to the labor and the load" (Lenski, 1943, p. 457). This real dissonance is what scripture teaches. All true Christians experience the inner battle and conflict against their own sin and weakness (Romans 7; Galatians 5).

The challenge in Christ's words, however, seems to come in his offering a "yoke" upon us to give us rest. Indeed, this "sounds like exchanging one load for another" (Lenski, 1943, p. 458). As Lenski points out, a yoke was placed on an ox so that the ox could be harnessed and pull a load (p. 458). Why is Jesus offering to put a yoke on us? The answer is because *his* yoke unites us not to a burden, but to *him*! This, of course, is amazing grace, because the only way it could happen was for the King of Kings, the Creator of Heaven and Earth, and the very Son of God to lower himself—taking on flesh (the *incarnation*)—and becoming *our* brother and *our* servant. This is the reason

Jesus says of himself, "I am gentle and lowly in heart." On account of his humiliation, we were served by him, and his service won for us rest—rest from sin, rest from guilt, from shame, from fear, and from death. In him, our burden is light—so light, in fact, that it carries us to know his strength in us. To borrow from another source, St. Paul says, "For the sake of Christ, then, I am content with weaknesses, insults, hardships, persecutions, and calamities. For when I am weak, then I am strong" (2 Corinthians 12:10).

Those served by Christian nurses find comfort not in one who is above them, but through one who is *like* them. Such nurses convey that they know what is needed of the ones whom they serve, because they (the nurses) have also been served this way. All of a sudden, by encountering such a nurse, the ones being served perceive that they are not alone. Such nurses are viewed as compassionate, and they are God's instrument for relieving the burdens of and extending rest to those weak and heavy laden.

Jeffrey A. Gibbs helps us to understand the broad scope—that is, the *inclusivity*—of Matthew 11:28-30. He writes that this text is "a stunning expression of universal mercy and divine grace, the Son of God speaks an all-embracing word of invitation, despite the rejection [he had] experienced from many in Israel. That invitation still holds true in our day" (Gibbs, 2010, p. 588). Gibbs further elaborates, "He invites to himself all who are weighed down by the changes and chances of life, and by their own sins . . . he invites all people, no matter how undeserving, to learn who *he* is . . . [as one] gentle and humble of heart (11:29)" (p. 593).

To know this Jesus is also to know the *exclusivity* of the Holy Gospel: that Jesus Christ is the one—and only one—whose blood was shed for the sins of the world. This is something no mere man could do, but only the **God-man** with all authority in himself who created all men (Colossians 1:16).

We also hear from the Christian faith—as we do in this case from R. T. France (2007)—that the "only requirement is that those who come to him must recognize their need for help and be willing to accept his yoke and learn from him" (p. 448). But such a condition should not be viewed as diluting the gospel with the law (i.e., as suggesting that God's love and mercy is contingent on our action and decision). On the contrary, God in His mercy leads us to see our need and His grace enables us to seek His healing. This is precisely one of the things that makes the field of nursing so special, because when people come for healing, God has already revealed to them —or is in the process of revealing to them—their considerable need. Vulnerability and mortality gain sharper focus. Nurses serve those individuals who are more likely to accept the yoke of the merciful Lord who offers them His yoke of rest, and all of this is made possible by the Lord's grace for all people. God works good through all circumstances for those who come to love Him and are called according to His purpose (Romans 8:28).

Finally, just what of this *rest*? The rest that Jesus provides is "to cause to cease"; it is a "cessation" or "interruption." The labor and heavy-laden condition stop. In "Mt. 11:28 the word comprehends the whole saving work of Jesus" (Kittel, 1964, p. 350). The whole saving work of Christ addresses the sin problem and all that sin brings with it, which includes all forms of suffering. In Christ, we receive cessation and interruption of the loss of hope that often accompanies our illnesses; on account of this rest-cessation, we know that we have received help (and will continue to receive help) in our time of need. Now, whether our healing comes sooner, or later in glory, it belongs to those yoked to Jesus. This is the gospel that all nurses in Christ bring with them in their holy service to God and to those whom the Lord directs them to serve. They can relate to these neighbors because the nurse in Christ also confesses: "I labor and am heavy laden, and I am yoked to Jesus!"

▶ The Scope and Attitude of Christ-Centered Nursing Ministry

The Christian faith is not to be confused with *universalism*. Universalism is the idea that regardless of what one believes, that God's salvation is given to all. That is, universalism believes in *everything* and, as a result, believes at the end of the day in *nothing*. To believe in *everything* includes believing—for example— that contrary statements are true in the same place and at the same time. Contrary statements and beliefs, however, cancel each other out. In the end, there is nothing. Universalism is therefore bankrupt and at the same time implies that everything Jesus Christ did and taught for salvation was unnecessary. For these reasons, Christians who confess the Word of God to be true while conveying truth (and while also warning against falsity) cannot and do not accept universalism. Instead, the Christian maintains that there is truth and there is error; there is right and there is wrong; there is good and there is evil; and there is death and there is life (also in their *eternal* versions— called "hell" and "heaven"—in accord with the Word of God). These truths are inherent in Christianity.

At the same time, the Christian faith is full of *universal* realities, which must never be confused with universalism. This distinction is immensely important for the belief and practice of the Christian faith. When we understand this both–and situation—that while universalism is wrong, the **universal truths** of the faith are adhered to—then God puts us in a position to effectively serve all people in diverse populations and of diverse faiths.

Understanding these aspects of universalism versus universal truths enables the Christian to know this actual state of affairs:

"While it matters what those whom I serve believe, no matter what they believe, they still have need for God's love and mercy that is for them." For this reason, it is important to have a lucid grasp of the universal truths of the Christian faith.

▶ Aware of Humanity's Universal Need

The first universal truth of the Christian faith is humanity's universal *need* of God's love and mercy. This basic theme has been inherent in everything considered thus far:

- God's very nature is mercy and love, and this is the God who created heaven and earth (Genesis 1:1) and therefore all people (Acts 17:24–27).
- The Biblical foundations demonstrate that God nourishes and carries those in need (and who is not needy?).
- The Christian Church itself is responsible for the first hospitals in society.
- Christ is the Good Samaritan and the one who invites all people who labor and are heavy-laden to Himself.

All of these insights assume *a universal need for the love and mercy of God.*

The universal need of all people, however, comes out in an even more straightforward manner in God's Holy Word. Some Christians call this article of the faith **original (hereditary) sin**, referring to the sin rooted in the origins of humanity that has been inherited by all people. It is properly understood as an internal condition rendering people helpless to save themselves from sin and death. In the Old Testament, Jeremiah 17:9 teaches, "The heart is deceitful above all things, and desperately sick; who can understand it?" Whose heart? Answer: The heart of *any* person with flesh and blood! Psalm 51:5 records the confession of the man described as a man after God's own heart (1 Samuel 13:14): "Behold, I was brought forth in iniquity, and in sin did my mother conceive me." David's confession describes our need from conception! The prophet Ezekiel cut to the chase: "The soul who sins shall die" (18:4, 20). The Old Testament teaching carries over into the New Testament: "for all have sinned and fall short of the glory of God" (Romans 3:23). And the results of sin are also universal and proven from observation: "For the wages of sin is death" (Romans 6:23a). Sin, as a spiritual disease, has a 100% mortality rate.

But we do not even have to quote scripture to realize that there is a universal problem and malady that inherently implies the need for God's love and mercy. The great C. S. Lewis, in his masterpiece *Mere Christianity* highlights the "Law or Rule about Right and Wrong used to be called the Law of Nature" (2001, p. 4). Everyone knows—innately—that there is morality ingrained in humanity, and we cannot try to deny it by saying right and wrong is determined by culture or country. Lewis wrote:

Men have differed as regards what people you ought to be unselfish to—whether it was only your family, or your fellow countrymen, or every one. But they have always agreed that you ought not to put yourself first. Selfishness has never been admired. (2001, p. 6)

Lewis goes on to argue that this *oughtness* residing in the conscious—that we *should* do what is right and that we *should not* do what is wrong (whether or not we do it)—is within people universally. But there is more to what Lewis is saying here. He also wrote, "None of us are really keeping the Law of Nature" (2001, p. 7). And this leads to this summary realization: "[There is] Something . . . directing the universe, and which appears to me as a law urging me to do right and making me feel responsible and uncomfortable when I do wrong" (p. 25).

Universally, people know guilt—they have a sense of having *committed* wrong. Universally, people know shame—they have a sense that something is flawed in *who and/ or what they are*. Universally, people know fear—they have a sense that the consequences of their guilt and shame are beyond *their* ability to repair. Every person served by the Christian nurse, regardless of his or her background, religion, culture, worldview, and experience, can relate to other human beings who grapple with sin and its ensuing manifestations: guilt, shame, and fear. And as a result, all people grapple with what these lead to: death. These things the Christian nurse must recognize as the great equalizers, as the "common language" that all people speak and know. For these reasons, all people need God. By being mindful of these universal needs, the Christian nurse begins to bring down the barriers between diverse populations and faiths and begins to see that they have more in common with all people than perhaps first realized.

We cannot overestimate the importance of this first universal truth. First, if we understand this universal need, then it should be impossible for Christians to try to justify the idea that some people might be better than others. Universal sin is the great equalizer of humanity. We are all in the same boat. We are all dying. All people have need of God's love and mercy. The practical ramifications are tremendous.

One of those practical ramifications is that Christian nurses do not have to worry about conducting a negative apologetic (giving reasons as to why other worldviews and faiths are *wrong*), but may rather begin with God's compassion regarding the great need that all people have in common. This is what love does first: It does not find a reason for *avoiding* another (possibly with a different faith or religion), but rather sees the reason for *drawing near*, because the person God puts before the nurse is a person in need.

▶ Committed to Christ's Universal and Inclusive Ministry

The second universal truth that brings down walls between diverse populations and faiths is the great truth of the gospel of Jesus Christ. It is summarized in what is probably the best-known verse in the New Testament, John 3:16: "For God so loved the world, that he gave his only Son, that whoever believes in him should not perish but have eternal life." The key word for our purposes of knowing the great universals of the faith is "world" (*kosmos*), which has an obvious implication: Christ gave his life to save *all people*. This interpretation is consistent with other scriptures. For example, 1 Timothy 2:4 says, "[God] desires all people to be saved and to come to the knowledge of the truth."

This universal truth—once again—is not to be confused with universalism. The Biblical concept known as **universal atonement** certainly teaches that Christ's blood covers the sins of all people, but John 3:16 also maintains that the benefits of this universal truth can only be personally received through faith ("that whoever believes in him should not perish but have eternal life"). That is, the fact that Christ died for the sins of the world does not mean that all people are *automatically* saved, but it does mean that God's grace and mercy have certainly been won for all people. That is, God's salvation is now *objectively accomplished* for all people. What is left is for individual persons to come to saving faith—to subjectively trust in—what has been objectively secured for them.

Nafzger, Johnson, Lumpp, and Tepker (2017) give further insights into how we can understand the universal atonement of Christ: "Only the vicarious (substitutionary) satisfaction of Christ has caused God to lay aside his anger against humanity and become reconciled to the world (2 Cor 5:19)" (p. 474). **Vicarious satisfaction** is another way of

saying that because Christ took the place of all people on the cross of Calvary (2 Corinthians 5:21 teaches that he became sin for us; Galatians 3:13 teaches that he became a curse for us) and gave his atoning blood for all people on the cross (for the whole world, 1 John 2:2), what is left for us is God's anger set aside. On account of Christ, God's disposition toward us is one of love and mercy. He now looks at all people with compassion. But how does the necessity of personal faith come into play?

In his book *Faith That Sees Through the Culture*, Espinosa (2018) points out that the universal gospel *itself* is what God uses to generate saving faith within the hearts of people. That is, Christian nurses should simply continue to live in God's unconditional love and mercy both for themselves and for others (and if the Lord opens the door to share the gospel in words, then Christian nurses should walk through that door and tenderly share the gospel to the one in need, permitting the witness). Espinosa attributes the creation of **subjective faith** to the **objective gospel**:

> Based on this state of affairs, God's love is unconditional even in the face of any personal circumstances and details in the lives of people today. It is unconditional precisely because it is already accomplished. God loves your neighbor across the street, your co-worker, your classmates, your relatives, and everyone else in your life. This is certain. There is no doubt about it. Salvation has been won for each and every one.
>
> Some people get nervous about this teaching and inherently challenge the universal grace of God (where *grace* means "God's undeserved love and mercy in Christ"): "But doesn't a person 'have' to have faith in order to be saved?" The answer is, "Yes, of course," but this is the part that many people don't understand. It is this

very characteristic of the inclusive, accomplished Gospel that makes it so powerful. When the Gospel is proclaimed, those who hear it are already assured that their forgiveness and salvation are firm. Faith in this Gospel does not make the Gospel effective; rather, the Gospel gives faith and makes faith effective. The Gospel—by the Holy Spirit who works through it—leads a person to grasp its inclusive guarantee. The person who hears it has the chance to see what makes the Gospel so wonderful: *It is for me and has already been done for me!* (Espinosa, 2018, p. 132)

Faith That Sees Through the Culture © 2018 Alfonso Espinosa, published by Concordia Publishing House. Used with permission. www.cph.org.

The implications for Christian nurses and how they serve those in their care are both liberating and profound. The objective Gospel accomplished in Christ absolutely guarantees God's unconditional love and mercy upon those whom they serve. Christian nurses are called, therefore, to treat those whom they serve this way. These nurses are set free from the need for judgment that Bonhoeffer warned about. No matter people's background or current position or worldview, they are completely loved by God in Christ. Christians do not wait until a person jumps through this or that hoop, gives such and such an expression of sincerity or worthiness, or expresses a confirmation of faith. No, the objective love and mercy of God in Christ is already in place. For this reason, Jesus said from the cross of Calvary, "It is finished" (John 19:30). All that had to be done for salvation to be won for all people was completed. It is now the call of the disciple of Jesus to live out this reality and serve others in the completed reality of the gospel.

God has planned these things for us. When we are faithful to these universal truths, God takes over. When by God's spirit nurses

are made low to see that they need the Lord as much as anyone to cease their labor and receive Christ's rest, then those whom they serve will be drawn to one like them. The feeling that someone relates grants great comfort to the suffering soul that he or she is not alone. And then, when by God's spirit we are filled with the love of Christ—His unqualified mercy—people, regardless of what they believe, will be drawn again to the servant of God who loves unconditionally. What does such a milieu of humility and grace produce? It produces open hearts eager to learn more. "Why does this nurse treat me this way?" It is at this juncture that Christian nurses are invited to say more, and that is when the Gospel may be clearly articulated.

▶ Disinterested in Status, Stereotypes, or Stigmas

In his inspired work, Garth Ludwig presents a fantastic summary of Jesus's manner while conducting His healing ministry:

We are moved by [Jesus's] sensitivity to those who were in pain, the gentleness of his demeanor to the outcasts of society. Once a man with leprosy approached Jesus with the plea, "Lord, if you are willing, you can make me clean" (Matt. 8:2–4). According to Levitical law (Lev. 13:46), Jesus ought not to have gone near him, let alone touch him. Yet Matthew underscores the love by which Jesus dealt with the sick: "Jesus reached out His hand and touched the man. 'I am willing,' He said, 'Be clean!'"

. . . [S]ickness in the Old Testament bore with it the stigma of shame. Yet Jesus broke through this barrier of shame in order to reach out to the rejected masses of His day. It was especially those who were labeled "unclean" by the church authorities and refused entrance into the temple that galvanize His attention. Jesus seems to have gone out of His way to heal the lame, the blind, and the dumb.

What etches itself on the modern reader's mind is that Jesus demanded no spiritual pre-condition of those He healed. He accepted all who came to him for healing and turned no one away for reason of station in life, moral failure, or spiritual maturity. (Ludwig, 1999, p. 90)

Order restored: A Biblical interpretation of health medicine and healing © 1999 Concordia Publishing House. Used with permission. www.cph.org.

The consideration of a person's worthiness or background was a nonfactor to Jesus. His disciples are called to be like their Master. In the first chapter of St. Matthew's Gospel, the apostle revealed Jesus's genealogy. In it, certain women—great-grandmothers of Jesus—are intentionally mentioned. They include Tamar (Matthew 1:3), Rahab (1:5), Ruth (1:5), and "the wife of Uriah," a clear reference to Bathsheba (1:6). So what? St. Matthew was making a point: Jesus is not ashamed to be the friend, son (great-grandson, and so on), and Savior of sinners. Tamar—whose husband had died—presented herself as a prostitute to deceive her father-in-law and sleep with him so that her family lineage would be preserved; Rahab was actually a prostitute and God worked through her to help the Israelite spies within Jericho; Ruth was a Moabitess considered an unclean outsider and idolater by God's people; and Bathsheba was the woman with whom King David had committed adultery. To anyone else, such a detailed genealogy would have been a great embarrassment. Not for Jesus, because he deliberately came through sinners for sinners.

The examples of Christ paying no attention to humanmade distinctions and barriers make for a long list. In Matthew 9, Jesus calls Matthew the tax collector to be one of his apostles. At the time, tax collectors were known as notorious sinners and robbers of the people. Jesus didn't care: He called Matthew anyway. Jesus compliments a Roman centurion for his great faith in Luke 7. This was viewed by Jews as scandalous, because the Romans were considered pagans committed to their polytheistic ways. Luke 15 tells the story of the prodigal son; what we learn in the process is that it is the love of God that is *prodigal* (so overflowing to seem as excessive because this shameful son was fully restored). In John 4, Jesus does what no good Jewish rabbi should ever do: speak to a woman alone in broad daylight. What made it worse was that this woman was a Samaritan, and Samaritans were considered unclean by the people of God. Again, to make the situation go from bad to worse in prejudiced eyes, this woman had been married five times and the man she was currently living with was not her husband. Again, Jesus didn't care: He shared God's love and the holy gospel with her. As a result, she became a witness to Christ.

Christian nurses are called to become experts at *never judging a book by its cover*. They take the eyes of Christ and the heart of Jesus. They learn by the grace of God to serve with God's love regardless of status, stereotypes, and/or stigmas. All that counts is faith working itself out in love (Galatians 5:6).

▶ The Adjustment and Sacrifice of Christ-Centered Ministry

When we say that Jesus did not care about what might otherwise be considered reasons for disqualifying a person from God's love and mercy, we do not mean to say that background details are not important in all respects. In fact, they are important to learn so that nurses can be considerate toward those served from diverse populations and faiths (see **TABLE 10.1**). The main motivation in this context is to avoid generating unnecessary offense

TABLE 10-1 Comparison of Cultural Groups

	American Indian	Hispanic and Latino	African American	Native Hawaiian/Pacific Islanders
Abuse incidence and type (if noted) [White 77%] [National Center for Elder Abuse (NCEA) percentage of all cases]	0.6% neglect; financial	10.5%	21.2%	0.7% spousal and child; ignored
Advance directives	Develop trust relationship before asking	Involve family; trust physician; complex	Less likely; God is ultimately in charge	Reluctant
Decision makers	Clan leaders; matriarchs; patriarchs; religious; or medicine	Nuclear and extended family; fictive kin (nonrelatives); friends; church members	Loved ones; fictive kin; long-standing family relationships	*Ohana:* family
Dementia deaths [White 25.4%] [Health, U.S. 2011]	11.4%; rare	15%; lower rates	19.7%; vascular dementia; higher rates	8.9%; Guam, Parkinsonism dementia [lytico-bodig]; lower rates
Education [all older adults: 76.5% high school; 20.2% bachelor's degree or higher]	All ages: 77% high school; 13% bachelor's degree; 4.5% advanced degree; doing rather than talking	All ages: 60.9% high school; 12.6% bachelor's degree or higher; Cubans: higher levels	Older adults: 44% high school; 7% bachelor's degree or higher	All ages: 85.3% high school; 49.7% bachelor's degree or higher

End-of-life/dying	Death is a natural part of life; home care; family may not visit—spiritually bad for living and dying; death rituals: dressing and positioning body, burning herbs and grasses, funerals and burials	Protect from cancer diagnosis; more likely to use heroic measures; *El Dia de Los Muertos* (Day of Dead) celebrates and honors lives; *dicos*—sayings about God; hospice less likely; die at home	Death rates higher until crossover; reluctant to participate due to mistrust; certain diseases and prognoses withheld	Keep at home; hospice; home care; *Ohana*: family stay at the side of the sick; *uwe*: death chant, wailing to express grief; money and cards given at funerals
Family system	Extended; mixed tribal heritage; many single-parent homes	Live with children; *familismo*; fictive kin (*compadres*)	Dependent care from children, grandchildren, or fictive kin; many raising grandchildren	Importance of group; multigenerational; value society; revere elders; defer to judgment of adult children; men live alone
Folklore/folk healers	558 tribes/nations; allopathic medicine, but "healer" used first; chanting to promote healing and remove evil; do not cut hair	Over-the-counter; home remedies, *curanderos* (general practitioners); *yerbistas* (herbalists); *sobadores* (massage); *empacho*: locked bowels	Herb and root doctors; *conjurer*: place a hex or ward off evil; spiritual healers; natural illness—physical cause; occult illness—supernatural forces/evil spirits; spiritual illness—willful violation of sacred beliefs or sin	*Kahuna lapa'au*: priest heals with medicines; tattoos denote significant achievement in rank; illness is seen as a curse; *noni*: plant to heal bowel problems and menstrual cramps; *lokahi triangle*: physical body along with environment, relationships with others, and mental and emotional states; *poi*: taro root used for illness; talking about illness hastens death

(continues)

TABLE 10-1 Comparison of Cultural Groups *(continued)*

	American Indian	Hispanic and Latino	African American	Native Hawaiian/Pacific Islanders
Functional status	Assess if they have ever performed activities of daily living (ADLs) first; self-care limitations and health-related mobility problems	More disabilities; fear of admitting one's dependence; report greater activity limitations; need more help with personal and routine activities, and more use of assistive devices for walking; women appear to be at higher risk than are men	Higher rates of walking difficulties and higher rates of activity limitations	Higher level of physical limitations
Health disparities	Diabetes; heart disease; gallbladder disease; poor survival rates with all types of cancer; low incidence of brain cancer; kidney disease; liver disease; tuberculosis; rheumatoid arthritis; hearing and vision problems	Border medications; complementary and alternative medicine; heart disease; cancer; cerebrovascular disease; respiratory disease; increased hip fractures, specifically in Mexican Americans	Diabetes; prostate cancer; Hypertension; blindness, specifically glaucoma; John Henryism: making it because of sheer determinism against overwhelming odds	Obesity; diabetes and lower-extremity infections; hypertension; tuberculosis death; rheumatic fever and heart disease; women: high rates of HIV; Samoan men: cancer; rehabilitation less likely; *Vog:* respiratory disease from volcano smoke
Historical events	Indian Self Determination and Education Act 1975; Indian Health Service	1910: Mexican revolution; 1940: Mexicans for labor (Cesar Chavez); 1996: welfare reform; Puerto Rico: overcrowding; Cuba: Fidel Castro, Bay of Pigs, Mariel Boatlift	Exploitation: South—legalized discrimination, North—covert discrimination; suspicious of healthcare providers (see Tuskegee experiment)	Distrust: confiscated land, mistreated; harbor resentment toward whites

Languages [Whites: 78.9 years]	106 Indian dialects; Indian sign language; limited English proficiency	Spanish; limited English proficiency	English	English; Hawaiian; Pidgin
Life expectancy	72.6 years	81.3 years; centenarians by 2050 = 19%	75 years; shorter "crossover phenomenon" (reversal in average life expectancy after age 80)	68.3 years; lowest
Long-term care	No provision in Indian Health Service; 12 tribally run nursing homes, but are a long distance for most families; social adult day care (ADC) centers	Less likely; cultural aversion hypothesis: myth of aversion to long-term care and "they take care of own"	Less likely; remain at home with support of family, church-paid home caregivers; higher among persons older than age 85	Half the rate of white elders; last resort
Mental health	Increased rate of major depression—Indian Depression Scale is highest among the Apache tribe, with 1.5 times the average suicide rate; "bad spirits"	Depression (women); Geriatric Depression Scale (GDS) less valid	Depression usually not treated	Decreased suicide rate; many homeless; drug abuse

(continues)

TABLE 10-1 Comparison of Cultural Groups

(continued)

	American Indian	Hispanic and Latino	African American	Native Hawaiian/Pacific Islanders
Nutrition	Food is an expression of taking care of people; high fat, high sugar, processed food, corn	*Tapas:* snacks; *sobremesa:* sitting after meal and talking; wine with meals; coffee is important with meals: *café con leche* (coffee with milk), *café solo* (coffee without milk), or *café cortado* (coffee with some milk); *churros:* twisted doughnut sprinkled with sugar or dunked in hot chocolate; large lunch; *arroz:* rice with meals; *chimichangas:* large, deep-fried burritos; spices in food and drinks	"Soul food": during slavery, had to cook with leftovers; okra, collard greens, black-eyed peas, and sweet potato; pigs feet, chicken livers, beef neckbones, and chitterlings (cleaned pig intestines); fried fish and chicken; corn as cornbread and grits	Rice; *musubi:* spam, rice, and seaweed wrap; barbecue; meats, macaroni salad; soda
Organ transplant need and donations [*Whites: 45% need; 68.2% donors*]	Do not desire; end-stage renal disease possibly; 1% need; 0.4% donors	18% need; 13.4% donors: decreased donors; mistrust of the medical profession; religious acceptance concern; perceptions of inequity in the distribution of donated organs; women more likely than men	Largest group in need of transplants: 29%; 14% donors	0.5% need; 0.2% donors; decreased donors

Pain	Withstand the pain; survival	Stoic; folk beliefs and nondrug remedies; do not understand pain scales	Higher pain intensity	Stoic; use massages, relaxation, and prayer
Religion	Indian spiritual beliefs and Christianity	*Espiritismo* (Puerto Rican): belief that good/evil spirits can affect well-being; *santeros* (Cuban faith healers)	Protestant, Catholic, Muslim; part of life's fabric; church community plays an important role	Catholic, Latter-Day Saints, Baptist, Pentecostal; worship god and goddesses, nature, human spirit; *Mana*: spiritual essence of protection
Respect	Listening; calmness; slow down; nondirect eye contact; may be guarded; modesty and privacy; obtain permission	Early attention to build rapport; use titles and last name	Titles: Mr./Mrs.	Revere elders; filial piety; indirect communication; negativity is not expressed; females: *Aunties*
Utilization of health care *[Whites: 11.7% uninsured]*	29.2% uninsured; Indian Health Service; limited English proficiency is a concern; cautious about nontribal health care	30.7% uninsured; limited English proficiency is a concern	20.8% uninsured	17.4% uninsured

Reproduced from Mauk, K. L., Shannon, M., & Hassler, L. (2018). Culture and spirituality. In K. L. Mauk (Ed.), *Gerontological Nursing: Competencies for Care* (4th ed., pp. 711–762). Burlington, MA: Jones & Bartlett Learning. Used with permission.

that might interfere with Christian nurses' efforts to serve in all the ways described here. That is, to ignore unique cultural, religious, and personal details pertaining to those we serve is to undermine efforts for engendering trust and respect. If we do not invest in people to the extent that we do no learn what makes them who and what they are, then love will be shallow, and any witness will be overgeneralized. Love, however, cares enough to get to know people as much as possible. Good pastors, for example, become experts in knowing not only the Word of God, but also the people whom God calls them to serve. The same basic principle should be true for the Christian nurse.

St. Paul's Missionary Strategy: Becoming All Things to All People (1 Corinthians 9:19–23)

Even though nurses certainly represent God's fundamental ministry of love and mercy, and nourishing care expressed through bearing and carrying in all tenderness and compassion, they are neither therapists nor pastors. That is, their time investment in getting to know those whom they serve is limited. Having said this, it should never be assumed that one cannot get to know a person surprisingly well in a relatively short period of time.

Regardless of the amount of time available to know those who are served, nurses should make every effort to capitalize on every opportunity to gain better insight *precisely for the sake of extending love and mercy.* This is not a tactic, but rather the expression of true compassion. This kind of service to another is the expression of love; such love extends itself to serve. Here, we do not speak of any love, but of the highest love—*agape.* This is the kind of love mentioned in John 3:16. It is *sacrificial* love; it is costly. Recall that in the church's early history, many gave up their lives for the nourishing care of others. This is the greatest love. It is God's love.

This sort of context is where the effort to know those whom we serve must take place. Such an investment extends the heart and mind of the servant of God to wrap around the needs of the person, but the needs of the person can be known only if the person is known. This kind of concern and interest is shown to the extent of being willing to suffer for another. Recall that Galatians 6:2 refers to such service as "bears one another's burdens." This bearing is costly. Ludwig (1999) leads us to consider Jesus to understand what "knowing the one whom we serve" means for those who serve:

> We can illustrate this cost by noting that the exercise of compassion is emotionally hurtful to the Healer. Luke, for example, describes the response of Jesus when He saw the pain of the widow of Nain whose only son had just died: "When the Lord saw her, His *heart went out to her* and He said, 'Don't cry'" (Luke 7:13).
>
> The Greek word here—*splangnidzomai*—refers to being moved in one's intestines, considered to be the seat of compassion and affection. Today we might say in the vernacular, "guts." Thus, a paraphrase of this passage would make it to read, "When the Lord saw her, He *hurt in His guts for her.* (p. 94)

So, to invest in truly serving is to invest in truly knowing, and to truly know is to be affected by the suffering of the sufferer. Such service comes at a cost. Thus, the investment to know those served involves more than just checking off a box for a pragmatic strategy, but rather permitting the other person to enter your "guts," and this is God's strategy for making true love and mercy known. St. Paul wrote at Romans 12:15: "Rejoice with those who rejoice, weep with those who weep." If we truly weep with those who weep, it will come at a cost, but it will also be a blessed work through which the Living Lord Jesus extends himself to another through the faithful ministry of one of his disciples.

It is in this vein that we now consider an invaluable text in the Holy Scripture that focuses precisely on how we effectively serve others by getting to know them to the extent that we authentically empathize and genuinely relate. Here is the text, 1 Corinthians 9:19–23:

> For though I am free from all, I have made myself a servant to all, that I might win more of them. To the Jews I became as a Jew, in order to win Jews. To those under the law I became as one under the law (though not being myself under the law) that I might win those under the law. To those outside the law I became as one outside the law (not being outside the law of God but under the law of Christ) that I might win those outside the law. To the weak I became weak, that I might win the weak. I have become all things to all people, that by all means I might save some. I do it all for the sake of the gospel, that I may share with them in its blessings.

St. Paul is here demonstrating the emulation of Jesus who didn't come to be served, but to serve and to give his life as a ransom for many (Matthew 20:28). Note the correlation: To serve is connected to *giving* one's life, and this is costly. St. Paul was not describing a chameleon's game; he is not prescribing a facade. Instead, to live out what St. Paul describes here, there must be a willingness to step into the life of the one being served.

It is important to note how St. Paul could even begin to become open to this level of investment in those whom he served. His own mentality—and that of his colleagues—was that they were bond-servants/willing slaves for Jesus's sake (2 Corinthians 4:5; Lockwood, 2000, p. 311). In his commentary, Lockwood describes St. Paul's strategy in terms of conducting a thorough consideration of those whom the Lord

put before him. He studied them and sought to identify natural connections and points of contact. "Accordingly he was careful never to cause them unnecessary offense" (p. 312). All the while, "Paul's flexibility in accommodating himself to all people was governed by one overriding purpose: 'that I might by all means save some' (1 Corinthians 9:22)" (p. 313).

By doing this, "Paul showed himself a model of missionary adaptability to the language and thought-forms of his hearers" (Lockwood, 2000, p. 314). Lockwood also reminds us that Paul did not, however, change the gospel itself "to suit people's religious or cultural tastes," but continued to be faithful to God's unchanging Word (p. 314). In other words, for St. Paul, his investment in relationships was expressed in a twofold commitment: (1) to do all he could to know those to whom he ministered and to serve them according to their unique perspectives and (2) to do so in such a way as to never compromise the saving faith or the Word of Christ.

It is helpful to consider St. Paul's general principle of becoming all things to all people placed within a kind of conceptual framework that might be useful for Christian nurses. On a practical level, what sorts of things might nurses seek to observe so that they may know those whom they serve? How might they make the most of their limited time to optimally know those whom they serve so that nurses are in position to truly invest in the relationship for the sake of showing Jesus? Simply asked, how do we become "all things to all people," one person at a time? There are five areas—think of them as concentric circles (starting on the outside with the largest circle and working inward toward the smallest circle)—that we may use for systematic analysis characterized by true compassion and therefore genuine interest (**FIGURE 10-1**).

First, nurses should take note of outward symbols attached to or around those whom they serve (e.g., a necklace, a tattoo, or a picture on the nightstand). These can—though not always—reflect what is in the heart and soul of a person. For example, a cross or

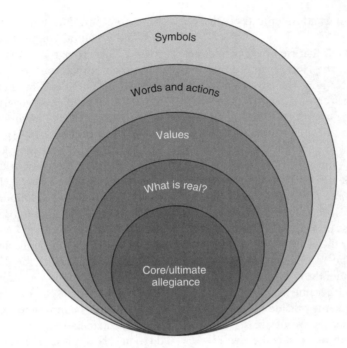

FIGURE 10-1 Diagnostic of those served.

crucifix may indicate that the individual holds to the Christian faith or, alternatively, that the person enjoys religious jewelry while possibly viewing it superstitiously. The nurse cannot know for sure. However, any signs and symbols that people obviously make public, in the sense that they make them visible for others to see, should be construed as a ready starting point for conversation. Because Christian nurses genuinely care about those whom they serve, they should try to find out if the external signs reveal something more.

Second, what comes out of a person in the form of words and actions speaks volumes about the person. Consider Christ's words recorded in Luke 6:45: "The good person out of the good treasure of his heart produces good, and the evil person out of his evil treasure produces evil, for out of the abundance of the heart his mouth speaks." Citing this scripture should not elicit thoughts of moral judgment,

which would contradict everything suggested so far in this chapter. Rather, gaining such insight about the person's heart puts the nurse in a better position to consider the best approach in forming a relationship.

Third, the nurse wants to try to understand the person's values. What does the individual consider to be right and wrong?

Fourth, if possible, the nurse should try to ascertain what the person considers to be real. Does the person show any indication, for example, of believing in the presence of angels and/or demons—that is, of believing in God's created, invisible realm? Does he or she hold to certain animistic, mystical, or ancestral beliefs?

Fifth, what is at the core of the one being served? What is the person's ultimate allegiance? What guides the individual's life and determines his or her decisions? What does the person live for?

These five concentric circles are easy to learn and make for an interesting way to get to know those whom we serve. Of course, the Christian nurse might also take a significant shortcut by boldly asking a question, which might sound something like this: "It's my privilege to serve you. Do you mind me asking if you hold to any religion or worldview? I want to be as considerate of your needs as possible." If the person is willing to share this information, then the concentric circles can be understood almost instantaneously. For example, if the person is a devout Muslim, then all five concentric circles can be known without further elaboration. This understanding would then enable the nurse to be more effective in serving the person. Keep in mind, however, that all faiths and worldviews have both devout believers and nominal adherents. Those who choose to identify themselves with key words and labels while maintaining a nominal commitment to that identifiable marker may not even be aware of the basic tenets of their faith.

St. Paul's teaching strategy is found in Acts 17:

> So Paul, standing in the midst of the Areopagus, said: "Men of Athens, I perceive that in every way you are very religious. For as I passed along and observed the objects of your worship, I found also an altar with this inscription, 'To the unknown god.' What therefore you worship as unknown, this I proclaim to you. The God who made the world and everything in it, being Lord of heaven and earth, does not live in temples made by man, nor is he served by human hands, as though he needed anything, since he himself gives to all mankind life and breath and everything. And he made from one man every nation of mankind to live on all the face of the earth, having determined allotted periods and the boundaries of their dwelling place, that they should seek God, in the hope that they might feel their way toward him and find him. Yet he is actually not far from each one of us, for 'In him we live and move and have our being'; as even some of your own poets have said, 'For we are indeed his offspring.' Being then God's offspring, we ought not to think that the divine being is like gold or silver or stone, an image formed by the art and imagination of man. The times of ignorance God overlooked, but now he commands all people everywhere to repent, because he has fixed a day on which he will judge the world in righteousness by a man whom he has appointed; and of this he has given assurance to all by raising him from the dead." Now when they heard of the resurrection of the dead, some mocked. But others said, "We will hear you again about this." So Paul went out from their midst. But some men joined him and believed, among whom also were Dionysius the Areopagite and a woman named Damaris and others with them.

To put it mildly, this is an astounding record and extremely valuable in informing how Christian nurses can serve diverse populations and faiths (**BOX 10-1**). Note that St. Paul did not go into the Areopagus to tell the Athenians that they were wrong and in error. While it is true that the Athenians held to false beliefs, St. Paul was wise in his approach. He used any fact available to him for truth-statements that would facilitate gaining the Athenians' attention. For example, St. Paul tells the Athenians that he perceived they were "in every way . . . very religious." This was not flattery, but fact.

St. Paul also did not agree for a second with the Athenians' polytheism, but he established common ground. Like the people of Athens, St. Paul was a religious person. In the broad sense, to be religious means to have a

St. Paul's Evidence-Based Practice: Acts 17:22–34

While *evidence-based practice* is a contemporary term, St. Paul in Athens at the Areopagus is a true-to-life *and* Biblical case study exemplifying this concept. Research may be applied through the testing of the following criteria represented by these questions:

1. Have negative and alienating remarks been avoided toward the one being served?
2. Have signs or symbols been identified for generating genuine engagement?
3. Has some level of common ground been established?
4. Is the Christian witness welcomed and being initiated and presented through the area of common ground?
5. Has the basic response to the witness—be it rejecting or open or accepting—been noted for the purposes of evaluation and follow-up?

serious worldview that shapes and directs life. This was true of the Athenians—it was a fact. St. Paul was actively taking inventory of what was true for those to whom he spoke. This step is significant because it conveys a basic message: "What you think and believe in is significant, it matters, and I care about it enough to know it." This is the foundation for building mutual respect.

At the same time, St. Paul looked for an "in." That is, as he approached this unique situation, he had asked himself—certainly even before he opened his mouth—"How can the Christian faith be introduced in this setting?" He observed and found his opening. The Athenians were polytheists and were thorough in that practice. In case they had inadvertently left out a deity, they permitted an altar with the inscription, "To the unknown god." St. Paul realized that this was his golden opportunity.

As St. Paul began to witness to the faith, he did *not* begin with the Gospel (the saving life, death, and resurrection of Jesus Christ for all people), but instead began to speak about *creation*. Here again was another ingenious move on the part of St. Paul. Creation was certainly also debatable (Aristotle taught that the universe was eternal), but was also a serious philosophical and logical option. For example, it is complementary to the law of cause and effect. This approach probably enhanced St. Paul's engagement with the Athenians and most likely served his legitimacy in their view of him.

Why did St. Paul think such an insertion would be permissible and accepted? As he elaborated upon creation, he was certainly aware that some of the Athenians' poets had made related statements about humanity's relationship to a sustainer and perpetuator of life. These ideas share similarities with the Christian article of creation. Again, St. Paul was building bridges and making the most of common ground.

After demonstrating a seamless logic and coherence, St. Paul shifts to the will of the Creator-God that every man should know Him and that this Creator-God has appointed "a man" with authority to judge and who was raised from the dead. Jesus was proclaimed. Was this roundabout process worth it? Undoubtedly. Three reactions toward St. Paul are recorded in Acts 17: (1) Some mocked; (2) some wanted to hear more later; and (3) some followed St. Paul. St. Paul invested in the Athenians and some of them came to faith. Even for those who mocked him, who knows what the Word planted in them might have led to?

▶ Conclusion

It is easy to see how the Christian nurse who nourishes the weak and needy can benefit

BOX 10-2 Research Highlight

The researchers in this study used a retrospective, qualitative, phenomenologic approach to explore student experiences and attitudes toward elderly patients having cognitive or physical challenges. The student participants were in a BSN course that had a service-learning component. "Themes included initial attitudes of anticipation, apprehension, anxiety, and ageist stereotypes. Final attitudes included a 'completely changed perspective' of caring, compassion, and respect indicative of a rewarding, 'life-changing' experience. Participants cited enhanced learning, especially in the areas of patient-centered care, collaboration, communication, advocacy, empathy, assessment skills, and evidence-based practice" (p. 29). Using a service-learning strategy resulted in less fear of the elderly, an increased openness to working in gerontological nursing, and transformed attitudes of students.

BOX 10-3 Outstanding Nurse Leader: Ninette DeYoung, RN

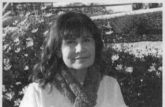

Ninette DeYoung was trained as an emergency room (ER) nurse and has been serving in the field professionally for 15 years. She has served in the ER primarily and is now working for the state of California. Ninette is a baptized disciple of the Lord Jesus Christ, and she lives out her faith in the Lord as naturally as she breathes. I have witnessed her spirit of compassion on many occasions, but especially when my mother of sacred memory, Josephine Espinosa, was in her last days. Ninette volunteered to travel out of town during her very busy schedule to serve my mother and make her more comfortable before she went to heaven. I saw Ninette epitomize nourishing care, the bearing and caring of one who serves not only with skill but also with God's heart. She came alongside my mother and extended Christ's presence to her.

from this object lesson: The unconditional love of God leads the servants of the Lord to avoid telling those whom we serve how wrong they are and how right we are (**BOX 10-2**). Instead, we seek truth-statements that will build mutual respect; we seek common ground that is readily available through the natural knowledge of God (such as creation/cause and effect); and we seek to find anything within the worldview of those to whom we speak that might naturally support and buttress the articles of the Christian faith (**BOX 10-3**). Finally, we look for the right time to share what is most important: that Jesus Christ is the God who nourishes, who carries, who puts up with, who nurses; that Jesus is the Good Samaritan; that Jesus invites everyone to him who labors and is heavy laden; that Jesus loves and saves unconditionally; that Jesus covers all sin with his blood; that he puts no pre-conditions upon those whom he heals and helps; that he is deeply moved in his guts with compassion toward the one who needs healing; and that he sends out his servants, including Christian nurses serious about receiving from Jesus and then giving to others what they have received.

▶ Clinical Reasoning Exercises

Goal

The Biblical image of *nurse* is of a person who is actively nourishing, bearing, and carrying. What does this look like in the modern setting?

1. Recall that these characteristics are marked by compassion. In what practical ways can compassion be expressed and demonstrated?

2. "To nourish" especially impacts the soul that labors and is heavy laden. Such nourishment finds a way to help the one being served approach rest (the cessation of laboring). How does the nurse lighten the load of the sufferer?

3. "To bear" and "to carry" relate to the idea of God putting up with His people. We are also mindful of the applicable form of love that is agape, sometimes translated as "long-suffering." That is, nurses in the image of Christ put up with those whom they serve by extending love that suffers with the other. Recall the word *splangnidzomai*, which means to be moved in the guts, such that compassion and affection are genuinely extended. This is the kind of long-suffering compassion Christ has for people. How does the Christian nurse begin to reflect this kind of bearing and carrying? Asked a different way, how do Christian nurses *suffer with* those they serve?

Malady

It helps to know what exactly we are being compassionate *toward* within those served.

That is, exactly what is the sufferer laboring with and burdened by?

1. Guilt emanates from those patients who are convinced that their struggle has been brought on by what they've done, as if they believe God is punishing them. How might this be diagnosed?

2. Shame is an expression of the conviction that there is something wrong with one's person—that one is a bad person, a cursed person, a defective or abandoned person. How might this be diagnosed?

3. Fear covers hope and brings a sense of imminent doom. The person who feels this way has the sense that life is out of control, as anxiety and depression fill his or her heart. How might this be diagnosed?

Means

To apply our insights about bringing nourishment and compassionate carrying and bearing for those filled with guilt, shame, and/or fear, we must consider how the person being served is unique among those within the diversity of populations and faiths.

1. In accord with St. Paul's missionary strategy described in 1 Corinthians 9, which approaches might be taken to identify with the one served as much as possible?

2. In Acts 17, we see an example of how the Apostle Paul found an entry point for beginning the process to relate to and then find common ground with those whom he served. How can the nurse emulate St. Paul when serving those heavy laden with guilt, shame, and/or fear?

3. We discussed the five concentric circles that may be used to try to

understand those whom we serve. Which kinds of indicators might help the nurse fill in each of the concentric circles for the person being served?

▶ Personal Reflection Exercises

Christ is *the* Nourisher and Bearer. How do you need him to nourish you and bear your burdens? More importantly, what does *he* prescribe that you need from him? How are his resources of word and sacrament, prayer, mutual encouragement/fellowship, and private confession and absolution made available to you? How are you seeking them out? How are you applying them?

Christ provides his church to care for its members. Who are the real people whom you consider to be a part of your support network? Be bold in thinking in terms of having a personal support team. Among these people, what are their distinctive roles in supporting you? It is commendable to be able to identify one or two or three close friends (no more than a few), a coach, a therapist/counselor, a doctor, and a pastor.

Christ is *the* Good Shepherd. He helps those people who are weak, like the man in the parable of the Good Samaritan who was beaten and left for dead. As we consider this picture of our great spiritual need, how do we experience Christ as coming to bind up our wounds and pouring on oil and wine, and as setting us on his animal to be brought to an inn to be cared for? How are we established in this care for the long term since Christ has paid and arranged for it?

These questions create a powerful visualization of our present need to receive Christ's healing gifts and his ongoing care expressed through his church. One healing gift in particular should be considered—namely, the gift of private or individual confession and absolution. Ideally, we should have a pastor or priest to whom we may go for pastoral care, or a fellow Christian whom we trust with hearing our burdens and our confession, and who is unafraid of bearing them with us and is able to clearly proclaim upon us God's love and mercy for us in Christ.

Who might you ask to do this for you? This is one of those things that is extremely easy to put off, but to employ this gift is to receive a great blessing from God. James 5:16: "Therefore, confess your sins to one another and pray for one another, that you may be healed."

References

Bauer, W. (1979 [1957]). *A Greek–English lexicon of the New Testament and other early Christian literature* (4th ed.), trans. W. F. Arndt & F. W. Gingrich. Chicago, IL: University of Chicago Press.

Bonhoeffer, D. (1955). *Ethics*, ed. E. Bethge. New York, NY: Macmillan.

Espinosa, A. (2016). God's nature as merciful God. In R. E. Johnson & J. T. Pless (Eds.), *The mercy of God in the cross of Christ: Essays on mercy in honor of Glenn Merritt* (pp. 211–221). Saint Louis, MO: Lutheran Church—Missouri Synod.

Espinosa, A. (2018). *Faith that sees through the culture.* St. Louis, MO: Concordia Publishing House.

France, R. T. (2007). *The new international commentary on the New Testament: The Gospel of Matthew.* Grand Rapids, MI: William B. Eerdmans.

Gibbs, J. A. (2010). *Concordia commentary: Matthew 11:2–20:34.* Saint Louis, MO: Concordia Publishing House.

Green, J. B. (1997). *The new international commentary on the New Testament: The Gospel of Luke.* Grand Rapids, MI: William B. Eerdmans.

Harris, R. L., Archer, G. L., & Waltke, B. K. (Eds.). (1980). *Theological wordbook of the Old Testament* (Vol. 2). Chicago, IL: Moody Press.

Just, A. A. (1997). *Concordia commentary: Luke 9:51–24:53.* Saint Louis, MO: Concordia Publishing House.

Keller, T. J. (1997 [1989]). *Ministries of mercy: The call of the Jericho road* (2nd ed.). Phillipsburg, NJ: P & R.

Kittel, G. (Ed.). (1964). *Theological dictionary of the New Testament* (Vol. I), ed. and trans. G. W. Bromiley. Grand Rapids, MI: William B. Eerdmans.

Lenski, R. C. H. (1943). *The interpretation of St. Matthew's Gospel.* Minneapolis, MN: Augsburg.

Lewis, C. S. (2001 [1952]). *Mere Christianity* (first HarperCollins paperback edition). New York, NY: HarperCollins Publishers.

Liddell, H. G., & Scott, R. (Comp.) (1968 [1843]). *A Greek–English lexicon* (9th ed.), ed. H. S. Stuart & R. McKenzie. Oxford, UK: Clarendon Press–Oxford University Press.

Lockwood, G. J. (2000). *Concordia commentary: 1 Corinthians.* Saint Louis, MO: Concordia Publishing House.

Ludwig, G.D. (1999). *Order restored: A Biblical interpretation of health medicine and healing.* Saint Louis, MO: Concordia Publishing House.

Luther, M. (1957). *Luther's works* (American ed., Vol. 31), ed. H. J. Grimm & H. T. Lehmann. Philadelphia, PA: Fortress Press.

Nafzger, S. H., Johnson, J. F., Lumpp, D. A., & Tepker, H. W. (Eds.). (2017). *Confessing the Gospel: A Lutheran approach to systematic theology* (Vol. 1). Saint Louis, MO: Concordia Publishing House.

Olson, J. E. (1992). *One ministry many roles: Deacons and deaconesses through the centuries.* St. Louis, MO: Concordia Publishing House.

Uhlhorn, G. (2007 [1883]). *Christian charity in the ancient church* (reprint by Lutheran Church—Missouri Synod). New York, NY: Charles Scribner's Sons.

Recommended Readings

Bennett, R. H. (2016). *Afraid: Demon possession and spiritual warfare in America.* Saint Louis, MO: Concordia Publishing House.

Bonhoeffer, D. (2003) *Discipleship.* Minneapolis, MN: Fortress. (Published in 1949 as *The Cost of Discipleship.*)

Brown, F., Driver, S. R., & Briggs, C. A. (Eds.). (1979). *The new Brown—Driver—Briggs—Gesenius Hebrew and English lexicon.* Peabody, MA: Hendrickson.

Corduan, W. (2006). *Pocket to world religions.* Downers Grove, IL: InterVarsity Press.

Craig, W. L. (2008). *Reasonable faith: Christian truth and apologetics.* Wheaton, IL: Crossway Books.

Evans, C. S. (2002). *Pocket dictionary of apologetics and philosophy of religion.* Downers Grove, IL: InterVarsity Press.

Keller, T. (2008). *The reason for God: Belief in an age of skepticism.* New York, NY: Riverhead Books.

Lewis, C. S. (1961). *A grief observed.* New York, NY: Bantam Books.

Lewis, C. S. (1962). *The problem of pain.* New York, NY: Macmillan.

McGrath, A. E. (1993). *Intellectuals don't need God and other modern myths.* Grand Rapids, MI: Zondervan.

Montgomery, J. W. (2002). *History, law and Christianity.* Calgary, Canada: Canadian Institute for Law, Theology, and Public Policy.

Nichols, L. A., Mather, G. A., & Schmidt, A. J. (2006). *Encyclopedic dictionary of cults, sects, and world religions.* Grand Rapids, MI: Zondervan.

Olson, R. E., Atwood, C. D., Mead, F. S., & Hill, S. S. (Eds.). (2018 [1951]). *Handbook of denominations in the United States* (14th ed.). Nashville, TN: Abingdon Press.

Poole, M. (2009). *The "new" atheism: 10 arguments that don't hold water?* Oxford, UK: Lion Book.

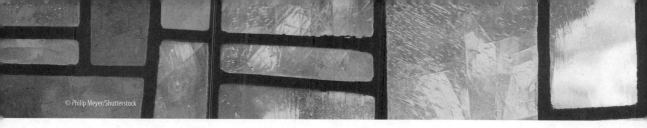

CHAPTER 11

Spiritual Gifts in Nursing Ministry

Rick Yohn, DMin, ThM

LEARNING OBJECTIVES

At the end of this chapter, the reader will be able to:

1. Understand the concept of spiritual gifts.
2. Explore the dangers and myths of spiritual gifts.
3. Identify the source and purpose of spiritual gifts.
4. Foster one's spiritual gifts in nursing while serving others in everyday life.
5. Implement one's spiritual gifts to impact and contribute to the lives of others.

KEY TERMS

Fruit of the Spirit	Service	Spiritual gifts

Why would a text on nursing include a chapter on spiritual gifts? After all, isn't it more important for nurses to learn about anatomy, chemistry, clinical skills, and other science-oriented topics? It is certainly true that a nursing student needs to be familiar with all of these fields, but the Christian nurse also has access to the spiritual realm, where spiritual battles are fought. Although you have much in common with other nurses, as a Christian nurse you possess several unique and distinctive characteristics. This chapter addresses those special capabilities.

▶ The Nurse and Spiritual Gifts

The Apostle Paul introduces us to this realm as he states, "For our struggle is not against flesh and blood, but against the rulers, against the authorities, against the powers of this dark world and against the spiritual forces of evil in the heavenly realms" (Ephesians 6:12). Along with an understanding of spiritual warfare, the Christian nurse has direct access to the One who provides the victory within that spiritual landscape. The writer of the Hebrews pens the following encouragement: "Let us then approach the throne of grace with confidence, so that we may receive mercy and find grace to help us in our time of need" (Hebrews 4:16). As an added blessing to guide the believing nurse toward making a significant impact in the lives of others, God has added to the nurse's arsenal some special abilities known as "spiritual gifts."

This chapter focuses on the significance of **spiritual gifts**, exploring how they can help a nurse make a significant contribution to the team, the patient, and one's personal life. The content provides an understanding of what a spiritual gift is, presents the dangers and myths of spiritual gifts, and then moves into the personal discovery, development, and deployment of spiritual gifts in everyday life.

Spiritual Gifts

A gift is something that is not earned. Instead, it is a blessing that one person wants to give another. It may take the form of a promotion, money, opportunity, or something special for a specific occasion. When we observe how the Bible identifies a spiritual gift, we discover that it is a significant ability given to us by God, which enables us to serve and equip others.

How does a spiritual gift differ from a talent or natural ability? The latter comes through the genes of our parents or other relatives, whereas the former is given by God only to believers. In his letter to the Church at Corinth, the Apostle Paul wrote, "Now to each one the manifestation of the Spirit is given for the common good" (1 Corinthians 12:7). Consider a few observations that can be made based on this statement. First, every

believer possesses at least one spiritual gift; no believer is excluded. Second, these spiritual gifts have been given to us by the Holy Spirit. Third, the spiritual gift may have been given to you at your birth or at some point after having received Jesus Christ as your personal Savior. The significant difference is that once you become a believer, you are motivated to use that gift for the sake of others, rather than for yourself. Furthermore, you will be using your spiritual gift under the guidance and power of the Holy Spirit, rather than depending on yourself.

Two individual nurses may possess a love for people and a desire to help them get better physically and even emotionally. The nurse who engages his or her spiritual gift, however, will include a spiritual dimension into his or her ministry of nursing. Such a nurse will not see nursing as a mere occupation. Instead, the nurse demonstrates a spiritual motivation to minister to the whole person: body (the physical dimension), soul (the emotional and mental aspect), and spirit (the spiritual make-up of the individual).

Along with spiritual gifts, specific types of ministries are possible, as well as differing results. The Apostle Paul informed the believers in Corinth, "Now there are varieties of gifts, but the same Spirit; and there are varieties of service, but the same Lord; and there are varieties of activities, but it is the same God who empowers them all in everyone" (1 Corinthians 12:4–6).

Varieties of Spiritual Gifts

First notice that spiritual gifts come in a variety of forms, which Paul lists in Romans 12:6–8 and Ephesians 4:11–13. The Apostle Peter also mentions some spiritual gifts in 1 Peter 4:10. You will also discover spiritual gifts in the Old Testament, such as the gift of craftsmanship (Exodus 31:1–11), prophecy (Deuteronomy 18:20–22), and music (the Psalms are hymns, many of which were written by David, the musician).

Varieties of Ministries

Along with the spiritual gifts comes a range of **service**. The original word used for "service" is the Greek *diakonia*, from which we derive the terms *deacon* and *ministry*. Your spiritual gifts will be significantly enhanced when you use them in a ministry where you will shine rather than fail. You may misdiagnose your spiritual gift if you experience poor results in a specific ministry—that is why it is essential to get involved in various types of ministries and learn where you best fit.

For instance, when I first entered the ministry, I was in charge of the adult ministries in the church I served. Early in that ministry, I was also given the task of teaching seventh-grade boys and girls. I soon discovered that my gift of teaching was far more effective when working with adults than with middle school kids. If I had attempted to determine my gift of teaching in the context of my interactions with middle school children, I would have concluded that I did not have the gift of teaching. Don't assess your gift based on your failure in a specific arena of serving the Lord. Instead, be willing to serve the Lord in some other capacity where you can find more success.

Similarly, nurses may think that the top of their career ladder reaches an administrative position over a department or hospital. But when they eventually reach that "top position," they soon discover that though they are skilled caregivers, they may not be gifted administrators, which the position demands, and frustration rapidly consumes them. As this example suggests, the spiritual gift must be linked with the proper area of service.

Varieties of Results

A variety of results when applying spiritual gifts are possible. Two people may possess the same spiritual gift, but that does not mean they will experience the same results with their gift.

Consider this scenario: Two young men entered seminary around the same time and soon became friends. They both chose the same major, had the same professors, and eventually graduated. Each became an associate in a church and then went on to become the teaching pastor of a church. God opened doors for both men to have a radio ministry, speaking ministry, and writing ministry. However, one young man became nationally famous for his writing and speaking, whereas the other had a much smaller impact. God used both men to change lives, but the far-reaching results differed. Did that produce jealousy in the pastor whose ministry was not as widespread? Not at all, for each man recognized that just as the gifts and ministries come from God, so do the results and the impacts on the lives of others.

The Lord has His plan for our lives and has given us spiritual gifts, specific ministries, and eventually His desired results in what we are able to accomplish. As we continue to walk with Him and allow Him to guide us to the ministries in which He wants us to serve, God will bring His intended results into being, based on His purpose for each person.

▶ The Dangers of Spiritual Gifts

As great and helpful as spiritual gifts are, we need to avoid some dangers along our spiritual journey. First, let's consider a problem we can call "gift-projection." In other words, we may have the tendency to think that everyone should have our spiritual gift and operate the way we do.

Gift-Projection

Consider this scenario: One nurse, who has the gift of mercy, loves to spend her time with people who are hurting and need special attention. Another nurse wants to devote most of her attention to making sure everything is done correctly and by the book. Her focus is less on the patient than it is on the process. The nurse who is more of a caregiver might be greatly tempted to mentally criticize the nurse who loves and is meticulous about the process, and to conclude that she does not care about people. As a result, tensions could develop between the two nurses as each mentally judges the other.

Gift-Envy

Another danger is that of gift-envy. You and a friend may graduate from the same school of nursing, having taken the same courses and studied with the same professors, but how would you feel if your friend advanced much faster than you did? With all of the responsibilities facing both of you, she may excel and even may want to accept more challenges, whereas you might struggle to just keep up with what comes across your plate. And as the years pass, your friend could continue to outpace you. Why would that be? Consider the following possibilities: (1) She has some gifts that you do not possess, or perhaps (2) the Lord has a very different purpose for her than He has for you.

This situation could lead to envy, jealousy, and even a strained relationship between the two of you. But none of that is truly necessary. Once you recognize that even what you do possess is a gift from God to be used in conjunction with His plan for your life, your feeling toward those who have been given greater praise in various ways will become more an attitude of encouragement and happiness for their success. God does not hold you responsible for what you do not possess.

Although he is now with the Lord, Cliff Barrows remains a great example of this principle. Cliff, who was known best for leading large choirs at the Billy Graham Crusades, was once a young preacher and had an active preaching ministry. One evening Cliff and his wife attended a Youth for Christ rally to hear the young evangelist Billy Graham. However, a problem arose when the man who was to lead the choir had to go to Chicago and could not

fulfill his responsibility that evening. Someone suggested to Billy that one of the attendees was not only a preacher but also a musician and might be willing to fill in for that evening. Billy agreed, and Cliff became that evening's choir director. Later, the famed evangelist asked Cliff if he would be willing to join him as his song leader. Cliff and his wife wrestled with the idea for a while, because Cliff had planned to go to seminary and later begin his ministry as a preacher. Eventually, he told Billy that after much prayer and discussion, he and his wife Billie became convinced that he should join the Billy Graham team. Therefore, Cliff put aside his love for preaching and accepted the responsibility of gathering millions of people all over the world to sing in his great choirs for the Billy Graham Crusades.

And how did Billy Graham view Cliff Barrows? Graham said this about his friend: "Sometimes he could just step up and preach a lot better sermon than me because God gave him the gift—not only of organization and music but also of preaching and teaching." He added, "We have a little conference center near my home where I would go to hear him when he was there, and he certainly was a powerful speaker." Both of these men of God had the gift of preaching, but Cliff was also a gifted musician, which Billy wasn't. And yet God used both of these men to bless the lives of literally millions of people worldwide.

Gift-Restraint

The third danger of spiritual gifts is thinking you should operate only in the area of your giftedness. In any occupation, you would be exposed to and expected to carry out responsibilities that you neither enjoy nor feel particularly qualified to perform. In such a case, thinking "Well, that's not my gift, so I should not have to be expected to do that," is to fall into the gift-restraint pit. As believers, we have responsibilities whether we are gifted in those areas or not. You may not have the gift of giving, but God expects you to use your financial resources for His purposes. You may not have the gift of mercy, but God expects you to be merciful to others. You may not have the gift of leadership (**BOX 11-1**), but sometimes you may be expected to lead a group in completing some project. At all costs, you will want to avoid the danger of gift-restraint.

Gift-Exaltation

The fourth danger of spiritual gifts is to conclude that the gift you possess is more important than the gifts that others possess. For example, during my seminary days I had the privilege of working with what was then called Campus Crusade for

---

BOX 11-1 Outstanding Nurse Leader: Grace Peterson, PhD, RN

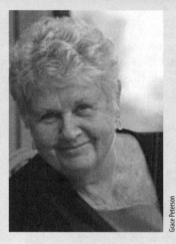
Grace Peterson

Dr. Grace Peterson always demonstrated her passion for Christ and utilized her spiritual gifts daily in her relationships with others. She loved working with others, and she enjoyed positive relationships with administrators, colleagues, faculty members, teachers, and students alike. Peterson was an excellent nursing professor, servant leader, and encourager who always gave to others and showed mercy when things did not go as planned. When asked to provide a reflection on her leadership, she immediately was there to assist in this project. She stated:

I have been searching for an article on "In Search of Excellence" that Tom Peters wrote in 1982. Since then, others have reworked [his ideas] on leadership. I just read an interesting article by two Swedish professors. These ideas are from a business-oriented model. I have applied some of the original authors' thoughts to my leadership. The newest article quotes a Toyota production system. What impressed me was their thought that the top identified priority was the Philosophy of the company. The second idea they identified was Process and how to create a flow when problems surface. This is an open model system. The third idea was People and Partners. They have subtitles of respect, challenge, and [growing] them. The fourth idea was Problem solving and learning, which is always continuous.

As I thought about my leadership at Concordia University Wisconsin (CUW), I accepted my position because of their Christ-centered approach to education. Their philosophical base was mine as well. I believe the nursing faculty brought problems to the table to solve. We respected each other and challenged each other. I challenged the faculty to get into a doctoral program and allocated funds for continuing education (CE). I believe we made decisions in our nursing school by consensus considering options.

Dr. Grace Peterson originally received her nursing diploma from Swedish Covenant Hospital School of Nursing in Chicago in 1962 and a BSN from North Park University in Chicago in 1964. She completed her MSN from the University of Wisconsin–Oshkosh in 1990, where her thesis was titled "An Investigation of the Relationship Between Nursing Students' Perception of Invitational Teacher Behaviors and Self-Esteem." Peterson received her PhD from Marquette University in 1997, where her doctoral dissertation was on "Nursing Perceptions of the Spiritual Dimension of Patient Care: The Neuman Systems Model in Curricular Formations."

Currently, Peterson is Professor Emeritus at CUW and an Emeritus member of the American Association of Colleges of Nursing. When she taught nursing, her specialty fields were legal/ethical aspects of nursing, professionalism, nursing theory, cultural nursing, and primary health care. She holds certification in parish nursing and is a parish nurse educator. She has been a consultant for

(continues)

the Commission of Collegiate Nursing Education (CCNE) and the Wisconsin State Board of Nursing, and was appointed to the Hearing Committee for CCNE in Washington, DC. Peterson also served on professional boards such as the Wisconsin Association of Colleges of Nursing and Ozaukee County Board of Health, and was president of the CUW Nursing Honor Society.

Peterson enjoys Bible studies, participating in church, being active with her grandchildren, and traveling in the United States. She has led mission trips to Costa Rica and Belize with nursing students in the past. Her mission as a Christian nurse has been a true vocation and calling to serve God, and she has utilized her spiritual gifts to serve others around her fully.

Christ (Cru). My friend Swede Anderson and I would travel from Dallas to Denton, Texas, each Friday and spend the day on campus. We would walk through the dorms, go into the cafeteria, or sit out on a bench and share Christ's message with the students at North Texas State University. Whereas Swede would see some students come to Christ each week, I would lead one or two to Christ in a month. At first, I thought there was something spiritually wrong with me. After all, we both had the same message sharing orientation—known as the "Four Spiritual Laws"—but we achieved different results.

At first, I became discouraged because I had seen so few people come to Christ under my ministry. But that feeling began to change during the Friday evening Bible studies. During these meetings I would see some people come to Christ, but more often noticed the believers showing great interest in the Bible. Swede could have looked down on me and said, "Because you are not as successful as I am in leading students to Christ, you may not belong in this organization." Instead, Swede would encourage me and tell me that my gift was one of teaching. In fact, he believed in my teaching so strongly that many years later he told his friend, Bill Armstrong, former president of Colorado Christian University, that I was his choice for becoming Dean of Biblical and Theological Studies at the university in the College of Adult and Graduate Studies.

Why are gift-projection, gift-envy, gift-restraint, and gift-exaltation so dangerous? All of these problems can prevent you from becoming all that God wants you to be and will promote an attitude that will result in ineffective relationships with coworkers. But when you understand the source and purpose of your spiritual gifts, you can avoid falling into these traps. Now let's look at some myths people have concerning spiritual gifts.

▶ The Myths of Spiritual Gifts

One significant concern that the Apostle Paul had with the believers in Corinth was their ignorance of spiritual gifts. Various unbiblical opinions and attitudes had arisen there and were hurting the church body at large. Recognizing this problem, Paul wrote, "Now about spiritual gifts, brothers, I do not want you to be ignorant" (1 Corinthians 12:1). Ignorance had nothing to do with the Corinthians' intellectual ability, but everything to do with their propensity to jump to conclusions without any evidence. Consider the following perspectives that some people have about spiritual gifts.

Myth 1

The more gifts you possess, the greater your spiritual life. Spiritual gifts and one's spiritual life are two different issues. Our spiritual life deals with our relationship with the Lord, whereas our spiritual gifts focus on what we do. The former reveals character, and the latter demonstrates what we can contribute when serving others. Too often, people use their spiritual gifts in ways that exalt themselves rather than the Lord, or they use their gifts in an unloving and uncaring manner. The believers in Corinth possessed all the gifts, but they lacked character and were seen as "carnal" or living under the influence of their sinful nature. The depth of your walk with the Lord will determine the effectiveness of your spiritual gifts.

Myth 2

Public gifts are more important than private gifts. A public, or "up-front," gift may include leadership, teaching, music, and evangelism. The people with these gifts are often the ones who stand in front of an audience and receive praise from their followers. Now consider the gifts of mercy, wisdom, serving, giving, and administration: They often go unnoticed and unappreciated. Paul, however, informs his readers that every gift is essential for the building up of the Body of Christ.

Think about this: When it comes to selling a house, who is most important? The designer of the house? The manufacturer of the materials for the house? The builder? The realtor? Most people neither know nor ever meet the first three. Instead, they only come in contact with the realtor. And yet, all of these individuals are essential for selling a house. Therefore, whatever gift you have, be thankful for what God has given you and put it to good use. Remember these words from the pen of the Apostle Paul: "What, after all, is Apollos? And what is Paul? Only servants, through whom you came to believe—as the Lord has assigned to each his task. I planted the seed. Apollos watered it, but God made it grow. So, neither he who plants nor he who waters is anything, but only God who makes things grow" (1Corinthians 3:5–7).

Myth 3

Spiritual gifts must be discovered before you get involved with people. One of the best ways

of discovering your spiritual gifts is to get involved in the lives of others and to learn what you do well, what you do naturally, and what you do that so many appreciate and about which they give you compliments. Just keep doing what seems to come naturally to you, because that is one of the best indicators of how God has gifted you.

Myth 4

There are male and female spiritual gifts. The spiritual gifts of the Holy Scripture are given to both men and women. The way or place where the gift is used might be more gender-related, but many women are gifted with leadership, teaching, singing, and administration. Also, some men are gifted with serving, mercy, giving, and helping. Remember also that both men and women may have the same spiritual gift but may use it in different venues.

Myth 5

God will miraculously show you your spiritual gift. Most of us have discovered our spiritual gifts by getting involved in some ministry or work of service. We might think that we would be good at a specific job and accept the responsibility. However, after a few months, we might discover that it is not an area of our strength and has caused us more frustration than pleasure. This is why the Bible places so much emphasis on beginning to serve. Find a need that you can meet and start the process of meeting that need. You will soon discover areas of strength and weaknesses. The areas of strength will indicate where you are most likely gifted.

Myth 6

You should serve God only in the areas of your spiritual gifts. This issue was addressed earlier in regard to gift-restraint, one of the dangers of spiritual gifts. But you may want to think through a what-if situation, such as the parable of the Good Samaritan. Recall that the

Samaritan saw the man who was robbed, lying in his blood and covered with bruises. There would be no parable if that Samaritan said to himself, "If only I had the gift of mercy, I would help this poor guy in such bad condition. But since mercy isn't my gift, I'll just pray that someone else comes along and helps him." Whether we have the gift of mercy or the gift of helping, when someone is in need, and we can meet that need, it is time to help, gifted or not. Now let's consider the source and purpose of spiritual gifts.

▶ The Source and Purpose of Spiritual Gifts

You have so many resources at hand that have equipped you to be effective in the calling to nursing that God has given you. You have God's Holy Spirit living within you. You also possess the spiritual gifts He has given you. In addition, God has given you the Scriptures that equip you for spiritual warfare and provide a Biblical worldview to help you interpret life around you. Finally, there is the power of prayer that He makes available to you. Let's consider each one of these individually.

Gift 1: The Holy Spirit

You possess the Holy Spirit, which means that God lives within you and you have become His *temple*. In fact, consider these words from Paul as he writes to the Corinthian believers: "Do you not know that your body is a temple of the Holy Spirit, who is in you, whom you have received from God? You are not your own; you were bought at a price. Therefore, honor God with your body" (1 Corinthians 6:19–20). When Paul refers to your body as a temple, recall that there were two parts of the temple in Jerusalem: the temple proper, and the "Holy of Holies" or "the Most Holy Place." That is where

the Ark of the Covenant was placed, along with the "mercy seat." The word Paul chooses in this passage refers to the "Holy of Holies." In other words, because your body houses the very presence of God, as did the Ark of the Covenant, your body is the present-day "Holy of Holies." This is the only body through which we can serve the Lord. Therefore, keep it clean, pure, and honoring to God.

Second, along with the Holy Spirit comes the *supernatural power* to do the things that you usually could not or would not do in the power of the flesh. When Jesus was preparing to ascend into heaven after his resurrection, he told his disciples this fundamental truth: "It is not for you to know the times or dates the Father has set by his own authority. But you will receive power when the Holy Spirit comes on you; and you will be my witnesses in Jerusalem, and in all Judea and Samaria, and to the ends of the earth" (Acts 1:7–8). For you, that power may take the form of wisdom, courage, insight, physical energy, love for the unlovely, care for the uncaring, understanding, or many other guises.

Third, *you belong to God* and not to yourself. You were once a slave to sin, but now you are a bond slave to God. In the Biblical days, some slaves served their masters against their own will. Other "bond slaves" willingly served their masters; that is, their masters showed them respect and provided well for their needs, although they were still slaves. Likewise, as a bond slave to Christ, who delivered you from the terrible slavery to sin, you serve him because you love him. He provides and protects us. He cares for us. And we love because he first loved us.

Fourth, God is your *illuminator*. The Holy Spirit is a gift from both the Father and the Son. One of his responsibilities is to make the scriptures understandable. This is why it is so important not just to open your Bible and read, but first to seek the guidance of the Holy Spirit as you read. Ask for enlightenment about what the writer meant. Then expect the Holy Spirit to meet that need, according to Jesus's promise:

"But the Counselor, the Holy Spirit, whom the Father will send in my name, will teach you all things and will remind you of everything I have said to you" (John 14:25–26).

Gift 2: Spiritual Gifts

The Holy Spirit gives spiritual gifts to believers. First, he gives spiritual gifts to "each one" (1 Corinthians 12:7a). Don't ever excuse yourself by thinking that you have nothing to contribute to this life and to other people who need what only you can offer. If Christ lives in you, you are spiritually gifted. There are no exceptions in the family of God.

Second, he gives spiritual gifts "for the common good" (1 Corinthians 12:7b). In other words, you have something that others need. If your gift is showing mercy, then humanity waits for you to exercise that gift. If it is doing research, the demand is high. If it is helping to solve the cure for specific diseases, your input is needed.

Third, the Holy Spirit gives these gifts "just as he determines" (1 Corinthians 12:11). How does the Spirit of God determine which gifts you should possess? He does so according to his plan for your life. You are not on earth accidentally, but rather by God's design, whether it was your parents' choice or not. You exist because God wants you to exist. He has a plan for your life made up of many opportunities. Likewise, He has gifted you according to His plan. Although you are responsible for discovering and developing the gifts that God has given you, you are already fully equipped to carry out whatever door He opens for you. Really? Yes, really!

Gift 3: The Word of God

Not only have you been equipped with the Holy Spirit and spiritual gifts, but you also possess the Bible, the very words of God (Romans 3:2). It is the Bible that becomes your compass to navigate through life. It provides a worldview that you will find nowhere else—but not a narrow worldview or a self-seeking worldview. The Bible will help you interpret the events of life by what it tells you about God. Too often people interpret God based on the events of life. For example, some might say, "There is no God to allow such tragedy to occur," while others say, "If God allows mankind to be so cruel, He must not be a good and merciful God."

The more you learn about the God of the Bible, the more you will come to realize that there is a real devil who seeks to steal people's happiness and does everything in his power to make people's lives miserable and to destroy whatever he can. Moreover, you will discover that God is slow to anger, merciful, loving, quick to forgive, and the ultimate promise keeper. So, when bad things occur in life, rather than blame God, you will recognize that God did not cause the event and that He can bring order out of chaos and joy out of suffering. That is why Joseph was able to say to his brothers who hated him and sold him into slavery, "You intended to harm me, but God intended it for good to accomplish what is now being done, the saving of many lives" (Genesis 50:20).

Gift 4: Prayer

Along with the Holy Spirit and the Bible, you are equipped with prayer. Prayer includes both speaking to God and listening to God. Many of us like to talk to Him, but too often we don't spend the time to listen. He speaks to us through His Word, which is why reading the Bible is not enough. That is, we must also meditate (pause and consider) on what we are reading. We must invest the time to study the Word of God so that we understand its meaning and application to our lives.

But it is prayer that brings us before the throne of grace. "Let us then approach the throne of grace with confidence, so that we may receive mercy and find grace to help us in our time of need" (Hebrews 5:16). You can be confident that the Lord will listen to your prayer and will respond to you according to your need. That is indeed a powerful gift that you possess. If you need wisdom, He will provide it. If you need courage to speak or to confront, it is yours for the asking.

Now that you have realized you indeed are fully equipped to do well in school and make a significant impact in the lives of others with these powerful blessings from God, consider the purpose of those spiritual gifts.

▶ The Purpose of Spiritual Gifts: To Serve and Equip

Serving

The Apostle Peter informs his readers, "Each one should use whatever gift he has received to serve others, faithfully administering God's grace in its various forms" (1 Peter 4:10). Peter then mentions some of the forms that God's grace takes, such as using the gifts of speaking and serving. The Apostle Paul mentions seven other types of God's grace—namely, prophesying, serving, teaching, encouraging, contributing to the needs of others, leadership (governing), and showing mercy (Romans 12:6–8). Furthermore, Paul includes the gifts of wisdom, knowledge, faith, healing, miraculous powers, prophecy, distinguishing between spirits, speaking in different tongues, interpretation of tongues, apostles, prophets, teachers, and administration (1 Corinthians 12:7–11, 28).

Equipping

The Apostle Paul identifies another purpose of spiritual gifts—"to equip" others for serving the Lord. Consider what he told the believers in Ephesus: "It was he who gave some to be prophets, some to be evangelists, and some to be pastors and teachers, to prepare God's people for works of service" (Ephesians 4:11–12). In this passage, Paul uses an interesting

Greek word, katartismos, that the New International Version (NIV) translates as "prepare." It can be used in a nautical sense—"to mend torn nets" (Matthew 4:21). The same word can also be used in a medical sense—"to set broken bones." Finally, it can be used in a military sense—"to equip or outfit a soldier." Basically, it refers to providing a person with whatever is needed to equip him or her to serve the Lord wholeheartedly.

There are traditional ways in which you can use your gifts, but you may also consider some creative means by which to apply those gifts to bless others. God is never limited to the circumstances of life or human traditions. He can place original thoughts into your mind that you had never previously imagined.

For example, I am no longer a pastor or the Dean of Biblical and Theological Studies. In those positions, I had a great platform to reach out and bless many people with my gifts of speaking and teaching. But today, my ability to use my gifts to bless others is limited, owing to my lack of a platform. Therefore, I've had to be creative to continue to bless through teaching.

Likewise, after many years of not writing, I've begun to write again, including blogs and my latest book, *A Love Story from God*, which takes the reader through an overview of the Bible and provides an answer to how we know that what we have today was written back then. Since my son is a pastor, I do have the opportunity to speak in his church a few times a year. I've also spoken for the Seed Company (an offshoot of the Wycliffe Bible Translators) on the Dead Sea Scrolls at the Denver Museum of Natural Science. But such opportunities are few and far between.

However, the Lord has recently opened up two other means by which I can use my gift of teaching and my love for photography. Every day I post a photograph on Facebook and, at times, include a scripture reference to match the photo. Based on the feedback I've received, it seems that many people have been blessed and encouraged by the photos.

The age of technology has greatly changed what happens when pastors retire today. In the past, they were generally limited to either taking a pastoral internship in a small church community or teaching a Sunday School class. Others thought that their "ministry days" were over, so they spent their time playing golf or getting involved in some other hobby. But today, retirement is recognized as a time for realizing one's creativity under the guidance of the Holy Spirit. So, think in terms of using your gifts creatively, both in your job and outside the confines of the building where you work. Recognize that some spiritual gifts remain active throughout your lifetime, whereas others are very effective during a specific time frame.

▶ Discover Your Spiritual Gifts

The primary question with which we all wrestle is, "What are my gifts?" How do we know what we possess? This is an excellent question and must be addressed if we are to be effective in blessing and serving others. You can take various "Spiritual Gift Tests," and they may help you discover your gifts. In most cases, however, they primarily confirm what you've already been thinking. It's not very often that people take such a test and conclude, "Wow, I never knew I had that gift!" Here, we'll consider a common-sense approach to discovering your spiritual gifts. Few of us are a "jack of all trades." Instead, most of us are limited in what we can do well and are aware of the many things we can't do very well. So, rather than focus on what we don't have or cannot do, let's consider how to discover what we can do well and experience success in life.

Awareness

The first thing you want to do is to become aware of the needs all around you. Those needs may surface as you see certain things lacking among your friends, whether Christian or non-Christian. The needs may arise through announcements at church, or perhaps the Holy Spirit may prompt you to ask some specific questions to your friends or to people at church, in the classroom, or in the workplace. In turn, the answers to those questions may direct you to get involved in an area you had never considered because you did not realize that the need existed.

A second step is to become aware of which gifts are listed in the Bible. I've had many people tell me that they never realized that craftsmanship was a spiritual gift. For some it is an inherited gene from a parent, but for others it is a spiritual gift. For instance, when Moses was told to build furniture for the Tabernacle, he was responsible for getting the job done, but he was not a craftsman. His first 40 years of life were lived in a world of privilege in the household of Pharaoh. Everything was built for him, rather than by him. Moses's second 40 years were spent as a shepherd in the back desert of Midian. Thus, when God told him to build the furniture for the Tabernacle, he had to surround himself with those that were gifted in craftsmanship.

How do I know that this was a spiritual gift in the Old Testament? Listen to the account in the Book of Exodus. Whereas Moses asked the people to select those who were skilled in making the materials for the Tabernacle, God actually chose the two men to create artistic designs for work in gold, silver, and bronze; to cut and set stones; to work in wood; and to engage in all kinds of craftsmanship (Exodus 4–5).

> Then the Lord said to Moses, "See, I have chosen Bezalel, son of Uri, the son of Hur, of the tribe of Judah, and I have filled him with the Spirit of God, with skill, ability and knowledge in all kinds of crafts to make artistic designs for work in gold, silver and bronze, to cut and set stones, to work in wood, and to engage in all kinds of craftsmanship." (Exodus 31:1–5)

Meanwhile, Oholiab was chosen by God and then given the Holy Spirit, who gave Oholiab the spiritual gift of craftsmanship: "Moreover, I have appointed Oholiab, son of Ahisamach, of the tribe of Dan, to help him. Also, I have given skill to all the craftsmen to make everything I have commanded you" (Exodus 31:6).

Common Sense

Today we live in an era when common sense sometimes seems as scarce as hen's teeth. So many decisions and actions are based on emotion, which results in both logic and common sense flying out the window. Discovering your spiritual gifts should not be some long, arduous process. Use your common sense by asking yourself five simple questions.

Natural Interests and Desires

"What do I enjoy doing?" You may want to begin with your responsibilities as a nurse. Which part of nursing do you think you will most enjoy? Which part of that profession seems to come naturally, and which role do you think might become more a drudgery? For instance, you may love the patient relationships, but may be concerned about all of the detail reporting or any administrative responsibilities that come with the job—or vice versa.

Another possibility might be that you really enjoy anything that deals with research, but when it comes to people skills, you would rather leave that responsibility to others. This preference does not make you less of a nurse than those who love to spend their time with patients: It just means that you might want to look for openings that involve more research projects than patient responsibilities.

Dr. Barbara White is the Dean of the School of Nursing for the College of Adult and Graduate Studies at Colorado Christian University. She spear-headed the development of the entire bachelor's, master's, and doctoral programs for the School of Nursing. Although she is a trained nurse, she has not been involved in a hospital with patients for many years. Her giftedness lies more in the area of design and development of excellent nursing programs and working with a team than in the realm of taking care of patients. She "equips" others to serve in the hospitals and clinics, along with "equipping" her staff to administer the programs of the university.

Ask yourself whether you would rather be in "patient ministry" than in an administrative role. Would you rather have the responsibility of developing new techniques and new systems? Or is your greatest desire meeting face to face with those who need physical, emotional, or spiritual help?

Needs

"Which needs do I see that no one is meeting, and can I meet those needs?" Although many nurses work in hospitals and doctors' offices, they don't always focus on the same needs. One nurse will notice patient needs, whereas another will mentally be reorganizing the nursing staff, and another will wonder why the facilities look so sterile. We tend to see needs according to our spiritual gifts.

When my wife and I go to a restaurant, we notice different things. If the service is not very good, I will be thinking about what I would do differently if I were the manager of the restaurant. Meanwhile, my wife will notice a man sitting by himself and inform me that I should go over and talk with him because she is confident that he is a widower and needs encouragement. If a friend of ours happens to be sitting with us, she will be mentally redecorating the entire restaurant. Which needs come to the mind that cause you to want to change something or to contribute to it mentally?

Past Success

"Which types of ministry have I enjoyed and in which have I been successful?" There are likely some responsibilities that you enjoy and handle very well, and other responsibilities that you wish you could delegate to others. The question you need to answer for yourself is, where do I shine? What have others told me that I do well? In which areas do others look to me as a mentor or have I demonstrated knowledge and competency? You will shine in the field of your giftedness and will become less motivated in those areas in which you have a responsibility, but you may work from an attitude of "ought" rather than one of "love" and "enjoyment."

Confirmation of Others

"Which abilities have others seen in me? What have other people told me that I do well?" Although you are taking the same classes as your classmates, all of you will not end up in the same type of nursing career. Some of you will head toward administrative duties. Others will seek the opportunity to do more research. Still others will love being with patients in the hospital or clinic. Which type of feedback are you receiving from your classmates, friends, and relatives? What can they envision for you when you graduate? It's not where you begin that is so important, but rather where you end your life as a nurse.

Flexibility

"Am I willing to be flexible to attempt something new, or do I enjoy the routine of what I am presently doing?" Some individuals enjoy "going with the flow" and adapt quickly to the changes around them. For others, change is frightening; they like things as they are, and routine is their friend. Where do you fit into this picture? Does change scare you or challenge you? Are you more or less likely to try something new? If you are willing to venture into a new area of nursing, you may discover a spiritual gift that you never realized even existed. As you find out how God has gifted you, don't stop there. Put your discovery to use so you can develop your gifts.

▶ Developing Your Spiritual Gifts

It is one thing to know how God has gifted you, but quite another to understand how you should develop your gift. A gifted musician is useful only as he continues to craft his gift of music, whether it be singing, playing an instrument, or composing songs. When people stop developing the gifts they have, those gifts can begin to atrophy. You have been taught anatomy and have learned how the body will begin to decline when specific muscles are not put into use. Moreover, the aging process exacerbates that degeneration. So it is with spiritual gifts: If they are not put to use, they will also atrophy.

Education

With technology advancing in so many areas, you have ample opportunities to take advantage of online classes in a specific area where you are gifted, or to enroll in seminars or courses. So many options are available today that, no matter what your spiritual gifts may be, you can almost certainly discover a venue that will suit your interest, budget, and time.

Reading

Every year, thousands of self-help books go on the market, covering many fields of interest. In fact, once you undertake a web search for some area of interest, don't be surprised to be inundated with ads for classes, seminars, apps, or something to purchase. One nice thing about reading is that you can do it digitally, in hard or soft cover, or even through audio as you drive to work. In addition, numerous self-help videos are available for free—so money should be no object as you begin to develop your gifts. Indeed, help is often a bookstore or a computer-click away.

Conferences

Attending conferences for gift development purposes is usually most helpful after graduation, when you are in your first employment position. At this point, you are already in the process of using what you've learned in school and through on-site experience, but a conference can be of great benefit for honing the tools that God has given you to use for the equipping of and serving others. Such a meeting may deal with administrative procedure, leadership, organizational skills, or just ways to serve others more effectively.

Organizations

Consider joining a Christian Nurses Group, such as the Nurses Christian Fellowship, where you can share ideas, insights, new skills, and other subjects that will enhance your gifting.

On a personal note, I was recently visiting a friend in hospice. As we talked, a woman with a guitar over her shoulder came up to my friend and asked him to introduce her to me. As we talked, I discovered that she was a musical therapist; earlier that day, she had played hymns and sang for my friend. I thought, "What a great way to minister to those who are incapacitated or preparing to meet Jesus!" The woman was a gifted musician who used her gift to encourage and serve others through music.

When you are working in a hospital, you will soon discover those who truly know the Lord and those who do not. Both types will need your smile, words of encouragement, and physical touch—but allowing the believer to know that you, too, have a personal relationship with God can create a special bond that believers alone can understand. Hospitals have their own rules for what a nurse can and cannot do when it comes to religious matters, but your smile, kind words, and presence at a patient's bed may be the best opening to share Christ, especially if the patient wants to know more about you and why you may seem different from other nurses.

Putting It to Use

The best way for most people to develop their spiritual gifts is to put them to use. You've often heard the phrase, "Use it or lose it"—it also applies when it comes to your spiritual gifts. When something is not used, it is easy to get into the habit of neglect. The Apostle Paul encouraged Timothy to "fan into flame the gift of God, which is in you through the laying on of my hands" (2 Timothy 1:6). On another occasion, he told Timothy, "Do not neglect your gift which was given you through a prophetic message when the body of elders laid their hands on you" (1 Timothy 4:14). Timothy was young and intimidated by others, so Paul had to continually remind him that he was a gifted young man and needed to sharpen his gift and put that gift to use.

Up to this point, you have learned how to discover and develop your spiritual gifts, but now consider the matter of deploying your gifts for the benefit of others.

▶ Deploy Your Spiritual Gifts

Don't wait until you graduate to deploy your gifts. Put them to work in your classes, during your internship, in your church, and in your Bible study group. A gift is not something to be used "later," but rather should be deployed as you are in the process of learning, growing, and serving. Ask yourself questions such as "Is there a need in my church that I could meet now?"; "Is there someone who could use a friend to come alongside them and just listen to where they are in their life's journey, as well as to what they are experiencing physically, mentally, emotionally, or even spiritually?"; "What need do I see that I could meet?"; "What opportunities lie before me for which I could volunteer?"; and "What has to be done that no one else is willing to try?" Such questions will help you to focus on how God has wired you.

▶ A Nurse's Perspective on Spiritual Gifts

Eckerd (2017) introduces "the Agape Model, based on the agape love and characteristics of Christ, upon which Christian nurses may align their practice to provide Christ-centered care" (p. 124). Within this model, initially the nurse must be dedicated to his or her Christian faith. A commitment to Christ must be in place to be his follower. As a Christian nurse, you believe that Jesus Christ is your Savior, and that he died for you on the cross to save you from your sins. According to Eckerd, "the calling into the nursing profession underscores the kingdom nurse's dedication to excellence in the profession and fulfills a God-given purposeful life" (p. 127). Many nurses feel called to their profession, and nursing is a vocation designed by God to serve others.

Nurses should always be in a state of professional growth. Provision 5 of the Code of Ethics for Nurses states, "The nurse owes the same duties to self as to others, including the responsibility to promote health and safety, preserve wholeness of character and integrity, maintain competence and continue personal and professional growth" (Fowler, 2015, p. 73).

Following this, the nurse utilizes prayer, the Holy Spirit, and his or her spiritual gifts. As a nurse caring for a patient who is critically ill, it is important to recognize that some individuals will welcome prayer and others will

not. After assessing the wishes of the patient, the nurse should either pray or not pray for the patient depending on his or her request. Nurses must be respectful to all patients. Prayers may be often said on the way to work and during work, and then possibly a prayer of thanksgiving may be said after work that all went well during patient care. Communicating with God and the Holy Spirit can bring a sense of peace for the nurse, a sense of trust that God will provide, and it can build a trusting patient relationship. It is like standing on holy ground when you bring the Holy Spirit to the bedside, and anywhere else, because you are asking for God's guidance in the use of your knowledge, skills, and spiritual gifts (see **BOXES 11-2** and **11-3**).

Finally, the nurse will use the **Fruit of the Spirit** at the point of care, when interacting with family, and when interacting with all colleagues on the healthcare team. The Fruit of the Spirit is described in Galatians 5:22–23 as "love, joy, peace, patience, kindness, goodness, faithfulness, gentleness, self-control; against such things there is no law." As a nurse demonstrating these attributes of the Holy Spirit, you are defining the compassionate care that Jesus demonstrated so well. Thus, as a nurse, it is vitally important for you to demonstrate the Fruit of the Spirit as well as employ your spiritual gifts.

▶ Conclusion

Always remember that you are unique in the eyes of God. He has fully equipped you to be useful as a person and as a nurse. Learn everything you can about nursing, but always remember that as a Christian nurse, you have access to spiritual resources. You possess the Holy Spirit, spiritual gifts, the Word of God, and the opportunity to talk to the Creator at any time of day or night. So, as you are in the process of getting that nursing degree, employ your spiritual gifts and observe how God is using you to impact and contribute to the lives of others.

BOX 11-2 Research Highlight

In this 2013 research study, Tomlinson describes seven motivational gifts: perceiving, serving, teaching, encouraging, giving, ruling, and mercy. The study focused on these motivational gifts, found in Romans 12:3–8, among nurses and their relationships with job satisfaction and person–job fit. The author utilized three surveys and a demographic questionnaire to gather data to assess and analyze motivation and gifts, job satisfaction, and person–job fit (p. 174). The demographic characteristics examined gender, unit or department (e.g., emergency, medical, pediatric), and generation (the Silent Generation, Baby Boomer, Generation X, and millennial). The study established that knowing the nurse's motivational gifts can impact recruitment, job satisfaction, and person–job fit. Additionally, the study found that nurses scored higher in serving, mercy, and encouraging.

Modified from Tomlinson, J. C. (2013). Do motivational gifts impact nurses' job fit and satisfaction? *Journal of Christian Nursing, 30*(3), 172–178.

BOX 11-3 Evidence-Based Practice Focus

According to Kofoed (2011), the importance of reflective practice in nursing is necessary. Nursing is both an art and a science, but in order to transform your thinking and knowledge as an RN, she proposes that reflection can transform your present and future nursing care. Kofoed notes the importance of "reflection-within-the-moment," which can lead nurses toward "mindful practice" in which they think critically and provide high-quality care and safety for their patients (p. 133). Additionally, the author describes the Christian nurse as asking himself or herself, "What would Jesus do?", and saying a simple prayer for an answer or guidance in patient care. In this article, Kofoed speaks about the relationship between reflection and evidence-based practice, and describes how it may influence education and nursing practice changes in the future.

Modified from Kofoed, N. A. (2011). Reflective practice for personal and professional transformation. *Journal of Christian Nursing, 28*(3), 132–138. doi:10.1097/CNJ.0b013e31821cbb92

▶ Clinical Reasoning Exercises

You are working the night shift in a busy intensive care unit (ICU) with three other registered nurses (RNs). At the beginning of your shift, an assigned patient coded. During the past two weeks, you have provided care to this patient, Jacob, who was suffering from congestive heart failure. You know the patient's spouse, Susan, and his family very well. You call them at 3:00 a.m. to let them know that their loved one passed away a few minutes ago. Susan starts screaming at you on the phone, criticizing you for not calling earlier and letting her and the family know that Jacob was not doing well. Susan is annoyed and requests that Jacob's body not be removed from his room until they visit him.

As the nurse, you are actively listening to Susan's comments. You know the unit has been very busy with codes and admissions since the beginning of the shift and two nurses called in sick. You also know that the nursing administration will be angry as well, as the outcomes for this patient will most likely be negative because Susan and her family are quite upset with the nurse and the care provided. You also know that the ICU bed is needed immediately for another patient who is now in the emergency room following a multiple-vehicle accident that led to several causalities.

1. Which spiritual gifts will you, as the RN, use while talking to Susan on the phone?
2. As a Christian nurse, how do you respond to Susan and her family when they arrive at the ICU?
3. How will you respond to their anger when they realize that you moved Jacob to room 234 because the bed was needed for another critical patient?
4. Which spiritual gifts will you use while being with the family and their loved one?

The next morning, while you are sleeping, the nursing director and the nursing manager of the ICU call you, after speaking with several family members early that morning. They ask you what happened with Jacob, Susan, and the family last night, and why you called them so late.

5. Which spiritual gifts will you use when speaking with the director of nursing and the manager of the ICU?
6. How will you care for yourself, given that you know you did the best job possible as a Christian nurse but everyone is angry and upset?
7. Which resources will you gather for the family before their arrival to the ICU?
8. Which resources will you use after being accused of not monitoring your patient more closely and not notifying the family in a timely manner that the patient status had changed?

▶ **Personal Reflection Exercises**

According to Dameron (2015), "As Christian nurses, we bring our natural talents, education, and experiences, coupled with the work of the Holy Spirit, for a unique and powerful ministry in nursing" (p. 143). Christian nurses can receive spiritual gifts from the Holy Spirit as they practice the art and science of nursing. These spiritual gifts are recorded in 1 Corinthians 12:4–11:

> Now there are varieties of gifts, but the same Spirit; and there are varieties of service, but the same Lord; and there are varieties of activities, but it is the same God who empowers them all in everyone. To each is given the manifestation of the Spirit for the common good. For to one is given through the Spirit the utterance of wisdom, and to another the utterance of knowledge according to the same Spirit, to another faith by the same Spirit, to another gifts of healing by the one Spirit, to another the working of miracles, to another prophecy, to another the ability to distinguish between spirits, to another various kinds of tongues, to another the interpretations of tongues. All these are empowered by one and the same Spirit, who apportions to each one individually as he wills.

Additionally, Romans 12:6–8 affirms the significance of spiritual gifts that we receive by grace from the Holy Spirit:

> Having gifts that differ according to the grace given to us, let us use them: if prophecy, in proportion to our faith; if service, in our serving; the one who teaches, in his teaching; the one who exhorts, in his exhortation; the one who contributes, in generosity; the

one who leads, with zeal; the one who does acts of mercy, with cheerfulness.

Ephesians 4:11–13 asserts, "And he gave the apostles, the prophets, the evangelists, the shepherds, and teachers, to equip the saints for the work of ministry, for building up the body of Christ." As Christian nurses, we need to open up our hearts and minds to the Holy Spirit that his will be done and that we glorify his holy name in our service as nursing in ministry (see **CASE STUDY 11-1**).

Reflect on the following questions so as to understand your ministry in nursing.

1. What are the spiritual gifts that God has given to you?
2. What role do your spiritual gifts play during your nurse practice?

3. How might a Christian nurse demonstrate his or her spiritual gifts on the nursing unit? With fellow colleagues and nurses? With patients? List three ways for each.
4. Complete a free online survey to understand your spiritual gifts at https://www.gifttest. org/gifts-explained/ or https:// spiritualgiftstest.com/ (you will be prompted to create an account to take this test).
5. After completing the spiritual gifts survey, were there any surprises in the list of your spiritual gifts? If so, reflect on this spiritual gift, including how it has impacted you in the past and how it might change your nursing practice.

🔍 CASE STUDY 11-1

Given the many challenges of nursing today, the nurse is called to effectively and efficiently provide high-quality care and safety for all assigned patients with positive patient care outcomes. Many nurses are comfortable following the medical model and providing for patients' physical needs. However, providing holistic care requires additional assessment of the person's emotional, social, and spiritual well-being. According to Murphy and Walker (2013), "the foundation of Spirit-guided care is how the nurse uses him or herself as Christ's hands and presence as he/she engages in nursing care" (p. 149). Additionally, "Spirit-guided care is the act of removing one's self as the motivating force and allowing Christ, in the form of the Holy Spirit, to flow through us and guide us in our care" (p. 150).

Jane, an RN, is going into the medical ICU for her second 12-hour shift in a row. Working from 7 a.m. to 7 p.m. meshes well with her family needs, and she is able to get the proper sleep needed for the care of high-acuity patients.

Yesterday afternoon, Jane admitted a 61-year-old female in septic shock for an unknown etiology. When this woman came to the emergency room by ambulance, she had a very low blood pressure and a weak, thready pulse. She is highly sedated and intubated. She is receiving several strong-acting antibiotics that are given frequently along with IV fluids. The patient is the color of a pumpkin, has 4+ pitting edema, and is in liver and renal failure with lab results that are not within the normal limits. The patient is accompanied by her husband, two sons, and one daughter-in-law; they do not have any medical background and are very frightened and anxious, yet speechless.

This morning, the patient's brother and her mother are present in the patient's room, and many other friends and family members are in the waiting room. This family belongs to a church in town, and they have been very strong believers and supporters of the church for many years.

As a Christian nurse, you speak with the family at the bedside and answer their questions, along with providing an update on the patient's status overnight. You have reassured the family and asked them to leave the room so that you can complete your morning assessment and care. The family requests to be notified if any physicians visit her.

The physician, a nurse practitioner (NP), and several specialists come in the room while Jane is providing the morning care. As the patient's nurse, you go out to the waiting room and allow two of the family members back in the room to ask questions of the doctor, NP, and specialists. These healthcare providers have no answers as to why the patient was in septic shock upon admission, and many of the healthcare providers did not believe this patient would survive initially.

Jane talked with the family members and explained the care that she was providing the patient. Before suctioning the patient, you noticed how the nurse held her hand and explained what would happen next. All her physical care was explained and provided well. When Jane had time, she sat down by the bedside and held the patient's hand and read from the Bible. She allowed family members to come and go as long as they were quiet. She actively listened to the family's questions and was present at the bedside most of the day. Jane was calm, had a smile on her face, and was never in a hurry. Before she would leave for the day, she would pray with the patient, speaking softly while holding her hand.

Questions

1. How did Jane provide spiritual holistic care?
2. Which unique spiritual gifts did Jane demonstrate at the bedside?
3. Did Jane employ her spiritual gifts during her care and with family members? Which ones?
4. Do you believe that this nurse was utilizing Holy Spirit–guided care?
5. What impact did this nurse have on the family and patient through her Holy Spirit–guided care?

References

Dameron, C. M. (2015). Spiritual gifts in nursing. *Journal of Christian Nursing, 32*(2), 143. doi:10.1097/CNJ.0000000000000191

Eckerd, N. (2017). A nursing practice model based on Christ: The agape model. *Journal of Christian Nursing, 35*(2), 124–130. doi:10.1097/CNJ.0000000000000417

Fowler, M. D. M. (2015). *Guide to the code of ethics for nurses with interpretive statements: Development, interpretation, and application* (2nd ed.). Silver Spring, MD: American Nurses Association.

Murphy, L. S., & Walker, M. S. (2013). Spirit-guided care: Christian nursing for the whole person. *Journal of Christian Nursing, 30*(3), 144–152. doi:10.1097/CNJ.0b013e318294c289

Recommended Readings

Janzen, K., Reimer-Kirkham, S., & Astle, B. (2018). Nurses' perspectives on spiritual caregiving: Tending to the sacred. *Intervarsity Christian Fellowship,* 1–7. doi:10.1097/CNJ.0000000000000575

McMillan, K. (2016). Employee spiritual care: Supporting those who care for others. *Journal of Christian Nursing, 33*(2), 98–101. doi:10.1097/CNJ.0000000000000258

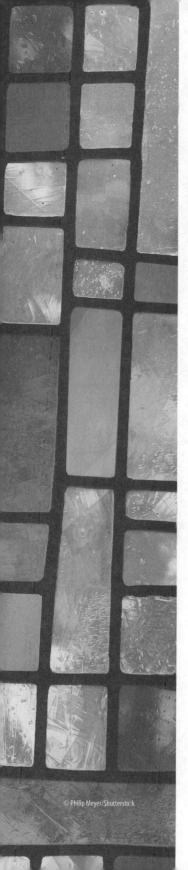
© Philip Meyer/Shutterstock

UNIT IV

Nursing as Ministry at Home and Abroad

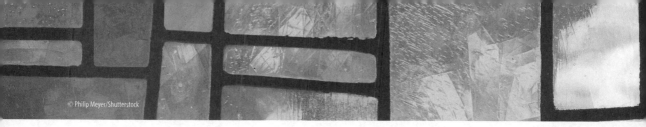

© Philip Meyer/Shutterstock

CHAPTER 12

Caring for Vulnerable Older Adults Across Settings

Christina Mulkey, DNP, RN, AGNP-C

LEARNING OBJECTIVES

At the end of this chapter, the reader will be able to:

1. Describe the transitional care model of nursing care for vulnerable elders transitioning across settings.
2. Implement evidence-based practice techniques to address specific conditions pertinent to vulnerable elders.
3. Understand the relationship between a Biblical worldview and the nurse's responsibility when caring for vulnerable elders.
4. Assess a vulnerable elderly client for spiritual needs in any setting and be prepared to meet those needs.
5. Create a plan of care for a vulnerable elderly client that incorporates Biblical principles.

KEY TERMS

Advance care planning	Malnutrition	Self-neglect
Alcohol use disorder (AUD)	Polypharmacy	Substance use disorder (SUD)
Assistive technology	Post-hospital syndrome (PHS)	Transitional Care Model (TCM)
Dementia	Presbycusis	Vulnerable elder
Elder abuse	Presbyopia	

And now, behold, the Lord has kept me alive, as He said, these forty-five years, ever since the Lord spoke this word to Moses while Israel wandered in the wilderness; and now, here I am this day, eighty-five years old. As yet I am as strong this day as on the day that Moses sent me; just as my strength was then, so now is my strength for war, both for going out and for coming in. Now therefore, give me this mountain of which the Lord spoke in that day; for you heard in that day how the Anakim were there, and that the cities were great and fortified. It may be that the Lord will be with me, and I shall be able to drive them out as the Lord said. (Joshua 14:10–12, New King James Version [NKJV])

Spoken by Caleb from the Bible, this passage is a reminder that our strength comes from the Lord, even as we age. Caleb reminds the Christian nurse that members of the elderly population have lived long lives filled with rich experiences from which we can learn. The physical body decays and wears down, back to dust, but the elderly often have difficulty accepting that reality, which is why the care and compassion of a Christian nurse is an invaluable component of the journey as health begins to fail.

Ben Carson's views complement Caleb's perspective on caring for the elderly. Dr. Carson (2014), a well-known neurosurgeon, author, and public speaker, writes in his book *One Nation* that the elderly should be cared for in a respectful manner. When the elderly require full-time care, two options are usually available: family members or nursing homes. One complicating factor with family members providing full-time care is that they might have jobs that require them to leave the home for several hours a day, leaving the elder alone. But what if the elder cannot be alone and unsupervised for safety reasons? More often than not, the older adult who meets this description would be placed in the care of a nursing home. Carson suggests another innovative answer that was developed out of necessity: adult daycare programs. Adult daycare programs can be very cost-effective, providing social interaction and sharing resources in a safe environment. The government cannot provide full-time care for the elderly due to the financial burden, so encouraging innovations such as adult daycare programs is crucial to finding solutions to this problem (Carson, 2014).

Our society must place a higher priority on, and take responsibility for, caring for the elderly, anticipating that the time will come when finances and resources will be devoted to that effort. If we prepare, we can do a better job of caring for the elderly (Carson, 2014). Caring for one's family is a moral obligation, and it falls on nurses to fill in the gaps when it comes to caring for the health and wellness of older adults.

▶ Background

Nursing care of the **vulnerable elder** is a unique calling that can be distinguished from all other areas of nursing. The American Nurses Association's (ANA) expert workgroup of gerontological nurses (Bikford, 2018) defines this calling:

> Gerontological nursing is an evidence-based nursing specialty practice that addresses the unique physiological, social, psychological, developmental, economic, cultural, spiritual, and advocacy needs of older adults. Gerontological nursing focuses on the process of aging and the protection, promotion, restoration, and optimization of health and functions; prevention of illness and injury; facilitation of healing; alleviation of

suffering through the diagnosis and treatment of human response; and advocacy in the care of older adults, careers, families, groups, communities, and populations. (p. 48)

Because the aging process itself leads to an increased risk of chronic illness, all nurses should have a working knowledge of the special needs associated with vulnerable elders. Approximately 50 million U.S. citizens are age 65 and older, representing 16% of the current population, and that proportion continues to increase (Kaiser Family Foundation, 2019). The Christian nurse needs to understand a few foundational principles to be prepared to care for this growing elderly population.

First, the aging process is inevitable and irreversible: "And as it is appointed for men to die once" (Hebrews 9:27a). A nurse who is a Christian has a different perspective on aging and death than the rest of the world does, based on the Bible and knowledge of life after death. The aging process is different for each individual, but the goal is that the elderly will retain their mental and physical functions throughout the life span (ANA, 2010). The changes that occur with aging require adaptation, yet the elderly still desire fulfillment and interaction in life.

Second, vulnerable older adults deserve the same rights in regard to their health care as any other population, including the right to informed decision making, especially at end-of-life. The elderly are considered vulnerable because of their multiple chronic comorbidities, which often interact, and their atypical responses, which are often slow or lead to inaccurate assessments during their care (ANA, 2010). As life expectancy increases, nurses must be prepared to provide cost-effective, prevention-focused medical care to vulnerable elders, teaching them self-management of their chronic diseases, improving their quality of life, and incorporating their family caregivers.

▶ Transitional Care Model

Collaboration is Standard 11 in *Gerontological Nursing: Scope and Standards of Practice* (ANA, 2010). Collaboration requires thorough communication among vulnerable elders, family members, healthcare providers, and the community across all settings. The **Transitional Care Model (TCM)** is an evidence-based, nurse-driven model that targets vulnerable elders in an effort to reduce poor outcomes and costs as these patients move across settings (Hirschman, Shaid, McCauley, Pauly, & Naylor, 2015). The holistic approach of the TCM has been refined to nine key components, which are illustrated in **FIGURE 12-1**.

The first component of the TCM is *screening*. Screening can occur in the emergency department, hospital, or outpatient setting, but its purpose is always the same: to recognize vulnerable elders who are at risk for poor outcomes (Hirschman et al., 2015). Some of the risk factors that are a part of screening include (1) recent fall, (2) multiple chronic comorbidities, (3) mental health concerns, (4) cognitive impairment or dementia, (5) inability to complete basic activities of daily living (ADLs), (6) hospitalization within the past 30 days, and (7) two or more hospitalizations within the past 6 months.

The second component is *staffing*. Staffing suggests that this is a team approach, led by nurses.

The third component of the TCM is *maintaining relationships*. A trusting relationship between the nurse and the patient and family members is developed and maintained in person and over the phone; consistency and availability are important (Hirschman et al., 2015). The nurse also develops a relationship with all other healthcare providers and community partners, once again illustrating the team-based approach to care for the elderly.

The fourth component is *engaging patients and family caregivers*. By tailoring the

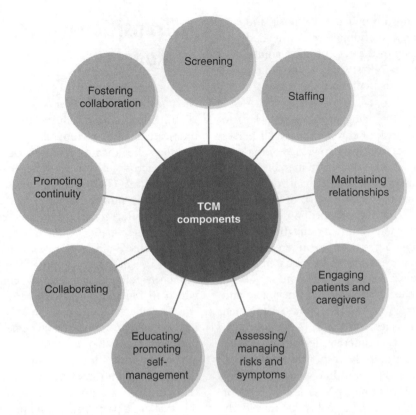

FIGURE 12-1 Transitional Care Model.

Reproduced from University of Pennsylvania, New Courtland Center for Transitions & Health, School of Nursing. About the TCM: Research, practice and policy.
Retrieved from https://www.nursing.upenn.edu/ncth/transitional-care-model/about-the-tcm/index.php

patient's care plan to his or her personalized goals, the nurse can elicit buy-in. The nurse should include the patient and family caregivers in all team meetings. Engagement in the process will grow as the patients see their values and preferences being honored in the plan of care (Hirschman et al., 2015).

The fifth component is *assessing and managing risks and symptoms*. A comprehensive assessment includes all of the factors listed in **TABLE 12-1**.

The sixth component of the TCM is *educating and promoting self-management*. Chronic disease self-management requires an ability to detect worsening symptoms early to prevent exacerbations; the nurse uses various techniques to teach the patient how to do that. Additionally, the nurse fosters medication management

TABLE 12-1 Transitional Care Model: Comprehensive Assessment of Risks and Symptoms

■ Functional status	■ Polypharmacy
■ Cognition	■ Use of high-risk
■ Mental health	medications
■ Physical symptoms	■ Continence
■ Perceived health	■ Nutrition
■ Quality of life	■ Pain
■ Family caregiver	■ Skin integrity
needs	■ Substance
■ Fall risk	abuse

Modified from Hirschman, K., Shaid, E., McCauley, K., Pauly, M., & Naylor, M. (2015). Continuity of care: The transitional care model. *Online Journal of Issues in Nursing, 20*(3). doi:10.3912/OJIN .Vol20No03Man01

BOX 12-1 Evidence-Based Practice Focus

Applying the Transitional Care Model to Reduce Hospital Readmissions and Incorporating the Christian Faith

In the past 10 years, hospitals have been tasked with reducing their readmission rates. The population with the highest readmission rates has two things in common: advanced age and multiple chronic conditions. By utilizing screening methods and assessment skills and managing risk factors and symptoms within the TCM, a nurse can predict which patients are at an increased risk for readmission. The collaboration, continuity, engagement, trusting relationships, and promoting self-management components of the TCM have all been studied and proven to reduce hospital readmission rates.

Faith community nurses (FCNs) are registered nurses with extra training to provide holistic care with a specific focus on spiritual aspects. FCNs believe that addressing spiritual needs allow the patient to better cope with his or her illness.

FCNs are in an excellent position to illustrate and implement the TCM. While a patient is in the hospital, a referral is made to the FCN, and the FCN is able to develop a trusting relationship and participate in discharge planning. After the patient's discharge, the FCN visits the patient's home to perform an assessment and to provide education. Throughout this process, the FCN is always approachable and available, and attends appointments with the patient and other healthcare providers. Incorporating resources is crucial during this time period, not only with regard to the faith community but also home health care, meals on wheels, transportation, and medication assistance as needed. The goal is for the patient to be ready for self-care by 60 days post discharge. FCNs applying the TCM offer patients holistic care while reducing hospital readmission rates.

Modified from Ziebarth, D., & Campbell, K. (2016). A transitional care model using faith community nurses. *Journal of Christian Nursing, 33*(2), 112–118. doi:10.1097/CNJ.0000000000000255

to promote adherence based on education and understanding (Hirschman et al., 2015). A written care plan is provided to the patient and updated regularly.

The seventh component is *collaborating*. Collaboration for the purposes of the TCM refers to the use of technology to communicate the patient's care plan to the entire team.

The eighth component is *promoting continuity*. For the first few months of the TCM, the same nursing provider follows the patient across all settings to avoid breakdowns in care (Hirschman et al., 2015).

The ninth and final component is *fostering coordination*. The nursing providers are the foundation that integrates hospital, post-acute, and community-based care. The nurse is able to determine which services the elderly patient needs in each setting, ensuring timeliness and easy transitions. When the time is right, palliative and hospice care can be added as another layer of support (Hirschman et al., 2015).

Thus, the TCM focuses on the vulnerable elder who is chronically ill and places an emphasis on the role of the nurse in coordinating health care (see **BOX 12-1**). This evidence-based approach to care increases access while reducing poor outcomes and cost. As vulnerable older adults may be found in multiple settings, this chapter is organized around those various places, starting with independent living.

▶ Independent Living

Many health conditions accompany aging; the Christian nurse has a unique Biblical perspective to aid understanding and care for the vulnerable elder with these types of conditions.

An attitude of compassion is absolutely necessary when caring for the elderly. Jude 1:22 states, "And on some have compassion, making a distinction." According to the National Council for Aging Care (2018), elderly persons do not want to give up their freedom and will choose independent living a majority of the time in comparison to other options. Three of the challenges discussed here that the vulnerable elder faces in independent living are hearing and vision loss, technology, and substance abuse.

Hearing and Vision Loss

Hearing Loss

Hearing—one of the five senses—often becomes impaired with aging. Indeed, hearing loss affects more than half of the elderly population, making it a public health issue. **Presbycusis** is defined as progressive hearing loss due to age-related changes. **TABLE 12-2** lists age-related ear changes. Hearing loss negatively impacts communication ability, which can lead to social stress, family frustration, and a decreased perception of quality of life (Kozakova, Tobolova, & Zelenikova, 2018; Moser, Luxenberger, & Freidl, 2017). If the hearing loss is serious, it can also impair the elder's ability to independently complete ADLs.

The Christian nurse can take a few approaches to provide compassionate care for the vulnerable elder with hearing loss. Kozakova et al. (2018) found that both the elderly patient and their family members reported a decreased quality of life due to the loved one's hearing loss. Moser et al. (2017) suggested that social support is the best way to improve quality of life for elders with hearing loss. Communicating slowly, while looking straight at the elderly patient and using clear pronunciation, may enhance verbal interaction, but the nurse will also need to incorporate writing, pictures, and gestures for the hearing-impaired patient to have the best experience. In addition, the nurse can provide noise-reducing headphones, offer assistance with hearing aids if the patient uses those devices, or use a personal amplification device. These interventions show vulnerable elders that communication is a priority.

Vision Loss

Vision loss has been associated with earlier death, due to the heavy impact it has on independence and ADLs (Christ et al., 2014). In **presbyopia**, a condition that starts when individuals are in their 40s, the eyes no longer focus or accommodate appropriately for several reasons. **TABLE 12-3** lists other age-related eye changes. Other complications of vision that are common with age include the following:

- Cataracts, a stiffening and clouding of the lens
- Macular degeneration, loss of central vision from changes in the retina
- Glaucoma, intraocular fluid buildup causing increased pressure and damage to the optic nerve
- Diabetic retinopathy, leakage and breakage of tiny vessels in the eye (Eliopoulos, 2018)

Because visual loss is directly associated with functional decline and disability, it is a

---

TABLE 12-2 Age-Related Changes in the Ear That Affect Hearing	
- Loss of hair cells - Decreased blood supply - Reduced flexibility of basilar membrane - Degeneration of spiral ganglion cells	- Reduced production of endolymph - Higher frequencies lost first - Inability to understand some speech frequencies - Increased cerumen (wax) production

Modified from Eliopoulos, C. (2018). *Gerontological nursing* (9th ed.). Philadelphia, PA: Wolters Kluwer.

TABLE 12-3 Age-Related Changes in the Eye That Affect Vision

- Reduced elasticity of the lens
- Decreased ability to adapt to light
- Visual field narrows/loss of peripheral vision
- Alterations in the blood supply of the retina and retinal pigmented epithelium
- Pupillary sphincter hardens
- Pupil size decreases
- Opacification of the lens (leads to cataracts)
- Distorted depth perception
- Less efficient reabsorption of intraocular fluid
- Ciliary muscle atrophies
- Reduced lacrimal secretions (dry eye)
- Corneal sensitivity diminished

Modified from Eliopoulos, C. (2013). *Gerontological nursing* (9th ed.). Philadelphia, PA: Wolters Kluwer.

promising area in which preventive medicine might facilitate independence in the elderly. Peres et al. (2017) found that vision loss in the elderly limits their mobility, ADLs, instrumental activities of daily living (IADLs), and activity participation; however, if prevention efforts focus on vision, they can help to reduce dependency. A compassionate nurse can adapt care for the vulnerable elder with vision loss by providing literature in large print or with a magnifying device, making sure the lighting is adequate, and using contrasting colors. If the patient's hearing is more intact than his or her vision, audio books and talking computers may be more enjoyable. To deal with the loss of depth perception, the environment can be made safer by removing tripping hazards in the home and issuing warnings when approaching curbs and stairs.

Biblical Application

Now Barzillai was a very aged man, eighty years old. And he had provided the king with supplies while he stayed at Mahanaim, for he was a very rich man. And the king said to Barzillai, "Come across with me, and I will provide for you while you are with me in Jerusalem." But Barzillai said to the king, "How long have I to live, that I should go up with the king to Jerusalem? I am today eighty years old. Can I discern between the good and bad? Can your servant taste what I eat or what I drink? Can I hear any longer the voice of singing men and singing women? Why then should your servant be further burden to my lord the king? And why should the king repay me with such a reward? Please let your servant turn back again, that I may die in my own city, near the grave of my father and mother." (2 Samuel 19:32–37a)

What can the Christian nurse learn from Barzillai? As an 80-year-old man, Barzillai had lost his senses of taste and hearing, and he felt like a burden to King David. He wanted to remain in his own home (independent living) until he died. These honest confessions from Barzillai open our eyes to some of the real experiences of the vulnerable elders for whom we care and allow us to see their perspective.

Technology

Technology can be a huge area of frustration for vulnerable elders due to the incredible changes that have occurred over their lifetime; at the same time, it can also increase access to health care, improve communication with loved ones, and promote independence. **Assistive technology** is defined as a mechanical aid that can support or improve a physical or mental impairment (Mauk, 2018). Lifeline alert systems are a good example of a technological advancement for elders who live alone and are at risk for falls. With such systems, at the push of a button, they can call for help. As this technology has improved, it has become able to detect changes in gait and balance, predicting those persons who need early intervention to prevent falls (Ory, Smith, & Dahlke, 2016). Taking matters one step further, "smart homes" now exist that can be monitored remotely, and that can alert caregivers to changes in the resident's habits and patterns. A smart home uses technology to create a safe environment and to facilitate the completion of ADLs and IADLs (Mauk, 2018). Technology can also be used to help with wandering, a common issue for elders with dementia, by utilizing equipment with Global Positioning System (GPS) capabilities.

Technology can be linked directly to healthcare providers, reporting vital signs and medication adherence from digital medication-dispensing devices. Peetoom, Lexis, Joore, Dirksen, and De Witte (2015) found that a combination of technological monitoring systems can detect changes in ADLs, worsening health status, and falls, thereby improving efficiency and cost of care and delaying the move into an institution. **TABLE 12-4** lists some examples of these monitoring systems.

One concern with monitoring the elderly is privacy, but it has to be balanced with a consideration for safety. Some other barriers that nurses and caregivers may encounter with the vulnerable elder and technology include the training needed, the elder's confidence level,

---

TABLE 12-4 Technological Monitoring Systems for the Elderly

▪ Passive infrared motion sensors	▪ Sound recognition
▪ Body-worn sensors	▪ Smart homes
▪ Video monitoring	▪ Multicomponent
▪ Pressure sensors	

Modified from Peetoom, K., Lexis, M., Joore, M., Dirksen, C., & De Witte, L. (2015). Literature review on monitoring technologies and their outcomes in independently living elderly people. *Disability and Rehabilitation: Assistive Technology, 10*(4), 271–294. doi:10.3109/17483107.2 014.961179

the need for personalization, and acceptance of the technology (Arif, El Emary, & Koutsouris, 2014). When it comes to the elderly and technology, the Christian nurse must exercise patience, as advised in 1 Timothy:

> Do not rebuke an older man, but exhort him as a father, younger men as brothers, older women as mothers, younger women as sisters, with all purity. But if any widow has children or grandchildren, let them first learn to show piety at home and to repay their parents; for this is good and acceptable before God. (I Timothy 5:1, 2, 4)

Substance Abuse

Substance abuse in the elderly is increasing in prevalence; the number of older Americans with a **substance use disorder (SUD)** or **alcohol use disorder (AUD)** is expected to rise to 5.7 million by 2020 (Mattson, Lipari, Hays, & Van Horn, 2017). Here is a relevant example from the Bible:

> And Noah began to be a farmer, and he planted a vineyard. Then he drank of the wine and was drunk, and became uncovered in his tent. And Ham, the father of Canaan, saw the nakedness of his father, and told his two brothers outside. But Shem and Japheth took a garment, laid it on both their shoulders, and went backward and covered the nakedness of their father. Their faces were turned away, and they did not see their father's nakedness. (Genesis 9:20–23)

This situation with Noah and his abuse of alcohol garnered two reactions: One reaction was to gossip about the situation and shame the person involved, whereas the other, Godly reaction was to respect the individual yet handle the inappropriate behavior.

Nurses and caregivers can watch for certain changes in behavior that may indicate an elder with SUD (**TABLE 12-5**). The substances most commonly abused by the elderly population are, in order, (1) alcohol, (2) marijuana, and (3) cocaine. The substances that the elderly population have been found to be using when admitted for treatment are (1) alcohol, (2) heroin or other opiates, (3) cocaine, and (4) marijuana. Finally, in order of prevalence, the following substances are the cause of emergency room visits for substance misuse in the elderly: (1) pain relievers, (2) benzodiazepines, (3) alcohol with other drugs, (4) antidepressants/antipsychotics, (5) cocaine, (6) heroin, (7) marijuana, and (8) illicit amphetamines or methamphetamine (Mattson et al., 2017).

For older adults, alcohol remains the most commonly abused substance; therefore, the rest of this section will focus on alcohol. The vulnerable elder is at an increased risk of harm from alcohol use for a few reasons. First, the liver cannot process alcohol as it did when the person was younger, causing higher blood alcohol concentrations. Second, the blood–brain barrier is more permeable, and neuronal receptors are more sensitive to alcohol, leading to a higher level of impairment (Kuerbis, Sacco, Blazer, & Moore, 2014).

Because SUD is more difficult to diagnose in the elderly, Kuerbis et al. (2014) developed risk categories to aid providers in identifying individuals at elevated risk for such disorders. One instrument that can be used for screening is the Comorbidity Alcohol Risk Evaluation Tool, shown in **TABLE 12-6**.

The Christian nurse should handle SUD in the vulnerable elder with love and respect. Most importantly, the nurse should not ignore this condition. When addressing SUD, a gentle, supportive approach will help to avoid

TABLE 12-5 Changes in Behavior That May Be Signs of Substance Abuse

- Changes in mood
- "Losing" prescriptions
- Nodding off
- Excessive sleeping
- Memory loss or confusion
- Messy house or appearance
- Two or more doctors filling the same prescription
- Preferring to be alone
- Lying about simple things
- Smelling of alcohol
- Frequently being late to work

TABLE 12-6 Comorbidity Alcohol Risk Evaluation Tool (CARET)

Item	Amount of Drinking Considered "At-Risk"
Alcohol Use and Behaviors in the Last 12 Months	
Number of drinks and frequency of drinking	≥5/day at any frequency, 4/day at least 2 times/month, 3/day at least 4 times/week
Four or more drinks on one occasion (binge drinking)	At least 1 time/week
Driving within 2 hours of drinking 3 or more drinks	Any frequency

(continues)

TABLE 12-6 Comorbidity Alcohol Risk Evaluation Tool (CARET)	*(continued)*
Item	**Amount of Drinking Considered "At-Risk"**
Alcohol Use and Behaviors in the Last 12 Months	
Someone concerned about participant's alcohol use	Any amount
Someone concerned about participant's alcohol use more than 12 months ago	≥4/day at any frequency, 2–3/day at least 4 times/week
Alcohol Use and Medications Taken at Least 3–4 Times per Week Currently	
Medications that may cause bleeding, dizziness, or sedation	≥4/day at any frequency, 2–3/day at least 4 times/week
Medications used for gastroesophageal reflux, ulcer disease, or depression	≥4/day at any frequency, 2–3/day at least 4 times/week
Medications for hypertension	≥5/day at any frequency, 4/day at least 2 times/week, 3/day at least 4 times/week
Alcohol Use and Comorbidities in the Past 12 Months	
Liver disease, pancreatitis	Any amount
Gout, depression	≥4/day at any frequency, 3/day at least 2 times/week, 2/day at least 4 times/week
High blood pressure, diabetes	5/day at any frequency, 4/day at least 2 times/month, 3/day at least 4 times/week
Sometimes have problems with sleeping, falling, memory, heartburn, stomach pain, nausea, vomiting, or feeling sad/blue	≥5/day at any frequency, 4/day at least 2 times/month, 3/day at least 2 times/week
Often have problems with sleeping, falling, memory, heartburn, stomach pain, nausea, vomiting, or feeling sad/blue	≥4/day at any frequency, 2–3/day at least 2 times/week

Republished with permission of Springer Science and Business Media B V from Barnes, A. J., Moore, A. A., Xu, H., Ang, A., Tallen, L., Mirkin, M., & Ettner, S. L. (2010). Prevalence and correlates of at-risk drinking among older adults: The project SHARE study. *Journal of General Internal Medicine*, *25*(8), 840–846. Permission conveyed through Copyright Clearance Center, Inc.

confrontation. Interventions to treat SUD in the older adult include motivational interviewing, normative feedback, psychotherapy, pharmacologic treatment, and self-help groups such as Alcoholics Anonymous (AA). Although SUD in older adults is a challenging issue, positive outcomes are possible, and even more likely, when approached from a Biblical worldview. Additional information on substance abuse appears in the *Integration of a Biblical Worldview and Substance Abuse* chapter.

▶ Assisted Living/Living with Family

When the vulnerable elder is no longer able to live alone, independently, the next options may be an assisted living facility (ALF) or living with family, both of which offer some unique opportunities for the Christian nurse to help the patient and family. As the elderly take their first steps away from independence, acceptance may be difficult.

Although living with family has the potential to be a loving arrangement, it can also lead to caregiver burnout and compassion fatigue. A shared living arrangement is also associated with a higher risk for most types of elder abuse or mistreatment. One solution to preventing burnout in caregivers is an adult daycare program, as discussed at the beginning of this chapter, which can relieve caregiver strain.

ALFs are another option when the elder does not need around-the-clock skilled nursing care or monitoring but can no longer live alone. ALFs are a safe environment developed for the elderly or disabled; services at such a facility may include medication management, meals, personal care assistance, social activities, housekeeping, transportation, and exercise classes (Mauk, 2018).

Whether in the ALF or when living with family, three worrisome conditions that may arise are elder abuse; depression and anxiety; and poor appetite, weight loss, and malnutrition. These risks are discussed next.

Elder Abuse

Elder abuse and self-neglect are often difficult to detect and frequently under-diagnosed because vulnerable elders rarely have contact with anyone outside of the situation. Additionally, the abuse and neglect often occur to elders with cognitive impairment, who may not be able to report the situation (Halphen & Burnett, 2014). Therefore, healthcare providers are frequently in the best position to evaluate for elder abuse and self-neglect. **Elder abuse** is defined as a caregiver or trusted person causing psychological or physical harm by intentional or negligent treatment of a vulnerable elder older than age 65 (Olson & Hoglund, 2014). The types of elder abuse are listed in **TABLE 12-7**. **Self-neglect** occurs when

TABLE 12-7 Types of Elder Abuse	
Financial exploitation	Theft, fraud, misuse of money or assets
Neglect	Abandonment or failure to provide for basic needs
Psychological/emotional	Intentional social isolation; verbal statements or threats that cause fear or distress
Physical	Physical force that causes bodily harm, whether threat or actual infliction
Sexual	Forcing sexual acts or physical contact without consent

Modified from Olson, J., & Hoglund, B. (2014). Elder abuse: Speak out for justice. *Journal of Christian Nursing, 31*(1), 14–21.

vulnerable elders have impairments that cause them to be unable to meet basic needs or perform personal care.

Elders identified to be in situations of abuse or self-neglect have a higher rate of mortality (Halphen & Burnett, 2014). The following risk factors increase the chance of elder abuse:

- Social isolation/lack of social support
- Female
- Age 80 or older
- Low income
- Dementia
- Mental health conditions
- Poor physical health
- Immobility
- Reliance on caregivers for ADLs and IADLs (Olson & Hoglund, 2014)

The prevalence of elder abuse is difficult to determine because it is under-reported; some resources say 1 in 10 elders, 11% of the elderly population, or anywhere from 1 to 2 million elders are abused (Olson & Hoglund, 2014).

One example of a standardized assessment tool for elder abuse is the Hwalek–Sengstock elder abuse screening test (**BOX 12-2**). Healthcare providers should become familiar with the questions on this screening tool so that they can be prepared to act when they suspect elder abuse. **TABLE 12-8** lists the signs and symptoms of elder abuse.

Many nursing diagnoses exist that are appropriate for cases of elder abuse, such as powerlessness, social isolation, self-neglect, and compromised human dignity. Some of the nursing interventions for these diagnoses would include placement into a safer environment, counseling, and consulting a financial advisor or someone trusted for all financial decisions. Several spiritual nursing diagnoses

---

BOX 12-2 Hwalek–Sengstock Elder Abuse Screening Test

Purpose: Screening device useful to service providers interested in identifying people at high risk of the need for protective services.

Instructions: Read the questions and write in the answers. A response of "no" to items 1, 6, 12, and 14; a response of "someone else" to item 4; and a response of "yes" to all others is scored in the "abused" direction.

1. Do you have anyone who spends time with you, taking you shopping or to the doctor?
2. Are you helping to support someone?
3. Are you sad or lonely often?
4. Who makes decisions about your life—like how you should live or where you should live?
5. Do you feel uncomfortable with anyone in your family?
6. Can you take your own medication and get around by yourself?
7. Do you feel that nobody wants you around?
8. Does anyone in your family drink a lot?
9. Does someone in your family make you stay in bed or tell you you're sick when you know you're not?
10. Has anyone forced you to do things you didn't want to do?
11. Has anyone taken things that belong to you without your OK?
12. Do you trust most of the people in your family?
13. Does anyone tell you that you give them too much trouble?
14. Do you have enough privacy at home?
15. Has anyone close to you tried to hurt you or harm you recently?

Neale, A., Hwalek, M., Scott, R., & Stahl, C. (1991). Validation of the Hwalek-Sengstock elder abuse screening test. *Journal of Applied Gerontology, 10*(4), 406–415. Copyright © 1991 by SAGE Publications. Reprinted by permission of SAGE Publications, Inc.

TABLE 12-8 Signs and Symptoms of Elder Abuse	
■ Several injuries in different stages of repair ■ Delays in seeking treatment ■ Injuries that cannot be explained ■ Contradictory explanations of injuries ■ Bruises, burns, welts, restraint marks ■ Poor hygiene ■ Depression, agitation, withdrawal ■ Dehydration, malnutrition ■ Decubitus ulcers	■ Signs of medication misuse ■ Pattern of missed or cancelled appointments ■ Frequent changes in healthcare providers ■ Missing prosthetic devices ■ Discharge or pain in the rectum or vagina ■ Not allowed to make decisions ■ Unsafe/unsanitary living conditions ■ Forgery of signature ■ Sudden or unexplained changes in finances

Modified from Olson, J., & Hoglund, B. (2014). Elder abuse: Speak out for justice. *Journal of Christian Nursing, 31*(1), 14–21; Mauk, K., & Benton, S. (2018). Elder abuse and mistreatment. In K. L. Mauk (Ed.), *Gerontological nursing: Competencies for care* (4th ed., pp. 779–796). Burlington, MA: Jones & Bartlett Learning.

are also pertinent, including hopelessness and spiritual distress. If appropriate, the Christian nurse can link a vulnerable elder to a faith community, as the faith community can really help to combat social isolation through visitation and support groups.

As Christians, Proverbs 23:22 tells us, "Listen to your father who begot you, and do not despise your mother when she is old." As humans, we are prone to embarrassment, frustration, and anger—but when dealing with vulnerable elders, we must exercise patience, be respectful, and know our limits. The Christian nurse is obligated to speak up in situations of elder abuse, to defend the weak, and to allow the elders their dignity. "Open your mouth for the speechless, in the cause of all who are appointed to die. Open your mouth, judge righteously, and plead the cause of the poor and needy" (Proverbs 31:8–9). By developing a trusting relationship with elderly patients and demonstrating true caring, the nurse can help them to open up. If the vulnerable elder describes a concerning situation, accurate documentation is imperative. Moreover, the nurse is obligated to report elder abuse or self-neglect to Adult Protective Services (APS). As an advocate for the vulnerable elder, healthcare providers can raise awareness of elder abuse in the community and educate the public.

Depression and Anxiety

Depression

Depression is a condition in which a person experiences sadness, emptiness, or irritability that results in physical and cognitive changes that affect the person's ability to function, with the condition having a minimum duration of two weeks (Hajjar, Nardelli, Gaudenci, & Santos, 2017). Depression in the elderly can be attributed to two main factors: multiple chronic comorbidities and physical inactivity. Additionally, reduced income, retirement, changing role or loss of roles, and death of loved ones may be contributing factors to depression in the elderly. **TABLE 12-9** lists symptoms of depression. As much as 30% of the elderly population struggles with depression (Eliopoulos, 2018). A tool such as the Geriatric Depression Scale: Short Form can be used to assess for depression.

Treatment for depression typically includes psychotherapy and antidepressants, but sometimes the elderly population requires a different sort of treatment. Jesus handled depression in the Bible by ensuring that the individuals would not be alone, as seen in John 19:25–27:

> Now there stood by the cross of Jesus His mother, and His mother's sister, Mary the wife of Clopas, and Mary Magdalene. When Jesus therefore saw

TABLE 12-9 Symptoms of Depression in the Elderly

- Altered patterns of sleep or appetite
- Fatigue
- Reduced concentration
- Neglecting personal hygiene
- Decreased self-esteem
- Feelings of worthlessness
- Loss of interest or joy
- Isolation/avoiding social interaction

Modified from Hajjar, R., Nardelli, G., Gaudenci, E., & Santos, A. (2017). Depressive symptoms and associated factors in elderly people in the primary health care. *Revista da Rede de Enfermagem do Nordeste, 18*(6), 727–733. doi:10.15253/2175-6783.2017000600004

TABLE 12-10 Potential Manifestations of Anxiety in the Elder

- Rigidity in thinking and behavior
- Insomnia
- Fatigue
- Hostility
- Increased frequency of voiding
- Fidgeting with clothing or utensils
- Changes in appetite
- Restlessness/pacing
- Fantasizing
- Confusion
- Increased dependency
- Increase in vital signs
- Difficulty concentrating

Modified from Eliopoulos, C. (2018). *Gerontological nursing* (9th ed.). Philadelphia, PA: Wolters Kluwer.

His mother, and the disciple whom He loved standing by, He said to His mother, "Woman, behold your son!" Then He said to the disciple, "Behold your mother!" And from that hour that disciple took her to his own home.

Anxiety

Anxiety in the elderly is twice as common as dementia and four to six times more common than depression, affecting as much as 50% of the elderly population (Koychev & Ebmeier, 2012). Anxiety and depression often occur together in the older adult. **TABLE 12-10** lists potential manifestations of anxiety in the elder. Many of the symptoms may mimic other disorders, but vulnerable elders are at an increased risk of developing anxiety if they have had a recent loss, traumatic event, fall, frailty, chronic pain, or chronic illness. Anxiety is defined as worrying that is excessive, difficult-to-control worrying about anything in life, accompanied by physical symptoms, and lasting more than six months. The FEAR questionnaire can be used to assess the elderly for anxiety (see **TABLE 12-11**).

Frequent follow-up, reassurance, pharmacotherapy, and cognitive-behavioral therapy (CBT) are indicated treatments for anxiety disorder. Nursing interventions for anxiety include all of the following:

- Allow adequate time for all activities.
- Encourage and respect the patient's decisions.
- Prepare the patient for anticipated activities.
- Provide basic explanations.
- Adhere to routines.
- Use familiar objects.
- Control the number of different people interacting with the patient.
- Prevent overstimulation of the senses. (Eliopoulos, 2018)

If the nurse implements these interventions in every encounter with a vulnerable elder, the encounters are much more likely to go smoothly and calmly.

Biblical Worldview

What can the Christian nurse do to provide care that is a step above the usual for a

TABLE 12-11 FEAR Questionnaire		
Main Question	**Follow-up Question**	**Scoring**
In the past month, have you felt so fidgety or restless that you couldn't sit still?	If yes: Do you know what brought it on? Was it worry, fear, or something else?	Score 1 if restlessness caused by worry/fear/anxiety
Do you take anything to help you relax?	What about sedative tablets or alcohol?	Score 1 if taking medication or alcohol to relax
How often, if at all, have you worried in the past month?		Some days: score 0 Most days: score 1
Have you felt on edge, strung up, or mentally tense in the past month?		Some days: score 0 Most days: score 1
A score of 2 or more predicts anxiety.		

Koychev, I., & Ebmeier, K. (2016). Anxiety in older adults often goes undiagnosed. *Practitioner, 260*(1789), 17–20.

vulnerable elder with depression or anxiety? First, creating a nonjudgmental environment will be very beneficial to all encounters. The nurse should encourage the patient to express his or her feelings, either verbally or written, and take the time to actually listen without minimizing the patient's feelings. Next, the nurse can ensure that all of the patient's physical needs are met so that the individual can better work through his or her depression. The nurse can facilitate the development of a positive self-concept by setting realistic goals and celebrating all successes. Finally, the Christian nurse can offer hope: "Now may the God of hope fill you with all joy and peace in believing, that you may abound in hope by the power of the Holy Spirit" (Romans 15:13).

Poor Appetite, Weight Loss, and Malnutrition

Now it came to pass, when Isaac was old and his eyes were so dim that he could not see, that he called Esau his older son and said to him, "My son." And he answered him, "Here I am." Then he said, "Behold now, I am old. I do not know the day of my death. Now therefore, please take your weapons, your quiver and your bow, and go out to the field and hunt game for me. And make me savory food, such as I love, and bring it to me that I may eat, that my soul may bless you before I die." (Genesis 27:1–4)

As Isaac illustrated, even at an advanced age, he loved savory food. Even today, many major life events revolve around eating. Unfortunately, several changes occur in the vulnerable elder that can lead to poor appetite, weight loss, and even malnutrition (**TABLE 12-12**).

The caloric needs of an older adult are reduced because of lower activity levels, decreased metabolism, and increased adipose tissue (Eliopoulos, 2018), making it difficult to define **malnutrition** for the

TABLE 12-12 Factors That Contribute to Poor Appetite and Weight Loss

- Decreased taste and smell sensations
- Reduced mastication capability
- Slower peristalsis
- Medication side effects
- Decreased hunger contractions
- Reduced gastric acid secretion
- Less absorption of nutrients in the intestine
- Poor lifelong eating patterns

Modified from Eliopoulos, C. (2018). *Gerontological nursing* (9th ed.). Philadelphia, PA: Wolters Kluwer.

TABLE 12-13 Nutritional Challenges and Potential Interventions for the Elderly

Challenges	Interventions
Indigestion Decreased stomach motility, slower gastric emptying time Food intolerance Dysphagia Constipation	Sit upright while eating and for 30 minutes after meals; avoid fried foods Eat several small meals a day Eliminate specific foods from the diet Referral to speech pathologist; take small bites; allow sufficient time for eating; consume thickened liquids Increase fluid and fiber intake; take Senna

elderly. Nevertheless, the consensus is that malnutrition is insufficient energy intake, resulting in weight loss from a combined loss of muscle mass and fat, leading to weakness and decreased functional capacity (Laur, McNicholl, Valaitis, & Keller, 2017). Other signs of malnutrition include delirium, depression, visual disturbances, dermatitis, hair loss, pallor, delayed wound healing, lethargy, and fatigue (Eliopoulos, 2018). The prevalence of malnutrition ranges from 15% to 85%, depending on the elder's environment (Crogan, 2018).

TABLE 12-13 identifies some interventions the nurse can employ when engaging a vulnerable elder with nutritional challenges. Additionally, the nurse can educate vulnerable elders on the importance of protein and vitamin D to their nutritional status, and adding liquid caloric supplements such as protein shakes in addition to meals may be beneficial. An educational tool, the U.S. Department of Agriculture's MyPlate graphic (**FIGURE 12-2**), may help the elderly visualize portion size for healthy eating.

▶ Acute Care/Hospital

Many risks are associated with vulnerable elders once they enter acute care, whether it is just time spent in the emergency department

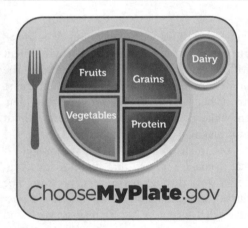

FIGURE 12-2 U.S. Department of Agriculture's MyPlate graphic.

Reproduced from USDA Center for Nutrition Policy and Promotion. 2019. ChooseMyPlate.gov

(ED) or an overnight admission stay in the hospital. When an elderly person goes into the hospital, the stay is typically for a serious illness requiring acute care, an acute injury, or an exacerbation of a chronic illness that cannot be managed in the outpatient or clinic setting. The vulnerable elder demographic has the highest rate of hospitalization and a longer length of stay when compared to others (Eliopoulos, 2018). In general, the major risks associated with acute care for the elderly are nosocomial (hospital-acquired) infections and iatrogenic complications, which are unintentionally caused by providers, medical treatments, or procedures. After hospitalization, elderly patients often experience a decline in function that nurses can try to prevent; in addition, nurses can help prepare the family and caregivers, and assist with discharge planning.

Post-Hospital Syndrome

Krumholz first wrote about **post-hospital syndrome (PHS)** in 2013, defining it as "an acquired condition of vulnerability." According to this author, the focus of care in an acute setting tends to be the cause of the hospitalization, with relatively less attention being paid to the fact that these patients are now at increased risk for many other adverse health events. During the 30-day period after an acute care stay, the lingering effects of the acute condition may continue to affect the body, and the older person's body is not prepared to handle any further health threats. More than 2.6 million elderly individuals, or 20% of elderly population who have been hospitalized, experience another hospitalization in that 30-day period, often for reasons not directly related to the first hospitalization or diagnosis (Krumholz, 2013). **TABLE 12-14** lists several causes of readmission.

TABLE 12-14 Common Causes of Readmission in the Elderly

▪ Heart failure	▪ Gastrointestinal conditions
▪ Pneumonia	
▪ Chronic obstructive pulmonary disease (COPD)	▪ Mental illness
	▪ Metabolic dysfunction
▪ Infection	▪ Trauma

Modified from Krumholz, H. (2013). Post-hospital syndrome: A condition of generalized risk. *The New England Journal of Medicine, 368*(2), 100–102. doi:10.1056/NEJMp1212324

Many stressors occur during hospitalization and cause impairment for the following 30 days, including sleep deprivation, disruption of normal circadian rhythms, poor nourishment, pain and discomfort, mentally challenging situations, medications that alter mental and physical function, and weakness from bed rest or inactivity (Krumholz, 2013). Imagine the complications that these stressors invoke in the vulnerable elder!

The Christian nurse can do two things to capitalize on this newfound awareness of the risks associated with PHS. First, early recognition of these stressors while in acute care and intervention whenever possible will better prepare the elder for discharge and reduce the chance of readmission in the first 30 days. Performing a thorough assessment of the patient that goes far beyond the conditions for which the patient was admitted for is necessary to prevent PHS. The vulnerable elder is highly likely to leave the acute care setting with cognitive and physical functioning impairments—maybe temporary, but perhaps permanent—for which planning will be key. The risk of PHS decreases if interventions are in place to promote sleep, nutrition, activity, and conservation symptom management (Krumholz, 2013). Second, the Christian nurse needs to have an arsenal of Bible verses ready to share with vulnerable, elderly patients in stressful, acute care situations. **BOX 12-3** gives several examples of excellent verses for stress relief. Writing a verse on your patient's whiteboard with permission or carrying a verse on a 3-by-5 card in your pocket are great ways to incorporate these verses in your day.

Advance Care Planning

Then they went up out of Egypt, and came to the land of Canaan to Jacob their father. And they told him, saying, "Joseph is still alive, and he is governor over all the land of Egypt." And Jacob's heart stood still, because he did not

> **BOX 12-3** Ten Bible Verses for Stress Relief
>
> Psalm 46:1–3 God is our refuge and strength, a very present help in trouble. Therefore, we will not fear, even though the earth be removed, and though the mountains be carried into the midst of the sea; though its waters roar and be troubled, though the mountains shake with its swelling.
>
> Philippians 4:6–7 Be anxious for nothing, but in everything by prayer and supplication, with thanksgiving, let your requests be made known to God; and the peace of God, which surpasses all understanding, will guard your hearts and minds through Christ Jesus.
>
> 1 Peter 5:7 Casting all your care upon Him, for He cares for you.
>
> Luke 12:25–26 And which of you by worrying can add one cubit to his stature? If you then are not able to do the least, why are you anxious for the rest?
>
> John 14:27 Peace I leave with you, my peace I give to you; not as the world gives do I give to you. Let not your heart be troubled, neither let it be afraid.
>
> 2 Corinthians 12:9 And He said to me, "My grace is sufficient for you, for My strength is made perfect in weakness." Therefore most gladly I will rather boast in my infirmities, that the power of Christ may rest upon me.
>
> 2 Thessalonians 3:12 Now may the Lord of peace Himself give you peace always in every way. The Lord be with you all.
>
> Psalm 27:13–14 I would have lost heart, unless I had believed that I would see the goodness of the Lord in the land of the living. Wait on the Lord; be of good courage, and he shall strengthen your heart; wait, I say, on the Lord!
>
> Deuteronomy 31:8 And the Lord, He is the One who goes before you. He will be with you, He will not leave you nor forsake you; do not fear nor be dismayed.
>
> Psalm 55:22 Cast your burden on the Lord, and He shall sustain you; He shall never permit the righteous to be moved.

believe them. But when they told him all the words which Joseph had said to them, and when he saw the carts which Joseph had sent to carry him, the spirit of Jacob their father revived. Then Israel said, "It is enough. Joseph my son is still alive. I will go and see him before I die." (Genesis 45:25–28)

Jacob (Israel) is a great example of **advance care planning** because he knew he wanted to go see his son before he died, and he traveled a long way to do it. He died in a foreign country (Egypt), but he did not want to be buried there. Instead, Jacob made it very clear to his son Joseph, before he died, that he was to be buried with his fathers. Joseph honored that wish, giving us another great example, of a child honoring his father's end-of-life wishes.

Death is inevitable, but the uncertainty of when and how it will happen bothers many people, especially those who have no medical knowledge and those who are not Christians. A Christian nurse really has an advantage in advance care planning, combining medical knowledge and spiritual power. Advance care planning fulfills the call for advocacy, standard 16 in *Gerontological Nursing: Scope and Standards of Practice* (ANA, 2010): "The gerontological nurse advocates to protect the health, safety, and rights of the older adult." Advance care planning entails a conversation with patient and family members to help clarify their values and goals regarding end-of-life care and medical interventions; this conversation is documented so that everyone can be prepared for the time when the patient can no longer communicate.

If advance care planning is done correctly, it improves communication, decreases conflict, and may allow patients to die at home rather than in the hospital. Research has shown that 80% of Americans would like to die at home, but fewer than 25% of them actually get to do so (Volandes & Davis, 2017). One of the goals of advance care planning is to avoid burdensome treatment for those with a terminal illness; unfortunately, only one-third of Americans who should have an advance directive on file actually do.

Today, the context of advance care planning is changing from a legal matter, involving signing of advance directives and medical durable power of attorney (MDPOA), to a conversation. The key stakeholders in this conversation are patients, family members, caregivers, healthcare providers, and healthcare systems. **FIGURE 12-3** presents one current example of an advance directive that is signed by a provider and serves as a medical order. When patients are seen in the ED, one of the first questions they are asked is their resuscitation status; having an advance directive on file can clarify that issue. **BOX 12-4** highlights research regarding the experiences of patients and families with advance care planning in the acute care setting that the nurse can apply to practice.

▶ Rehabilitation and Home Health Care

The next step for a vulnerable elder after leaving acute care is often an inpatient rehabilitation facility (IRF) or home health care (HHC). The purpose of these services is to restore the patient to the best possible functional status and highest possible level of independence. Such services are interprofessional, and collaboration is key. Rehabilitation in a structured setting is often quite valuable, as the patients are required to fulfill a certain number of therapy hours every day or week and usually see great improvement; unfortunately, once the patients leave that setting, they do not always continue that progress at home. HHC services are similar in that once they end the patient may start to regress. A physician orders HHC,

and patients must meet specific criteria for homebound status for their insurance to cover these services. Nursing plays an important role in both of these settings, with a core component of that role being education to prevent the patient from regressing once the services end.

Functional Status, Falls, and Frailty

Falls are directly related to functional status and frailty in the elderly: Falls are not only common but also very detrimental to quality of life. Frailty is defined as "a medical syndrome with multiple causes and contributors that is characterized by diminished strength, endurance, and reduced physiologic function that increases an individual's vulnerability for developing increased dependency and death" (Laur et al., 2017, p. 393). According to Laur et al., frailty in the elderly increases the risk of death by more than 50%. The prevalence of falls in the elderly is as high as 40% annually, and the World Health Organization (WHO) projects that injuries from falls will increase 100% by 2030 if better interventions are not put in place (Halaweh, Willen, Grimby-Ekman, & Svantesson, 2016). Elderly patients with high physical functioning have less fear of falling and a lower incidence of falls. The major assessment question to ask an elderly patient is when his or her last fall occurred. If it was within the past year, that finding should raise a red flag for high fall risk.

Fall prevention and safety promotion are priorities of nursing care for elderly patients, and many nursing interventions can be implemented to help achieve these goals. In an inpatient setting, purposeful rounding, observation devices, and bed or chair alarms are utilized. Additionally, using nonskid socks, decluttering the room, and providing easy access to the toilet are necessary in the inpatient environment. If the patient experiences side effects or impairment from certain medications, the nurse can observe and ask the provider for a

---

HIPAA PERMITS DISCLOSURE OF POLST TO OTHER HEALTH CARE PROVIDERS AS NECESSARY

Physician Orders for Life-Sustaining Treatment (POLST)

First follow these orders, then contact **Physician/NP/PA**. A copy of the signed POLST form is a legally valid physician order. Any section not completed implies full treatment for that section. **POLST complements an Advance Directive and is not intended to replace that document.**

EMSA #111 B
(Effective 4/1/2017)*

Patient Last Name:	Date Form Prepared:
Patient First Name:	Patient Date of Birth:
Patient Middle Name:	Medical Record #: *(optional)*

A

Check One

CARDIOPULMONARY RESUSCITATION (CPR): *If patient has no pulse and is not breathing.*
If patient is NOT in cardiopulmonary arrest, follow orders in Sections B and C.

☐ **Attempt Resuscitation/CPR** (Selecting CPR in Section A **requires** selecting Full Treatment in Section B)

☐ **Do Not Attempt Resuscitation/DNR** (Allow Natural Death)

B

Check One

MEDICAL INTERVENTIONS: *If patient is found with a pulse and/or is breathing.*

☐ **Full Treatment** – primary goal of prolonging life by all medically effective means.
In addition to treatment described in Selective Treatment and Comfort-Focused Treatment, use intubation, advanced airway interventions, mechanical ventilation, and cardioversion as indicated.

☐ *Trial Period of Full Treatment.*

☐ **Selective Treatment** – goal of treating medical conditions while avoiding burdensome measures.
In addition to treatment described in Comfort-Focused Treatment, use medical treatment, IV antibiotics, and IV fluids as indicated. Do not intubate. May use non-invasive positive airway pressure. Generally avoid intensive care.

☐ *Request transfer to hospital only if comfort needs cannot be met in current location.*

☐ **Comfort-Focused Treatment** – primary goal of maximizing comfort.
Relieve pain and suffering with medication by any route as needed; use oxygen, suctioning, and manual treatment of airway obstruction. Do not use treatments listed in Full and Selective Treatment unless consistent with comfort goal. *Request transfer to hospital only if comfort needs cannot be met in current location.*

Additional Orders: _____

C

Check One

ARTIFICIALLY ADMINISTERED NUTRITION: *Offer food by mouth if feasible and desired.*

☐ Long-term artificial nutrition, including feeding tubes.   Additional Orders: _____

☐ Trial period of artificial nutrition, including feeding tubes. _____

☐ No artificial means of nutrition, including feeding tubes. _____

D

INFORMATION AND SIGNATURES:

Discussed with: ☐ Patient (Patient Has Capacity)   ☐ Legally Recognized Decisionmaker

☐ Advance Directive dated _____, available and reviewed →	Health Care Agent if named in Advance Directive:
☐ Advance Directive not available	Name: _____
☐ No Advance Directive	Phone: _____

Signature of Physician / Nurse Practitioner / Physician Assistant (Physician/NP/PA)
My signature below indicates to the best of my knowledge that these orders are consistent with the patient's medical condition and preferences.

| Print Physician/NP/PA Name: | Physician/NP/PA Phone #: | Physician/PA License #, NP Cert. #: |
| Physician/NP/PA Signature: *(required)* | | Date: |

Signature of Patient or Legally Recognized Decisionmaker
I am aware that this form is voluntary. By signing this form, the legally recognized decisionmaker acknowledges that this request regarding resuscitative measures is consistent with the known desires of, and with the best interest of, the individual who is the subject of the form.

Print Name:	Relationship: *(write self if patient)*
Signature: *(required)*	Date:	Your POLST may be added to a secure electronic registry to be accessible by health providers, as permitted by HIPAA.
Mailing Address (street/city/state/zip):	Phone Number:	

SEND FORM WITH PATIENT WHENEVER TRANSFERRED OR DISCHARGED

*Form versions with effective dates of 1/1/2009, 4/1/2011,10/1/2014 or 01/01/2016 are also valid

FIGURE 12-3 Physician Orders for Life-Sustaining Treatment (POLST) form.

HIPAA PERMITS DISCLOSURE OF POLST TO OTHER HEALTH CARE PROVIDERS AS NECESSARY

Patient Information

Name (last, first, middle):		Date of Birth:	Gender: **M** **F**

NP/PA's Supervising Physician	**Preparer Name** (if other than signing Physician/NP/PA)	
Name:	Name/Title:	Phone #:

Additional Contact   □ None

Name:	Relationship to Patient:	Phone #:

Directions for Health Care Provider

Completing POLST

- **Completing a POLST form is voluntary.** California law requires that a POLST form be followed by healthcare providers, and provides immunity to those who comply in good faith. In the hospital setting, a patient will be assessed by a physician, or a nurse practitioner (NP) or a physician assistant (PA) acting under the supervision of the physician, who will issue appropriate orders that are consistent with the patient's preferences.
- **POLST does not replace the Advance Directive.** When available, review the Advance Directive and POLST form to ensure consistency, and update forms appropriately to resolve any conflicts.
- POLST must be completed by a health care provider based on patient preferences and medical indications.
- A legally recognized decisionmaker may include a court-appointed conservator or guardian, agent designated in an Advance Directive, orally designated surrogate, spouse, registered domestic partner, parent of a minor, closest available relative, or person whom the patient's physician/NP/PA believes best knows what is in the patient's best interest and will make decisions in accordance with the patient's expressed wishes and values to the extent known.
- A legally recognized decisionmaker may execute the POLST form only if the patient lacks capacity or has designated that the decisionmaker's authority is effective immediately.
- To be valid a POLST form must be signed by (1) a physician, or by a nurse practitioner or a physician assistant acting under the supervision of a physician and within the scope of practice authorized by law and (2) the patient or decisionmaker. Verbal orders are acceptable with follow-up signature by physician/NP/PA in accordance with facility/community policy.
- If a translated form is used with patient or decisionmaker, attach it to the signed English POLST form.
- Use of original form is strongly encouraged. Photocopies and FAXes of signed POLST forms are legal and valid. A copy should be retained in patient's medical record, on Ultra Pink paper when possible.

Using POLST

- Any incomplete section of POLST implies full treatment for that section.

Section A:

- If found pulseless and not breathing, no defibrillator (including automated external defibrillators) or chest compressions should be used on a patient who has chosen "Do Not Attempt Resuscitation."

Section B:

- When comfort cannot be achieved in the current setting, the patient, including someone with "Comfort-Focused Treatment," should be transferred to a setting able to provide comfort (e.g., treatment of a hip fracture).
- Non-invasive positive airway pressure includes continuous positive airway pressure (CPAP), bi-level positive airway pressure (BiPAP), and bag valve mask (BVM) assisted respirations.
- IV antibiotics and hydration generally are not "Comfort-Focused Treatment."
- Treatment of dehydration prolongs life. If a patient desires IV fluids, indicate "Selective Treatment" or "Full Treatment."
- Depending on local EMS protocol, "Additional Orders" written in Section B may not be implemented by EMS personnel.

Reviewing POLST

It is recommended that POLST be reviewed periodically. Review is recommended when:

- The patient is transferred from one care setting or care level to another, or
- There is a substantial change in the patient's health status, or
- The patient's treatment preferences change.

Modifying and Voiding POLST

- A patient with capacity can, at any time, request alternative treatment or revoke a POLST by any means that indicates intent to revoke. It is recommended that revocation be documented by drawing a line through Sections A through D, writing "VOID" in large letters, and signing and dating this line.
- A legally recognized decisionmaker may request to modify the orders, in collaboration with the physician/NP/PA, based on the known desires of the patient or, if unknown, the patient's best interests.

This form is approved by the California Emergency Medical Services Authority in cooperation with the statewide POLST Task Force. For more information or a copy of the form, visit **www.caPOLST.org**.

SEND FORM WITH PATIENT WHENEVER TRANSFERRED OR DISCHARGED

FIGURE 12-3 *Continued*

Used with permission from EMSA.

BOX 12-4 Research Highlight

This article discusses a qualitative research study on the experiences of patients and families with advance care planning in the acute care setting. Several factors came to the forefront as influential in the process: (1) duty to care for the loved one, (2) past experiences in similar situations, (3) severity or impact of the critical illness, and (4) trust in the healthcare provider or healthcare system. The power of prior advance care planning discussions significantly reduced stress levels in the acute situation. Understanding these factors from a patient and family perspective allows the nurse to engage in advance care planning conversations therapeutically.

Modified from Rasmussen, K., Raffin-Bouchal, S., Redlich, M., & Simon, J. (2018). Duty to defend: Patient and family experiences of advance care planning conversations held prior to intensive care unit admission. *Canadian Journal of Critical Care Nursing, 29*(3), 19–25.

TABLE 12-15 Intrinsic Risk Factors for Falls

- Muscle weakness, decreased strength
- Cognitive impairment: Slow thinking, poor planning, memory loss; executive dysfunction issues
- Delirium: Acute cognitive impairment (reversible)
- Dementia: Chronic cognitive impairment (not reversible)
- Physical impairment or impaired mobility
- Use of assistive devices
- Gait and/or balance problems
- Age over 80 years
- Visual impairment
- Low body mass index
- Depression
- Foot problems
- Frailty
- Four or more medications
- Use of alcohol
- Use of pain or sleeping medications
- History of a fall in the past year
- Urinary or bowel problems (infection, incontinence, urgency)
- Sensory deficits, peripheral neuropathy, poor vision perception or peripheral vision

Zwicker, D. (2018). Falls in older adults. In K. L. Mauk (Ed.), *Gerontological nursing: Competencies for care* (4th ed., pp. 453–469). Burlington, MA: Jones & Bartlett Learning.

dose adjustment or change in agent. **TABLE 12-15** lists intrinsic risk factors for falls. In the home setting, a physical or occupational therapist with HHC can evaluate for hazards.

Above all else, it is imperative that functional status and mobility are maintained; as soon as the nurse notices any decline, early intervention is key. Jesus was our perfect example of how to treat a woman with frailty and poor functional status. He brought her near and was kind to her.

> And behold, there was a woman who had a spirit of infirmity eighteen years, and was bent over and could in no way raise herself up. But when Jesus saw her, He called her to Him and said to her, "Woman, you are loosed from your infirmity." And He laid His hands on her, and immediately she was made straight, and glorified God. (Luke 13:11–13)

Polypharmacy and Medication Nonadherence

Polypharmacy, defined as the use of five or more prescription medications daily, is one of the risk factors for falls. Many factors go into decision making when it comes to pharmacotherapy in the elderly. Choosing the correct medication and dosage for the indication is the first step. Monitoring the patient for effectiveness and providing education about adverse reactions then follows (Marques et al., 2018). Many of the clinical trials for medications are not generalized to the elderly, which is a problem because the elderly process medications differently than younger adults. Also, many people are taking over-the-counter (OTC) medications, vitamins, and supplements in addition to their prescriptions. These complexities, and more, make it very challenging for the healthcare provider to perform good medication management for the vulnerable elder.

The resource most commonly used to determine whether a medication is safe for the elderly is the Beers Criteria. Note that the Beers Criteria is a list of "potentially inappropriate medications" (PIM), rather than a list of "do not use" medications. **TABLE 12-16** lists risk factors for medication nonadherence in the elderly.

Nursing interventions for polypharmacy are very logical and methodical. First, make sure each medication taken by the patient can be matched with a diagnosis; there should be no medications without a good rationale for their use. Another way to weed out unnecessary medications is to discuss with the patient whether the pharmacotherapy was started out of need or want. If a medication cannot be removed, perhaps the dose can be decreased.

Second, nurses should provide medication education on names, dosages, purpose, and side effects, both verbally and written, and provide a written list of when to take them. Many patients take their pills by size and color, which is not safe because that is subject to change at any time.

Third, the nurse may be able to offer some alternative, holistic options to the patient, to be used instead of medications—with provider approval, of course. King David's caregivers illustrate a Biblical example of using holistic care for one of the common issues experienced by the elderly:

> Now King David was old, advanced in years; and they put covers on him, but he could not get warm. Therefore his servants said to him, "Let a young woman, a virgin, be sought for our lord the king, and let her stand before the king, and let her care for him; and let her lie in your bosom, that our lord the king may be warm." (1 Kings 1:1–2)

▶ Nursing Home

When the vulnerable elder can no longer live alone safely or needs more assistance than family or community can provide, he or she may need to move into long-term care (LTC) such as a nursing home. Nursing homes offer around-the-clock skilled nursing care and assistance with ADLs. Nurses play an incredible role in the nursing home setting, as they have the opportunity to care for loved ones, and to show them the love of Christ. Bowel and bladder incontinence and dementia are two areas that are often seen and addressed in the nursing home setting.

Bowel and Bladder Incontinence

> Even to your old age, I am He, and even to gray hairs I will carry you! I have made, and I will bear; Even I will carry, and will deliver you. (Isaiah 46:4)

Bowel and bladder incontinence are very frustrating and humiliating for the vulnerable elder; therefore, the Christian nurse can shine Jesus's light by showing patience, love, and compassion to individuals with these conditions.

TABLE 12-16 Risk Factors for Medication Nonadherence in the Elderly	
■ High cost	■ Accessibility
■ Motivation and beliefs	■ Relationships with healthcare providers
■ Perception of self-efficacy	■ Cultural or lifestyle factors

Modified from Mauk, K. (Ed.). (2018). *Gerontological nursing: Competencies for care* (4th ed.). Burlington, MA: Jones & Bartlett Learning.

BOX 12-5 Causative Factors for Urinary Incontinence

Menopause
Hysterectomy
Tumors
Obstruction
Enlarged prostate
Prostate cancer
Neurological disorders
Restricted mobility
Weak pelvic muscles
Medications

Data from Resnick, N. M. (1984). Urinary incontinence in the elderly. *Medical Grand Rounds, 3,* 281–290.

Protecting their privacy and allowing them dignity whenever and however possible are some ways to show respect. Bowel incontinence may affect as many as 25% of the elderly in nursing homes (Gillibrand, 2012). Urinary incontinence (UI) affects more than 70% of residents in nursing homes (Mauk, 2018).

The initial step for managing both disorders is a thorough assessment in an attempt to figure out the cause. **BOX 12-5** lists some of the causative factors of UI. If the cause cannot be corrected, the nurse has an opportunity to employ various care strategies.

For chronic fecal incontinence, relatively few management options exist. However, the focus of treatment of diarrhea is based on the cause, so proper and thorough assessment is needed. The patient with continued diarrhea should be referred to a specialist. Bowel management is imperative to avoid constipation, a more common problem in older adults, and hydration/fluid balance is required for both bowel and bladder incontinence improvement.

Many urinary continence products exist, but the patient will need education on how to use them and, more importantly, on how to protect the skin. In addition, many options are available for treating UI. Behavioral management includes use of a voiding schedule, diet counseling, and pelvic floor muscle exercise. Pharmacotherapy and surgery are available and effective for many patients. The nurse's role could be to assist the patient with bladder training. Bladder training starts with a bladder diary to assess for patterns, then voiding at a specific interval with gradual increases.

Although bowel and bladder incontinence can be disabling and have negative social and psychological impacts, nursing care is instrumental in helping these patients achieve an improved quality of life.

Cognition and Dementia

Changes in cognition for the elderly can vary quite widely, from age-related forgetfulness to mild cognitive impairment (MCI) to dementia. More than 50 million people in the world have **dementia**, and it is the seventh leading cause of death (Kennison & Long, 2018). Dementia is caused by progressive, irreversible neurodegeneration that negatively affects memory, learning, and mood. Risk factors for dementia include the following characteristics:

- Increasing age
- African American or Hispanic ethnicity
- Lower educational level
- Genetic factors
- Various health conditions: cardiovascular disease, diabetes, obesity, smoking, chronic inflammation, and prior head injury (Kennison & Long, 2018)

To date, the pharmacotherapies introduced to treat dementia have shown only limited efficacy. **BOX 12-6** provides a wonderful discussion of one nurse leader's views on nonpharmacologic interventions that a Christian nurse can utilize for persons with dementia.

BOX 12-6 Outstanding Nurse Leader: Elizabeth M. Long, DNP, APRN, GNP-BC, CNS, Faith Community Nurse

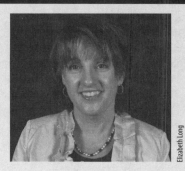

Elizabeth Long

As a registered nurse on the medical–surgical and critical care units, I frequently encountered patients who had dementia in addition to the primary reason for hospitalization. Most recently and extensively, as a gerontological nurse practitioner in long-term care facilities, I have encountered dementia in the majority of our residents.

Challenges

Caring for a person with dementia (PwD) poses several challenges.

Acceptance and Realistic Expectations

In all of the previously mentioned settings, acceptance and realistic expectations from family members has been a challenge.

Adjusting Misconceptions

The major misconception is that the PwD is only a "shell" or somehow "no longer themselves." In our culture, we have a tendency to define people by what they can or cannot do. The PwD is still his or her own person with needs and wants.

We Have Always Done It That Way

As I began to learn more about how to appropriately treat persons with dementia, I realized there was a lack of evidence-based information, and we were doing things because we had always done them that way. My first encounter with this challenge was with reality orientation. It seemed so cruel to keep making patients relive their diagnosis or the death of someone they had forgotten was dead. Fortunately, that is a thing of the past! A more current, yet prime example is the use of antipsychotics for agitation. There is no evidence to support this practice, yet it has been and still is, unfortunately, a common method of treatment.

Triumphs

Of course, there are also triumphs when caring for a PwD. The triumphs began with a simple change in perspective. I started to help loved ones look at who the person is now and who the person is becoming instead of only looking at who they had been.

The first triumph I can recall is when I realized I needed to tap into who the person identified himself or herself to be. I recall a gentleman who was a retired accountant. He was a challenge, aggressive, wandering, and verbally insulting to the staff. He was often placed at the nursing station in an effort to watch him more closely. One day, I had the idea to get him a ledger book and a pencil. I asked him to do my taxes. He sat there for about an hour with no outburst and wrote in the ledger book. This was an *aha* moment: If I could figure out what had meaning to a person, maybe that was a key.

The Music and Memory Program has been a certain triumph. Repeatedly, I have seen the benefits of personalized music for individuals with dementia. A PwD who had not spoken in

(continues)

BOX 12-6 Outstanding Nurse Leader: Elizabeth M. Long, DNP, APRN, GNP-BC, CNS, Faith Community Nurse   *(continued)*

more than a year burst into song, singing all the verses of "Tis So Sweet to Trust in Jesus." After a personalized music list was played for a resident who wandered around the facility and was aggressive with other residents, during dinner she began talking and telling us of her past. She was a waitress and worked extra hours to clean the tables at night before she could get home to her children. We realized she felt the need to clean the tables as she had years ago, so that she could "get home to her children." We gave her a cloth and some water and let her clean the tables—and the aggression was gone.

Considerations for a PwD in a Nursing Home Setting

A nursing home should be as home-like as possible (if the home situation was a good one). Provide person-centered care and tap into what is important to that individual. My grandmother was a good example of this need. She had lived alone for the last several years and was not interested in going to the dining room to eat. It took a lot of convincing for the facility to let her just eat in her room. Socialization is important, but it needs to be individualized.

Incorporating Scripture and Biblical Principles When Caring for PwD

I think we have to look at ourselves as nurses: Often we are the barrier to the PwD being able to express their faith. The PwD is waiting for our response. We need to ask, "What am I trying to accomplish spiritually with this PwD? What are my beliefs about how a PwD can worship? How do I create an atmosphere for expression of worship?"

For example, we can utilize redirection. Sometimes simply asking the person if we could read some Bible verses together or pray for a minute will help redirect behavior.

Another technique is remembering. I try to make a habit of remembering for patients or triggering a memory, never putting them on the spot to recall something. The senses often trigger memory.

Other ideas can be individualized:

- Visual prompts
  - Christian education materials from 1920 to 1950 (depending on the PwD's age)
  - Bibles
  - Hymnals
  - Crosses
  - Stained glass
- Auditory prompts
  - Bible readings using Bible translations like the King James Version (not new translations the PwD did not have when young)
  - Music that has meaning to the PwD
  - Music with an organ accompaniment (the guitar is nice, but most persons in this age group went to church with an organ)
  - Hymns
  - Prayers

- Tactile prompts
  - Touching or holding a cross
  - Touching or holding a Bible
  - Touching or holding a hymnal
  - Rosaries
- Gustatory prompts
  - Communion
- Olfactory prompts
  - Communion
  - Incense
- Ritual (if that ritual has meaning to the PwD)
  - Communion
  - Liturgy
  - Lord's Prayer
  - Apostle's Creed
  - Stained glass

▶ Conclusion

The vulnerable elder requires and deserves specialized care across all settings. The Christian nurse has an excellent understanding of the kindness, love, and compassion that Jesus Christ showed to all, and can pass that on to these patients. The TCM provides a foundation for effective care of the elderly transitioning across all settings, when coordinating care, and for keeping readmission rates down.

Each setting may present challenges for vulnerable elders, but nursing interventions can be implemented to overcome them (see **CASE STUDY 12-1**). A Biblical worldview coloring the perspective of care provided is the added layer that the vulnerable elder needs. As life expectancy lengthens, nurses will be on the forefront of providinz prevention-focused medical care to vulnerable elders, teaching them self-management of their chronic diseases and improving their quality of life.

🔍 *CASE STUDY 12-1*

Michael W. is a single 70-year-old Caucasian male who lives alone in a senior high-rise apartment building. His lack of family and friend support has always been a concern. He has a history of depression with several exacerbations over the years, insomnia, anxiety, chronic back pain due to a car accident and spinal fusion, hyperlipidemia, vitamin D deficiency, and diabetes mellitus type 2 (DM2). He chooses not to treat his DM2 against medical advice, saying, "It doesn't affect me that much, and I don't want to take more pills." He reports being on disability due to chronic back pain and depression. Michael's medication reconciliation includes the following information:

Medication Record					
Date: 07/15/2019 Patient name: Michael W. Allergies: Penicillins Pharmacy name: Community Pharmacy Phone: (333) 333-3333 Primary doctor name: Dr. Bongard Phone: (555) 555-5555					
Medication Name/Dose	**Medication Indication**	**Medication Frequency**			**Notes, Comments, or Questions**
		Morning	Noon	Evening	Bedtime	
Cyclobenzaprine 10 mg PO PRN TID	Muscle spasms					Only take if needed up to 3 times a day.
Oxycodone-Acetaminophen 5-325 mg PO daily PRN	Back pain					Only take once a day if needed.
Trazodone 100 mg PO once PRN at bedtime	Insomnia					Only take at bedtime for insomnia.

Questions

1. How might the nurse formally assess this patient for anxiety and depression?
2. Discuss four nursing interventions for anxiety and depression.
3. What are two community resources that might be helpful for Michael as he has no support system?

Michael faithfully attends appointments with his primary care provider (PCP), Dr. Bongard, once a year for medication refills. Dr. Bongard assesses these new complaints: fall within the past 6 months resulting in an injury to his left knee (never evaluated or treated), started using a cane, "persistent sinus infection," difficulty breathing, gaining "water weight," lower extremities and abdomen are twice what they should be, weight gain of 46 pounds, still not treating his diabetes. Vital signs: temperature, 97.5°F; respiratory rate, 16 breaths/minute; pulse, 45 beats/min; blood pressure, 128/78 mm Hg; oxygen saturation, 85% on room air. The physical exam also revealed a pale, generally unwell and uncomfortable appearance; depressed; lungs clear but diminished; anasarca, mainly abdominal distention and +2 pitting edema in both lower extremities; and heart sounds regular.

Questions

4. What do you think is wrong with this patient based on your assessment findings?
5. Write two priority NANDA-I nursing diagnoses based on your assessment.
6. Name two immediate interventions that the nurse can perform in the clinic.

Dr. Bongard is unable to treat Michael in the outpatient clinic at this point and advised him to go to the nearest hospital for further evaluation.

Questions

7. How should the nurse arrange for Michael to go to the nearest hospital?
8. If Michael refuses to go to the hospital, does he have the right to refuse? Include your rationale.

Michael went to the emergency department and was admitted to the hospital, where he received care for nine days. While he was there, he was diagnosed with heart failure (HF) and cardiomyopathy and treated with IV furosemide. An echocardiogram revealed an ejection fraction of 19%. His chest x-ray showed hypoexpanded lungs with small bilateral pleural effusions and mild bibasilar atelectasis. He was started on five new medications and was discharged to home health care (HHC) with instructions to follow up with his PCP and cardiologist on an outpatient basis.

Questions

9. Write out, in a word-for-word format, three discharge teachings that the nurse would want to educate Michael about prior to discharge.
10. How does his lack of social support play into Michael's discharge?
11. Is it appropriate for Michael to be discharged with HHC? Would Michael benefit from an alternate discharge plan such as rehabilitation?

(continues)

🔍 CASE STUDY 12-1 *(continued)*

Medication list upon discharge:

Medication Record
Date: 07/15/2019 Patient name: Michael W. Allergies: Penicillins Pharmacy name: Community Pharmacy Phone: (333) 333-3333 Primary doctor name: Dr. Bongard Phone: (555) 555-5555

Medication Name/Dose	Medication Indication	Medication Frequency				Notes, Comments, or Questions
		Breakfast	Lunch	Dinner	Bedtime	
Aspirin 81 mg daily	Antiplatelet and cardio protection	X				
Carvedilol 6.25 mg BID with meals	Heart failure	X		X		
Cyclobenzaprine 10 mg PO PRN TID	Muscle spasms					Only take if needed up to 3 times a day.
Furosemide 40 mg BID	Heart failure	X		X		
Lisinopril 5 mg at bedtime	Heart failure				X	
Oxycodone-Acetaminophen 5-325 mg PO daily PRN	Back pain					Only take once a day if needed.
Spironolactone 25 mg BID	Heart failure	X		X		
Trazodone 100 mg PO once PRN at bedtime	Insomnia					Only take at bedtime for insomnia.

Questions

12. Michael was prescribed new medications; do these new medications increase his fall risk? Include rationale.
13. What precautions can be taken to prevent future falls?

Eighteen days post discharge, Michael returned to the clinic to follow up with Dr. Bongard. On assessment, Michael was receiving HHC services from a nurse and a physical therapist. His post-hospital syndrome (PHS) was severe. He reported dizziness, extreme weakness, and productive cough with yellow sputum; his weight had gone down 68 pounds in less than a month.

Questions

14. Based on the details in the case study, why does Michael have severe PHS?
15. How can an acute care nurse advocate for Michael to prevent PHS?

Vital signs are temperature, 97.3°F; pulse, 116 beats/minute; respiratory rate, 14 breaths/minute; blood pressure, 70/42 mm Hg; and oxygen saturation, 97% on room air. The physical exam revealed exacerbated depression, anasarca resolved, and no edema noted. Michael reported taking his medications correctly as ordered. He is taking five new medications after the hospitalization, and he still wants refills for the three medications he was on prior to the hospitalization.

Questions

16. Is Michael dealing with polypharmacy? Include your rationale.
17. What is the nurse's role in identifying and preventing polypharmacy?

Michael had not been seen by the cardiology group yet, so Dr. Bongard set up his cardiology appointment for him before he left the office that day. Dr. Bongard also called and spoke with the HHC nurse to coordinate care, discuss concerns, and order some labs. Finally, Dr. Bongard asked the HHC team to set him up with remote technology monitoring for HF including daily weights, blood pressure monitoring, and medication adherence tracking.

Questions

18. Why is it imperative that Michael be seen by cardiology for his heart failure?
19. Which community resources would Michael benefit from to prevent another hospital admission for heart failure?

▶ # Clinical Reasoning Exercises

1. Watch the following videos about elder abuse:
   - Elder Abuse Training Video: https://youtu.be/mHKuA6iBQaY
   - Elder Abuse Case Study: https://youtu.be/EYQVIwVC48s

2. Referring back to the section on elder abuse, discuss the risk factors for abuse in each scenario.
3. Using Table 12-7, discuss what type or types of elder abuse are taking place in each scenario.
4. Using the Hwalek–Sengstock elder abuse screening test in Box 12-2, role-play screening with a partner using one of the scenarios (one person will be the nurse, one person will be the elder suffering abuse).

Transitional Care Model Component	Applications	Bible Verses to Support Applications
Screening	1. 2. 3.	
Staffing	1. 2. 3.	
Maintaining relationships	1. 2. 3.	
Engaging patients and caregivers	1. 2. 3.	
Assessing/managing risks and symptoms	1. 2. 3.	
Educating/promoting self-management	1. 2. 3.	
Collaborating	1. 2. 3.	
Promoting continuity	1. 2. 3.	
Fostering collaboration	1. 2. 3.	

Then discuss the possible signs and symptoms the nurse may find in the abused elder from Table 12-8.

5. Come up with two nursing diagnoses for your scenario (one should be spiritually related) and discuss nursing interventions for those diagnoses.

6. Review the Adult Protective Services (APS) website for your state to familiarize yourself with how to report elder abuse. Here is one example website: https://www.coloradoaps.com/.

▶ Personal Reflection Exercises

You have been educated on the Transitional Care Model for vulnerable elders. Think about an elderly figure in your life—your grandmother, mother, elderly neighbor, elderly patient, or friend. Using Figure 12-1, how does the Christian nurse apply each component of the TCM? Include three applications per category using the worksheet provided above. Include one Bible verse to support your applications.

References

American Nurses Association (ANA). (2010). *Gerontological nursing: Scope and standards for practice.* Silver Spring, MD: Author.

Arif, M., El Emary, J., & Koutsouris, D. (2014). A review on the technologies and services used in the self-management of health and independent living of elderly. *Technology and Health Care, 22,* 677–687. doi:10.3233/THC-140851

Bikford, C. J. (2018). A contemporary look at gerontological nursing. *American Nurse Today, 13*(6), 48.

Carson, B. (2014). *One nation.* New York, NY: Sentinel.

Christ, S., Zheng, D., Swenor, B., Lam, B., West, S., Tannenbaum, S.,... Lee, D. (2014). Longitudinal relationships among vision acuity, daily functional status, and mortality: The Salisbury eye evaluation study. *Journal of the American Medical Association Ophthalmology, 132*(12), 1400–1406. doi:10.1001/jamaophthalmol.2014.2847

Crogan, N. L. (2018). Dysphagia and malnutrition. In K. L. Mauk (Ed.), *Gerontological nursing: Competencies for care* (4th ed., pp. 577–600). Burlington, MA: Jones & Bartlett Learning.

Eliopoulos, C. (2018). *Gerontological nursing* (9th ed.). Philadelphia, PA: Wolters Kluwer.

Gillibrand, W. (2012). Management of fecal incontinence in the elderly: Current policy and practice. *British Journal of Community Nursing, 21*(11), 554–556. doi:10.12968/bjcn.2012.21.11.554

Hajjar, R., Nardelli, G., Gaudenci, E., & Santos, A. (2017). Depressive symptoms and associated factors in elderly people in the primary health care. *Revista da Rede de Enfermagem do Nordeste, 18*(6), 727–733. doi:10.15253/2175-6783.2017000600004

Halaweh, H., Willen, C., Grimby-Ekman, A., & Svantesson, U. (2016). Physical functioning and fall-related efficacy among community-dwelling elderly people. *European Journal of Physiotherapy, 18*(1), 11–17. doi:10.3109/21679169.2015.1087591

Halphen, J., & Burnett, J. (2014). Elder abuse and neglect: Appearances can be deceptive. *Psychiatric Times.* Retrieved from https://www.psychiatrictimes.com/special-reports/elder-abuse-and-neglect-appearances-can-be-deceptive

Hirschman, K., Shaid, E., McCauley, K., Pauly, M., & Naylor, M. (2015). Continuity of care: The transitional care model. *Online Journal of Issues in Nursing, 20*(3). doi:10.3912/OJIN.Vol20No03Man01

Kaiser Family Foundation. (2019). Population distribution by age. Retrieved from https://www.kff.org/other/state-indicator/distribution-by-age/?current Timeframe

Kennison, M., & Long, E. (2018). The long journey of Alzheimer's disease. *Journal of Christian Nursing, 35*(4), 218–227. doi:10.1097/CNJ.0000000000000529

Koychev, I., & Ebmeier, K. (2016). Anxiety in older adults often goes undiagnosed. *Practitioner, 260*(1789), 17–20.

Kozakova, R., Tobolova, J., & Zelenikova, R. (2018). Perceived emotional and situational hearing handicap in the elderly and their family members. *Central European Journal of Nursing and Midwifery, 9*(1), 767–772. doi:10.15452/CEJNM.2018.09.0003

Krumholz, H. (2013). Post-hospital syndrome: A condition of generalized risk. *The New England Journal of Medicine, 368*(2), 100–102. doi:10.1056/NEJMp1212324

Kuerbis, A., Sacco, P., Blazer, D., & Moore, A. (2014). Substance abuse among older adults. *Clinics in Geriatric Medicine, 30*(3), 629–654. doi:10.1016/j.cger.2014.04.008

Laur, C., McNicholl, T., Valaitis, R., & Keller, H. (2017). Malnutrition or frailty? Overlap and evidence gaps in the diagnosis and treatment of frailty and malnutrition. *Applied Physiology, Nutrition & Metabolism, 42*(5), 449–458. doi:10.1139/apnm-2016-0652

Marques, G., de Rezende, D., da Silva, I., de Souza, P., Barbosa, S., Penha, R., & Polise, C. (2018). Polypharmacy and potentially inappropriate medications for elder people in gerontological nursing. *Revista Brasileira de Enfermagem, 71*(5), 2440–2446. doi:10.1590/0034-7167-2017-0211

Mattson, M., Lipari, R., Hays, C., & Van Horn, S. (2017, May 11). A day in the life of older adults: Substance use facts. *CBHSQ Report.* Rockville, MD: Center for Behavioral Health Statistics and Quality, Substance Abuse and Mental Health Services Administration.

Mauk, K. (Ed.). (2018). *Gerontological nursing: Competencies for care* (4th ed.). Burlington, MA: Jones & Bartlett Learning.

Moser, S., Luxenberger, W., & Freidl, W. (2017). The influence of social support and coping on quality of life among elderly with age-related hearing loss. *American Journal of Audiology, 26*(2), 170–179. doi:10.1044/2017_AJA-16-0083

National Council for Aging Care. (2018). Independent living is the top choice for seniors today. Retrieved from https://www.aging.com/independent-living-is-the-top-choice-for-seniors-today/

Olson, J., & Hoglund, B. (2014). Elder abuse: Speak out for justice. *Journal of Christian Nursing, 31*(1), 14–21.

Ory, M., Smith, M., & Dahlke, D. (2016). Technological solutions for extended independence. *Aging Today, 37*(6), 7–8.

Peetoom, K., Lexis, M., Joore, M., Dirksen, C., & De Witte, L. (2015). Literature review on monitoring technologies and their outcomes in independently living elderly people. *Disability and Rehabilitation: Assistive Technology, 10*(4), 271–294. doi:10.3109/17483107.2014.961179

Peres, K., Matharan, F., Daien, V., Nael, V., Edjolo, A., Bourdel-Marchasson, I.,... Carriere, I. (2017). Visual loss and subsequent activity limitations in the elderly: The French three-city cohort. *American*

Journal of Public Health, 107(4), 564–569. doi:10.2105/AJPH.2016.303631

Volandes, A., & Davis, A. (2017). Advance care planning leads to wished-for care. *Health Progress, 98*(6), 41–45.

Recommended Readings

Gawande, A. (2014). *Being mortal: Medicine and what matters in the end.* New York, NY: Metropolitan Books.

Kalanithi, P. (2016). *When breath becomes air.* New York, NY: Random House.

National Council on Aging. (2012). Older American behavioral health: Alcohol misuse and abuse prevention. Retrieved from https://www.ncoa.org/resources/issue-brief-2-alcohol-misuse-and-abuse-prevention/

Substance Abuse and Mental Health Services Administration. (2010, August). Talking with your adult patients about alcohol, drug, and/or mental health problems: A discussion guide for primary health care providers. Retrieved from https://store.samhsa.gov/product/Talking-with-Your-Adult-Patients-about-Alcohol-Drug-and-or-Mental-Health-Problems/sma15-4584

Thomas, W. (2006). *In the arms of elders: A parable of wise leadership and community building.* St. Louis, MO: VanderWyk & Burnham.

Zitter, J. (2017). *Extreme measures: Finding a better path to the end of life.* London, UK: Penguin.

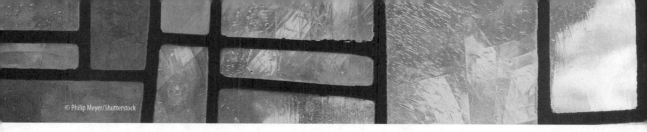

© Philip Meyer/Shutterstock

CHAPTER 13

Nursing as Ministry for Those in Prison

Rev. Mel Mertens and **Eileen Mertens**, RN

LEARNING OBJECTIVES

At the end of this chapter, the reader will be able to:

1. Appreciate the implications of statistics related to U.S. prisoners on their health and suicide risk.
2. Understand why and how a person becomes a prisoner.
3. Analyze how a prisoner thinks.
4. Demonstrate compassion for the incarcerated.
5. Empathize with the journey of a prisoner.
6. Appreciate the practice of nursing as ministry in the prison setting.

KEY TERMS

Correctional forensic nursing	Jails	Prisoners
Incarcerated	Prison	

▶ The Prison Problem

Valleta (2017) gives some staggering statistics about the U.S. **prison** system: "The nation's hefty inmate population is spread across 1,719 state prisons, 102 federal prisons, 901 juvenile correctional facilities, 3,163 local **jails**, as well as military prisons, immigration detention facilities, civil commitment centres and prisons in the US territories" (para. 1). More than 2.3 million Americans were **incarcerated** in 2017. Even though the United States represents only about 5% of the world's population, it houses approximately 25% of the world's **prisoners**, having more prison facilities than any other country globally (**FIGURE 13-1**).

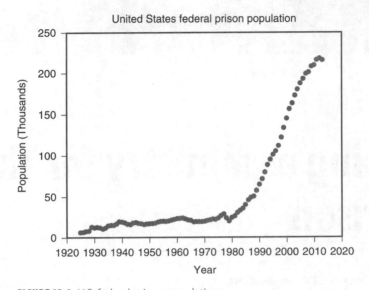

FIGURE 13-1 U.S. federal prison populations.

10 staggering statistics about the US prison system. SBS. Retrieved from https://www.sbs.com.au/guide/article/2017/12/06/10
-staggering-statistics-about-us-prison-system

A significant proportion (more than 75%) of prisoners return to prison within five years after their release, and the prison system costs the United States approximately $80 billion per year (Valleta, 2017). African Americans and men (versus women) are more likely to be imprisoned than others.

Much of the crime associated with those sentenced to time in prison is related to drug abuse and mental illness. Health care in the prison system is a constant challenge for both care providers and chaplains. In 2013, 89% of deaths in U.S. prisons was from illness, but suicide rates have risen as well (Bureau of Justice, 2017). Consider this alarming news:

> According to the Justice Department, approximately a dozen inmates die behind bars each day, or roughly 4,400 per year. In state and federal prisons, most deaths are health-related—the leading illnesses being cancer or heart disease. In local prisons, the top cause is suicide, making up a third of all deaths and usually occurring within the first month of incarceration. Tragically, more than 70 percent of those suicides eventuate before conviction. (Valleta, 2017, para. 8)

Prisons, jails, detention facilities, and the like are places where nurses may encounter the most broken of people. **Correctional forensic nursing** is a challenging field, filled with needy souls who have strayed from a righteous path. This chapter introduces nursing students and nurses to the realities of prison ministry and provides some strategies for working with those who are incarcerated. The authors—a pastor and his wife, a nurse, both experienced in this area—provide some insights into nursing as ministry with this unique population.

▶ The Prisoner's Journey: A Pastor's Perspective

"For I was hungry, and you gave Me something to eat; I was thirsty, and you gave Me drink; I was a stranger, and you invited Me in; naked, and you clothed Me; I was sick, and you visited Me; I was in prison, and you came to Me." Then the righteous will answer Him, saying, "Lord, when did we see You hungry, and feed You, or thirsty, and give You drink? And when did we see You a stranger, and invite You in, or naked, and clothe You? And when did we see You sick, or in prison, and come to You?" And the King will answer and say to them, "Truly I say to you, to the extent that you did it to one of these brothers of Mine, even the least of them, you did it to Me." (Matthew 25:35–40, New American Standard Bible)

In his book entitled *Forty Chances*, Howard Buffett, son of the multibillionaire Warren Buffett, makes the argument that not all people are given the same chance in life (Buffett & Buffett, 2013). Some are born into wealth, some into poverty. Some are born into loving families, some into very dysfunctional families. Buffett argues, quite forcefully, that one's birth and early years determine to a large extent what kind of life an individual will have.

Given what we have experienced and seen in prison, we are convinced that Buffett is not very far off the mark. Statistics have proven time and again that the vast majority (80% to 90%) of incarcerated men grew up in fatherless homes or homes where the father may have been present "physically" but absent in all ways that count (Sedlak & Bruce, 2016). As a pastor, Rev. Mel Mertens's personal experience of more than 20 years of jail and prison ministry bears that out. Most men in prison had neither one of their biological parents in their lives as they grew up; many were raised by a grandmother.

Most prisoners have been "hardened" early in life and have been in trouble with those in authority over them for most of their lives. Many have been in so many jails, youth detention centers, probation alternative programs,

and the like, that they have lost count of these experiences. In my early days in jail ministry, I worked with a young man in his early 30s. He told me that since the age of 12, when he was first sentenced, he had been in 32 different institutions. "Johnny" (not his real name), was sent to a Colorado Correctional Center, where he finished the sentence he was currently serving when I was working with him. I picked him up the day he got released, took him to see his parole officer, worked with him to get a good job with a landscape company, and paid his first month's rent. Johnny wasn't out for more than about a month when he went to a bar, got in a fight, and violated his parole—and back to prison he went.

It is difficult for someone who has not "been there" to understand the life of a prisoner; I still don't understand it after all these years of tending to prisoners. For most people, to spend even one week behind bars with hardened criminals is unimaginable; it would be one of the most frightful experiences they could have. For other people, prison is what they know best and desire more than being "on the outside." Prison officials from another Colorado Correctional Center (a very minimum security facility with no fences) reported, "Some guys, when they are getting close to their release date, will walk outside of the prison boundary and sit on the hillside till they are picked up by the guards." By taking this action, they ensure that they get an additional five years for an "attempted escape."

Most prisoners eventually "find their way to prison" over a period of time. To be sure, some commit a very serious crime as their first offense and become incarcerated for a long period. The majority of prisoners, however, have engaged in criminal activities for years before they get sentenced to prison. When I was first starting prison ministry in the mid-1990s, I remember taking volunteer training with prison staff. They explained that few prisoners get sentenced to prison as first-time offenders. Instead, as one of the prison guards said, "by the time they get here, they have had a lot of experiences and been given a lot of chances to get it right." They have grown up not being taught what is right and wrong. They have not had a good example of living modeled to them.

That description applies to a prisoner's life before incarceration. But what about their life during and after sentencing and incarceration? This chapter provides some general statements about the process the prisoners face; the case study presented later in the chapter goes into more detail. Between being arrested and being sentenced, a prisoner has probably spent one to three years in a county jail waiting to be worked through the judicial system. Unless prisoners can gain their release on bond between court appearances, they will sit in a county jail during this span. The time served during this process will count toward fulfillment of their eventual sentence. During this time, the prisoner will be talking with lawyers, going to court sessions, perhaps discussing plea deals, and in general doing a lot of just sitting and waiting. In a county jail, there is little to keep one's time occupied. An actual prison setting differs in that respect. In prison, there are jobs, classes, places to work out, televisions, community rooms, workshops, and maybe even basketball groups, among other options.

If a plea deal hasn't been worked out ahead of time, the day of the jail inmate's trial eventually arrives. A trial is a very emotional and nerve-racking experience for all to go through—the prisoner as well as his or her family and friends. The person on trial will usually sit in the courtroom and listen to all the evidence, through the entire trial, which may last for days. In the evenings, he or she will return to the cell in the county jail.

Once a verdict has been issued and the prisoner has been found guilty, he or she goes back to jail to await sentencing. The day of sentencing is also a very anxious time for all involved. Usually, the decision is in the hands of the presiding judge. What will he or she decide? How long will the sentence be? This must be an incredibly difficult part of a judge's duties. Johnny (the prisoner mentioned earlier)

BOX 13-1 The Diagnostics Center

In some communities, a Reception and Diagnostic Center is an intake and classification facility. Offenders will not be housed there permanently; the facility will process the inmate into the department of corrections system by [physically and mentally evaluating the inmate]. It is at this point that the staff will determine what programs the inmate may benefit from. An educational and skills testing will take place, which will further classify the offender's needs. From all these factors the staff will determine which facility is best to house the inmate at permanently.

---

and I were together "outside of the walls" one day when we passed, on the sidewalk, the judge who had sentenced him. The comment he made about the judge surprised me but indicates a little about the mindset of the prisoner: "He is a good man; he was very fair to me."

After sentencing, the prisoner goes back to jail again to wait for arrangements to be made with the Department of Corrections (DOC) in the state where the sentence will be served. The first part of an inmate's "time" spent in the DOC will be in a diagnostics center (DC) (see **BOX 13-1**). The time spent in the DC, which is a lock-up facility, may last anywhere from 30 to 60 days. During this time, the inmate is allowed limited visitation rights. Clergy may also be allowed on a limited basis at this point.

Life in Prison

Once an inmate is housed permanently, as determined by the DC process, day-to-day prison life starts. Much of a prisoner's day is spent in some kind of work at the prison, in classroom studies, or in programs designed to address the needs of the individual prisoner. Most inmates serve on some kind of work detail around the prison, for which they get paid by the state. Examples of jobs are housekeeping, laundry, mending clothing, groundskeeping, kitchen duties (yes, they handle knives and cook), and chaplain's assistant. At some of the less secure prisons, supervised work crews are actually sent out into the community. There is actually competition among inmates for some of the more "prized" jobs.

Wages earned by any prisoner are minimal—perhaps $150 per month. But the jobs keep prisoners busy, give the prisoners personal money to spend at the "canteen," and save the state money. While $150 per month might sound like a lot of spending money, prisoners pay the same price as anyone on the outside would for, say, a Pepsi or a postage stamp. Some of the "lucky" ones have family on the outside who will send them money. Jobs also give prisoners a sense of purpose and may help build self-worth. Prisoners widely report that working is a positive thing.

Prisoners are limited in what they can have in their possession; physical space in their cell is limited. They are restricted to keeping only a certain number of books. Their clothing is all furnished by the state, although if they have money, they can usually buy such things as tennis shoes. But everything has to be bought through the canteen, and styles are very limited—and for good reason. Prisoners usually value "their stuff" highly, even to the point of guarding their own coffee grounds. This sense of possessiveness is an example of their desire to have some control over their life.

Research shows that prison can negatively affect the mental health of adult inmates. However, for those who can think positively about the experience, serving a prison sentence can be a time of respite and even safety (Goomany & Dickinson, 2015).

Many prisons have worked out programs with local colleges whereby college classes are offered free of charge or for very minimum fees to prisoners; these classes, if passed, count toward college degrees. Many prisoners do not have a high school diploma. There are always some working on getting their General Education Development (GED) certificate, and at some institutions, inmates have to obtain a GED as a condition of release. I once gave the "commencement address" at a GED awards ceremony: It was an honor. I got a chance to see firsthand that some people really want to improve their lot in life and will work hard for it.

The Mindset of a Prisoner

This section explores the "mindset" of a prisoner. For full transparency, we note that this information is solely gleaned from the authors' personal experiences and is explored further in **CASE STUDY 13-1**.

It is very difficult to tell if a prisoner is being honest with you. Many, although not all, prisoners have grown up in an environment where truth-telling was not a highly valued virtue. Usually a prisoner has learned to get what he or she wants by deception and manipulation. In fact, prisoners are often experts at it.

Of course, many people on the "outside" are not much better! I have been lied to by prisoners more times than I care to imagine, but as a pastor in the parish, sometimes my interactions with non-prisoners weren't a whole lot different. So, while prisoners, by the standards of those on the outside, seem much different and are often perceived as "bad" or "worse" than anyone else, that may be an unfair judgment.

Prisoners have a difficult time with trust. Many of them have grown up not being able to trust anyone, even those closest to them. I was told by prison fellowship trainers in my early days of training, "They are going to look at you as if you were a fish in a fishbowl." You, at all times, will be "watched" by prisoners, looking for a weakness in you they can exploit. Anyone working with prisoners must be aware of this reality for two reasons. First, if you promise a prisoner something and don't follow through, that person will not trust you again. If someone has lost all individuality and had

🔍 CASE STUDY 13-1

This case is an experience the chapter authors had with a young woman. We will call her Angie to protect her identity, and her story is a real-life example of much of what many prisoners have experienced both prior to and after incarceration. This experience extended over a period of six years. This young woman was not related to us and was unknown to us prior to this experience. We became involved with her shortly after she was arrested and continued that involvement through county jail, court trials and hearings, her sentencing, her incarceration in a state prison, and her release from prison on parole.

The crime for which Angie was imprisoned was child neglect leading to death, a class 2 felony. Angie's 2-year-old child was murdered by the child's father, and Angie did not do enough to protect that child, according to the determination of the courts. She received a sentence of 12–22 years, with her first chance at parole being at the conclusion of serving 6 years. Angie was 26 years old when I, as pastor, first visited her. She was the mother of four children; the second youngest was the victim of the crime. Her mother and father were jailed at county jails close by, and her other three children were in custody of the Social Services department.

Angie had been the victim of sexual abuse at the hands of her brother starting at 5 years of age. She was verbally and emotionally abused by both her parents from age 5 onward. Her father was a very strict disciplinarian who used the Bible as a weapon of control. Angie grew up fast, she grew up hardened, and she grew up knowing how to lie and manipulate people to get what she wanted. At 17 years of age, she left home, which was a camper shell on the back of a pickup, and joined the army.

In the army, Angie was sexually abused by the majority of men in her unit; however, by now, it was somewhat a voluntary thing. She received a less-than-honorable discharge after one year, and her life went on a downward spiral. Sexual and emotional abuse continued at the hands of her husband.

After Angie was incarcerated, my wife and I went to see her about every three weeks for four years. It took a long time for her to trust us—especially me, as a man. We had been seeing her for almost a year when the following incident happened. During visitation at the prison, inmates sat facing their visitors, separated by a distance of 1–2 feet. We were talking with Angie about forgiveness, about the love of Christ for her, and about her feelings of unworthiness.

At one point in our conversation (my wife was seated right beside me), I reached out and touched Angie's knee with my hand—and that was all it took. Our visit was over shortly after that, and we received a letter from her in the mail the following week: Angie did not ever want to see us again! Her actions may simply have been a matter of not trusting us (which it probably was to an extent), but may also have been her way of manipulating us to get a little control in her life.

During our ministry, we had to be constantly on the alert for many of the things described in this chapter, including the warnings and the advice to future nurses. Many times we failed to see the warning signs ourselves because we got too emotionally involved and we got taken advantage of. This case demonstrates them all.

There were certainly frustrations in our relationship with Angie. Each time we planned to see Angie, I communicated with her ahead of time to make sure she would want a visit. One week we made the 1½-hour drive, only to be told at the check-in desk that Angie did not want to see us. Often she would tell us one thing on a particular visit, and then the next time she might tell us something totally contradictory. After almost every visit, we would talk on the way home about what we thought we could believe and what we thought we could not believe. Over the years, Angie shared much with us about her past. But what could we believe and what could we not believe? We never really knew if we were being told the truth.

Angie finally got paroled out of prison in May 2018. We were there to celebrate with her. It was a big day for her and us. She lived two states away from us, so we saw very little of each other after her release; we don't even talk on the phone much anymore. In prison, we extended an incredible amount of grace to Angie because of the environment she was in and her past experiences in life. We gave her money and overlooked a lot of things in how she spent that money, and how little gratitude was expressed for anything done for her. But once Angie got on the outside, things did not get better, but only worse. She became demanding that we do things for her, always on her terms. Sadly, this story does not have a happy ending: Angie still struggles with many issues and doesn't appear to want to change.

Questions

1. How would you have approached this situation with Angie in showing her the love of Jesus?
2. How did you feel about Angie being partially responsible for her own small child's death? Did this fact color your view of her?
3. Which events in Angie's life influenced the adult that she became? How do you reconcile God allowing the evil things that happened to Angie?
4. What are three ways you could show your love to someone like Angie who is in prison?
5. Is there anything in this case study that you would have done differently than the authors? If so, what?
6. If you had to predict the outcome of Angie's life, what do you think would happen to her?

everything precious taken away by the system, how can that person trust anyone after that?

Second—and most important—prisoners *know the rules*. They know what they can and cannot do; they also know what you can and cannot do. I, as a volunteer at a prison, may not receive anything from a prisoner, not even a note. In turn, I cannot give a prisoner anything, not even a piece of paper, unless I first get it approved by the prison personnel. One time I was chatting with a couple of inmates after class and another inmate "brushed by me" and slipped a drawing he had done on top of my Bible. It happened rather fast and I didn't even catch who had done it; I never figured out whether the two guys I had been talking with were "working with" the third guy. In any event, I filed a report of what had happened and gave the drawing to the guard present as evidence.

The following incident actually happened in a Colorado prison, and is a good example of manipulation at the hands of a prisoner. An inmate talked a guard into "breaking the rules" and giving the inmate something the guard was not to give him. At that point, the inmate "had the guard." All the inmate had to do from that point forward was to use the threat of reporting the guard to the authorities to get whatever he wanted. This particular inmate actually coerced the guard into giving him an entire guard uniform, including shoes. The inmate planned to use the uniform in an escape attempt. His plan was discovered before the escape attempt occurred; however, the guard lost his job and faced criminal charges himself.

Prisoners are masters at manipulation (**BOX 13-2**). If they can get you to break a rule, just by a "little bit," they will continue to "work you" for more and more. It is a game that some of them play, and they are good at it. Some prisoners have a lot of spare time on their hands and being able to manipulate someone is a way of "winning" something. For example, a handshake is the extent of physical contact that a volunteer is allowed with any prisoner. If a person violates any of these rules, he or she can be released from volunteer status.

Some prisoners also struggle with unworthiness—another topic addressed in Case Study 13-1. They have done bad things,

BOX 13-2 Research Highlight

Correctional facility nurses, also called correctional forensic nurses, need to have a unique set of skills to work in detention facilities. The research question for this article was "How do correctional nurses describe their working experience in prisons? What issues emerged?" Using a qualitative, descriptive study, the authors used purposive sampling to conduct five focus groups ($N = 31$) with correctional nurses in seven prisons in northern Italy. Five themes were identified: "(1) prisoners' healthcare needs, (2) negotiation between custody and care, (3) satisfaction of working in prisons, (4) obstacles to quality care and (5) safety" (p. 393). Manipulation was a common theme throughout the study. There was high turnover among nurses due to ethical dilemmas and distress with prison staff. The authors recommend that specific education interventions related to restorative nursing be required of all those who work in the prison systems in an effort to resolve ethical problems and reduce moral distress.

Modified from Sasso, L., Delogu, B., Carrozzino, R., Aleo, G., & Bagnasco, A. (2018). Ethical issues of prison nursing: A qualitative study in Northern Italy. *Nursing Ethics, 25*(3), 393–409.

and they have hurt people badly, even killed in some instances. All but the most hardened individuals know this in their mind. They may not show their guilt on the outside, but they know inside that they have "messed up" badly. If we do something we know is not right, our conscience haunts us until we repent and receive forgiveness. And even then, we sometimes have problems forgiving ourselves.

When we are on the "outside," we can talk with others and cry with others as we work through these kinds of issues. Prisoners don't have this luxury. A prison environment is not conducive to anyone publicly admitting his or her sin. A prisoner cannot "shed the tears" necessary to work through forgiveness issues.

A prisoner cannot be sympathetic toward and/or protect another inmate who is struggling hard with an issue. Even if allowed limited phone privileges, the prisoner cannot and will not admit any guilt, since such conversations are monitored. If a prisoner breaks any of these "prison rules," he or she will pay for it!

What happens to those prisoners who need to "spill their guts" or "cry it out"? They bottle it up, put on a tough guy image and live with it, and rot away inside. David spoke well in Psalm 32:3–4: "When I kept silent about my sin, my body wasted away through my groaning all day long. For day and night Thy hand was heavy upon me; my vitality was drained away as with the fever heat of summer." Remember, the prisoners with whom you are working and treating no doubt have all sorts of "stuff" that may well be a contributing factor to their illnesses.

Finally, most prisoners are very self-centered. To go along with this attitude, many are in desperate need to feel some control over their life. When a person "checks in" to a prison, he or she "checks out" of control over everyday living. The person goes to bed with lights out on the prison's time schedule. The person wakes up in the morning on the prison's timetable. The person eats at the appointed time determined by the prison or doesn't eat at all.

Day-to-day decisions made regarding regular activities of daily living, unlike on the outside, are not available to the prisoner. Outside prison walls, people can decide to go to a movie at 1:00 in the morning and then go out to breakfast at 3:30, then go home and sleep the day away after calling in sick for work, if they want. It might not be the ethical thing to do and there may be consequences for that kind of behavior, but they can do it, if they want. A prisoner doesn't have that option. On the outside, a person can decide to do a crazy thing like spend $400 for a pair of super-exclusive basketball shoes. In contrast, a prisoner would have access to maybe two different kinds of sneakers, the same ones worn by everyone else.

This loss of control experienced by prisoners helps explain some of the other characteristics of prisoners. Lying, deception, and manipulation are ways that prisoners can be in control of something. They often will play the "victim" card. They will tell you whatever story they think you want to hear, always making themselves appear as a victim for the purpose of moving you to do something for them. Christians are easy prey, because of the commands of Jesus to love our neighbor. Reread Matthew 25, quoted at the beginning of this chapter. You may love your neighbor, but if that expression of love becomes something that enables someone to continue in an irresponsible, dangerous, and destructive lifestyle, then it ceases to be love.

The inability to trust completely what a prisoner shares is probably the most difficult part of working with prisoners. For example, if you ask a prisoner what his or her pain level is on a scale of 1–10, you may not be able to trust the answer, because the majority of prisoners have a history of substance abuse and may give a response to ensure they are prescribed certain pain medications.

Everything discussed in this section about the life of the prisoner—all the emotions, all the feelings, all the characteristics, all the losses—help explain why a prisoner acts the way he or she does. A big loss is the loss of communication with the outside world: Most prisoners never receive a visit or a letter or a birthday card. Some others may have a family member or two who continue to keep in touch, hoping for a major life change. Many others have been "written off" by their families after years of lying, stealing, manipulation, substance abuse, and a hurricane of destruction they left behind. Throw in a big dose of anger, and the result is an individual who is very different from any person whom we might encounter on the outside. For one working with the prisoner, a measure of the Fruit of the Spirit is helpful—particularly patience.

▶ The Need for Nursing as Ministry in the Prison Setting

The preceding discussion raises an obvious question: "Since I know how prisoners think; since I know how they act; since I know they are eyeing me with the intent to somehow use me to their advantage—why would I want to even bother with prisoners? Let someone else take care of them. Let someone else be taken advantage of." That is the normal human reaction, and it is certainly the world's response. But God has called Christians out of the world and set them aside for a special work. What work is that? To serve Him. And how do we serve God—after all, He is God, so what does He need? We serve Him by serving our neighbors. This chapter opened with that well-known passage from Matthew 25: "For I was hungry, and you gave Me something to eat; I was thirsty, and you gave Me drink . . . I was in prison, and you came to Me."

But what about your life's work, your calling to a vocation of nursing as ministry? In the discussion that follows, I will draw on a book entitled *Luther on Vocation* by Gustaf Wingren (1957). He states, "A vocation is a station in life, which is by nature helpful to others, if it be followed. All stations are so oriented that they serve others" (p. 4). All Christians have several and various vocations at any one time: husband/wife, parent, child, grandparent, sibling, and so on. Vocations are also marked by our work or careers: pastor, bookkeeper, farmer, nurse, and so on.

For this chapter, the focus is on the vocation of the nurse. Wingren (1957) says, "In his vocation, one is not reaching up to God, but rather bends oneself down toward the world. When one does that, God's creative work is carried on" (p. 7). In other words, in your vocation as a nurse, God is reaching down to earth, through you, and ministering to your patient. In my years in the parish as pastor, whenever I made a hospital call I always reminded those under my spiritual care: "Look at these doctors, anesthesiologists, aides, and nurses as an extension of God's hands. He has given those who need it calm hands to do surgery, intelligent minds to know what needs to be done, and compassionate nurses to care for you."

If we all could have this outlook on all of our vocations in life, how would it change us? If we could all look at those whom we serve and see nothing but a human being God has created, maybe there wouldn't be a need for so many prisons! A nurse once told me of her days doing rotations during her training. In one of her rotations, she was assigned a patient who was to give birth in the near future. She was to do preliminary visitations prior to birth, be at the bedside during birth, and then do follow-up visits after birth. At the conclusion of this rotation, the nurse was interviewed by her instructor and asked this question: "How was it for you being assigned a black patient?" Evidently the nurse, in all seriousness, looked at her instructor and said: "You mean, my patient was black?" She hadn't even noticed!

We all have our faults. None of us is perfect. All have sinned and fallen short of God's glory (Romans 3:23). There has only been one perfect man to ever live, and he died on a Roman cross more than 2000 years ago. By his blood all believers are washed clean of all sin and imperfection, thereby freeing us for God's service to His creation, all done in His Name. The human being who is a prisoner was also created in the image of God before falling into sin. Those in prison may be the "least of these," but Jesus extends his grace and love to them as well, and you may be the only representation of God's love they ever see.

Although many of the characteristics of prisoners discussed in this chapter seem negative, I encourage you to not immediately assume the worst about such a patient. Just because a person is or has been a prisoner,

that status does not in and of itself mean that person is a bad person. Look for the best in people. In many ways, you and the prisoner are much alike. I have never met a prisoner who told me that he or she did not love his or her children. Almost all will say, "My children are the most important thing in my life." They understand they have not shown that love properly in the past, but they all are determined to make the future different. Almost all married male prisoners will tell you that they do love their wives; they may not know how to express that love in the proper way, but they do love their wives. Those who have divorced almost always understand clearly their part in that divorce, and are sorry for it, and will do what they can to make the future different and to work with their ex-spouse to do the right thing for their children.

I have never met prisoners who were happy for all the evil things that had happened around them, and in which they played a part. They all regret doing the bad they have done. I have met few prisoners who did not want their future to be better than their past. They want the best for their future; they might be clueless as to how that can become a reality, but they still do want the best.

Consider this: How many prisoners, especially those close to your age, would have a common interest with you in such things as music, movies, reading, hobbies, and dreams? How many prisoners may well share with you common experiences from the past, such as growing up in a blended family, or growing up in a single-parent household, or being involved in similar high school sports or activities? How many prisoners may share with you a love of skiing, or gardening, or the Holy Scriptures? Yes, I believe you and the prisoner have more in common than you might initially think.

Of course, you and the prisoner are also significantly different! That difference, however, is not an acceptable excuse for not giving prisoners the same professional care you would give someone who has never been in prison. Many prisoners have been in places that they would wish you never go. Most have been involved in activities that they would not wish you to be involved in. Most have done things in the past that they would plead with you not to mimic.

Many prisoners have done irreversible damage to their bodies with alcohol and drugs; you probably have not been there or done that. Prisoners would advise you to stay away from such substance abuse. Most prisoners have not grown up in a loving, Christ-centered home as you may have; you have something in this regard other than medical care you can give them. Most prisoners have never experienced true, Biblical grace. If you have, pass it on.

So, how do you treat the prisoner? This next section suggests some strategies for ministering to the incarcerated patient.

▶ Strategies for Care of the Incarcerated Patient: A Nurse's Perspective

Treat prisoners the same way that you would treat your best friend. Address them by their name; they may be known only by their five-digit inmate number in the prison system. How detached is that? If their name is not on their clothing, ask them for it, and use it.

Treat prisoners as you would like to be treated. Follow "the Golden Rule." If I were to go into a hospital for surgery, I would expect the nurse assigned to me to treat me according to the professional standards expected of all nurses. Guard yourself against giving the prisoner anything less than your best.

Having said that, always be on your guard with prisoners. Remember some of the things you have read here. Don't forget: They know the rules they have to follow. They also know the rules you have to follow and may well try to persuade you to relax those rules. Don't tolerate such games; call them on it. If a prisoner does or says something inappropriate, report him or her. Prisoners will always be accompanied by at least one corrections officer, so notify that officer and maybe hospital personnel as well. You can be assured the officer will write up a report when he or she gets back to the prison—and inmates do not like to be written up, because there will be consequences for them.

Remember that prisoners have often learned to manipulate others for control. In the care of prisoners, use caution in a rapport-building conversation. The approach to care is always professionalism. Keep a watchful eye for any situation that could compromise your safety or the safety of others around you. Don't allow your sympathetic side to lead to any compromise. The same rules from volunteer training—to not accept anything from prisoners or give anything to prisoners—apply when those prisoners are inside a hospital or clinic setting. Examples would include asking you for an extra can of pop "for the road," or handing you a picture the prisoner drew, or asking for your full name. Unless patients choose to share that information, you may never know the offenses for which they were incarcerated. In the post anesthesia care unit (PACU) where one of the authors worked, for added protection, we always had two nurses present in addition to the guards.

As a registered nurse (RN) working in the PACU (**BOX 13-3**) and caring for incarcerated patients, I was thankful for some exposure to the inside of the correctional facility. It helped me remember that these patients were people and provide compassionate care. The differences I most frequently noted in care of prisoners were, to put it bluntly, related to their outward appearance. Many prisoners are covered with tattoos and appear both big and strong (see **BOX 13-4**).

Another difference was their high requirement for pain medications. Many had a history of drug addiction so their pain tolerance

BOX 13-3 Outstanding Nurse Leader: Eileen Mertens, RN

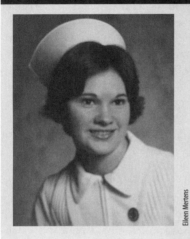

Eileen Mertens

I graduated from a diploma RN program in the late 1970s, when professionalism was drilled into nurses as part of our education. Those were the "white dress, white shoes, nursing cap" attire days, and the RN was accorded automatic respect and expected to take command in any situation.

In most circumstances, the nurse has a relatively good idea of the surrounding environment and has learned to adapt to any changes in that setting in a fairly quick time frame. Building a rapport with the patient during assessments and care is beneficial and enjoyable, and a step built into the daily routine. However, when your patient is accompanied by two guards, who may be armed, and in most cases doesn't appear to be a "routine" patient, it causes some anxiety and, even if brief, a moment of consideration. As an RN, the majority of my experience in caring for patients who were also prisoners came while working in the post anesthesia care unit in a small Midwestern town.

In the PACU setting, our patients would arrive to our unit just out from anesthesia, so the immediate care was to establish a clear airway and make assessments. This trumped any other concerns. But as the prisoner patient became more awake and the vital signs stabilized, the nurse's awareness noted the differences. The patient would always wear an ankle or wrist device locked to the bedframe. In our hospital, one guard would sit at the bedside at all times. It was a natural thing to wonder why the person was imprisoned. In spite of these differences, the role for the nurse was always to provide excellent care for the patient. In this situation, your nursing education and experiences must override any fear, and you must provide kind, caring, compassionate, and professional care.

My husband began prison ministry in the 1990s. Some of the first times he went to the state correctional facility to lead a Bible study, I stayed home and prayed—I guess my mind felt that he was going into an unknown and risky situation. After approximately six months, I went through training so that I could accompany him on special occasions. Much of this training focused on awareness and safety. There were rules for the volunteers to follow, and we were informed of the rules the prisoner was expected to follow.

I remember my first time going into the correctional facility quite clearly. We passed through the metal detector and were patted down, and then a guard accompanied the volunteers back through several locked doors, which clanged shut behind us before the next door opened. We walked through the yard in route to the educational building in the center of the quads. The prison was a men's facility, and I saw darkness and hardness in the faces of many inmates whom we passed. I was relieved to discover much friendlier and kind faces in the classroom.

The invisible church is the body of Christ known to our Lord alone, and in this facility this body of Christ was present and freed on the inside, even while being imprisoned on the outside. It changes you to see men in prison green singing from their hearts, listening to God's Word, and praying. Over the years, I returned several more times with my husband and saw the tears and heard the concerns of young men, husbands, fathers, and grandfathers—men loved by God, men serving out their sentences.

BOX 13-4 Evidence-Based Practice Focus

As described in this article, the researchers used focus groups for the second phase of a study examining the Rediscovery of Self-Care (RSC) model, part of *A Care Intervention for Persons with Incarceration Experience*, which served as the framework for this study. Participants from three county jails in Massachusetts expressed the importance of self-care, defining this mainly in terms of physical needs (such as exercising or healthy eating). Self-care to this group also included addressing mental health and substance abuse issues with counseling interventions (p. 126). The results of the study supported the RSC model constructs and may be used to direct future research with this population.

Modified from Maruca, A. T., Dion, K., Lobelo, A. A., Ampiah-Bonney, O., Chen, C., Sanger, K., & Zucker, D. (2017). Self-care management in corrections: Perspectives from persons with an incarceration experience. *Journal of Forensic Nursing, 13*(3), 126–134.

---

was low, but many also were keenly aware that a constant cry of pain would bring more narcotics. This became an interesting balance, in which the PACU nurses relied on one another to help navigate and assess real needs.

Another difference was that outpatient prisoners would almost without exception request a cola drink and a roast beef sandwich before discharge. Apparently, they were rarely served beef at the prison. Finally, prisoners would try almost anything to delay returning to the facility.

Even while frequently testing us and pushing limits, most prisoners who received treatment in the PACU were still respectful, appreciative, and courteous. For those patients who were not, we learned to address the problem quickly, by stating that their behavior was not acceptable and letting the guards handle the non-nursing "stuff."

Nurses who feel called to prison ministry should be given a thorough orientation to the position of a nurse working in corrections and the culture of prison life, as this type of work can affect the nurse positively or negatively (Choudhry, Armstrong, & Dregan, 2017). Nurses working in the prison system are highly autonomous, providing health assessments, dispensing medications, running the infirmary, and responding to emergencies (Holwick, 2018). Nurse practitioners

have additional responsibilities for managing the complexities of chronic illness in a closed setting with members of a population who are generally forgotten, have higher rates of mental illness and substance abuse, may be going through withdrawal from addiction while imprisoned, and have higher rates of suicide. All of this care takes place in an environment that can be scary, threatening, and sometimes violent for the caregiver, the inmates, the staff, and the public. Certainly, God's grace is needed in extra measure for nurses called to this ministry.

In addition to understanding the background of this patient population, nurses called to serve those who are incarcerated should remember that they work with a vulnerable population. Prisoners cannot repay caregivers for kindness shown. They may not deserve the care they receive, and they may not ever show any appreciation. Even so, each person in jail, prison, or juvenile corrections/detention is someone's son or daughter, husband or wife, mother or father. Family members who once had high hopes for their loved ones now grieve, and they continue to feel the pain and stigma of these negative events for years to come.

A background in mental health and/or emergency nursing is helpful if one wishes to work as a correctional forensic nurse

(International Association of Forensic Nurses, 2019). No special certification is required, although certifications are available.

In providing care for those in prison, remember the words of the Lord in the beginning of this chapter: "if you have cared for the *least* of these, you have done it unto me." Several strategies for care have been recommended by nurses to those working in this setting (Parrish, 2016, p. 62):

- Make eye contact.
- Listen actively.
- Reaffirm you hear what the patient is saying.
- Pay attention to details—that is, what is said as well as what is not said.
- Let the patient finish speaking.
- Smile when appropriate to show you are human.
- Monitor your own voice tone and facial expressions.
- Advocate for the well-being of your patient.
- Remember that kindness and reassurance may be all that is needed.
- Speak in terms that the patient can understand.
- Maintain your patience.
- Be nonjudgmental. It is not necessary to know a patient's crime to provide care.
- Remind yourself this is a person who deserves to be treated with respect.
- Practice true self-reflection: If you questions whether boundaries were crossed, they probably were.

In the vocation of nursing, you are given a unique opportunity to be the hands and feet of our Lord Jesus, serving in compassion and love, speaking the Gospel always even if not using words. To prisoners, receiving care in a professional, caring, and loving manner may be the first or perhaps rare opportunity they have to experience Christ's love through you.

▶ Clinical Reasoning Exercises

1. Where are the prisons in your county? In your state? How many inmates do they hold and what is the level of security?
2. What role do nurse practitioners play in the prisons in your state? If you don't know, find out and share this information with your peers.
3. When considering nursing as ministry, how are inmates a vulnerable population? Why did they become vulnerable?
4. If you were to work in a prison, what would be your biggest challenge in showing love and compassion in this setting?
5. If you were conducting research with prisoners, what are some of the major ethical points you would need to consider? What about protection of human subjects with this group?

▶ Personal Reflection Exercises

1. Have you ever personally known someone who was in prison? What were the circumstances? How did you feel about it?
2. Have you ever done clinical experiences in a prison? Visited someone in prison? How did this experience make you feel?
3. How would you feel if a close relative, such as a father, brother, mother, sister, or cousin, was

incarcerated? What would be most difficult for you in this situation?

4. Have you ever considered working in a prison as your nursing job? If so, what prompted you to consider this as a place of employment?

5. Do you have any personal challenges to working with those in prison? For example, do you have biases that you need to explore related to persons who are being punished for criminal activities of certain types? Where do you think these biases stem from?

References

Buffett, H. G., & Buffett, H. W. (2013). *40 chances: Finding hope in a hungry world.* New York, NY: Simon and Schuster.

Bureau of Justice. (2017). Mortality in local jails and state prisons, 2000–2013: Statistical tables. Retrieved from https://www.bjs.gov/index.cfm?ty=pbdetail&iid=5341

Choudhry, K., Armstrong, D., & Dregan, A. (2017). Prison nursing: Formation of a stable professional identity. *Journal of Forensic Nursing, 13*(1), 20–25.

Goomany, A., & Dickinson, T. (2015). The influence of prison climate on the mental health of adult prisoners: A literature review. *Journal of Psychiatric and Mental Health Nursing, 22*(6), 413–422.

Holwick, A. (2018). Correctional nursing: Caring for the least of these. *Journal of Christian Nursing, 35*(1), 44–45.

International Association of Forensic Nurses. (2019). Correctional nursing. Retrieved from https://www.forensicnurses.org/page/CorrectionalNursing

Parrish, S. (2016). Can nurses care within these walls? *American Jail, 30*(4), 61–63.

Sedlak, A. J., & Bruce, C. (2016). *Survey of youth in residential placement: Youth's characteristics and backgrounds. SYRP Report.* Rockville, MD: Westat.

Valleta, E. (2017). 10 staggering statistics about the US prison system. Retrieved from https://www.sbs.com.au/guide/article/2017/12/06/10-staggering-statistics-about-us-prison-system

Wingren, G. (1957). *Luther on vocation.* Eugene, OR: Wipf & Stock.

Recommended Readings

Barnwell, W. H. (2016). *Called to heal the brokenhearted: Stories from Kairos Prison Ministry International.* Jackson, MS: University Press of Mississippi.

Carrasco-Baún, H. (2017). Prison nursing: Legal framework and care reality. *Revista Espanola de Sanidad Penitenciaria, 19*(1), 3–12.

Dickinson, T., Mullan, A., Lippiatt, K., & Owen, J. A. (2018). Nursing people in prisons, forensics and correctional facilities. In J. C. Santos & J. R. Cutliffe (Eds.), *European psychiatric/mental health nursing in the 21st century* (pp. 211–222). New York, NY: Springer.

Drake, S. A., Koetting, C., Thimsen, K., Downing, N., Porta, C., Hardy, P.,... Engebretson, J. (2018). Forensic nursing state of the science: Research and practice opportunities. *Journal of Forensic Nursing, 14*(1), 3–10.

Jackson, R. (2017). *Voice for the voiceless: Developing a resource ministry that addresses the holistic needs of returning citizens.* Richmond, VA: Virginia Union University.

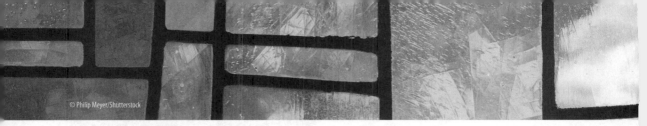
© Philip Meyer/Shutterstock

CHAPTER 14

Poverty and Homelessness

Margaret Barnes, DNP, RN, PMHNP-BC

LEARNING OBJECTIVES

At the end of this chapter, the reader will be able to:

1. Analyze the concepts of poverty and homelessness.
2. Assess consequences of poverty and homelessness from a holistic perspective.
3. Evaluate federal, state, and local responses to poverty and vulnerability, including trends and concerns facing uninsured and underinsured populations.
4. Describe strategies that nurses can use to improve the health status and decrease health disparities in poor and homeless individuals.
5. Apply ethical principles when caring for the poor and the homeless.

KEY TERMS

Crisis poverty
Distributive justice
Generational poverty
Homelessness

Neighborhood poverty
Poverty
Social justice
Social poverty

Spiritual poverty
Working poor

▶ Concept of Poverty

Often poverty is a matter of perspective. Those who grow up with very little may not consider themselves poor if all of their friends and classmates are in the same financial condition. In contrast, those who are brought up in homes where there is increased stress over finances may consider themselves poor even if the family income is well above the federal poverty level. Escobar (2005) shared a story about how as a child she wondered if a friend was poor. When her mother asked her why she thought the child was poor, she said, "'Because her socks were dirty'" (p. 47). Escobar's parents were illegal immigrants living in a small apartment and fearing deportation; however, Escobar did not consider herself poor because she was able to wear clean clothes.

In this chapter, you will have the opportunity to consider different types of poverty as well as the healthcare concerns that often accompany poverty and homelessness. Have you ever been at a place in your life where you were not sure how you would be able to afford food, housing, utilities, medications, or other necessities? To whom did you turn for assistance? Many individuals living in poverty have a limited social support system, particularly if they feel isolated due to their poverty.

▶ Defining and Understanding Poverty

When we think about **poverty**, we immediately tend to think in terms of a lack of financial resources, which makes it difficult to cover the cost of food, clothing, housing, utilities, health care, and other necessities. Every year, the U.S. Department of Health and Human Services (DHHS, 2019) calculates poverty guidelines to be used for determining financial eligibility for federal programs such as Head Start, the Supplemental Nutrition Assistance Program (SNAP), the National School Lunch Program, the Low-Income Home Energy Assistance Program (HEAP), and the Children's Health Insurance Program (CHIP). **TABLE 14-1** presents these poverty guidelines for 2019.

Demographics

According to Fontenot, Semega, and Kollar (2018), 39.7 million people in the United States were living in poverty in 2017, based on information from the U.S. Census Bureau. As these authors indicated, poverty levels would be higher if adult children were not living in their parents' home contributing to the household

TABLE 14-1 Department of Health and Human Services Poverty Guidelines, 2019

2019 POVERTY GUIDELINES FOR THE 48 CONTIGUOUS STATES AND THE DISTRICT OF COLUMBIA

Persons in Family/ Household	Income Level
For families/households with more than 8 persons, add $4420 for each additional person.	
1	$12,490
2	$16,910
3	$21,330
4	$25,750
5	$30,170
6	$34,590
7	$39,010
8	$43,430

Department of Health and Human Services. (2019). Poverty guidelines. Retrieved from https://aspe.hhs.gov/poverty-guidelines

income. **TABLE 14-2** outlines the poverty status of people by family relationship, age, and race based on 2017 U.S. Census Bureau statistics (Fontenot et al., 2018).

Types of Poverty

Poverty can come in all shapes and sizes. Persistent poverty, also called **generational poverty**, is passed down from parents to children to grandchildren, often as a result

	All People	Families	Female Head of Household/No Husband Present	Age (Years)		
				0–17	18–64	65 and Older
Asian	10.0%	7.7%	15.7%	11.3%	9.5%	10.8%
White	10.7%	8.7%	25.8%	15.2%	9.9%	7.8%
Hispanic	18.3%	16.9%	34.3%	25.0%	15.0%	17.0%
Black	21.2%	19.0%	32.9%	29.0%	18.3%	19.3%

TABLE 14-2 Poverty Status of People by Family Relationship, Age, and Race, 2017

Compiled from data in Tables B-1 and B-2. Fontenot, K., Semega, J., & Kollar, M. (2018). Income and poverty in the United States: 2017. Retrieved from www.census.gov/library/publications/2018/demo/p60-263.html

of learned behavior as well as the lack of resources to pull out of the cycle of poverty. When a neighborhood consists of several families living in persistent poverty with no hope of change, it can result in **neighborhood poverty**. In neighborhood poverty, often homes become run-down because of insufficient funds to maintain the home or landlords who are unresponsive to calls to maintain the home. Because of psychosocial factors, such neighborhoods can become unsafe. According to Sackett (2016), violent crimes are more prevalent in neighborhoods with high poverty rates, neighborhoods that are racially or ethnically segregated, and neighborhoods characterized by income inequality.

Not all impoverished individuals started out poor. Edwards (2015) defined **crisis poverty** as a short, isolated period of poverty. Crisis poverty occurs when an individual suddenly loses all he or she has. This loss can be the result of a fire, tornado, hurricane, or some other natural disaster, or it can be the result of a motor vehicle accident or other cause of injury that means the individual or family

suddenly does not have the resources to cover their food, shelter, and/or medical expenses.

Even those who work 40 or more hours/week may be living in poverty. According to the DHHS (2019), a family of four does not meet the federal guidelines for poverty if their income is greater than $25,750/year. If both parents are working 40 hours/week at minimum-wage jobs, their income may exceed $25,750/year, rendering them ineligible for food stamps, Medicaid, low-income housing, and other types of assistance. This, in turn, may make it difficult for them to feed and clothe their family. The cost of housing may consume as much as half of their income. These individuals are considered the **working poor**. According to U.S. Legal (n.d.), "Working poor is a term used to describe individuals and families who remain as poor even though they have regular employment. The working poor are distinct from paupers, poor who are supported by government aid or charity" (para. 1).

A lack of social support can be a form of **social poverty**. When adult children move away from their extended family due to jobs, college, or relationships, they lose the resources associated with having friends and family to call upon in times of need, which can result in a sense of social poverty. The elderly can experience social poverty as well when they become isolated as family move away and friends die.

Hopelessness can result in **spiritual poverty**. When people have no sense of meaning or purpose, or when they cannot sense the love and forgiveness of God and/or others, they may become acutely aware of the emptiness that comes with a lack of relationship with God. In the medical setting, patients may experience spiritual poverty when they are separated from their religious community or they feel overwhelmed by illness or injury and question God's love for them.

▶ Consequences of Poverty

Physiological

Adults living in poverty are at increased risk for chronic diseases, such as diabetes, heart disease, and chronic obstructive pulmonary disease (COPD); communicable illnesses such as human immunodeficiency virus (HIV) infection, acquired immunodeficiency syndrome (AIDS), sexually transmitted diseases, and tuberculosis; and high-health-risk behaviors, injuries, accidents, homicide, drug-related mortality, teenage pregnancy, and disability (Price, Khubchandani, & Webb, 2018; Schroeder, 2016). In addition, the poor are at increased risk for obesity (Bratanova, Loughnan, Klein, Claassen, & Wood, 2016; Schroeder, 2016). According to Bratanova, Loughnan, Klein, Classen, and Wood (2016), when people see themselves as poor, their caloric intake increases due to a sense of social inequity and social anxiety. Unfortunately, when overeating is due to psychological factors such as food insecurity or social anxiety, people are less likely to change their diet as a result of an educational intervention.

Individuals living in poverty often forgo preventive care as well as treatment for illness due to concerns over the cost of care (Academy of Oncology Nurse and Patient Navigators, 2017). Cornelius et al. (2017) reported on the lack of adherence to antiretroviral therapy to treat HIV infection due to the cost of the medication, because housing, food, and transportation costs may take precedence over the cost of the medications for HIV. Levitz et al. (2015) found that unmarried women forgo preventive care as well as cancer treatments due to the inability to absorb the direct and indirect costs associated with health care. As a result of the lack of preventive care and follow-through with treatments ordered for disease, the rate of hospitalization is higher for individuals living in poverty. According to Singer et al. (2017), survival rates for persons with cancer are shorter for those individuals who live in poverty regardless of the stage at which the cancer is diagnosed and the use of alcohol and tobacco.

Children living in poverty are also at increased risk of prematurity, low birth weight, birth defects, increased infant mortality, nutritional deficits, iron-deficiency anemia, and elevated lead levels. "Children of the working poor . . . are less likely to receive care, and when they receive care, it is more likely to be of limited quality" (Price et al., 2018, p. 172). In addition, according to Schroeder (2016), the risk of teenage pregnancy is greater in girls who are poor.

Psychological

Adults and children living in poverty are at increased risk of depression and low self-esteem due to the stigma and culture of poverty. Inglis (2016) reported on an attitudes survey completed in the United Kingdom, in which 56% of the respondents stated that if people wanted to work, there are jobs available for them. In the survey, 23% of the respondents believed that people who are poor are lazy. In medical settings, adults tend to be acutely aware of negative attitudes displayed by healthcare providers when they say they are on Medicaid or do not have insurance.

According to Price et al. (2018), "children in poverty are more likely to experience . . . acute and chronic psychological stressors including family conflict, child abuse, single-parent families, and violence" (p. 171), resulting in emotional and behavioral problems. Chamberlain et al. (2016) also indicated that children living in poverty are at higher risk for mental illness. However, there is hope for improved mental health. Ljungqvist, Topor, Forssell, Svensson, and Davidson (2016) completed a study in which they provided monthly supplemental income to individuals with severe mental illness. Compared to a control group not provided with the monthly supplemental income, those who received the funds displayed less anxiety and depression, improved social networks, and an improved sense of self.

Sociocultural

Persons living in poverty typically have poor access to health care due to a lack of insurance, maldistribution of providers, transportation difficulties, inconvenient clinic hours, and (potentially) language barriers. Children in these situations may also experience decreased opportunities for education, income, and occupational alternatives. According to Leadley and Hocking (2017), childhood poverty leads to decreased opportunities for leisure activities, play, and socialization, which can impact occupational choices later in life. In addition, such children are at increased risk of death due to violence and/or trauma.

Spiritual

Among older adults, Polson, Gillespie, and Myers (2018) reported that spirituality is an important source of strength and resilience. Meraviglia, Stuifbergen, Morgan, and Parsons (2015) evaluated health-promotion behaviors among low-income cancer survivors.

They found low compliance with proper nutrition, exercise, and stress management, yet 75% of the participants reported a spiritual connection to God was a source of strength for them. Kim, Harty, Takahashi, and Voisin (2018) found that increased religious involvement among African American adolescents resulted in better school engagement, reduced risky sexual activity, and lower drug usage rates.

Developmental

According to Tran, Luchters, and Fisher (2017), children who grow up in impoverished families are at risk of not being able to reach their developmental potential as a result of "intrauterine growth restriction, child undernutrition, micronutrient deficiencies, infectious diseases and environmental exposures; and psychosocial factors including early childhood education, parenting practices and exposure to violence" (p. 415). Schubert and Marks (2016) noted that brain development is permanently affected when children experience "toxic stress" during the first few years of life (p. S21). Likewise, Chamberlain et al. (2016) used the term "toxic stress" when referring to delayed childhood development. According to Chaudry and Wimer (2016), child outcomes are worse when poverty is experienced early in life, when it is ongoing, and when there is a high concentration of poverty in the community. According to Lee and Jackson (2017), there is a strong association between low socioeconomic status and negative effects in relation to cognitive achievement.

Often, when caring for patients, nurses tend to focus on the immediate physical needs that caused the patients to enter into the healthcare system; however, it is essential that nurses complete a holistic assessment that looks at the psychological, sociocultural, spiritual, and developmental consequences of poverty if their goal is to improve the health of this population on a long-term basis. These consequences of poverty are not likely to change given the lack of social and political power experienced by those living in poverty. Individuals living in poverty need nurses who will provide a voice and advocate for their needs. In addition, when nurses care for patients who live in poverty, they need to be aware of resources in their community to which they can refer patients. What resources are available in your community?

▶ Homelessness

Another consequence that may be faced by those in poverty is **homelessness**. Often when we think of homelessness, we think of individuals living on the street, in tents, on park benches, under bridges, in their cars, or in other areas outside, or living in homeless shelters. The U.S. Department of Housing and Urban Development (HUD, 2018), however, defines the homeless as an "individual or family who lacks a fixed, regular, and adequate nighttime residence" (p. 5). This definition includes individuals who are living with friends or relatives on a short-term basis as a result of having no home of their own.

Causes of homelessness vary widely. Some individuals have experienced a job loss due to a layoff or factory closing and are no longer able to afford housing; others become homeless due to divorce, domestic violence, or other family disputes. Some are homeless as a result of aging out of the foster care system and being kicked out of the foster home once money is no longer being paid for their care. Others have experienced a fire or natural disaster that destroyed their home. Some have recently been released from prison and no longer have family ties, whereas others are veterans who have no place to go. According to Weber and Mulvihill (2017), due to the soaring cost of rental apartments, many low-income individuals and families cannot afford housing today. Many individuals live from paycheck to paycheck and are only one or two paychecks away from not having the money to pay for basic living expenses. If they were to lose their job or become unable to work, they could be in danger of becoming homeless.

Demographics

Each year, HUD oversees a "point-in-time" count of the homeless, in which localities across the United States are asked to count all of the sheltered and unsheltered homeless persons within their communities on one night between January 22 and January 31 (Dunton et al., 2014). In January 2018, this count identified 552,830 people who were experiencing homelessness (HUD, 2018, p. 13). **TABLE 14-3** provides a breakdown of these numbers. According to Dunton et al., the sheltered homeless include individuals or families living in homeless shelters, transitional housing, and hotels or motels paid for by the federal, state, or local government or a charitable organization. The unsheltered homeless are those who are found sleeping in "a car, park, abandoned building, bus or train station, airport, or camping ground" (p. 8).

The homeless population includes children, teenagers, single men and women, family groups, and veterans. According to the National Alliance to End Homelessness (n.d.a), "over the course of 2016, roughly half a million people in families stayed at a homeless shelter or transitional housing program—292,166 were children, and 144,991 were under the age of six" (para. 1). Homeless children face insecurity that may result in emotional and behavioral problems. Some may attend several different schools over the course of a school year, leading to deficiencies in their education. Their health and safety can also be affected due to the close living quarters within homeless shelters or transitional housing.

Marginalized youth are at higher risk for homelessness (National Alliance to End Homelessness, n.d.c). These populations include persons who identify as lesbian, gay, transgender, bisexual, or unsure of their sexual identity or preference. **TABLE 14-4** provides

TABLE 14-3 Total Number of People Experiencing Homelessness by Type, 2018

	Total	Unsheltered	Percentage	Sheltered	Percentage
Overall	552,830	194,467	35.2%	358, 363	64.8%
Individuals	372,417	178,077	47.8%	194,340	52.2%
People in families	180,413	16,390	9.1%	164,023	90.9%
Chronically homeless	88,640	57,886	65.3%	30,754	34.7%
Veterans	37,878	14,566	38.5%	23,312	61.5%
Unaccompanied youth	36,361	18,350	50.0%	18,011	50.0%

Compiled data from Housing and Urban Development. (2018). State of homelessness. Retrieved from https://www.hudexchange.info/resources /documents/2018-AHAR-Part-1.pdf

TABLE 14-4 Demographic Summary of People of Experiencing Homelessness by Gender, 2018

	Total	Sheltered	Percentage	Unsheltered	Percentage
Female	216,211	160,024	74.0%	56,187	26.0%
Male	332,925	197,025	59.2%	135,900	40.8%
Transgender	2521	1108	44.0%	1413	56%
Do not identify as female, male, or transgender	1173	206	17.6%	967	82.4%
Total	552,830	358,363	64.8%	194,467	35.2%

Compiled data from Housing and Urban Development. (2018). State of homelessness. Retrieved from https://www.hudexchange.info/resources /documents/2018-AHAR-Part-1.pdf

a demographic summary of homelessness by gender based on the 2018 HUD survey, and **TABLES 14-5** and **14-6** give demographic summaries by race and ethnicity, respectively (HUD, 2018). The 2017 HUD survey revealed that 20% of homeless individuals (111,902) had severe mental illness, 16% (89,333) experienced chronic substance abuse, 16% (87,329)

TABLE 14-5 Demographic Summary of People Experiencing Homelessness by Race, 2018

	Total	Sheltered	Percentage	Unsheltered	Percentage
White	270,568	156,673	57.9%	113,895	42.1%
Black or African American	219,809	168,716	76.8%	51,093	23.2%
Asian	6643	3588	54.0%	3055	46.0%
Native American	15,414	7628	49.5%	7786	50.5%
Pacific Islander	8039	4177	52.0%	3862	48.0%
Multiple races	32,357	17,581	54.3%	14,776	45.7%
Total	552,830	358,363	64.8%	194,467	35.2%

Compiled data from Housing and Urban Development. (2018). State of homelessness. Retrieved from https://www.hudexchange.info/resources/documents/2018-AHAR-Part-1.pdf

TABLE 14-6 Demographic Summary of People Experiencing Homelessness by Ethnicity, 2018

	Total	Sheltered	Percentage	Unsheltered	Percentage
Hispanic/Latino	122,476	78,180	63.8%	44,296	36.2%
Non-Hispanic/non-Latino	430,354	280,183	65.1%	150,171	34.9%
Total	552,830	358,363	64.8%	194,467	35.2%

Compiled data from Housing and Urban Development. (2018). State of homelessness. Retrieved from https://www.hudexchange.info/resources/documents/2018-AHAR-Part-1.pdf

were victims of domestic violence, and 2% (10,171) had HIV or AIDS.

According to HUD (2017), 7% of veterans (40, 056) were homeless during the point-in-time survey. Veterans at the highest risk of becoming homeless are those who served in Vietnam, Afghanistan, and/or Iraq (National Alliance to End Homelessness, n.d.c). The Department of Veterans Affairs has been working to end veteran homelessness, but it is an ongoing process.

Chronic homelessness is defined as homelessness lasting for at least a year, or repeatedly experiencing homelessness (National Alliance to End Homelessness, n.d.b). Often, those persons who are chronically homeless have serious mental illness, a physical disability, or a substance use disorder. Approximately 16% (88,640) of the homeless are chronically homeless (HUD, 2018).

▸ Consequences of Homelessness

Physiological

Homeless persons are at increased risk for COPD, peripheral vascular disease, hypertension, tuberculosis (TB), diabetes, HIV/AIDS, musculoskeletal problems, increased emergency room (ER) utilization, hypothermia, infestations, pneumonia, malnutrition, nutritional deficits, poor dental health, and poor skin integrity as well as a lack of preventive care. According to the Centers for Disease Control and Prevention (2018), individuals who have been homeless are five times more likely to contract TB in the course of a year than are those who have not experienced homelessness. In addition, the prevalence of hepatitis C among the homeless ranges from 22% to 53% (Dan, 2017). Treating the homeless for hepatitis and TB can be challenging because of their transient lifestyle and the lack of a consistent place to keep their belongings, including medications, secure, clean, and dry.

Psychological

Depression, increased incidence of mental/psychological illnesses, alcohol abuse, and substance abuse are more commonly seen in the homeless. Kim (2017) reported on a study by the National Institute of Mental Health (NIMH) that found 45% of the homeless population has a history of mental illness, with 20% to 25% being severely mentally ill (compared to 6% of the general population).

Mental illness can be a cause as well as a result of homelessness (Kim, 2017).

Sociocultural

Homeless individuals are at increased risk of trauma. They often have decreased access to care, and they live in an environment that is potentially detrimental—physically and socially—for both children and adults. According to Kim (2017), homeless individuals are more likely to be physically assaulted, raped, and incarcerated if they suffer from mental illness. Forty percent of prison inmates were homeless at some point in their lives prior to being incarcerated (Kim, 2017).

Spiritual

BOX 14-1 highlights some of the spiritual concerns associated with homelessness.

BOX 14-1 Research Highlight

The authors of this article performed a thorough review of the literature on the relationship between income, poverty, and well-being of children. "Poverty and low income are causally related to worse child development outcomes, particularly cognitive developmental and educational outcomes" (p. S23). Factors related to negative outcomes via poverty included material hardship, stress in the family, parental input, and the environment. Early experiences of poverty were associated with worse child outcomes. Persistent or chronic poverty in childhood, as well as extreme poverty, was associated with poorer health outcomes in both adolescents and adults. This evidence gives clear guidelines for early childhood interventions, where nurses can impact families and communities affected by poverty and make a different in their lives.

Chaudry, A., & Wimer, C. (2016). Poverty is not just an indicator: The relationship between income, poverty, and child well-being. *Academic Pediatrics, 16*(3), S23–S29. https://doi.org/10.1016/j.acap .2015.12.010. Copyright © 2016, with permission from Elsevier.

Developmental

According to Anthony, Vincent, and Shin (2018), as many as 2.48 million children may experience homelessness over the course of a year, and more than half of these homeless children are younger than the age of six. Children who are homeless may experience developmental regression such as bedwetting, behavioral issues, confusion, sadness, anxiety, depression, withdrawal, anger, overeating as a result of food insecurity, or weight loss as a result of becoming picky eaters (Anthony et al., 2018).

Nott and Vuchinich (2016) compared attitudes of homeless youth with the attitudes of youth involved in 4-H, who mainly came from two-parent households. They found homeless youth tend to be more self-reliant and self-aware. When asked about their strengths, the homeless youth identified internal qualities such as being a good leader, being creative, being compassionate, and being honest (Nott & Vuchinich, 2016). By contrast, children and teens who participated in 4-H tended to identify activities that brought them positive recognition, saying their strengths were sports, music, working with animals, and so on. Thus, homeless youth have some notable strengths as a result of their situation in life.

▶ Federal, State, and Local Responses to Poverty and Vulnerability

Distributive Justice

According to Reamer (2015), **"distributive justice** involves the use of ethics concepts and criteria to determine how scarce resources should be divided among people, groups, organizations, and communities" (para. 5). A related term is **social justice**, a type of justice that recognizes the worth in all individuals and encourages that all members of society be treated fairly. According to the American Nurses Association (ANA, 2015), social justice is "the analysis, critique, and change of social structures, policies, laws, customs, power, and privilege that disadvantage or harm vulnerable social groups through marginalization, exclusion, exploitation, and voicelessness" (p. 63). These terms imply that society is responsible for ensuring that all persons have their basic needs met, including for housing, nutrition, education, and health care.

Price et al. (2018, p. 173) described several federal and state programs that benefit the poor and the homeless, including the following:

- Medicare, Medicaid, the Child Health Insurance Program, Social Security programs for the elderly and the disabled, federally funded health centers, and Veterans Administration hospitals to improve healthcare access
- "Section 8," fair housing initiatives, public housing, and energy assistance programs to assist the poor and homeless with housing needs
- The Supplemental Nutrition Assistance Program (SNAP); the Women, Infants, and Children (WIC) program; and school breakfast and lunch programs to provide food for the poor
- Federal financial aid programs for college students including grants and loans, National Institute of Health loan repayment programs, and Health Resources and Services Administration workforce programs
- Earned income tax credits, and Temporary Assistance for Needy Families (TANF)
- The Federal Emergency Management Agency (FEMA), individual/household and crisis counseling programs, and disaster relief in the event of major disasters

- Head Start and foster care/adoption services
- Poisoning prevention programs
- Unemployment insurance, the Uniformed Services Employment and Reemployment Rights Act (USERRA), the Veterans' Employment and Training Service (VETS), and the Disabled Veterans Outreach Program (DVOP)

Despite the broad scope of the governmental programs, there remains a need for advocacy (**BOX 14-2**). Many of these programs have expiration dates. Our congressional leaders need to be contacted to renew these programs when they are set to expire. In addition, in our local communities, we need to ensure there are no laws enacted that harm the poor and/or homeless.

In 2014, 21 cities had a law prohibiting feeding the homeless (Barclay, 2014). Two years later, 71 cities had made it illegal to feed the homeless (Cole, 2016). The thought is that handing out food will encourage people to remain homeless rather than trying to better themselves. The idea of making it a crime to help homeless individuals is alarming.

BOX 14-2 Outstanding Nurse Leader: Sister Ann John

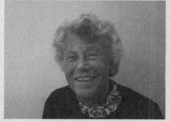

In 1989, Sister Ann John followed God's calling to open a clinic for the homeless. She has a deep love for those who are served by the clinic. She started the clinic single-handedly at the local community center. She invited men to come over to her and have their blood pressure checked. They were reluctant at first, but she began offering them a pair of socks if they consented to a blood pressure check. From that meager start, the program expanded and eventually moved to a larger location.

For several years, Sister Ann recruited volunteer physicians and medical residents to staff the clinic on Mondays. On Wednesdays, the medical director for the clinic saw patients. On Fridays, the clinic was staffed with both an adult nurse practitioner and a psychiatric mental health nurse practitioner. Many of the homeless have foot problems, so the clinic hosted foot clinics once a month providing foot care as well as shoes.

The clinic sees individuals between the ages of 18 and 70. Prior to the enactment of the Patient Protection and Affordable Care Act, none of the patients had insurance, so Sister Ann saw 17 to 27 patients on Friday mornings when there was a mental health provider as well as an adult health provider available. On Monday and Wednesday, 8 to 10 patients were seen.

Sister Ann works with a local pharmacy to make sure patients are able to afford any medications ordered. Currently, many patients are on Medicaid, but for the first 24 years, the registered nurse (RN) staff spent their time arranging for drug assistance programs (DAPs) to supply medications for patients who were seen on an ongoing basis. Medications not available from DAPs were purchased through grant monies received by Sister Ann John. These grant funds also pay for lab testing and x-rays as needed. The RNs schedule follow-up appointments with specialists in the area and, if needed, supply patients with a bus pass or a taxi cab ride.

The clinic continues to give socks to patients who come in to be seen by a provider. In addition, patients receive a snack and have the opportunity to look through donated clothing and donated toiletries to obtain supplies they need. The clinic gives away toothbrushes, toothpaste, combs, disposable shavers, and deodorant as well as small toiletries such as those received at hotels.

(continues)

BOX 14-2 Outstanding Nurse Leader: Sister Ann John *(continued)*

According to Sister Ann, some patients have been coming to the clinic for 3 to 5 years; others have been coming for as long as 10 years. Sister Ann occasionally sees patients who started coming to the clinic more than 25 years ago and who are still homeless or have become homeless again.

The biggest challenge that Sister Ann has seen with this population is a lack of follow-up. Patients may go several months without their medications because they do not return when they run out of medications. The homeless clinic provides tuberculin (TB) tests annually because TB is so common among the homeless population; however, some patients do not return to have the test read. As an incentive to encourage them to return, patients are given the opportunity to pick a prize from a cabinet that contains clothing items, toys that the homeless may give to their children, and other items donated to the clinic.

The clinic accepts donations. In addition, it sponsors the "Hopebox Derby," an annual soapbox car race in which several area organizations compete with one another, sponsoring a car in the race and aiming to win the Derby. Thousands of dollars have been donated through this fundraising event. Also, each year the clinic sponsors a Christmas party for the patients, providing them with new gloves, hats, scarves, sweatshirts, boot socks, thermal underwear, toiletries, food items, and other donated gifts.

In the Old Testament, one of the complaints God had against the people of Israel was lack of compassion for the poor and oppressed. A few examples of these scriptures can be found in Deuteronomy 5:7–8, Isaiah 58:6–10, Jeremiah 22:3–5, Ezekiel 16:49, and Amos 4:1–2. Christian nurses need to be mindful of the command to have compassion for the poor. We need to be aware of what is happening in our communities, and fight against laws such as those against feeding the homeless.

According to Schroeder (2016), politicians are less responsive to the needs of the poor due to lower voter turnout among this population. Moreover, to fund their expensive campaigns, politicians tend to cater those who can contribute to their reelection campaigns—which leads them to overlook the needs of the poor. The poor and homeless need nurses to serve as advocates on the local, state, and national levels to promote justice for their needs.

Trends and Concerns Related to Uninsured and Underinsured Populations

The Patient Protection and Affordable Care Act (also known as the Affordable Care Act)

encouraged states to expand their Medicaid programs to cover the poorest of the poor. In addition, marketplace insurance plans were developed so that lower-income individuals could purchase insurance. According to Amadeo (2018), depending on the amount of income individuals make in comparison to the federal poverty level, their premium under the Affordable Care Act ranges from 2% to 9.5% of their income for the silver plan. However, with the silver plan, patients are still responsible for paying 30% of the medical costs they accrue (Amadeo, 2018). Therefore, even though insurance for all was mandated by the Affordable Care Act, many individuals chose not to purchase insurance because it was too expensive (Goldman, Woolhandler, Himmelstein, Bor, & McCormick, 2018).

For those who are able to purchase insurance through their employer, there has been a push toward high-deductible healthcare plans (HDHPs) under which insured individuals and families pay the first $2000 to $5000 of their healthcare expenses. After that deductible is met, the insurance begins to pay a portion of the cost. Many individuals who have HDHPs avoid seeking medical care, as they will be responsible for 100% of the cost of the care with no insurance assisting them to pay the bill.

Currently, Medicare recipients face a similar coverage gap— referred to as the "donut hole"— once they have spent $3820 in out-of-pocket costs for medications until they reach $5100 in out-of-pocket costs (Medicare, n.d.). The increased cost of medications during this period can be a major burden for the elderly living on a fixed income. Under the Affordable Care Act, the donut hole will be eliminated by 2020.

▶ The Role of Nursing When Caring for Poor and Homeless Individuals

When caring for poor and/or homeless individuals, nurses need to seek to understand what life is like for these individuals. A complete assessment is needed, including physiological, psychological, sociocultural, spiritual, and developmental needs. It is important to assess whether these patients will have the resources they need to retain their health after they leave the nurse. Specifically, nurses need to determine whether patients have the financial resources to purchase the medications and treatment supplies that will be ordered. They also need to speak with patients about their home situation. Is it safe? Is it healthy? If concerns are identified, it is important to contact case management or social services as early in the process as possible. In addition, nurses may need to speak with the healthcare provider to see if lower-cost medications and treatments are an option so the patient is able to afford the medications and treatments ordered.

Wise and Dreussi-Smith (2018) discussed the differences between caring for middle class patients and impoverished patients. According to these authors, poor patients tend to see a healthcare provider only when there is a problem; however, if the healthcare provider develops a trusting relationship with poor persons, they are more likely to follow up and consider preventive care and health-promotion strategies. Health literacy may be low among this population, so it is essential to avoid medical terminology and to not expect patients to read and understand forms. According to Wise and Dreussi-Smith, lower-income patients tend to be storytellers: They are apt to take their time describing their symptoms and situations. It is important to take the time to listen, as they may feel devalued if they are not allowed to speak. Listening is needed to create a trusting relationship.

Nurses should maintain a resources list including agencies in the local community to which they can refer patients. This list may include local food pantries, soup kitchens, homeless shelters, battered women shelters, drug and alcohol rehabilitation facilities, community mental health clinics, and free and sliding-scale clinics and dental offices. In addition, nurses should have phone numbers for the local health department, WIC program, food stamps office, legal aid, early childhood services, transportation services, Council on Aging, Meals on Wheels, and whatever other services may be pertinent to the populations whom they serve.

Nurses also need to assess for spiritual concerns (**BOX 14-3**). Many spiritual assessment tools are available for nurses to use, including the FICA, HOPE, and SPIRIT instruments (Dameron, 2005). Such spiritual assessment tools use brief, easy-to-remember acronyms to help healthcare providers obtain appropriate, patient-centered information related to the spiritual state of those for whom they are caring (LaRocca-Pitts, 2012). FICA provides guidance for asking questions about patients' spirituality, the importance of their religious or spiritual beliefs, connections they have to a religious or spiritual community, and how their faith may affect the care they receive in the healthcare setting (LaRocca-Pitts, 2012). HOPE directs the healthcare provider to ask about patients' source of hope, whether they participate in an organized religion, how they put their spirituality into practice, and the effect their faith has on their feelings about health care and end-of-life concerns (Anandarajah & Hight, 2001).

BOX 14-3 Evidence-Based Practice Focus

Spirituality and Religion in the Homeless

Often, a stigma surrounds the homeless, which leads to the erroneous assumption that they are all drug addicts or alcoholics who are not interested in God. In 2016, Hurlbut and Ditmyer completed a qualitative research study that refuted these assumptions. These authors interviewed 14 women living in a homeless shelter and found that 71% of the women stated that their belief in God helped them to make better lifestyle choices—for example, avoiding smoking and the use of drugs and alcohol, exercising, eating right, and taking medications as prescribed. Many of the women (78%) identified with a formal religion and desired to attend religious services. They felt their spirituality brought them encouragement and hope, and increased their resilience in the face of the difficulties of homelessness. Hurlbut and Ditmyer stressed the need for nurses to complete a spiritual assessment and to provide spiritual care by providing quiet time for meditation and prayer, providing religious music and reading materials, providing the opportunity to attend religious services, and being open to talking about spirituality with the homeless. The negative effects of homelessness were mitigated by assessing the importance of spirituality in these homeless women and providing appropriate support.

Modified from Hurlbut, J., & Ditmyer, M. (2016). Defining the meaning of spirituality through a qualitative case study of sheltered homeless women. *Nursing for Women's Health, 20*(1), 52–62. https://doi.org/10.1016/j.nwh.2015.12.004

Nurses should have spiritual resources available to support and encourage spiritual health in the patients they serve. These resources may include a Bible, Christian literature, and Christian music as well as a phone number for local clergy or chaplains, among other resources. Eye contact and touch can be meaningful spiritual interventions for the homeless as well as for those who live in poverty. Often, those who are homeless feel invisible because people tend to avoid eye contact and touch.

▶ Ethical Principles: Adopting an Empathetic View of Poor and Homeless Individuals

As nurses, we seek to live up to the ANA's (2015) Code of Ethics. Provisions of the Code of Ethics require us to treat people with compassion, respect, and dignity, recognizing their worth and their uniqueness. In addition, the Code of Ethics requires us to advocate for our patients, protecting their rights and safety. We are accountable for our nursing practice, and need to take our responsibility seriously as we promote the health of our communities and provide optimal care to our patients (ANA, 2015).

One of the ethical principles we uphold is recognizing the autonomy of our patients. Each person/patient is created in the image of God and is worthy of dignity and respect. God gave each of us a free will, and we need to allow our patients to express their free will by allowing them autonomy in their decision making. As nurses, we may believe that we know what is best for our patients; however, we need to respect their autonomy even when they are poor and/or homeless.

We practice beneficence—doing what is good for our patients—as well as nonmaleficence—not doing anything that would harm them. However, are we doing enough? James 2:14–16 says:

What good is it, my brothers and sisters, if someone claims to have faith but has no deeds? Can such faith save them? Suppose a brother or a sister is without clothes and daily food. If one of you says to them, "Go in peace; keep warm and well-fed," but does nothing about their physical needs, what good is it? (New International Version [NIV])

Are we sending homeless individuals back to the streets without assuring they have information and resources they need to meet their needs—simply saying "keep warm and well-fed"?

In addition, to show beneficence and nonmaleficence, we should not simply focus on the physical condition of the patient and the medications, treatments, and diagnostic tests ordered by the physician. When Jesus approached people in need of healing, He considered their emotional, sociocultural, and spiritual concerns as well as their physical needs. Matthew 8:2–3 says:

A man with leprosy came and knelt before him and said, "Lord, if you are willing, you can make me clean." Jesus reached out his hand and touched the man. "I am willing," he said. "Be clean." Immediately, he was cured of leprosy.

In Jesus's day, lepers were outcasts. Lepers were not allowed to live with their families, but rather lived in caves. Their only contact was with other lepers. When they went to an area where there were people without leprosy, they were required to shout, "Unclean," so that people would know not to come near them. The practice had to be very psychologically distressing. Lepers were not allowed to go to the temple to worship because they were considered unclean. The man mentioned in Matthew 8 went to Jesus with a physical need, but he needed sociocultural healing, psychological healing, and spiritual healing as well.

Jesus provided healing for these needs by touching this man.

Touch is powerful for anyone who is hurting, but for those who have not been touched in years because of their disease, it is even more significant. We need to be willing to attend to our patients' physical needs, as well as their developmental, sociocultural, psychological, and spiritual needs. Facing the stigma of poverty and homelessness, many of those living in poverty or homelessness may not have been touched with care in a long time. How can we meet their emotional, social, and spiritual needs?

According to Thompson et al. (2008), "A review of the empirical literature on nurse–patient communication revealed that nurses tend to offer advice and provide information but pay little attention to the subjective experiences of their patients" (p. 15). Have you spent time talking with a homeless person or someone who is impoverished to discover what his or her life is like? How did that affect your perspective on this population? It is important for nurses to understand the patients for whom they care, particularly when the needs are as diverse as those seen in patients who live in poverty and in patients who are homeless. Complete care cannot be provided without in-depth understanding of these populations (**CASE STUDY 14-1**).

▶ Clinical Reasoning Exercises

1. Explore the National Alliance to End Homelessness website at https://endhomelessness.org/.
2. Discuss with another student the causes of poverty and homelessness.
3. What biases are common among healthcare providers with regard to the homeless and/or with regard to patients who are on Medicaid?

🔍 CASE STUDY 14-1

Read the following case study and answer the subsequent questions based on your understanding of the needs of impoverished and/or homeless individuals.

You work as a nurse on a medical–surgical unit. One of your patients today is Ms. Jones, a 42-year-old African American woman with diabetes, hypertension, hyperlipidemia, and cellulitis of her right lower leg. Her blood pressure is 168/104 mm Hg, her temperature is 99.6°F, her pulse is 78 beats/minute, her respiratory rate is 18 breaths/minute, and her pulse oximetry reading is 95%. She is 5 feet 4 inches tall and weighs 190 pounds, and body mass index (BMI) is 32.6. Her right leg is swollen, reddened, and warm and tender to the touch, with a centrally located abscess that is draining yellow exudate. Upon admission, Ms. Jones's labs were as follows: HbA$_{1c}$: 8.6; glucose: 260 mg/dL; cholesterol: 248 mg/dL; non-HDL (high-density lipoprotein): 150 mg/dL; LDL (low-density lipoprotein): 130 mg/dL; HDL: 40 mg/dL, WBC (white blood cells): 16.8 × 10^3/mcL. Her other lab results were unremarkable. Ms. Jones has no history of smoking or alcohol use.

Ms. Jones's routine medications include metformin 1000 mg BID, metoprolol 50 mg BID, atorvastatin calcium 40 mg QD, aspirin 81 mg Qhs, and ciprofloxacin 400 mg Q12h intravenously to treat her cellulitis. In addition to IV therapy, the interventions follow the HAMMMER acronym: hydration, analgesia, monitor temperature, mark the area to assess for spreading of the infection and complete a vascular assessment, measure the limb circumference, elevate the limb, and record assessment findings (Hanson, Langemo, Thompson, Anderson, & Swanson, 2015).

When completing her assessment, you learn Ms. Jones has been homeless for the last three months since she left her abusive husband. She has been living in a "tent city" in the back of a local park. The clothing she was wearing when she was admitted is tattered and soiled. She states that she has only two sets of clothing she was able to bring with her when she left her husband, and she has no money. She has been eating one meal per day at the soup kitchen, and is occasionally able to get food from the local food pantry. She has no means of transportation. Ms. Jones has not seen her primary care physician for two years due to a lack of insurance and money. She stated she has not had the money to buy prescriptions in more than a year.

Ms. Jones has no family in this area other than her husband. Her daughters are married, and they moved out west with their husbands and her grandchildren several years ago. In the past, she worked as a nursing assistant at a local nursing home, but she injured her back on the job and has not been able to work for the last four years. Ms. Jones used to attend a Missionary Baptist church; however, her husband prohibited her from attending over the last three years. She spends most of her day alone and does not see much hope for the future.

Questions

1. Spirituality is a source of strength for many women who are homeless. How will you approach Ms. Jones's spiritual assessment? Which spiritual interventions might be helpful for Ms. Jones in order to renew her sense of hope?
2. Which referrals might you make to ensure Ms. Jones is able to obtain her medications and treatment supplies after discharge?
3. As you look ahead to discharge, which resources are available in your community to assist Ms. Jones with being able to live in a clean environment that will support her?
4. Where can Ms. Jones go to receive follow-up care?

▶ Personal Reflection Exercises

1. Have you ever considered yourself or your family to be poor?
2. Do you believe people would not be poor if they took responsibility for themselves and got a job? Why do you feel some individuals have difficulty breaking out of the cycle of poverty?
3. Have you ever been approached by a homeless individual asking for money? How did you respond? Why did you respond in this way?
4. Have you ever volunteered at a soup kitchen, food pantry, or homeless shelter? What were your thoughts about that experience? Would you consider volunteering on a regular basis?
5. What is the role of the nurse in response to the needs of impoverished individuals and homeless individuals?

References

Academy of Oncology Nurse and Patient Navigators. (2017). Cancer health disparities among low-income populations. *Journal of Oncology Navigation & Survivorship, 8*(1), 38–39.

Amadeo, K. (2018, November 1). How much will Obamacare cost me? Retrieved from https://www.thebalance.com/how-much-will-obamacare-cost-me-3306054

American Nurses Association (ANA). (2015). *Code of ethics for nurses with interpretive statements*. Silver Spring, MD: Author.

Anandarajah, G., & Hight, E. (2001). Spirituality and medical practice: Using the HOPE questions as a practical tool for spiritual assessment. *American Family Physician, 63*(1), 81–89. Retrieved from http://www.aafp.org/afp/2001/0101/p81.html

Anthony, E. R., Vincent, A., & Shin, Y. (2018). Parenting and child experiences in shelter: A qualitative study exploring the effect of homelessness on the parent–child relationship. *Child & Family Social Work, 23*(1), 8–15. doi:10.1111/cfs.12376

Barclay, E. (2014, October 22). More cities are making it illegal to hand out food to the homeless. Retrieved from http://www.npr.org/blogs/thesalt/2014/10/22/357846415/more-cities-are-making-it-illegal-to-hand-out-food-to-the-homeless

Bratanova, B., Loughnan, S., Klein, O., Claassen, A., & Wood, R. (2016). Poverty, inequality, and increased consumption of high calorie food: Experimental evidence for a causal link. *Appetite, 100,* 162–171. doi:10.1016/j.appet.2016.01.028

Centers for Disease Control and Prevention. (2018, July 2). TB in the homeless population. Retrieved from https://www.cdc.gov/tb/topic/populations/homelessness/default.htm

Chamberlain, L. J., Hanson, E. R., Klass, P., Schickedanz, A., Nakhasi, A., Barnes, M. M.,... Klein, M. (2016). Childhood poverty and its effect on health and well-being: Enhancing training for learners across the medical education continuum. *Academic Pediatrics,* S155–S162. doi:10.1016/j.acap.2015.12.012

Chaudry, A., & Wimer, C. (2016). Poverty is not just an indicator: The relationship between income, poverty, and child well-being. *Academic Pediatrics, 16*(3), S23–S29. doi:10.1016/j.acap.2015.12.010

Cole, S. (2016, November 29). No giving Tuesday here: Is your city trying to make feeding the homeless illegal? Retrieved from https://thefreshtoast.com/culture/are-you-living-in-one-of-the-cities-thats-trying-to-make-feeding-the-homeless-illegal/

Cornelius, T., Jones, M., Merly, C., Welles, B., Kalichman, M. O., & Kalichman, S. C. (2017). Impact of food, housing, and transportation insecurity on ART adherence: A hierarchical resources approach. *AIDS Care, 29*(4), 449–457. doi:10.1080/09540121.2016.1258451

Dameron, C. M. (2005). Spiritual assessment made easy... with acronyms! *Journal of Christian Nursing, 22*(1), 14–16. doi:10.1097/01.CNJ.0000262323.59843.2e

Dan, C. (2017, July 18). Viral hepatitis in the news: Fighting hepatitis C by providing treatment at homeless shelters. Retrieved from https://www.hhs.gov/hepatitis/blog/2017/07/18/fighting-hepatitis-c-by-providing-treatment-at-homeless-shelters.html

Department of Health and Human Services (DHHS). (2019). Poverty guidelines. Retrieved from https://aspe.hhs.gov/poverty-guidelines

Dunton, L., Albanese, T., D'Alanno, T., Buron, L., Silverbush, M., & Barker, K. (2014). Point-in-time count methodology guide. Retrieved from https://www.hudexchange.info/resources/documents/PIT-Count-Methodology-Guide.pdf

Edwards, A. (2015, May 2). Crisis, chronic, and churning: An analysis of varying poverty experiences [U.S. Census Bureau SEHSD Working Paper Number 2015-6]. Retrieved from https://www.census.gov/content

/dam/Census/library/working-papers/2015/demo/SEHSD-WP2015-06.pdf

Escobar, J. (2005). Overcoming cultural barriers in health-care. In J. M. Burger (Ed.), *Perspectives on poverty and health care*. Indianapolis, IN: Precedent Press.

Fontenot, K., Semega, J., & Kollar, M. (2018). Income and poverty in the United States: 2017. Retrieved from https://www.census.gov/library/publications/2018/demo/p60-263.html

Goldman, A. L., Woolhandler, S., Himmelstein, D. U., Bor, D. H., & McCormick, D. (2018). Out-of-pocket spending and premium contributions after implementation of the Affordable Care Act. *JAMA Internal Medicine, 178*(3), 347–355. doi:10.1001/jamainternmed.2017.8060

Hanson, D., Langemo, D., Thompson, P., Anderson, J., & Swanson, K. (2015). Providing evidence-based care for patients with lower-extremity cellulitis. *Wound Care Advisor, 4*(3), 24–29.

Housing and Urban Development (HUD). (2017). HUD 2017 continuum of care homeless assistance programs homeless populations and subpopulations. Retrieved from https://www.hudexchange.info/resource/report management/published/CoC_PopSub_NatlTerrDC _2017.pdf

Housing and Urban Development (HUD). (2018). The 2018 Annual Homeless Assessment Report (AHAR) to Congress: Part 1: Point-in-time estimates of homelessness. Retrieved from https://www.hudexchange .info/resources/documents/2018-AHAR-Part-1.pdf

Inglis, G. (2016, October 19). The stigma of poverty. Poverty Alliance. Retrieved from https://povertyalliance .wordpress.com/2016/10/19/the-stigma-of-poverty/

Kim, D. H., Harty, J., Takahashi, L., & Voisin, D. R. (2018). The protective effects of religious beliefs on behavioral health factors among low income African American adolescents in Chicago. *Journal of Child & Family Studies, 27*(2), 355–364. doi:10.1007/s10826-017-0891-5

Kim, M. (2017, July 31). Mental illness and homelessness: Facts and figures. Retrieved from https://www.hcs.harvard.edu/~hcht/blog/homelessness-and-mental-health-facts

LaRocca-Pitts, M. (2012). FACT, a chaplain's tool for assessing spiritual needs in an acute care setting. *Chaplaincy Today, 28*(1).

Leadley, S., & Hocking, C. (2017). An occupational perspective of childhood poverty. *New Zealand Journal of Occupational Therapy, 64*(1), 23–31.

Lee, D., & Jackson, M. (2017). The simultaneous effects of socioeconomic disadvantage and child health on children's cognitive development. *Demography, 54*(5), 1845–1871. doi:10.1007/s13524-017-0605-z

Levitz, N. R., Haji-Jama, S., Munro, T., Gorey, K. M., Luginaah, I. N., Bartfay, E.,... Holowaty, E. J. (2015). Multiplicative disadvantage of being an unmarried and inadequately insured woman living in poverty with colon cancer: Historical cohort exploration in California. *BMC Women's Health, 15*(1), 166. doi:10.1186/s12905-015-0166-5

Ljungqvist, I., Topor, A., Forssell, H., Svensson, I., & Davidson, L. (2016). Mental illness: A study of the relationship between poverty and psychological problems. *Community Mental Health Journal, 52*(7), 842–850. doi:10.1007/s10597-015-9950-9

Medicare. (n.d.). The Part D donut hole: Medicare Part D costs. Retrieved from https://www.medicare interactive.org/get-answers/medicare-prescription-drug -coverage-part-d/medicare-part-d-costs/the-part-d -donut-hole

Meraviglia, M., Stuifbergen, A., Morgan, S., & Parsons, D. (2015). Low-income cancer survivors' use of health-promoting behaviors. *Medsurg Nursing, 24*(2), 101–106.

National Alliance to End Homelessness. (n.d.a). Children and families. Retrieved from https://endhomeless ness.org/homelessness-in-america/who-experiences -homelessness/children-and-families/

National Alliance to End Homelessness. (n.d.b). Chronically homeless. Retrieved from https://endhomelessness.org /homelessness-in-america/who-experiences-homeless ness/chronically-homeless/

National Alliance to End Homelessness. (n.d.c). FAQs. Retrieved from https://endhomelessness.org /homelessness-in-america/homelessness-statistics /faqs/

Nott, B., & Vuchinich, S. (2016). Homeless adolescents' perceptions of positive development: A comparative study. *Child & Youth Care Forum, 45*(6), 865–886. doi:10.1007/s10566-016-9361-2

Polson, E. C., Gillespie, R., & Myers, D. R. (2018). Hope and resilience among vulnerable, community-dwelling older persons. *Social Work & Christianity, 45*(1), 60–81.

Price, J. H., Khubchandani, J., & Webb, F. J. (2018). Poverty and health disparities: What can public health professionals do? *Health Promotion Practice, 19*(2), 170–174. doi:10.1177/1524839918755143

Reamer, F. G. (2015). Eye on ethics: The challenge of distributive ethics. Retrieved from https://www.social-worktoday.com/news/eoe_011515.shtml

Sackett, C. (2016, Summer). Neighborhoods and violent crime. Retrieved from https://www.huduser.gov/por-tal/periodicals/em/summer16/highlight2.html

Schroeder, S. A. (2016). American health improvement depends upon addressing class disparities. *Preventive Medicine, 92*, 6–15. doi:10.1016/j.ypmed.2016.02.024

Schubert, K. B., & Marks, J. S. (2016). The cost of poverty and the value of hope. *Academic Pediatrics*, S21–S22. doi:10.1016/j.acap.2016.02.012

Singer, S., Bartels, M., Briest, S., Einenkel, J., Niederwieser, D., Papsdorf, K.,... Krauß, O. (2017). Socio-economic disparities in long-term cancer survival-10 year follow-up with individual patient data. *Supportive Care in Cancer, 25*(5), 1391–1399. doi:10.1007/s00520-016-3528-0

Thompson, N. C., Hunter, E. E., Murray, L., Ninci, L., Rolfs, E. M., & Pallikkathayil, L. (2008). The experience of living with chronic mental illness: A photovoice study. *Perspectives in Psychiatric Care, 44*(1), 14–24. doi:10.1111/j.1744-6163.2008.00143.x

Tran, T. D., Luchters, S., & Fisher, J. (2017). Early childhood development: Impact of national human development, family poverty, parenting practices and access to early childhood education. *Child: Care, Health & Development, 43*(3), 415–426. doi:10.1111/cch.12395

U. S. Legal. (n.d.). Working poor law and legal definition. Retrieved from https://definitions.uslegal.com/w/working-poor/

Weber, C., & Mulvihill, G. (2017, December 6). America's homeless population rises for the first time in years. Retrieved from https://www.usnews.com/news/us/articles/2017-12-06/us-homeless-count-rises-pushed-by-crisis-on-the-west-coast

Wise, B., & Dreussi-Smith, T. (2018). The primary care provider and the patient living in poverty. *Journal of the American Association of Nurse Practitioners, 30*(4), 201–207. doi:10.1097/JXX.0000000000000036.

Recommended Readings

Adamson, E., & Dewar, B. (2015). Compassionate care: Student nurses' learning through reflection and the use of story. *Nurse Education in Practice, 15*(3), 155–161. doi:10.1016/j.nepr.2014.08.002

Alicea-Planas, J. (2016). Listening to the narratives of our patients as part of holistic nursing care. *Journal of Holistic Nursing, 34*(2), 162–166. doi:10.1177/0898010115591396

Balint, K. A., & George, N. M. (2015). Faith community nursing scope of practice: Extending access to healthcare. *Journal of Christian Nursing, 32*(1), 34–40. doi:10.1097/CNJ.0000000000000119

Christopher, A. S., Himmelstein, D. U., Woolhandler, S., & McCormick, D. (2018). The effects of household medical expenditures on income inequality in the United States. *American Journal of Public Health, 108*(3), 351–354. doi:10.2105/AJPH.2017.304213

Community nursing improving health care for homeless people. (2014). *Journal of Community Nursing, 28*(5), 10.

Donohoe, M., Hoffman, J., & McKeon, L. (2015). Simulation of living in poverty: An innovative program designed to transform nursing practice for vulnerable populations. *Tennessee Nurse, 78*(1), 7.

Gerber, L. (2014). Caring for the homeless: An underserved population. *Florida Nurse, 62*(2), 19.

Kagan, S. H. (2016). Embracing our own vulnerability for more effective and compassionate care. *Geriatric Nursing, 37*(5), 401–403. doi:10.1016/j.gerinurse.2016.08.010

Morton, J. (2017). Down but definitely not out. *Nursing Standard, 31*(29), 35.

National Academies of Sciences, Engineering, and Medicine. (2018, October 8). Health literacy: A prescription to end confusion [Videofile]. Retrieved from http://www.nationalacademies.org/hmd/Reports/2004/Health-Literacy-A-Prescription-to-End-Confusion/Video-4.aspx

National Alliance to End Homelessness. (n.d.). Health. Retrieved from https://endhomelessness.org/homelessness-in-america/what-causes-homelessness/health

National Alliance to End Homelessness. (n.d.) Housing. Retrieved from https://endhomelessness.org/homelessness-in-america/what-causes-homelessness/housing/

National Alliance to End Homelessness. (n.d.). Income. Retrieved from https://endhomelessness.org/homelessness-in-america/what-causes-homelessness/income inequality/

Paavola, A. (2018, February 14). Nurse at Jackson Health System establishes clothing closet for discharged homeless patients. Retrieved from https://www.beckershospitalreview.com/patient-engagement/nurse-at-jackson-health-system-establishes-clothing-closet-for-discharged-homeless-patients.html

Wittenauer, J., Ludwick, R., Baughman, K., & Fishbein, R. (2015). Surveying the hidden attitudes of hospital nurses' towards poverty. *Journal of Clinical Nursing, 24*(15/16), 2184–2191. doi:10.1111/jocn.12794

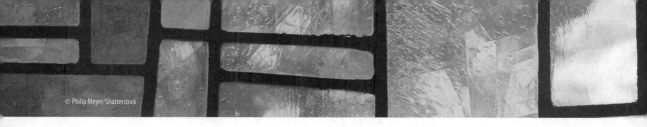
© Philip Meyer/Shutterstock

CHAPTER 15

Integration of a Biblical Worldview and Substance Abuse

Steven Hobus, BA, MEd, and **John Schreiber**, MA, MS, RN

LEARNING OBJECTIVES

At the end of this chapter, the reader will be able to:

1. Explain the importance of nursing assessment of the substance abuse issue.
2. Differentiate between the different diagnoses of substance abuse disorder (SAD).
3. Analyze the plan and the testing methods to assist individuals with SAD.
4. Prioritize the treatment plan to help individuals overcome SAD.
5. Evaluate the success of overcoming SAD.
6. Create an individualized plan to maintain competency in your knowledge and attitudes about SAD.

KEY TERMS

Cannabidiol (CBD)
Cannabinoids
Cannabis

Delta-9-tetrahydrocannabinol (THC)
Marijuana

Medical marijuana programs (MMPs)
Substance abuse disorders (SAD)

"On March 29, 2017, President Donald J. Trump signed an Executive Order establishing the President's Commission on Combating Drug Addiction and the Opioid Crisis" (Christie et al., 2017, para. 1). In the United States, 115 deaths occur each day from opioid overdose, whether from prescription drugs or heroin. Substance abuse is a life-threatening national crisis that must be dealt with on both national and local bases. The national financial burden is $78.5 billion per year for opioid addiction alone (National Institute on Drug Abuse [NIDA], 2017; Volkow, Baler, Compton, & Weiss, 2014). **Substance abuse disorders (SADs)**—whether they involve illegal drug use, **marijuana** abuse, or alcohol abuse—cost Americans more than $820 billion each year. This figure, large as it is, does not even include health care, lost revenue, or criminal costs due to substance abuse (Buddy T, 2018).

The illicit drug crisis in the United States has a major impact on its citizens, with approximately 52,000 fatalities from drug overdoses occurring each year, and this phenomenon is emerging as one of the leading nonmedical causes of death in the United States (Mack, Jones, & Ballesteros, 2017). The United States has responded in a variety of ways, such as with increased enforcement and incarceration (Lassiter, 2015). Substance use disorders among college and high school students, along with subsequent poor academic achievement and incarceration, are major issues facing U.S. schools (Hussong, Ennett, Cox, & Haroon, 2017). Schools suffer as students drop out, underperform, and cause discipline problems related to drug abuse (Reboussin, Ialongo, & Green, 2015).

Substance abuse is a major problem in the United States, and sometimes the people who have this addiction are seen as lacking moral principles or willpower. But looking at these people from our Biblical worldview tells us that they still are made in the image of God. Genesis 1:26 (New International Version [NIV]) reads, "Let us (the triune God) make man in our image, after our likeness." Even people with SADs are made in the image of God and, therefore, deserve dignity and respect. This essential Biblical truth must be considered whenever we discuss SADs. The path to SAD "begins with the act of taking drugs. Over time, a person's ability to choose not to take drugs is compromised.

Protracted drug use affects the brain which in turn affects behavior. Addiction, therefore, is characterized by compulsive drug craving, seeking, and use that persists even in the face of negative consequences" (NIDA, 2016, para. 2). Sometimes it is difficult to remember that someone who is addicted was made in the image of God, due to his or her behaviors, but it is essential to remember this truth to help draw the person to God and to facilitate recovery.

This chapter covers the integration of the Biblical worldview concerning all persons being made in the image of God with relation to substance abuse, looking through the lens of the nursing process. Using the nursing process as our guide, this chapter reviews the following steps:

- Step 1: Assessment of the substance abuse issue
- Step 2: Diagnosis of the SAD problem
- Step 3: Plan to resolve SAD
- Step 4: Implementation of the plan to help overcome SAD
- Step 5: How to evaluate success in overcoming SAD

▶ Step 1: Assessment of the Substance Abuse Issue

According to the Monitoring the Future (MTF) survey, substance use affects a significant number of adults, who may in turn have comorbid mental illnesses, health problems, and an increased risk of death from overdose or car crashes (Volkow et al., 2014). As of 2017, the attitudes of society toward marijuana use appeared to have shifted, with 33 U.S. states passing laws allowing use of medical marijuana and 9 states passing laws permitting recreational marijuana use (Sarvet et al., 2018). Oregon, in fact, has passed a law decriminalizing possession of small amounts of methamphetamine, cocaine, and heroin in an attempt to guide users to treatment rather than incarceration. Sadly, many of the individuals who use such drugs are hooked for life (Lewis, 2017).

The passage of these medical and recreational marijuana bills was intended primarily to increase states' revenues, but all states are now dealing with increased costs of health and addiction issues of their citizens who choose to use drugs (Hasin et al., 2015). Schools have responded to the illicit drug crisis by developing drug intervention programs and increased use of drug testing to better educate students about the dangers of drug use, as well as to dissuade them from even starting to use drugs (DuPont, Merlo, Arria, & Shea, 2013). Many of these efforts have fallen short of their goal of decreasing drug use and initiation (Flynn, Falco, & Hocini, 2015).

Miech, Johnston, O'Malley, Bachman, et al. (2015) posited that decriminalization of marijuana could be considered a risk factor for future marijuana use and acceptance of usage. Likewise, Oregon's decriminalization of possession of small amounts of highly addictive methamphetamine, cocaine, and heroin is grave cause for concern. Concurring with this sentiment, D'Amico, Miles, and Tucker (2015) noted that with greater medical marijuana advertising, exposure to these messages led to high probability to use and strong intention to use one year after seeing the ads. When marijuana dispensaries pop up on almost every other street corner, it legitimizes the use of this drug as well as other drugs. In an adolescent's mind, if marijuana is accepted, then why not methamphetamine, cocaine, and heroin?

With the passage of its medical marijuana bill (S.B. 1449, California State Legislature, 2010), California decriminalized the use and possession of small amounts of marijuana, making such behaviors seem similar to an infraction warranting a parking fine. Compared to youths from other states, youths in California are significantly more likely to have tried marijuana in the last 30 days and have a much greater likelihood of using marijuana within

a year. California high school seniors demonstrate a statistically significant decrease in perceived harm from marijuana use and have lower levels of personal disapproval of regular marijuana use (Miech, Johnston, O'Malley, Bachman, et al., 2015). One may worry that "as California goes, so goes the nation."

Marijuana is not a safe recreational drug. The primary psychoactive (mind-altering substance) in marijuana is **delta-9-tetrahydrocannabinol (THC)**, but the plant actually contains more than 500 compounds. Research shows THC causes cognitive effects that induce behavioral reactions (Compton, 2017).

Colorado can be viewed as a test case in legalizing marijuana. For every dollar gained in tax revenue from legal marijuana sales, Coloradans spend approximately $4.50 to mitigate the effects of legalizing this drug. Obviously, the cost of use outweighs any superficial monetary gain.

The full scope of the costs of marijuana use also needs to be addressed as compared to any insignificant gain in revenues (**TABLE 15-1**). There are costs related to increased use of the healthcare system, costs from high school drop-outs, and costs from the low economic output of high users of marijuana. Research also shows a connection between marijuana use and the use of alcohol and other substances of abuse (Centennial Institute, 2018). Moreover, calls to poison control centers related to marijuana use have increased dramatically since legalization of medical marijuana and recreational marijuana. An estimated 15 people are severely burned as a result of marijuana use each year in Colorado.

People who use marijuana more frequently tend to be less physically active, and a sedentary or inactive lifestyle is associated with increased medical costs. Adult marijuana users generally have lower educational attainment than non-users. Research also suggests that long-term marijuana use may lead to reduced cognitive ability, particularly in people who begin using it before they turn age 18. Yearly out-of-pocket cost estimates

TABLE 15-1 Annual Costs Summary of Marijuana Use in Colorado		
Amount	**General Area**	**Notes**
Costs		
($381,915,043)	Health	Hospitalizations
($31,448,906)	Health	Treatment for cannabis use disorder
($593,924)	Health	Burn treatments
($697,036)	Health	Low-birth-weight babies
($54,833,218)	Health	Physical inactivity
($3,782,625)	Productivity	Cost to businesses for policy development
($3,401,300)	Productivity	Cost to employers for rehabilitation
($481,600)	Productivity	Cost to employees for rehabilitation
($423,362,337)	Productivity	K–12 drop-outs
($7,194,600)	Crime	Arrests
($18,565,226)	Crime	DUI court costs
($1,170,126)	Crime	Juvenile court filings
($3,484,282)	Crime	Adult court filings
($3,111,114)	Crime	Denver-only marijuana-related crime
($87,014,326)	Crime	Probationers going back for THC violation
($5,362,620)	Traffic	Fatal car accidents
($18,565,226)	Traffic	DUIs
($83,732,717)	Traffic	Car accidents from impaired drivers
($1,837,500)	Housing	Evictions due to marijuana use, cost to landlords
($130,500)	Tourism	Arrests crossing the border to Colorado
Total: ($1,130,684,226)		

Benefits		
$247,368,473	Tax Revenue	2017 only
$127,452,000	Housing	Increased value of homes in areas with legalized marijuana
Amount Spent on Marijuana		
$1,444,524,486		Collective income spent on marijuana
Lives Lost		
-139	Traffic	Fatal accidents caused by a driver using THC
-180	Health	Suicides where the victim had THC in his or her system

Reproduced from Centennial Institute (CI). (2018, November 15). Economic and social costs of legalized marijuana. Used with permission from Colorado Christian University.

for marijuana users are estimated at $2200 for heavy users, $1250 for moderate users, and $650 for light users.

Sixty-nine percent of marijuana users say they have driven under the influence of marijuana at least once, and 27% admit to driving under the influence on a daily basis. The estimated costs of driving under the influence (DUI) infractions for people who tested positive for marijuana in 2016 alone approached $25 million (Centennial Institute, 2018).

Many senior high students from the class of 2016 reported that they approved of drug use, with only 43.1% stating that they disapproved of this behavior (Miech, Johnston, O'Malley, Bachman, et al., 2015). Most indicated that they had tried marijuana once or twice. Surprisingly, drug disapproval among all grade levels decreased for most drugs, but an increase was noted in disapproval of cigarette smoking (1.3%). In addition, 91% of seniors disapproved of alcohol consumption of five or more drinks two times a weekend. The disapproval for trying marijuana once or twice was at its highest in 1992 (69.9%). Miech, Johnston, O'Malley, Bachman, et al. (2015) also noted that adolescent use of vaping (utilizing nicotine or marijuana oils) is a direct bridge

to teen cigarette use, and a growing concern among educators and health professionals.

Johnston et al. (2018) found that the perceived harmfulness of drug use for the 2016 senior high school classes increased slightly, with marijuana, Ecstasy, cocaine, heroin, drinking alcohol, and using electronic cigarettes (e-cigarettes) showing small increases in perceived harm. Comparing the class of 2016 to the class of 2015, perceived harm was lower for the use of LSD, bath salts, amphetamines, and barbiturates. Alarmingly, a 2.9% decrease in perceived harm was noted for amphetamine use. A disconcerting statistic was that an increasing number of high school seniors believed that marijuana and cocaine use was not harmful until regular use of the drug was demonstrated (Miech, Johnston, O'Malley, Bachman, & Schulenberg, 2016). This follows a pattern identified by Kilmer et al. (2006), who found that 98% of the college students they surveyed incorrectly believed that most students in general use marijuana at least once a year. Agreeing with this finding, Salloum, Krauss, Agrawal, Bierut, and Grucza (2018) found that the reciprocal nature of perceived risk and cannabis use demonstrate a strong association with drug use and lower subsequent perceived harm. This merits continuing monitoring for its actual cause.

Other troubling aspects of the general population's drug-related beliefs include the decreased perception of harm from occasional use of some drugs such as synthetic cathinones (bath salts), crack, and Vicodin. Methamphetamine, like cocaine, can induce lifetime addiction after only one use. It has been estimated that 2.1 million individuals in the United States suffered from prescription opioid abuse for pain in 2012, and an estimated 500,000 individuals were addicted to heroin (Volkow et al., 2014). With an increasing number of students in the 8th, 10th, and 12th grades believing that many drugs are not harmful, and the perceived lessening of disapproval of drug use, much more needs to be done to prevent illicit drug use (**FIGURE 15-1**).

In the analysis of research on marijuana use by employees and employers, most investigations have focused on the impacts on worker productivity and businesses' risk. Due to the long-lasting properties of marijuana compounds (such as THC), marijuana can remain in a user's system for as long as 30 days after use (Centennial Institute, 2018). General adverse effects of THC include increased heart rate, increased appetite, sleepiness, dizziness, decreased blood pressure, dry mouth/dry eyes, decreased urination, hallucination, paranoia, anxiety, impaired attention, memory, and psychomotor performance disturbance (Russell et al., 2018).

Federal limits on **cannabis** research prevent an adequate description of the adverse effects of products containing only **cannabidiol (CBD)**. Because no large-scale studies on the adverse effects of CBD have been completed, any description of these effects in a specific population cannot be generalized. A moderate- to high-quality study involving adults with schizophrenia and CBD use reported sedative effects. In a separate study of adolescents with epilepsy using CBD, "diarrhea, vomiting, fatigue, pyrexia, somnolence, and abnormal results on liver-function tests" were reported (Russell et al., 2018).

The adverse effects of cannabis reported by some participants across the various studies include fatigue, nausea, asthenia, vertigo, and suicidal ideation. The risk of suicide and cannabis use is a contentious area of study. Current findings are contradictory, and more research is needed to confirm any association between cannabis use and suicide risk while

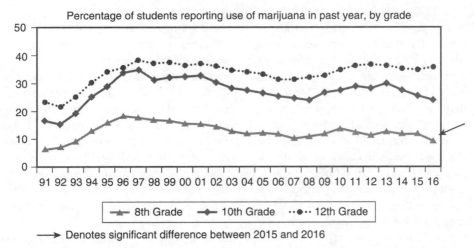

FIGURE 15-1 Trends in marijuana use and annual prevalence of marijuana use: 8th, 10th, and 12th graders.

University of Michigan, Monitoring the Future Survey 2016.

controlling for numerous confounding variables. Individuals with a greater risk of psychological disturbances and suicidal ideation should take precautions when utilizing cannabis as therapeutic (Russell et al., 2018).

▶ Step 2: Diagnosis of the SAD Problem

Drug use among students is an alarming problem across the United States, with almost one-third of graduating high school seniors reporting that they have used marijuana or other illicit drugs (Miech, Johnston, O'Malley, Bachman, et al., 2015). According to Wong, Zhou, Goebert, and Hishinuma (2013), there is a strong correlation between drug use during adolescence and later mental illness issues. Drug use in adolescence is a critical factor influencing subsequent drug use and the health and mental illness that may follow (Hall et al., 2016).

Individuals who are against decriminalization of marijuana point to these facts as delivering a message to youth that marijuana use is not harmful, which in turn increases youth acceptance and usage (Svrakic et al., 2011). Increased negative health outcomes such as respiratory inflammation and bronchitis (Hancox, Shin, Gray, Poulton, & Sears, 2015), increased probability of using "harder" drugs (Lynskey et al., 2003), and loss of IQ points (Meier et al., 2012) are all important factors to consider in allowing marijuana to become decriminalized and legal. Thus, the process of decriminalization has become known as a "signaling hypothesis"—that is, the notion that as drugs become decriminalized, more individuals will begin using drugs (DuPont & Voth, 1995). The prevailing mindset may be that if use of drugs is legal, they must be harmless. Also, as adolescents see adults using drugs, and as drugs become more readily available, that pattern makes all drugs appear more acceptable and normal.

All too often, individuals who are in favor of legalization indicate that decriminalization is not a risk factor and suggest that rates of marijuana use and acceptance will remain unchanged even in those states that have legalized marijuana use—which is a misconception (Cerda et al., 2018). Advocates of marijuana decriminalization focus on the high cost of arresting and prosecuting individuals who consume marijuana for their own use, stating that these costs are too high a penalty to pay, and that such arrests and prosecutions waste time that could be spent prosecuting other, more serious crime. In 2016, arrests for marijuana possession outnumbered all other arrests related to drugs, with more than 574,000 arrests being made (Federal Bureau of Investigation, 2016).

In the state of Colorado, which passed legislation that allows for recreational use of marijuana, a host of far-reaching complications have already been observed, such as decreased perception of risks about the use of marijuana in all age groups, and the incidence of daily use has increased drastically (Chilukuri, 2017). Colorado continues to have the top rate of marijuana use in the United States (NIDA, 2016), but also has experienced a 145% increase in the number of fatal crashes in which the driver tested positive for marijuana (Salomonsen-Sautel, Min, Sakai, Thurstone, & Hopfer, 2014). Moreover, in that state, chronic use of smoked marijuana, whether in cigarettes, bongs, or vaping, has been associated with increased risks of cancer, lung damage, bacterial pneumonia, and poor pregnancy outcomes (Wilkinson & D'Souza, 2014).

A recent issue that has arisen with regard to marijuana abuse is the development of mental disorders. Specifically, regular cannabis use is linked with chronic mental health risks (Degenhardt et al., 2013). For example, daily marijuana use among adolescents has been associated with higher incidence of anxiety disorder by the age of 29 than among peers who did not use marijuana. Because the marijuana available today is more potent than it was in the 1960s and 1970s, even first-time adolescent users of marijuana can become psychotic. In addition, Epstein et al. (2015) reported that users who begin use prior to age 14 tend to acquire more antisocial peers, have greater alcohol use, and have poorer academic achievement.

Besides marijuana, use of several other drugs has increased in recent years, according to the Monitoring the Future survey. Notably, use of alcohol, cigarettes, heroin, cocaine, methamphetamine, inhalants, and sedatives as reported by 12th-grade students has grown (Miech, Johnston, O'Malley, Bachman, et al., 2015). Interestingly, 8th- and 10th-grade students have demonstrated a five-year decline in use of these drugs, including a decline in marijuana use. According to Johnston, O'Malley, Miech, Bachman, and Schulenberg's (2016) summary of the Monitoring the Future survey results, high school seniors report that marijuana is readily available, with more than 81% stating that marijuana is very easy or easy to obtain—a 1.5% increase from the previous year's data. Similarly, Schuermeyer et al. (2014) suggest that with the legalization of marijuana in several states, perceived availability has increased.

In comparison to marijuana, cocaine and steroids have demonstrated a greater than 2% decrease in perceived availability compared to the previous year's survey findings (4.8% and 2.3%, respectively), and amphetamines have seen a 0.7% decrease in perceived availability (NIDA, 2017). Ten drugs were perceived to be easier to obtain in 2016, while only six drugs were perceived to be more difficult to get. While some drugs may be more difficult to obtain today, it is interesting to note that among 12th-graders, disapproval of drug use has decreased. Palamar (2014) contends that using an illicit drug over time may reduce an individual's disapproval of use of another hard drug. The disapproval toward drug use has in the past been a protective factor against drug use, but as the perceived attitude changes toward one of more tolerance, this factor's effectiveness will be mitigated (Palamar, 2014).

The impacts of marijuana on health have been the most widely studied, especially as the use of marijuana for medical therapies has increased. Although marijuana includes more than 400 known chemical compounds, analyses have focused on the two most prevalent chemical compounds known for their medical and psychoactive impacts: CBD and THC (Centennial Institute, 2018).

The impacts of unintentional marijuana use have also been studied, including ingestion of edible marijuana by children, overdosing on marijuana (especially through edibles, as overconsumption can easily lead to overdoses), and accidents related to marijuana use. Further assessments include the costs of addiction and treatment for marijuana use, the impact of hospitalizations and poisonings, and the impact of marijuana on specific populations, such as pregnant women and adolescents (Centennial Institute, 2018).

▶ Step 3: Plan to Resolve SAD

Nurses can advocate for persons and patients with SADs at the local, state, and national levels. Plans that could be put into effect through new legislation, and for which nurses could get involved in policy making, include the following:

- A national prescription drug monitoring programs for all opioids (Barry, 2018)
- Continuing Education (CE) requirement for pain management for prescribers (Keller et al., 2012)
- Grants for public education to include drug addiction teaching in schools (Miech, Johnston, O'Malley, Keyes, et al., 2015)
- A national policy for first responders to carry Narcan (naloxone) (Barry, 2018)

- National addictions treatment programs
- Research on developing non-opioid pain relievers and long-term effects of legalization of marijuana (O'Donnell, 2018)
- National addiction treatment in correctional facilities, with early parole if individuals successfully complete the program (Barry, 2018)

The drug and opioid crisis that is occurring in the United States has had an alarming impact on citizens, resulting in numerous drug overdoses (Mack et al., 2017). Many states have resorted to supplying the overdose remedy Narcan to police, first responders, and drug users' families in an effort to counteract the growing number of fatalities associated with opioid overdose (Schwartz et al., 2013). Unfortunately, the increased cost of health care and mental illness issues resulting from the increased drug use have affected the entire country (Hasin et al., 2015). U.S. schools now find themselves in the unenviable position of teaching students about the dangers of drug use while having to contend with the changing attitudes in society toward drug use (Das, Salam, Arshad, Finkelstein, & Bhutta, 2016).

The Joint Commission (2017) has developed New and Revised Pain Assessment and Management Standards that accredited hospitals must comply with to maintain their accreditation status. These new standards, which were developed in response to the U.S. opioid crisis, are intended to assist hospitals, physicians, nurse practitioners, and nurses by providing guidelines to improve patient care outcomes and decrease patients' pain, as well as decrease dependency on opioids (**BOX 15-1**).

Drug Testing

Drug testing is one component in developing a plan to decrease substance abuse. The impetus for drug testing emerged during the Vietnam War (1955–1975), when it was alleged that many active-duty soldiers had been using heroin and other illicit drugs; in consequence, the U.S. military initiated a drug testing program in 1971 (Bray, Marsden, Mazzuchi, & Hartman, 1999). The use of random drug tests in the military during this time resulted in a 90% reduction in self-reported drug use among active-duty military personnel (Bray et al., 1999). U.S. companies began drug testing

---

BOX 15-1 Evidence-Based Practice Focus

Snell, Hughes, Fore, Lukman, and Morgan focused on chronic nonmalignant pain (CNMP) in their 2019 research study by applying evidence-based practice and faith-based approaches to those suffering. In this research study, Snell et al. employed a three-phase needs assessment and evaluation of patients with CNMP that was conducted by a certified registered nurse anesthetist (CRNA) with extensive education in this field. The study utilized a descriptive quantitative design; the three phases included (1) pre-assessment, (2) assessment, and (3) post-assessment. The authors utilized the CREATION Health Model, which allows one to investigate holistic pain management. The study findings included concerns about the many variances in patient populations, the effects of CNMP in patients, and inadequate management of pain and appropriate interventions during patient care. The authors purported that the nurse must understand the patient population, which will influence high-quality patient care.

Modified from Snell, S., Hughes, T., Fore, C., Lukman, R., & Morgan, B. (2019). Treating chronic nonmalignant pain: Evidence and faith-based approaches. *Journal of Christian Nursing, 36*(1), 22–30. doi:10.1097/CNJ0000000000000569

their workers in the 1980s, especially for high-risk jobs, and this trend has continued to this day (Substance Abuse and Mental Health Services Administration, 2018). Nurses may be involved in facilitating and monitoring this type of testing as part of their job if they work in occupational health, the military, prisons, or corporate organizations.

Several tests can be used to prove whether someone is impaired by marijuana or another drug. Usually, blood or urine samples need to be taken and sent to the laboratory. In the past, the results from the laboratory might have taken days or weeks, but quicker turnaround times are now possible. There are benefits and costs with each test:

- Blood testing: Blood testing has been used the longest and is the most accurate type of testing. Yet, because of its intrusiveness, it cannot be used "in the field." Such tests are used at schools, hospitals, and other places where a blood draw can be done by a skilled phlebotomist.
- Oral fluid testing: Other bodily fluids could be used for drug testing, but sometimes a search warrant is required, making such samples difficult to get. Some field kits allow for sample collection by anyone to test for certain drugs and marijuana, but their accuracy is sometimes suspect.
- Sweat testing: This type of test is difficult to perform and cannot be widely used due to its inaccuracy.
- Hair testing: This type of test cannot prove the point of exposure and has accuracy problems. Nevertheless, hair follicle testing does give a longer-term picture of use with certain drugs and medications.
- Urine testing: Urine testing is well established, and samples are easy to obtain. This type of test can show that drugs and marijuana are present in the person's system, but cannot prove

that the drugs influenced the person's actions at the time of a purported crime. (Compton, 2017)

The first author of this chapter has had personal experience with a drug testing program, having worked in a Southern California high school in an administrative position. At the time, the school administration believed that a drug testing program should be implemented to combat a recent spate of expulsions for having drugs on campus that had occurred in the past year in the wake of the school's "zero tolerance" policy. Initially, a period of anxiety occurred as notification was sent out to parents, stating that they needed to sign a permission form that would allow the school to perform the drug testing. Surprisingly, only a few parents had additional questions of the school, due in part to the excellent notification campaign in which the school actively informed the parents of the upcoming change. The program was touted as a benefit to parents and their children: In addition to keeping students off drugs, it was expected to give students a "way out" when offered drugs by their friends.

Overall, the program was successful due to the positive atmosphere of the school and the positive effects on students of the drug-free campus culture. As time went on, however, this author began to be concerned about his role in drug testing students. As an administrator at the school, he was often put in awkward situations in dealing with students and parents who questioned the "randomness" of the drug testing and wondered if their student was being singled out because of animosity on the part of the school administration. This suspicion was difficult to combat and guard against, and this author began to communicate that the school should investigate and pursue the hiring of an outside firm to handle the drug testing program.

In his role as an administrator, the author had worked diligently to develop a "relational ministry" with the students and parents at the school. He found it very difficult to maintain this relationship, as his role had become more of an enforcer and less of a minister. Nurses may find themselves in similar situations if called to ministry where drug testing is used. Individuals in the medical profession should exercise caution in developing their "roles" with clients who are abusing drugs. A kind and caring counselor can work with the individual and make a great impact that stays with the client much longer than the threat of failing a drug test. When Sznitman and Romer (2014) compared the effects of positive school climate and student drug testing on changes in student substance abuse, they found that perceived student drug testing was not associated with changes in student's substance abuse. Although Sznitman, Dunlop, Nalkur, Khurana, and Romer (2012) found a positive correlation between lower substance abuse and positive school climate, it occurred only among female students. However, neither drug testing nor positive school climate effected a change in alcohol abuse rates among students (Sznitman & Romer, 2014). The call for a "people-centered" approach to drug policy (via harm-reduction policies) brings to bear not only empirical evidence of the therapeutic benefits of cannabis, but also an understanding of its associated health risks (Cousijn, Núñez, & Filbey, 2017).

Reviewing clinical guidelines for prescribing opioids could be one way to decrease their abuse. Other medications for pain management may potentially benefit patients who require treatment for chronic pain (Centers for Disease Control and Prevention [CDC], 2018). At the same time, those patients who are taking their opioids as prescribed should not be punished for their use. When a safer, more effective chronic therapy or pain treatment cannot be found for individuals who use opioids but do not abuse them, those patients should be allowed to continue to use the medications without incurring added cost or experiencing more difficulties in obtaining the medications. Prescribing recommendations focus on the use of opioids in treating chronic pain (pain

lasting longer than three months or past the time of normal tissue healing) outside of active cancer treatment, palliative care, and end-of-life care (CDC, 2018).

Many police academies train their new recruits how to detect and recognize impairment in drivers, including individuals driving under the influence of a drug (DUID). Unfortunately, knowing and proving impairment is a different matter. The 16-hour Advanced Roadside Impaired Driving Enforcement Program (ARIDE) is designed to give police the ability to apply information they have learned about DUID to make effective arrests that are based on probable cause and that provide the necessary evidence for prosecution (Compton, 2017).

▶ Step 4: Implementation of the Plan to Help Overcome SAD

In the past, some laws passed by the U.S. government have had a detrimental effect on patients who were suffering from SAD. A case in point was the Harrison Narcotic Act of 1914 (Public Law No. 223, 1914), which had unintended consequences. The legislation was intended to help control the use and distribution of opium products. This law sought to register and subject to taxation anyone who produced, imported, or manufactured opium products or derivatives; at that time, it was not considered a measure to prohibit narcotics. Even so, the Harrison Narcotic Act had dire consequences for people who were prescribed opium by their physicians and became addicted to it, and for those who were already addicted to opium. At the time, addiction was not considered a disease, but rather a curable condition. As a result of this law's interpretation, doctors were arrested and imprisoned for writing prescriptions for their patients who needed opium.

Almost immediately, a large number of these people became unable to obtain their opium through legal means and had to turn to illegal methods of obtaining it, leading to a black market for drugs of abuse (Courtwright, 2015).

Thus, less than a year after the Harrison Narcotic Act was enacted, drug addiction became one of the largest problems faced by the United States. The careers of numerous doctors were destroyed when they attempted to prescribe opium to patients who were addicted to it. Unable to obtain the drugs that they needed, users had to resort to crime and violence to obtain the money needed to purchase drugs from criminals, who sold these products at much higher prices than the legally prescribed drugs of the past (Musto, 1999). The result was the imprisonment of many desperate users, sometimes repeatedly, for attempting to obtain the drugs needed for their addiction. Three years after the passage of the Harrison Narcotic Act, a committee was formed to determine if the law should be amended. Rather than being repealed, the law was strengthened

in terms of the severity and length of prison sentences meted out to drug addicts (Courtwright, 2015). In the face of today's national epidemic, it is imperative that we develop sounder policies that will resolve the opioid crisis more compassionately.

Certainly, the opioid crisis will not be eliminated overnight. However, with a united front and changes being made across the nation as a whole, the country can achieve its goal of reducing the amount of opioid misuse (and the number of deaths) while still providing adequate pain control to patients (see **BOX 15-2**, New and Revised Pain Assessment and Management Standards).

In the late 1960s, drug prevention interventions began to be implemented at U.S. schools due to a perceived increase in student drug use (**CASE STUDY 15-1**) (Kearney & Hines, 1980). The programs that were implemented utilized "scare tactics," which created students who were increasingly distrustful of and cynical about those programs (Kearney & Hines, 1980, p. 127). Another approach provided the

---

BOX 15-2 New and Revised Pain Assessment and Management Standards

On January 1, 2018, The Joint Commission (TJC) implemented new and revised pain assessment and management standards for accredited hospitals. To receive TJC accreditation, hospitals will need to establish policies and procedures that address comprehensive clinical assessment of pain, treatment or referral for treatment, and reassessment for patients, based on patient population and scope of services provided. The standards include the following components:

- Establish a clinical leadership team.
- Actively engage medical staff and hospital leadership in improving pain assessment and management, including strategies to decrease opioid use and minimize risks associated with opioid use.
- Provide at least one nonpharmacologic pain treatment modality.
- Facilitate access to prescription drug monitoring programs.
- Improve pain assessment by concentrating more on how pain is affecting patients' physical function.
- Engage patients in treatment decisions about their pain management.
- Address patient education and engagement, including storage and disposal of opioids to prevent these medications from being stolen or misused by others.
- Facilitate referral of patients addicted to opioids to treatment programs.

Based on The Joint Commission: https://com-jax-emergency-pami.sites.medinfo.ufl.edu/files/2018/03/Joint-Commission-and-PAMI.pdf.

🔎 *CASE STUDY 15-1*

A school drug testing program was effective during the first few years after its implementation, but as time went on several students, who were passionate about their drug use, began to develop ways to cheat the drug test. One student, who had been allowed to return to the school after a previous expulsion, was under notice that he could be tested "on demand." The student had passed several previous tests, but the administration noticed several suspicious problems with his drug tests, such as the large volume of urine produced and the clear, colorless nature of the urine. The administrator on his next test added a chemical to the toilet water, and made sure the water in the lavatory was turned off and the cabinet to the water supply was locked. Upon reviewing the sample, the same clear, colorless sample was found. However, upon opening the sample jar, the unmistakable smell of the cleaning solution was readily apparent. The student was found to have adulterated the sample with toilet water in an attempt to mask his resumed drug use. He was expelled as a result of his choice to continue to use drugs. Ultimately, schools need to work together with parents and students to curb drug use initiation and better inform students of the dangers of drug initiation.

Questions

1. What is the role of the registered nurse in schools that test for substance abuse? Include elementary school, middle school, and high school concerns in your response.
2. What is the role of a school nurse when substance abuse issues occur with the children?
3. Are there any laws that a school nurse must understand?
4. How do you visualize working with the school administration, the local police and sheriff's department, and the families and children in the community in regard to school-based drug testing?

students with a plethora of information, which had the unintended consequence of developing more positive attitudes among students favoring the use of drugs (Swisher, Warner, & Herr, 1972). During the 1980s, the Drug Abuse Resistance Education (DARE) program received widespread support as a drug intervention. However, the DARE program, which was disseminated to more than half of all U.S. school districts, was later shown to be largely ineffective at preventing substance use behavior—though it has continued to be utilized because of the excellent community relations developed between communities, schools, students, and police departments through this intervention (Brownson et al., 2015).

Given the shortcomings in previous treatments of SAD, we must ask ourselves: What can nurses who minister in this area do to effect change?

Treatment

Not all religions believe in original sin, but Christianity does. The scriptures are a good place for faith-based nurses to start as various individual treatment options are considered. Genesis 3 tells us of the fall of mankind and how sin and death entered the world. Thus, from a Christian perspective, we have the answer for all psychological and mental illnesses, including drug addictions: They stem from original sin, other people's sin, and personal sin.

- The sin that causes death, which we all inherited—that is, original sin: Romans 5:12 describes how death entered the world: "Therefore, just as sin entered the world through one man, and death through sin, and in this way, death came to all people, because all sinned." Death perverted the nature of humans, penetrating all the way into their physical, mental, and spiritual being. Because of death entering the world, we have genetic defects, we have mental disorders, and we have sin. Romans goes on to say that death reigns because of one man's sin. Therefore, death dwells in our genes because of original sin. Smith (2011) writes, "It is a simple fact of life: There will be difficulty, setback and disappointment. For some there will be rejection; for others there will be tragic losses. For others—there is no other word for it—there will be suffering. No one is immune from pain; it is part of the package that comes with life. This is a broken and cruel world. GOD is good, but life is unfair" (p. 206).

■ The sin of others. This sin is evident when we see the abuse and neglect that occur directly from drug addiction and mental illness. Physical, sexual, emotional, and mental abuse can scar children for the rest of their lives. Addictive parents may be either abusive or neglectful. They love their addiction more than anything else in the world. They may or may not say with their mouths, "I love you," but with their actions they say they love the drugs or alcohol more. The sins of others can cause lifelong pain and suffering and lead them to sin as well (see **BOX 15-3**, Research Highlight).

■ Our own sinful nature. God gave us free will, and with that free will, we sin against our Creator. We cause our own troubles many times by our own actions. As the old saying goes, sometimes we are our own worst enemy. We believe what Romans 3:23 states: "all have sinned and fall short of the glory of God."

Thus, as Christians, we know that all addictions, all genetic defects, and all death come from original sin, the sins of others, or our own sins. But we have hope, and that hope is in Jesus the Messiah. Romans 5:15–17 reads:

But the gift is not like the trespass. For if the many died by the trespass of the one man, how much more did God's grace and the gift that came by the grace of the one man, Jesus Christ, overflow to the many! [16]Nor can the gift of God be compared with the result of one man's sin: The judgment followed one sin and brought condemnation, but the gift followed

---

BOX 15-3 Research Highlight

Romisher, Hill, and Cong expressed real caring concerns for infants born with neonatal abstinence syndrome (NAS). According to the authors' 2018 survey, the incidence of NAS in the United States is increasing dramatically. Working with infants who have NAS and their families can be challenging for healthcare providers. The method chosen for this research was an anonymous, cross-sectional survey study that used a researcher-developed questionnaire. The survey questionnaire included (1) 20 Likert scale questions focusing on nurses' attitudes, knowledge, and practice; (2) a case study with three questions; and (3) two open-ended questions. This survey was completed at a regional neonatal nursing conference. Nurses who cared for infants with NAS, advanced practice nurses, and leaders were invited to participate. A total of 54 participants completed the survey. According to Romisher et al., more research into nursing practices when providing care to infants with NAS is needed, along with additional education for nurses.

Modified from Romisher, R., Hill, D., & Cong, X. (2018). Neonatal abstinence syndrome: Exploring nurses' attitudes, knowledge, and practice. *Advanced Neonatal Care, 18*(2), E3–E11.

many trespasses and brought justification. [17]For if, by the trespass of the one man, death reigned through that one man, how much more will those who receive God's abundant provision of grace and of the gift of righteousness reign in life through the one man, Jesus Christ!

We have hope in Jesus Christ. Our hope for healing from an addiction lies in Jesus. For some reason, God heals some people all at once, but not all people. God seems to choose most people to be healthy, if they are healed, through progression in relationship to Him and others. Even Paul himself had a thorn in his side that God chose not to heal (2 Corinthians 12). But there still is hope in Jesus.

Our ability to make a difference for God in a broken world, in society, in the church, and in our vocation as nurses comes through our capacity to be life amidst death, to be people of hope in a discouraging world (Smith, 2011, p. 208). We all have limitations due to original sin, the sin of others, or our own sins, but we also have to come to the acceptance that God is God, and we are not—and that He allows evil and sin into our lives. Look at Job. Or, consider the most outrageous act of pure evil, the death of Jesus our Messiah—the sinless dying for the sinful. Whenever we ask the question "why," we can look to the cross. Why was I born into this horrible abusive family? Because we live in an evil/sinful world, but Jesus has overcome the world! Why was I born an addict? Because we live in an evil/sinful world, but Jesus has overcome the world! Sin in the world is painful. But we will not live with joy unless we learn to accept with grace the losses we experience and choose to live in peace within the limits of our lives (Smith, 2011, p. 215). Healing from addiction comes from God, but it most likely will not come spontaneously but rather in Christian community, with others who are on their way to healing and those whom God has trained to walk alongside the person toward healing.

Sometimes medications can also be helpful, but individuals should never be used to trade one addiction for another.

▶ # Step 5: How to Evaluate Success in Overcoming SAD

While research into substance abuse is ongoing, it remains to be seen how certain drugs, now purported to be a panacea or to offer a wealth of benefits, might eventually be shown to have potentially harmful effects. For example, the literature on marijuana includes a plethora of studies demonstrating harm, but relatively few touting the controversial therapeutic effects of THC or CBD. Therapeutic effects, such as reduced chemotherapy-induced nausea and vomiting, modest pain reduction, and moderate reduction of self-reported spasms in patients with multiple sclerosis, have been documented. Nevertheless, the overwhelming majority of research shows multiple harmful outcomes with prolonged marijuana use (Cousijn et al., 2017). With the increasing numbers of patients who use marijuana for recreational purposes as well as self-administer it for various medical symptoms, nurses need to be cognizant of the many implications of this usage.

Without evidence that is scientifically rigorous, statistically reportable, and based on patient populations, nurses will face increasing challenges concerning use of medical cannabis. To address the lack of guidelines for nurses when caring for individuals utilizing cannabis, the National Council of State Boards of Nursing's (NCSBN) Board of Directors appointed members to the Medical Marijuana Nursing Guidelines Committee. To create the requested guidelines and recommendations for education and care, a review of the relevant statistics, current legislation, scientific literature, and clinical research on cannabis as a therapeutic agent was required. The committee also consulted known experts in the area of medical marijuana, its use, its safety, and legislation (Russell et al., 2018).

Medical marijuana programs (MMPs) are likely to include many conditions qualifying patients for legally sanctioned marijuana use based on promising preclinical research for specific indications. To date, 57 qualifying conditions have been included in the various jurisdictional laws; **BOX 15-4** identifies the most common qualifying conditions across all MMPs. Some of these conditions are likely included only because of symptoms they share with better-studied conditions. A few broad qualifying conditions/symptoms—notably chronic pain, neuropathies, and nausea/vomiting—are the most researched and commonly posited to respond to medical cannabis.

BOX 15-4 Most Common Qualifying Conditions in Medical Marijuana Programs

- Alzheimer's disease
- Amyotrophic lateral sclerosis
- Arthritis
- Cachexia
- Cancer
- Crohn's disease and other irritable bowel syndromes
- Epilepsy/seizures
- Glaucoma
- Hepatitis C
- Human immunodeficiency virus (HIV)/ acquired immunodeficiency syndrome (AIDS)
- Nausea
- Neuropathies
- Pain
- Parkinson's disease
- Persistent muscle spasms (including multiple sclerosis)
- Post-traumatic stress disorder
- Sickle cell disease

Russell, K., Cahill, M., Gowen, K., Cronquist, R., Smith, V., Borris-Hale, C., … Sutton-Johnson, S. (2018, July). The NCSBN national nursing guidelines for medical marijuana. *Journal of Nursing Regulation, 9*(2), s2–s60.

In general, there is a dearth of randomized clinical trials that have compared the effects of cannabis and **cannabinoids** against those of other standard medications with clinically proven efficacy and regular use in clinical practice. When and if cannabis and cannabinoids show therapeutic effects, practitioners using evidence-based practice should not consider cannabis as a first- or second-line treatment. Indeed, when compared to standard first-line medical treatments for pain, nausea, and cachexia, cannabinoids were shown to underperform relative to megestrol acetate, ondansetron, and dihydrocodeine, and to have effects comparable to those of tramadol and pregabalin (Russell et al., 2018). Moreover, cannabis carries its own set of adverse effects that must be carefully considered, monitored, and recorded. More important is the possibility that patients may forgo effective standard medications in favor of cannabis. Therefore, the use of cannabis and cannabinoids is best considered for patients who could benefit from complementary use or when currently accepted first- and second-line medications or therapies show no or insufficient effect or demonstrate dangerous adverse events in selected patients (Russell et al., 2018).

The treatment of certain symptomology with cannabis might be attributed to the more general and well-known effects of cannabis—sedation, appetite stimulation, and euphoria—which may contribute to a subjective sense of well-being, instead of the cannabis actually treating underlying symptoms. This increase in subjective sense of well-being could improve self-reported quality of life in patients who have difficulty sleeping, chronic pain, and poor appetite. Studies such as those done by the Centennial Institute (2018) and Russell et al. (2018) have attempted to demonstrate the efficacy of these general effects as a treatment for neurodegenerative behavioral disturbances and sleep disturbances in individuals with multiple sclerosis. For diseases that cause irritability and agitation, cannabis is suggested as a method of reducing aggressiveness in patients with inhibited mental function (e.g., Alzheimer's disease, autism, Huntington's disease). However, a study of patients with dementia contradicted this claim by demonstrating that THC had no effect on objective scores of agitation, aggression, aberrant motor behavior, or other behavioral disturbances. The sedative effect of cannabis is not applicable to every condition (Russell et al., 2018).

▸ Conclusion

The societal costs associated with legalization of marijuana are likely to increase in the future, as the long-term health consequences of marijuana use become clearer. Like tobacco, commercial marijuana is likely to have health consequences that will not become fully evident for decades. Bottom line: The economic and social costs of ongoing marijuana use have intentionally been minimized by proponents of this drug's legalization, and the comprehensive costs are likely much higher (Centennial Institute, 2018).

To date, high-quality randomized controlled trials and experimental studies of marijuana use have shown mixed findings, depending on age, sex, route of administration, preexisting risk factors, and cannabis history, among other factors. Although the evidence base is underdeveloped for many health outcomes, we believe that substantial evidence shows that cannabis can have both positive (e.g., reducing pain, multiple sclerosis symptoms, and nausea) and negative (e.g., aggravation of existing respiratory problems, psychosis, motor vehicle accidents, low birth weight, and cannabis dependence) effects. The mixed effects of cannabis may, therefore, contribute significantly to the mixed evidence. The conclusion that cannabis can have both positive and negative effects has been drawn numerous times since the 1980s (Cousijn et al., 2017).

The substance abuse crisis will not be resolved overnight. However, with a united front and sweeping changes, the United States can achieve its goal of reducing the number of deaths related to substance abuse. Nurses should be at the forefront in leading reform efforts to promote health for those with substance abuse and mental health issues (**BOX 15-5**).

BOX 15-5 Outstanding Nurse Leader: Cynthia A. Russell, PhD, RN, FAAN, PCC, NBC-HWC

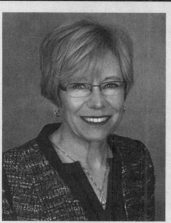

Dr. Cynthia A. Russell is dean and professor at Holy Family University (HFU) School of Nursing and Allied Health Professions. She received her BS in nursing and her MS in adult psychiatric mental health nursing from the University of Wisconsin–Madison, and her PhD in nursing with a focus on geriatric psychiatric practice from Rush University in Chicago. She was certified by the American Nurses Credentialing Center as a Clinical Specialist in Adult Psychiatric and Mental Health Nursing. In addition to teaching numerous undergraduate courses throughout her long and distinguished career, Russell has taught graduate courses in theory; advanced psychiatric mental health nursing; tertiary prevention in health care; ethical, legal, and spiritual dimensions of health care; all levels of psychiatric mental health nursing; and loss and grief.

Cynthia Russell

(continues)

BOX 15-5 Outstanding Nurse Leader: Cynthia A. Russell, PhD, RN, FAAN, PCC, NBC-HWC *(continued)*

Nationally board certified as a health and wellness coach, she has distinguished herself in these areas, receiving recognition as a Fellow in the American Academy of Nursing and being honored with numerous teaching awards. Prior to her time at HFU, she served as faculty and interim dean at Valparaiso University for several years, dean and then provost at Grand Canyon University, and senior vice president for academic programs for an innovative nurse education company. She is the author of several articles and book chapters, and coauthor of two books on promoting health in congregations. Of her philosophy as an educator, Russell says, "I think that you cannot separate teaching and learning. . . . This is not a simple process, but I believe the ultimate compliment is when the learners teach the teacher."

A mother of five children and stepchildren, she thoroughly enjoys being a grandmother. Russell also breeds, owns, and professionally shows championship Belgian Malinois dogs.

▶ Clinical Reasoning Exercises

You are a nurse working in the emergency department (ED) of an inner-city hospital. You are finding that since your state has passed a law to legalize marijuana, more people who are high are being dropped off by the police to the ED, because this practice means that the police do not have to do the paperwork on these individuals. If the person was driving, the police have a new breathalyzer they are piloting to determine if the person has marijuana in his or her system; if the individual tests positive, he or she is charged with driving while impaired (DWI).

When police drop off an impaired person at the ED, there are no clear directives about what to do with an individual who has used marijuana. So, the person just sits in the ED until someone can pick him or her up, thus wasting resources that could be used in other ways.

1. What should the ED personnel do when the police show up with those people who are high on marijuana?
2. Is this a good use of the ED resources?

3. Are there measures that the ED should take to protect these people?
4. Which types of directives should the ED have regarding people who come in high?
5. Should the ED test these people for marijuana, alcohol, and other drugs?

▶ Personal Reflection Exercises

1. Many inner-city hospitals in states that permit marijuana use do not even check for marijuana, stating they just assume all patients have used this drug. Do you think this is wise?
2. Do you think every state that has passed permissive marijuana laws should research the full impact of marijuana use in the state? Why or why not?
3. Now that many states are allowing marijuana use, do you believe other drug use will be decriminalized?
4. What do you believe will be the long-term effects on a society that permits marijuana use?

References

Barry, C. L. (2018). Fentanyl and the evolving opioid epidemic: What strategies should policy makers consider? *Psychiatric Services, 69*(1), 100–103. doi:10.1176/appi.ps.201700235

Bray, R. M., Marsden, M. E., Mazzuchi, J. F., & Hartman, R. W. (1999). Prevention in the military. *Prevention and Societal Impact of Drug and Alcohol Abuse, 345–367.*

Brownson, R. C., Allen, P., Jacob, R. R., Harris, J. K., Duggan, K., Hipp, P. R., & Erwin, P. C. (2015). Understanding mis-implementation in public health practice. *American Journal of Preventive Medicine, 48*(5), 543–551.

Buddy T. (2018, November 18). The cost of drug use to society. *Verywell Mind.* Retrieved from https://www.verywellmind.com/what-are-the-costs-of-drug-abuse-to-society-63037

California [S.B. 1449], (California State Legislature, 2010).

Centennial Institute. (2018, November 15). *Economic and social costs of legalized marijuana.* Lakewood, CO: Colorado Christian University.

Centers for Disease Control and Prevention (CDC). (2018). Opioid overdose: State information. Retrieved from https://www.cdc.gov/drugoverdose/states/index.html

Cerda, M., Sarvet, A. L., Wall, M., Feng, T., Keyes, K. M., Galea, S., & Hasin, D. S. (2018). Medical marijuana laws and adolescent use of marijuana and other substances: Alcohol, cigarettes, prescription drugs, and other illicit drugs. *Drug and Alcohol Dependence, 183,* 62–68.

Chilukuri, S. (2017). *The impacts of recreational marijuana legalization on Colorado policy analysis on Amendment 64.* Theses and Dissertations—Public Health (M.P.H. & Dr. P. H.), 168.

Christie, C., Baker, C., Cooper, R., Kennedy, P. J., Madras, B., & Bondi, P., (2017, November 1). The President's Commission on combating drug addiction and the opioid crisis. Office of National Drug Control Policy. Retrieved from https://www.whitehouse.gov/ondcp/presidents-commission/

Compton, R. (2017, July). *Marijuana-impaired driving: A report to Congress* (DOT HS 812 440). Washington, DC: National Highway Traffic Safety Administration.

Courtwright, D. T. (2015). Preventing and treating narcotic addiction: A century of federal drug control. *New England Journal of Medicine, 373*(22), 2095–2097.

Cousijn, A., Núñez, A. E., & Filbey, F. M. (2017, December 21). Time to acknowledge the mixed effects of cannabis on health: A summary and critical review of the NASEM 2017 report on the health effects of cannabis and cannabinoids. *Addiction Journal Club, 113,* 958–966. doi:10.1111/add.14084

D'Amico, E. J., Miles, J. N., & Tucker, J. S. (2015). Gateway to curiosity: Medical marijuana ads and intention and use during middle school. *Psychology of Addictive Behaviors, 29*(3), 613.

Das, J. K., Salam, R. A., Arshad, A., Finkelstein, Y., & Bhutta, Z. A. (2016). Interventions for adolescent substance abuse: An overview of systematic reviews. *Journal of Adolescent Health, 59*(4), S61–S71.

Degenhardt, L., Coffey, C., Romaniuk, H., Swift, W., Carlin, J. B., Hall, W. D., & Patton, G. C. (2013). The persistence of the association between adolescent cannabis use and common mental disorders into young adulthood. *Addiction, 108*(1), 124–133.

DuPont, R. L., Merlo, L. J., Arria, A. M., & Shea, C. L. (2013). Random student drug testing as a school-based drug prevention strategy. *Addiction, 108*(5), 839–845.

DuPont, R. L., & Voth, E. A. (1995). Drug legalization, harm reduction, and drug policy. *Annals of Internal Medicine, 123*(6), 461–465.

Epstein, M., Hill, K. G., Nevell, A. M., Guttmannova, K., Bailey, J. A., Abbott, R. D., Kosterman, R., & Hawkins, J. D. (2015). Trajectories of marijuana use from adolescence into adulthood: Environmental and individual correlates. *Developmental Psychology, 51*(11), 1650–1663.

Federal Bureau of Investigation. (2016). 2016 crime in the United States. Retrieved from https://ucr.fbi.gov/crime-in-the-u.s/2016/crime-in-the-u.s.-2016/

Flynn, A. B., Falco, M., & Hocini, S. (2015). Independent evaluation of middle school–based drug prevention curricula: A systematic review. *JAMA Pediatrics, 169*(11), 1046–1052.

Hall, W. D., Patton, G., Stockings, E., Weier, M., Lynskey, M., Morley, K. I., & Degenhardt, L. (2016). Why young people's substance use matters for global health. *Lancet Psychiatry, 3*(3), 265–279.

Hancox, R. J., Shin, H. H., Gray, A. R., Poulton, R., & Sears, M. R. (2015). Effects of quitting cannabis on respiratory symptoms. *European Respiratory Journal,* ERJ-02289.

Harrison Narcotic Act, Public Law No. 223, 1914.

Hasin, D. S., Saha, T. D., Kerridge, B. T., Goldstein, R. B., Chou, S. P., Zhang, H.,... Huang, B. (2015). Prevalence of marijuana use disorders in the United States between 2001–2002 and 2012–2013. *JAMA Psychiatry, 72*(12), 1235–1242.

Hussong, A. M., Ennett, S. T., Cox, M. J., & Haroon, M. (2017). A systematic review of the unique prospective association of negative affect symptoms and adolescent substance use controlling for externalizing symptoms. *Psychology of Addictive Behaviors, 31*(2), 137.

Johnston, L. D., Miech, R. A., O'Malley, P. M., Bachman, J. G., Schulenberg, J. E., & Patrick, M. E. (2018). *Monitoring the future national survey results on drug use, 1975-2017: Overview, key findings on adolescent drug use.* Ann Arbor, MI: Institute for Social Research, The University of Michigan.

Johnston, L. D., O'Malley, P. M., Miech, R. A., Bachman, J. G., & Schulenberg, J. E. (2016). *Demographic subgroup trends among adolescents in the use of various licit and illicit drugs, 1975–2016.* Monitoring the Future Occasional Paper Series, Paper 88. Ann Arbor, MI: Institute for Social Research, The University of Michigan.

The Joint Commission. (2017). Joint Commission enhances pain assessment and management requirements for accredited hospitals. *Perspectives, 37*(7), 1–3.

Kearney, A. L., & Hines, M. H. (1980). Evaluation of the effectiveness of a drug prevention education program. *Journal of Drug Education, 10*(2), 127–134.

Keller, C. E., Ashrafioun, L., Neumann, A. M., Van Klein, J., Fox, C. H., & Blondell, R. D. (2012). Practices, perceptions, and concerns of primary care physicians about opioid dependence associated with the treatment of chronic pain. *Substance Abuse, 33*(2), 103–113. doi: 10.1080/08897077.2011.630944

Kilmer, J. R., Walker, D. D., Lee, C. M., Palmer, R. S., Mallett, K. A., Fabiano, P., & Larimer, M. E. (2006). Misperceptions of college student marijuana use: Implications for prevention. *Journal of Studies on Alcohol, 67*(2), 277–281.

Lassiter, M. D. (2015). Impossible criminals: The suburban imperatives of America's war on drugs. *Journal of American History, 102*(1), 126–140.

Lewis, N. (2017, July 11). Oregon bill decriminalizes possession of heroin, cocaine and other drugs. *The Washington Post.* Retrieved from https://www.washingtonpost.com/news/post-nation/wp/2017/07/11/oregon-legislature-passes-bill-decriminalizing-heroin-cocaine-meth-possession-hoping-to-curb-mass-incarceration/?noredirect=on&utm_term=.6357f2623674

Lynskey, M. T., Heath, A. C., Bucholz, K. K., Slutske, W. S., Madden, P. A., Nelson, E. C.,... Martin, N. G. (2003). Escalation of drug use in early-onset cannabis users vs co-twin controls. *Journal of American Medical Association, 289*(4), 427–433.

Mack, K. A., Jones, C. M., & Ballesteros, M. F. (2017). Illicit drug use, illicit drug use disorders, and drug overdose deaths in metropolitan and nonmetropolitan areas of the United States. *American Journal of Transplantation, 17*(12), 3241–3252.

Meier, M. H., Caspi, A., Ambler, A., Harrington, H., Houts, R., Keefe, R. S.,... Moffitt, T. E. (2012). Persistent cannabis users show neuropsychological decline from childhood to midlife. *Proceedings of the National Academy of Sciences, 109*(40), E2657–E2664.

Miech, R. A., Johnston, L. D., O'Malley, P. M., Bachman, J. G., & Schulenberg, J. E. (2016). *Monitoring the future national survey results on drug use, 1975–2015: Volume I, secondary school students.* Ann Arbor, MI: Institute for Social Research, The University of Michigan.

Miech, R. A., Johnston, L., O'Malley, P. M., Bachman, J. G., Schulenberg, J., & Patrick, M. E. (2015). Trends in use of marijuana and attitudes toward marijuana among youth before and after decriminalization: The case of California 2007–2013. *International Journal of Drug Policy, 26*(4), 336–344.

Miech, R. A., Johnston, L., O'Malley, P. M., Keyes, K., & Heard, K. (2015). Prescription opioids in adolescence and future opioid misuse. *Pediatrics, 136*(5). doi:10.1542/peds.2015-1364d

Musto, D. F. (1999). *The American disease: Origins of narcotic control.* Oxford, UK: Oxford University Press.

National Institute on Drug Abuse (NIDA). (2016, February 11). *Understanding drug abuse and addiction: What science says.* Retrieved from https://www.drugabuse.gov/understanding-drug-abuse-addiction-what-science-says

National Institute on Drug Abuse (NIDA). (2017, May 31). *"All scientific hands on deck" to end the opioid crisis.* Retrieved from https://www.drugabuse.gov/about-nida/noras-blog/2017/05/all-scientific-hands-deck-to-end-opioid-crisis

O'Donnell, J. (2018, March 21). Feds work with drug makers to boost research into non-opioid painkillers, treatments. *USA Today.* Retrieved from https://www.usatoday.com/story/news/politics/2018/03/21/feds-work-drugmakers-boost-research-into-non-opioid-painkillers-treatments/440959002/

Palamar, J. J. (2014). Predictors of disapproval toward "hard drug" use among high school seniors in the US. *Prevention Science, 15*(5), 725–735.

Reboussin, B. A., Ialongo, N. S., & Green, K. M. (2015). Influences of behavior and academic problems at school entry on marijuana use transitions during adolescence in an African-American sample. *Addictive Behaviors, 41*, 51–57.

Russell, K., Cahill, M., Gowen, K., Cronquist, R., Smith, V., Borris-Hale, C.,... Sutton-Johnson, S. (2018, July). The NCSBN national nursing guidelines for medical marijuana. *Journal of Nursing Regulation, 9*(2), s2–s60.

Salloum, N. C., Krauss, M. J., Agrawal, A., Bierut, L. J., & Grucza, R. A. (2018). A reciprocal effects analysis of cannabis use and perceptions of risk. *Addiction, 113*(6), 1077–1085.

Salomonsen-Sautel, S., Min, S. J., Sakai, J. T., Thurstone, C., & Hopfer, C. (2014). Trends in fatal motor vehicle crashes before and after marijuana commercialization in Colorado. *Drug and Alcohol Dependence, 140*, 137–144.

Sarvet, A. L., Wall, M. M., Fink, D. S., Greene, E., Le, A., Boustead, A. E.,... Hasin, D. S. (2018). Medical marijuana laws and adolescent marijuana use in the United States: A systematic review and meta-analysis. *Addiction, 113*(6), 1003–1016.

Schuermeyer, J., Salomonsen-Sautel, S., Price, R. K., Balan, S., Thurstone, C., Min, S. J., & Sakai, J. T. (2014). Temporal trends in marijuana attitudes, availability and use in Colorado compared to non-medical marijuana states: 2003–11. *Drug and Alcohol Dependence, 140*, 145–155.

Schwartz, R. P., Gryczynski, J., O'Grady, K. E., Sharfstein, J. M., Warren, G., Olsen, Y., . . . Jaffe, J. H. (2013). Opioid agonist treatments and heroin overdose deaths in Baltimore, Maryland, 1995–2009. *American Journal of Public Health, 103*(5), 917–922.

Smith, G. T. (2011). *Courage and calling: Embracing your God-given potential* (rev. ed.). Downers Grove, IL: InterVarsity Press.

Substance Abuse and Mental Health Services Administration. (2018). *Key substance use and mental health indicators in the United States: Results from the 2017 National Survey on Drug Use and Health* (HHS Publication No. SMA 18-5068, NSDUH Series H-53). Rockville, MD: Center for Behavioral Health Statistics and Quality, Substance Abuse and Mental Health Services Administration.

Svrakic, D. M., Lustman, P. J., Mallya, A., Lynn, T. A., Finney, R., & Svrakic, N. M. (2011). Legalization, decriminalization and medicinal use of cannabis. *Missouri Medicine, 109*(2), 90–98.

Swisher, J. D., Warner, R. W., & Herr, E. L. (1972). Experimental comparison of four approaches to drug abuse prevention among ninth and eleventh graders. *Journal of Counseling Psychology, 19*(4), 328.

Sznitman, S., Dunlop, S., Nalkur, P., Khurana, A., & Romer, D. (2012). Student drug testing in the context of positive and negative school climates: Results from a national survey. *Journal of Youth & Adolescence, 41*(2), 146–155.

Sznitman, S. R., & Romer, D. (2014). Student drug testing and positive school climates: Testing the relation between two school characteristics and drug use behavior in a longitudinal study. *Journal of Studies on Alcohol and Drugs, 75*(1), 65–73.

Volkow, N. D., Baler, R. D., Compton, W. M., & Weiss, S. R. (2014). Adverse health effects of marijuana use. *New England Journal of Medicine, 370*(23), 2219–2227.

Wilkinson, S. T., & D'Souza, D. C. (2014). Problems with the medicalization of marijuana. *Journal of the American Medical Association, 311*(23), 2377–2378.

Wong, S. S., Zhou, B., Goebert, D., & Hishinuma, E. S. (2013). The risk of adolescent suicide across patterns of drug use: A nationally representative study of high school students in the United States from 1999 to 2009. *Social Psychiatry & Psychiatric Epidemiology, 48*(10), 1611–1620.

Recommended Readings

American Nurses Association. (2018). *The opioid epidemic: The evolving role of nursing* (pp. 1–14). Silver Spring, MD: Author.

Gilvarry, E. (2013). Limited evidence: Many pitfalls. *Addiction, 108*(5), 846–847.

Goudreau, K. A., & Smolenski, M.C. (2014). *Health policy and advanced practice nursing.* New York, NY: Springer.

Graham, K. M. (2006). Evaluating addictions treatment in light of scriptures. *Journal of Christian Nursing, 23*(2), 18–24.

Guohua, L., Brady, J. E., & Chen, Q. (2013). Drug use and fatal motor vehicle crashes: A case-control study. *Accident Analysis and Prevention, 60,* 205–210.

Hels, T., Lyckegaard, A., Simonsen, K. W., Steentoft, A., & Bernhoft, I. M. (2013). Risk of severe driver injury by driving with psychoactive substances. *Accident Analysis and Prevention, 59,* 346–356.

National Institute on Drug Abuse. (2018). Opioid summaries by state. Retrieved from https://www.drugabuse.gov/drugs-abuse/opioids/opioid-summaries-by-state

Welsh, J. W., Rappaport, N., & Tretyak, V. (December 2017/January 2018). The opioid epidemic: 7 things educators need to know. *Educational Leadership, 75*(4), 18–22.

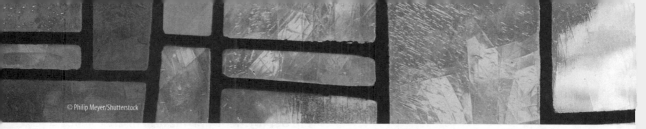

© Philip Meyer/Shutterstock

CHAPTER 16

The Role of the Nurse in Disaster Response

Jill McElheny, DNP, APRN, CPNP, ENP-BC

LEARNING OBJECTIVES

At the end of this chapter, the reader will be able to:

1. Describe the deployment process for disaster response nurses.
2. Discuss discernment of the call to work as a disaster response nurse.
3. Identify aspects of cultural accommodation necessary to provide relief in international medical disasters.
4. List teamwork skills necessary for all team members working in medical disasters.
5. Explain the process of prioritization of patients and tasks while working in a medical disaster.
6. Discuss the importance of sustainable relief when providing care in medical disasters.

KEY TERMS

Debriefing	Displacement	Triage
Deployment	Prioritization	
Disaster	Sustainable relief	

Nurses can minister to others in a variety of ways by working in disaster settings. A **disaster** can be defined by the acronymic paradigm developed by the American Medical Association to assist in organizing the response to a mass-casualty incident ("Disaster," 2012):

D: disaster

I: incident command

S: scene security and safety

A: assess hazards

S: support

T: triage and treatment

E: evacuation

R: recovery

Medical disasters may include the response by medical personnel to a natural disaster, such as an earthquake, fire, hurricane, or flood, as well as the response to an epidemic spread of disease.

The role of the nurse in a disaster response includes discernment in identifying the call for deployment, cultural accommodation for populations receiving care, teamwork, and prioritization skills to provide sustainable relief to vulnerable populations affected by disasters (**FIGURE 16-1**).

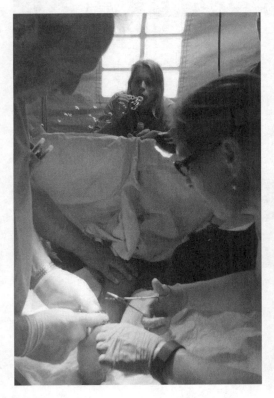

FIGURE 16-1 Teamwork is essential in medical missions: Donald Nixon, Maranatha Weeks, and Jill McElheny, Ecuador, 2016.

▶ Deployment

The **deployment** of a medical disaster team happens quickly, and it requires the nurse to be readily available to respond to the call (**FIGURE 16-2**). In most situations, relief organizations send an assessment team to the site of a disaster within 12 to 24 hours. The assessment team assesses the extent of the disaster and determines the immediate needs for relief. In developing countries, limited medical resources may be available to provide care for extensive injuries in the mass casualties accompanying a disaster. The assessment team works closely with government and health officials in countries affected by disasters to quickly develop a plan for medical relief. Depending on the type of disaster, a plan for deployment of medical professionals is developed.

A typical initial response team may consist of medical providers, anesthesia providers, surgical technicians, and nurses. Following the 2010 earthquake in Haiti, this author was deployed as part of one of the first medical disaster response teams within a few days of the earthquake. Due to the large number of orthopedic injuries, our team consisted of two orthopedic surgeons, two anesthesiologists, a

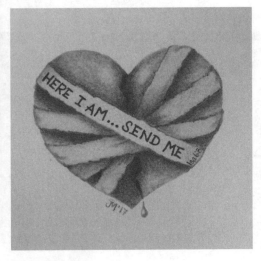

FIGURE 16-2 Deployment: the call.
Artwork by Joany McDougall.

family physician, two nurse practitioners, a paramedic, and five registered nurses. Our disaster relief organization partnered with a local hospital to provide care for hundreds of patients injured in the earthquake.

The Call

The deployment call for the disaster response nurse may come with little or no warning. Healthcare members who have special training in providing relief in disasters are included on a call list, and they may be placed on "standby" following a disaster. If the skills of a team member are deemed necessary for a specific disaster response, those members will receive a call to deploy, often within 24 hours or less. This type of call can be daunting, especially for nurses who have carefully scheduled lives. It is important for the nurse working in disaster response settings to prepare employers, family members, and others for the possibility that an unscheduled deployment for as long as 2 to 3 weeks may be necessary.

The Christian nurse receiving the call for disaster deployment must be able to quickly discern if he or she is called to serve in the specific disaster. In Luke 5:27, Jesus said to Levi, "Follow me." He does not say, "Follow me if . . ." or "Follow me when . . ." His simple instructions are to get up and go! This verse was revealed to me after I received my first disaster deployment call in 2010. I did not have the details arranged for my emergency department shifts to be covered, for my children to be picked up from school, or for any of my other responsibilities. Responding to the disaster required me literally to "follow Him," and to prayerfully trust in His divine foresight as I was called to serve for an undetermined length of time in the disaster-stricken country of Haiti.

Maranatha Weeks, a fellow disaster response nurse and team member with my disaster relief organization, describes her calling to disaster response nursing: "God's plan unfolds, and He transformed my heart. In Jeremiah 1:5, He told Jeremiah that He ordained him a prophet long before he was born. Paul was inspired to tell us to 'run the race that is set before us' (Hebrews 12:1), not the race that we set before us." Kelly Sites, also a fellow disaster team nurse, advises nurses to be "always abiding in Christ" so that they are ready to discern the call for medical disaster deployment.

▶ Cultural Accommodation

Cultural Care and Nursing Theory

Many disasters occur in foreign countries whose cultures differ in their beliefs, customs, and practices from the cultures of the teams deployed to provide medical disaster relief. It is essential to be aware of these cultural differences so as to provide the best care for populations affected by disasters.

Madeline Leininger's theory of culture care diversity and universality (Leininger, 1988) was developed to establish a substantive knowledge base to guide nurses in discovery and use of transcultural nursing practices (Smith & Parker, 2015). Leininger believed that differences in culture greatly affect the way that nurses are able to provide adequate care to patients with diverse beliefs and customs that differed from the nurses' own beliefs and customs. Fears, resistance to health personnel, misunderstandings, misdiagnoses, and frustrations are all too often observed as nurses care for patients of diverse backgrounds (Smith & Parker, 2015).

Leininger identified three nursing concepts that achieve culturally congruent care for patients: cultural preservation or maintenance, cultural care accommodation or negotiation, and cultural care repatterning or restructuring (Petiprin, 2016). Her culture care theory defines nursing as a profession that focuses on care to support patients in a culturally sensitive way (Petiprin, 2016). This theory closely aligns with the challenges encountered in the field while caring for patients in international disaster settings. In this chapter, the author will share some of her experiences, focusing on the cultural challenges faced while working in Haiti following the devastating earthquake in 2010.

On January 12, 2010, a 7.0-magnitude earthquake struck the Caribbean island of Haiti, resulting in catastrophic damage to most buildings and homes, an estimated 316,000 deaths, more than 300,000 injuries, and the displacement of more than 1.3 million Haitian people (DesRoches, Comerio, Eberhard, Mooney, & Rix, 2011). The country's infrastructure was severely compromised; many aspects of it had often been described as nonexistent even prior to the earthquake, which further compounded the effects of the disaster. With an unstable and unsupportive government, Haiti is the poorest country in the Western Hemisphere and home to some of the most dangerous slums in the world (DesRoches et al., 2011).

Our medical disaster teams were assembled and deployed within a few days after the initial disaster assessment. Because most of the hospitals in and around the capital city of Port au Prince were badly damaged, our teams began working in an undamaged hospital approximately 40 miles away on a mountain outside of the city. We were able to secure two operating rooms and approximately 100 inpatient beds in that hospital. Hundreds of injured patients were transported from Port au Prince to the hospital by the U.S. 82nd Airborne in military helicopters. Numerous strong aftershocks occurred in the days following the earthquake, making the rescue of trapped and injured individuals, along with the recovery of those killed, very difficult.

Cultural Challenges

Amidst the immediate trauma and unthinkable chaos of the disaster, our medical teams began the process of triaging and caring for earthquake victims. As we began the process of caring for hundreds of severely injured patients, we encountered multiple cultural challenges. The biggest and the most obvious challenge was a language barrier. Very few members of our team were able to speak Haitian Creole, the primary language in Haiti. While some members of our team spoke French, which is similar to Haitian Creole, none was fluent in the language.

Differences in religious beliefs also presented cultural challenges with regard to providing medical relief. Haiti is a country with deeply rooted voodoo beliefs. Most Haitians believed the earthquake was a punishment—part of a voodoo curse. The same beliefs existed regarding illness and injury, which often prevented Haitians from seeking medical care. Many Haitians believe illness and injury occur as a result of poor life choices.

Many of the patients we received and cared for at our hospital had severe crush injuries and fractures requiring amputation of one or more limbs. While we believed that our teams were performing life-saving surgeries, many of the Haitian patients were reluctant to allow us to perform surgeries for amputation. After learning more about the Haitian culture, we came to understand the reasons behind the objections to surgical amputation, even when it was a necessary life-saving procedure. One male Haitian patient explained to us that he could not carry the large buckets required for his job if he had a lower leg amputation. Without his job, he was unsure how he would support his family. Another female Haitian patient explained that the voodoo culture in Haiti teaches most people to shun people with disabilities, believing that disabled people are cursed.

Many of the severe injuries required blood transfusions for survival; however, Haitians were reluctant to accept blood products due to their voodoo beliefs. Most were afraid of being poisoned or becoming less pure by accepting unknown blood. Additionally, there was resistance to breastfeeding the infants of injured mothers out of fear of transferring the supposed curse. Mothers also believed they should not eat certain foods after delivery, such as eggs, chicken, fruits, and vegetables, because they feared those foods would cause the breastmilk to be "bad."

▶ Application of Leininger's Culture Care Theory

Madeline Leininger's culture care theory can be applied to nursing experiences caring for patients in international disasters.

My experiences working in other countries during disasters deepened my understanding of this theory by outlining the reasons for preserving, accommodating, and restructuring culture to provide appropriate care to patients of other cultures (**CASE STUDY 16-1**). These major concepts are discussed here.

🔍 *CASE STUDY 16-1*

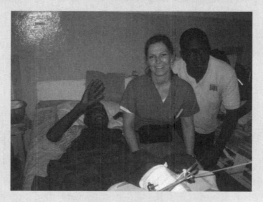

FIGURE 16-3 Jill McElheny, Haiti, 2010.

The medical disaster relief work in post-earthquake Haiti was the most difficult work that any of our teams had ever experienced. The conditions in Haiti, combined with the tremendous mass-casualty numbers, proved to be challenging for all team members.

I recall one day during my several weeks of working 18-hour days when I was completely physically, mentally, and emotionally exhausted. On this day, I was finding it difficult to be culturally sensitive to patients' needs. I felt as if I had "no more room" to hear any more of the personal horror stories or cultural accommodation requests of my patients. I believe I was working in a "survival mode" of my own, concentrating on the medically necessary skills needed to save lives that day. An older male Haitian patient and his son recognized my fatigue, and they called me to the bedside to pray for me (**FIGURE 16-3**). This act of kindness reminded me that our patients were cognizant of our efforts to accommodate them both medically and culturally.

Questions

1. What do you do when you feel you have nothing left to give to a patient, but you still need to be ministering the love of God?
2. How did you feel when reading about the act of kindness by the patient and his son who recognized Dr. McElheny's fatigue and burnout?
3. Does reading this account make you feel more or less inclined to consider international medical relief work?

Cultural Preservation/ Maintenance

Our medical disaster teams quickly recognized the need to preserve the culture of our Haitian patients as a means of respecting and maintaining their culture, fostering trust, and allowing our teams to provide the much-needed medical relief. Rather than forcing our patients to struggle with the English language, we employed several interpreters who spoke both Haitian Creole and English to assist us with communication as we worked. Most of the interpreters were former students of the university in Port au Prince who were unable to return to school after the university collapsed during the earthquake.

Cultural Care Accommodation/ Negotiation

In an effort to be sensitive to their strong voodoo beliefs and to build a relationship of trust with the Haitian patients whom our medical teams were treating, we remained respectful of their objections to medical treatments, such as blood transfusions and amputations. We explained through our Haitian Creole interpreters the necessity of blood transfusions, and all staff members on our team donated blood for transfusion purposes. We also shared our faith in Jesus Christ with these patients, and we explained that he was the reason for our medical relief efforts. Our teams ensured that all patients in our care heard the good news of the gospel, and many patients came to accept Jesus Christ as their Savior.

There was a critical shortage of blood in Haiti following the earthquake, and no refrigeration areas were available to store the blood supplied by nongovernmental organizations from outside countries. By donating and transfusing our own blood to our Haitian patients, we were able to accommodate the cultural fears regarding receiving blood, while also building trust with our Haitian patients.

Our medical teams also worked to accommodate Haitian patients who were fearful of amputation surgeries. We worked with prosthetic companies in the United States to supply prosthetic limbs for Haitians. Our lead orthopedic surgeon arranged for multiple prosthetic clinics to be held in the months following the earthquake to provide artificial limbs and, ultimately, to enable Haitians to resume working and provide for their families.

The nursing staff remained sensitive to the wishes of breastfeeding mothers by providing the specific foods requested. In extreme circumstances, when the breastfeeding mother was fearful of transferring a curse to her infant, our teams provided infant formula. This cultural accommodation was utilized only when the infant's life was endangered by lack of nutrition, as we realized that infants in Haiti were unlikely have formula consistently available to them.

Culture Care Repatterning/ Restructuring

In the weeks following the earthquake, patients were discharged from the hospital after their surgeries and other medical stabilization/ treatment. Hundreds of patients began building tent homes on the grounds around the hospital. Further investigation revealed that these patients were completely displaced. Patients reported that they had been airlifted hours away from their homes following the earthquake to receive care at our mountain hospital. Most of the patients had completely lost their homes, and their remaining possessions had been stolen by looters in the days following the earthquake. With no transportation available, and often with no homes left, patients resorted to camping out on the grounds of the hospital. They chose to stay near the hospital until their scheduled follow-up appointments and prosthetic clinics. Our organization began to employ these patients as cooks, housekeeping workers, supply room workers, and interpreters in an attempt to repattern or restructure their post-earthquake lives. Employing and supporting the surviving earthquake victims and allowing them to live and work near our hospital provided sustainable relief and encouraged appropriate follow-up health care and rehabilitation.

Our relief organization learned numerous lessons in Haiti regarding cultural care. We became more sensitive to the aftermath of our relief efforts, constantly evaluating the consequences of our efforts as we provided the initial medical disaster relief. While we were certainly focused on life-saving measures, we were also contributing to the displacement and difficult rehabilitation of our Haitian patients.

While these examples of the application of Leininger's culture care theory may be extreme, this theory can also be applied in multiple ways to nursing care in the United States. Many immigrants and culturally diverse populations seek and receive care in the United States, and healthcare providers can strive to provide cultural preservation, accommodation, and repatterning for these patients.

▶ Teamwork

Teamwork is essential to successful care following a medical disaster. All team members must have the flexibility to perform many different roles and to adapt to the rapidly changing conditions.

> Teamwork is critical when dealing with an already vulnerable population, in difficult conditions. Often on the field, we all seem to have a clear picture of what we are battling outside—whether Ebola or ISIS. There are no questions about the enemy in disaster, and therefore we run towards it. This is where the true enemy can lay seeds of bitterness, resentment, or jealousy in our hearts, as he tries to tear us down from within. Therefore, not only exhibiting Christ's love to others,

but being centered in His person, and walking in His Spirit is critical to successful teamwork. (M. Weeks, personal communication, 2018)

Skill Sets of Team Members and God's Assembly of the Team

When a disaster response team is deployed, efforts are made to assemble a group with the necessary skills to form a complete medical team. This process occurs quickly and depends on the availability of the team members on the disaster team call list. The assessment team arriving shortly after the disaster determines the medical needs of the disaster victims, and this information is communicated to the relief organization headquarters.

The necessity of teamwork becomes evident when the team arrives at the scene of a disaster (Figure 16-1). All members of the team arrive with different levels of experience and different skill sets, and all come from different clinical settings. The team members are usually unknown to each other, and they must quickly coordinate the functions of the team. God's hand is always evident in the assembly of the team: The skills of each team are divinely coordinated to perform the work needed to function as the hands and feet of Christ. "We need all experiences and backgrounds, just as we need the different members of the body." (M. Weeks, personal communication, 2018)

Revolving/Flexible Roles

All members of a medical disaster team must be willing to perform a variety of functions while working in a disaster setting. Although a nurse may have skills and experience in one area, he or she may be required to care for patients in a completely different clinical area during a disaster. Similarly, surgeons who are used to working in technologically sophisticated operating suites may be required to perform primary care duties or even basic patient care duties. A nurse who has spent the first several days of deployment working as a triage nurse may be asked to work in a medical–surgical ward or other area of the field hospital due to changes in patient flow.

Nurses as Coordinators and Leaders

Nurses working disaster settings serve as the coordinators of care and as leaders of the clinical care team. Their duties may include scheduling surgeries for the operating suite, organizing the medical staff, and reorganizing the field hospital daily based on patient flow. A charge nurse may be assigned for a longer deployment to organize the transition of medical teams on shorter deployments throughout a disaster response.

▶ Prioritization

One of the most important skills utilized in a disaster response is **prioritization** of injuries. The START (Simple Triage and Rapid Treatment) **triage** algorithm is a tool that is available to rescue personnel in case of a disaster or mass-casualty incident (Badiali, Giugni, & Marcis, 2017). **FIGURE 16-4** illustrates the elements of the START system and outlines the categories of triage injuries.

Difficult Decisions

Triage is an important management and decision-making concept in disaster settings but is often a difficult process to implement. The type of triage used in the START system was first introduced in the United States in the 1980s (Pouraghaei et al., 2017). Triage decisions can be emotionally difficult, as responders' efforts are directed toward those people who have a higher chance of survival,

leaving other, more-critical patients behind (Pouraghaei et al., 2017).

The START system is based on a color-coded system of sorting patients. The triage categories include the following:

- *Minor: green triage tag color.* Victim with relatively minor injuries; also known as "walking wounded."
- *Delayed: yellow triage tag color.* Victim's transport can be delayed; may include serious and potentially life-threatening injuries.
- *Immediate: red triage tag color.* Requires medical attention within minutes for survival (up to 60 minutes).
- *Expectant: black triage tag color.* Victim unlikely to survive given the severity of injuries, level of care available, or both; palliative care and pain relief should be provided.

Nurses working in disaster settings are faced with the difficult decision-making process of triaging patients according to these criteria. Following the earthquake of 2016 in Ecuador, multiple scenarios occurred in which decisions had to be made regarding patients in the "delayed" and "immediate" START categories. These patients required transport for higher-level or specialty care, but transport was difficult due to the road damage caused by the earthquake and its aftershocks.

Spiritual Support

Christian nurses can provide palliative care and spiritual support to patients who may fall into the "expectant" (black tag) category of triage. Joany McDougall, a registered nurse, recalls the process of caring for expectant patients in an emergency field hospital on the border of Mosul, Iraq:

> As patients arrive at the hospital, we use a color-coded triage system to determine the severity and numbers

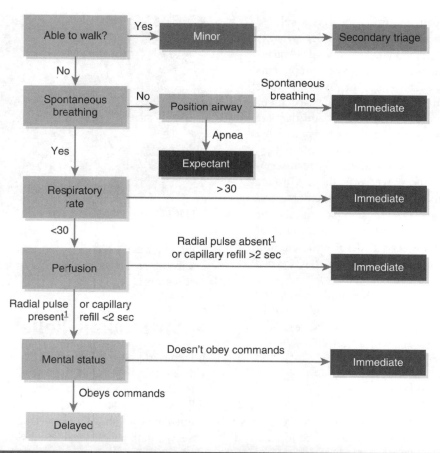

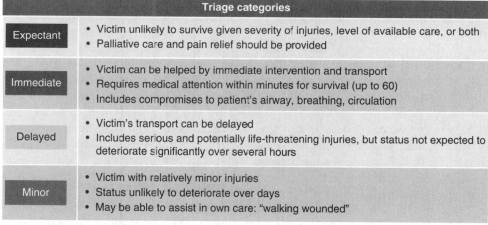

FIGURE 16-4 START algorithm for adults.

of patients. Everyone gets a colored ribbon tied around his/her wrist. A black ribbon means either dead on arrival or expectant. Expectant patients are still alive, but the severity of their wounds goes beyond our capacity or resources to treat them and they are expected to die. It was our policy that no matter what, no one in our hospital would die alone. We read scripture and prayed over them. We sang to them. We cried over them. We held them. These Muslim patients saw the light of Christ in us, and the hope that we carried despite the circumstances. We told them that we had simply come because we had Jesus in our heart. They understood, and many patients were overwhelmed by the love and respect they were shown. (Personal communication)

▶ Displacement

Victims of disaster are often moved quickly to different areas to receive care for their injuries and illnesses. This movement may result in **displacement**. The infrastructure of Haiti was minimal even before the earthquake, which exacerbated the effects of the displacement that occurred following this event. Specifically, without the necessary infrastructure, it was difficult for families to reunite following the disaster.

The youngest victims of disaster displacement are children (**FIGURE 16-5**). Thousands of children in Haiti became orphans because of the earthquake—many due to the deaths of their parents, but others because of displacement. Children who were at school at the time of the earthquake or younger children who had parents at work were never reunited in the chaos during the days and months that followed. Those who are declared orphans because the whereabouts of their parents is

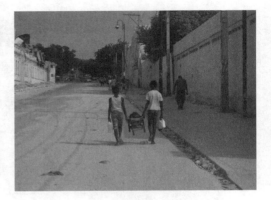

FIGURE 16-5 Displacement: orphans on the streets.

unknown after a disaster may continue to be disadvantaged, being unable to be adopted for that reason.

▶ Sustainable Relief

It is important for relief organizations to provide **sustainable relief** to victims of disaster. It is difficult for victims to continue to recover following a disaster if the care provided is only immediate care and does not support full recovery. Examples of sustainable relief may include both medical care and other types of support (**BOXES 16-1** and **16-2**). Patients who have received surgery or other types of care, such as sutures, casting, or medical device placement, may require follow-up care to ensure they have optimal chances of recovery. Victims of disaster who have lost their homes, jobs, and food supply may require construction, economic, and agricultural support to aid in their overall recovery.

Follow-Up Care

Medical care provided to victims during the days, weeks, and months following the disaster is essential. Diseases and epidemics can result in populations affected by disaster and subsequent displacement. Follow-up clinics in the aftermath of a disaster can provide much-needed

---

BOX 16-1 Research Highlight

The training of nurses for disaster relief is quite limited in China. These researchers interviewed 12 registered nurses (RNs) who participated in medical assistance teams after two earthquakes in China. Narrative inquiry methods were used to extract their individual stories and themes. "Five themes emerged: *unbeatable challenges*; qualities of a disaster nurse; *mental health and trauma*; poor *disaster planning* and co-ordination; and *urgently needed disaster education*" (p. 75). Participants noted the lack of preparedness of nurses to meet the challenges of mass casualties and disaster relief. They encouraged China to examine the need for nursing education in this specialized area.

Reprinted from Wenji, Z., Turale, S., Stone, T. E., & Petrini, M. A. (2015). Chinese nurses' relief experiences following two earthquakes: Implications for disaster education and policy development. *Nurse Education in Practice, 15*(1), 75–81. Copyright © 2015, with permission from Elsevier.

BOX 16-2 Evidence-Based Practice Focus

Nurses are often called upon to respond to mass disasters, whether natural or human-made. However, most nurses do not receive any formal education on this topic in their basic training. This article "presents a curriculum blueprint for nurse educators that provides readers with best practices for implementation while avoiding pitfalls and mistakes." Written by two disaster preparation nurse experts with many years of real-world experience, the curriculum aims to "help ensure that nursing students are prepared to respond to disasters, whether in their own neighborhoods or around the world, by giving nurse educators strategies and solutions for incorporating disaster preparedness" into their basic nursing education.

Modified from Veenema, T. G. (2016). Designing and integrating a disaster preparedness curriculum: Readying nurses for the worst. *Journal of Radiology Nursing, 35*(1), 65.

---

medical support for patients requiring post-surgical care. Education and prophylaxis to prevent the spread of disease can help thwart the onset of epidemics in nations whose infrastructure is damaged by disaster. The cholera epidemic following the Haiti earthquake is an example of how education could have prevented the rapid spread of a deadly disease.

▶ Debriefing

Nurses who work in disaster settings require **debriefing** to process their experiences. A debriefing session with a group of team members encourages those who have been exposed to stressful events to share their experiences and seeks to prevent long-term problems (Samaritan's Purse, 2015). Group debriefing should be a safe place for all members to share without criticism or judgment, and all shared information should remain confidential. Positive aspects of the disaster should be discussed along with the difficult topics.

The Multiple Stressor Debriefing (MSD) model was developed for debriefing of team members at the end of a disaster relief response (Samaritan's Purse, 2015). It includes four phases:

1. Disclosure of events: The purpose, rules, and phases of the session should be outlined; each member shares one or two distressing events.
2. Feelings and reaction: Discussion of thoughts and feelings.

3. Coping strategies: Discussion of coping strategies.
4. Termination: Discussion of the transition back to home life.

Although team members may be tempted to avoid debriefing after the conclusion of a disaster response or may discount this process, it is essential for team members to process events with other team members who have experienced similar situations and events during the disaster response. It is sometimes difficult to identify positive aspects of a disaster response, and nurses have often struggled to understand the purpose of mass casualty. A verse that speaks to this is Isaiah 55:8: "For my thoughts are not your thoughts, neither are your ways my ways."

▶ Conclusion

Nurses called to serve in disaster response can be assured that God will comfort them, just as they have comforted others (**BOXES 16-3** and **16-4**). This is an area of unique ministry, and one to which a nurse must feel decidedly called.

BOX 16-3 Outstanding Nurse Leader: Kristen Dirks, MSN, RN, FNP

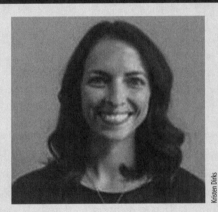
Kristen Dirks

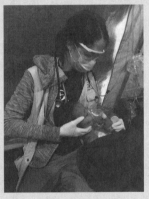
Kristen Dirks

Kristen served in a disaster field hospital in Iraq on the border of Mosul in 2018. She shares her account of the difficult decisions regarding prioritization of injuries and dealing with death in disasters.

The ER/trauma unit was busy as usual at 5 p.m. I walked in as a radio call went out that six children would be coming in. I heard a patient was being tagged black, which means death is imminent. I immediately went to the stretcher and saw it was a young girl: no name, about six or seven years old. She had a large shrapnel wound to her brain with no exit. I helped carry her to our area where patients are expectant. Another nurse and I made her as comfortable as we could and gave her medicine to help relax her breathing.

I heard, "We have another code black coming, Kristen." I looked on the other side of the curtain and they handed me a three-year-old child, about the same size as my three-year-old daughter. She also had an injury to the brain with no exit, as well as several other wounds. I held her, rocked her, and pushed her hair curls back. I tried to make her comfortable with medication.

The other nurse and I began singing over these two girls. As if out of thin air, a staff member produced a guitar and led us in singing worship songs over these two angels. The three-year-old passed quickly. We were told the two were sisters; the other four children were their cousins. We placed the three-year-old on the stretcher next to us, and then I helped hold the older sister. We continued singing praises over her. It felt surreal to have a lifeless child on one end of the stretcher and to be praying over her sister that Jesus would take her quickly. After more than two hours, she was still breathing. Several staff came by and told us to take a break, so we did. As soon as I stepped away, I felt everything hit me at once, what I was actually doing—ushering little souls into God's arms. We went back to the child, and she was still alive. We washed her and got her comfortable again. She passed away at 2:17 a.m. with myself and another nurse holding her.

My heart and head felt better after some rest. We had a debriefing and discussed how to walk through this experience. I can't help but think what the world has lost with each one of these deaths. I have had six patients die in my arms or in my care. What were they contributing in this world that we will no longer have? Who were those children going to grow up to be?

Pure evil has a face. It is dropping mortars on children and attempting to take innocent lives early. Evil wants the light of the world gone, and what better way than to wipe out a generation of hope that comes with children's dreams and laughter. But what prevails over darkness? LIGHT. We are the light in this dark place. Singing hymns over a dying child and ushering her into God's arms is looking at evil and not letting it win. It has no rule or reign within these walls.

BOX 16-4   Outstanding Nurse Leader: Joany McDougall, RN

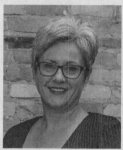

Joany McDougall

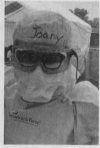

Joany McDougall

Joany served in the Ebola treatment center in the Democratic Republic of the Congo (DRC) in 2019. She shares her account of the cultural accommodations and difficult working conditions as she treated patients during the Ebola epidemic.

> Fear not fear, for I have redeemed you: I have called you by your name: you are mine. When you pass through the waters, I will be with you; And through the rivers, they shall not overflow you; When you walk through the fire, you shall not be burned; Nor shall the flame scorch you. (Isaiah 43:1–2)

Ebola is an ugly disease, and my prayer was that God would wipe it from the planet. But, if in His will, He chose not to eradicate the disease, then it was my fervent prayer that He would use me in some capacity to help the people of the DRC in their fight. It was a "Here I am, send me" moment. Our team would be running into the fire, and we would not be overcome, scorched, or burned.

Weighing heavily on my mind was the fact that I had not yet done a trial run of being in personal protective equipment (PPE) in the heat of the day. I was finding the heat and humidity almost unbearable under regular circumstances: How would I ever manage in full PPE? I would be a failure to what God had called me here to do, to my colleagues, and most importantly to those whom I had come to serve. It was a fear that I kept to myself; it would stay between God and me.

Finally, the day came. We would do a full PPE rehearsal, completing assigned tasks, and

(continues)

BOX 16-4 Outstanding Nurse Leader: Joany McDougall, RN   *(continued)*

then proceed to doffing as though it were the real thing. That morning, in devotions, we talked about how we all needed to be honest with ourselves about our doubts "in this, Ebola." We would all need to find ways for our faith to be strengthened. I remember praying, "Okay, God, this fear I have been carrying has been between You and me. Please, please, I know You have given me Your strength before. I need You to do it again."

Our rehearsal was challenging, but it went very well. I breathed a small sigh of relief—but that relief was to be short-lived. At noon, an ambulance arrived unannounced. Receiving an ambulance requires donning full PPE. There was much confusion from the driver as to who he had in the back of the ambulance. Once the doors were finally able to be opened, we found a family of five. It was determined that the four-year-old child was ill. Once we were able to get the family out of the ambulance, it became clear that this child was critically ill.

We had now been out in the direct high-noon sun for about 30 minutes. I was starting to feel unwell, and my fears were creeping in. We still had triage work to do and were still having difficulty communicating with the family. Waves of nausea started in me while we were negotiating who would stay with the child, explaining all the while that they were at significant risk if the child, in fact, did have

Ebola. I had to make a conscious effort to slow my breathing, and my heart rate was about 140. Again, the waves of nausea came and with them the fear that I might actually vomit in my suit.

We were able to get the child into a room and start the admission. I was able to get his armband on and then turned to get the blood draw bag ready. Again, the nausea returned. I was now becoming a risk to my coworkers and had no choice but to tap out and proceed to the doffing tent as quickly and carefully as possible. That was the longest, loneliest walk of my life. I was fighting the nausea with every fiber of my being, and panic was starting to set in. The first spray of chlorine in the doffing tent has an immediate cooling effect and the relief was welcomed, but I was in no way out of the woods. With each layer I removed came disappointment, failure, and tears. I had walked away from a dying child because I wasn't strong enough to handle the PPE in the heat. Another had to go in my place to do what I could not, and my heart was breaking for this dying child and his family. To use the words from the verse I had written on the day of my departure, I felt burned and scorched. The fear that I had kept between myself and God was now out there for all to see, and my heart was utterly shattered. My shift was now over and I would not get another opportunity, ever, to care for that child. He went into the arms of Jesus two hours later.

Praise be to the God and Father of our Lord Jesus Christ, the Father of compassion and the God of all comfort, who comforts us in all our troubles, so that we can comfort those in any trouble with the comfort we ourselves receive from God. For just as we share abundantly in the sufferings of Christ, so also our comfort abounds through Christ. If we are distressed, it is for your comfort and salvation; if we are comforted, it is for your comfort, which produces in you patient endurance of the same sufferings we suffer.

And our hope for you is firm, because we know that just as you share in our sufferings, so also you share in our comfort. (2 Corinthians 1:3–7)

▶ Clinical Reasoning Exercises

1.   How would you practice cultural accommodation when caring for patients in a disaster with special dietary preferences?

2. What level of triage would a patient be who arrives with an absent radial pulse and/or capillary refill more than 2 seconds?

3. What is the purpose of debriefing, and why is it important?

4. While working in an emergency field hospital following a disaster, you have developed an efficient system with other team members providing care in the medical–surgical ward. The charge nurse suddenly reassigns you to the operating suite due to the increased number of surgical patients that day. How do you respond?

▶ Personal Reflection Exercises

1. In what ways could you prepare your heart to hear the call for disaster deployment?

2. How can you provide spiritual support to patients of different religious beliefs?

3. Ponder these questions posed by Marantha Weeks (2018): "Do we do the best for the most amount of people, or do we close early and provide more quality care for less people? Do we pour limited resources into a child who may well not survive, or do we let him go after the first steps taken are not deemed successful? We have one ventilator left, and a mom and a 16-year-old boy who both need it. Their conditions are the same. Who gets it? The other may die."

4. How do you interpret this verse in the light of the serving in mass disasters: "Behold, he who keeps Israel will neither slumber nor sleep. The Lord is your keeper; the Lord is your shade on your right hand. The sun shall not strike you by day, nor the moon by night. The Lord will keep you from all evil; he will keep your life. The Lord will keep your going out and your coming in from this time forth and forevermore" (Psalm 121:4).

References

Badiali, S., Giugni, A., & Marcis, L. (2017). Testing the START triage protocol: Can it improve the ability of nonmedical personnel to better triage patients during disasters and mass casualties incidents? *Disaster Medicine and Public Health Preparedness, 11*(3), 305–309.

DesRoches, R., Comerio, M., Eberhard, M., Mooney, W., & Rix, G. J. (2011). Overview of the 2010 Haiti earthquake. *Earthquake Spectra, 27*, S1–S21. Retrieved from http://escweb.wr.usgs.gov/share/mooney/142.pdf

Disaster. (2012). In *Medical Dictionary for the Health Professions and Nursing*. Retrieved from https://medical-dictionary.thefreedictionary.com/disaster

Leininger, M. M. (1988). Leininger's theory of nursing: Cultural care diversity and universality. *Nursing Science Quarterly, 1*(4), 152–160.

Petiprin, A. (2016). Leininger's culture care theory. Retrieved from http://www.nursing-theory.org/theories-and-models/leininger-culture-care-theory.php

Pouraghaei, M., Tabrizi, J. S., Moharamzadeh, P., Ghafori, R. R., Rahmani, F., & Mirfakhraei, B. N. (2017). The effect of START triage education on knowledge and practice of emergency medical technicians in disasters. *Journal of Caring Sciences, 6*(2), 119.

Samaritan's Purse. (2015). Disaster assistance response team (DART) manual. Boone, NC: Author.

Smith, M. C, & Parker, M. E. (2015). *Nursing theories and nursing practice* (4th ed.). Philadelphia, PA: F. A. Davis Company.

Weeks, M. (2018). *From the plains of Nineveh: A nurse on the front lines of Mosul*. (n.p.): Author.

Recommended Readings

Bhalla, M. C., Frey, J., Rider, C., Nord, M., & Hegerhorst, M. (2015). Simple triage algorithm and rapid treatment and sort, assess, lifesaving, interventions, treatment, and transportation mass casualty triage methods for sensitivity, specificity, and predictive values. *American Journal of Emergency Medicine, 33*(11), 1687–1691.

Leininger, M. M., & McFarland, M. R. (2002). *Transcultural nursing: Concepts, theories, research and practice*. New York, NY: McGraw-Hill.

McFarland, M. R., & Wehbe-Alamah, H. B. (2014). *Leininger's culture care diversity and universality*. Burlington, MA: Jones & Bartlett Learning.

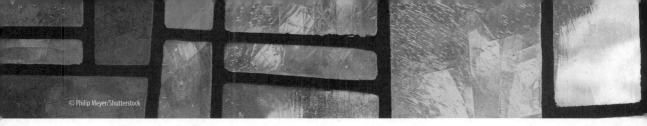

CHAPTER 17

Nursing Care at End-of-Life

Luana S. Krieger-Blake, BA, MSW, LCSW

LEARNING OBJECTIVES

At the end of this chapter, the reader will be able to:

1. Identify the options for care of a person who is at end-of-life.
2. Understand the various dynamics and adjustments that affect a patient who is dying.
3. Recognize the components of a hospice or palliative care team.
4. Appreciate the characteristics of a good death.
5. Evaluate one's interest in hospice nursing as a faith-based career.

KEY TERMS

Advance directives	Hospice care	Patient driven
Good death	Palliative care	Presence

I n my experience as a long-time hospice social worker, I encountered many nurses who said, upon becoming hospice nurses, something like this: "This is what I believe nursing is all about: holistic care in a setting that is conducive to quality patient care, with attention paid to not only the physical aspects of the patient's disease and care needs, but also their psychosocial and spiritual needs—and not just those of the patient, but also of the family." I also encountered many people from the community who often said, "It takes someone really special to work in hospice care."

I have come to believe that a certain degree of "special" truly is involved in being a good caregiver at end-of-life. This "special" includes a comfort with the concept of dying as a natural part of living, the ability to offer oneself as a **presence** to the dying patient and the family members and caregivers who are along on the journey, and the personal acquisition of a level of self-care and support that permits one to continue offering that presence over an extended period of time. Based on my more than 25 years in the field, my impression is that faith-based nurses are often (but not always) more comfortable with this type of work, leaning on their faith, which helps shape their concept of living and dying, and finding personal supports through people around them who share the faith and the belief in the "mission" that carries them from day to day.

This chapter discusses the options for end-of-life care, focusing specifically on hospice care. The nurse has a very important role in hospice care as the case manager.

▶ Care Options at End-of-Life

When faced with news that a medical condition is potentially life-ending, patients and families are required to make choices as to the focus and extent of the medical care sought. Medical personnel—doctors and nurses—are required to outline the treatments, side effects, and long-term expectations of each type of treatment.

Acute and Active Treatment

One option is to continue acute and active treatment for as long as possible. Some patients and their families want to be able to say that they "did all that could be done to save the patient's life." These care choices are focused on cure and "doing everything possible" regardless of outcome. This option frequently requires stays or visits at the hospital or treatment center/clinic care for a wide range of ongoing treatments. A patient may choose this option when he or she wants to be able to say, "I did everything I could to fight this illness!"

Palliative Care

Another option may be **palliative care**, which is often appropriate for both terminal and nonterminal conditions. Palliative care is usually provided to those patients with life-limiting illnesses who are not actively dying and not ready for hospice. Some define this period as roughly two years from end-of-life. Some of the diagnoses associated with palliative care include end-stage chronic obstructive pulmonary disease (COPD), end-stage dementia, cancers of certain types, congestive heart failure (CHF), end-stage renal disease (ESRD), amyotrophic lateral sclerosis (ALS), and Parkinson's disease.

Palliative care focuses on assuring the patient's comfort, with additional support of a team of medical professionals for the patient and the family/caregivers—including spiritual and psychosocial support. Treatment focuses not on a cure, but rather on comfort. It emphasizes the management of common symptoms such as pain, shortness of breath, anxiety, fatigue, nausea, constipation, trouble sleeping, and lack of appetite.

This type of professionally guided comfort care may sometimes be combined with ongoing curative treatment. For example, a patient in palliative care may receive antibiotics for pneumonia, or radiation to shrink a tumor if it relieves pain. However, whether palliative care is covered by Medicare or private insurance depends on one's treatment plan and benefit coverage, so certain restrictions will apply (National Institute on Aging, 2017). In contrast, hospice is covered by Medicare.

Palliative care is often chosen by the patient who says, "I am not ready to say 'no more treatments,' but I definitely need some improvement in my physical comfort as well as more support for my family." Palliative care can be hospital based or provided through clinic care, in facility-based programs such as a nursing home, or via in-home care programs (**BOX 17-1**). The focus is on improving quality of life. It is frequently used as a bridge between active/curative care and hospice care.

BOX 17-1 Research Highlight

The purpose of this study was to examine the effect of palliative care consultation (mainly done by nurse practitioners) on transitions at end-of-life. The authors looked at multiple outcomes in nursing home residents who died between 2006 and 2010. Those residents who had palliative care consultations had lower hospitalizations than the control group. Those participants who had initial palliative care consultations within 8 to 30 days before death had a significantly decreased hospitalization rate in the last week of life than those with initial consultations 61 to 180 days before death. The researchers concluded that palliative care consultations improve end-of-life care for nursing home residents by reducing hospitalizations and decreasing the burden of care transitions.

Modified from Miller, S. C., Lima, J. C., Intrator, O., Martin, E., Bull, J., & Hanson, L. C. (2016). Palliative care consultations in nursing homes and reductions in acute care use and potentially burdensome end-of-life transitions. *Journal of the American Geriatrics Society, 64*(11), 2280–2287.

Hospice Care

Hospice care is specialized care for persons who are living with a life-ending illness, with death expected to occur within six months if the illness takes its usual course. The focus is on comfort, not cure, and the patient and family/caregivers are considered the unit of care. Hospice patients forgo additional curative measures and hospitalizations, utilizing the additional supports of a hospice team to receive care at home—wherever home might be. Hospice may be provided in patient/family homes, extended-care facilities, assisted-living units, some prisons, and specialized hospice centers or units. Hospice care is covered by Medicare, Medicaid, and most other medical insurance plans. It is paid on a per-diem basis, versus a per-intervention charge. The remainder of this chapter focuses on hospice care.

When a cure is not possible, hospice is often the choice for end-of-life care. This decision can be made with confidence if the advance care discussions have been held and documents are in place stating the patient's desires for comfort care. In 2016, approximately 1.2 million Medicare recipients were admitted to hospice care and were served by 4382 Medicare-certified hospices (National Hospice and Palliative Care Organization [NHPCO], 2017). By comparison, approximately 1.7 million people all together

(Medicare and non-Medicare) received hospice care in 2015 (NHPCO, 2017). When the patient makes this choice, the family and caregivers also continue the journey right along with the patient and are formally recognized as the hospice "unit of care."

The National Hospice and Palliative Care Organization has developed a formally recognized philosophy of hospice care:

Hospice provides support and care for persons in the last phases of an incurable disease so that they may live as fully and as comfortably as possible. Hospice recognizes that the dying process is a part of the normal process of living and focuses on enhancing the quality of remaining life. Hospice affirms life and neither hastens nor postpones death. Hospice exists in the hope and belief that through appropriate care, and the promotion of a caring community sensitive to their needs that individuals and their families may be free to attain a degree of satisfaction in preparation for death. Hospice recognizes that human growth and development can be a lifelong process. Hospice seeks to preserve and promote the inherent potential for growth within individuals and families during the last phase of life. Hospice offers palliative care for all individuals and their families without regard to age, gender, nationality, race, creed, sexual orientation, disability, diagnosis, availability of a primary caregiver, or ability to pay.

Hospice programs provide state-of-the-art palliative care and supportive services to individuals at the end of their lives, their family members and significant others, 24 hours a day, seven days a week, in both the home and facility-based care settings. Physical, social, spiritual, and emotional care are provided by a clinically-directed interdisciplinary team consisting of patients and their families, professionals, and volunteers during the last stages of an illness, the dying process and bereavement period. (Reprinted with permission from NHPCO, 2000, para. 6)

▶ History of the Hospice Movement

The word *hospice* dates from medieval times, with its original meaning being "shelter and rest on a long journey for weary travelers." The term was first used to describe specialized care for dying patients by Dame Cecily Saunders in 1948. Dr. Saunders was first a nurse, then trained as a social worker, and then as a medical doctor. She founded the first hospice, St. Christopher's,

in London in 1967 to provide comfort care to the dying. Saunders promoted the principle of dying with dignity and maintained that death is a natural process that can be eased by sensitive nursing and effective pain control.

Saunders's pioneering work and philosophy of care brought her to Yale University in the United States in 1968, where she lectured about this new type of care to medical students, nurses, social workers, and chaplains. Her visit and the awareness that her ideology offered a better alternative for the terminally ill subsequently precipitated the founding of the first hospice in the United States by Florence Wald in 1974, in Hartford, Connecticut. This first program was developed by volunteers and included an interdisciplinary team. As the public began to accept the hospice concept of "a better way to die," the ideas spread nationwide (**BOX 17-2**).

In 1978, the U.S. Department of Health Education and Welfare determined that the hospice movement was worthy of federal support as part of an effort to provide more humane care for the dying, while possibly reducing costs of medical care at end-of-life. In 1986, the U.S. Congress included provisional coverage for hospice services as part of the Medicare program, for hospices certified to provide such care. This hospice benefit proved so successful that it was made permanent a year or two prior to the original target date. States were also given the option to provide hospice care under their Medicaid benefits. Hospice care was made available to nursing home residents in this banner year.

BOX 17-2 Facts About Hospice

- In 2007, a study in *Journal of Pain and Symptom Management* showed hospice patients lived an average of 29 days longer than comparable patients without hospice care.
- In 2007, another study in *Journal of Pain and Symptom Management* showed that hospices saved money for Medicare, while bringing quality care to patients and families.
- In 2016, the number of hospice volunteers continued to grow, with more than 550,000 people serving as volunteers in the United States.

In 1993, hospice was confirmed as a nationally guaranteed benefit, and an accepted part of the healthcare continuum.

▶ Advance Care Planning

Advance care planning is inherent to development of the patient-/family-driven plan of care found in hospice. Nurses and other professional care staff need to recognize that they may be involved in difficult discussions with patients and families related to disease progression and decline. They may also be required to educate patients and family members about choices for ongoing care.

Advance care planning entails making decisions about the care one would want to receive if one became unable to speak for oneself. The decisions are the patient's to make whenever possible and are based on personal values, preferences, and discussions with loved ones. Such decisions tell family, friends, and healthcare providers about the patient's wishes about continuing or withdrawing medical treatments at the end-of-life. Families are often in a state of confusion, perhaps denial, and general disarray when faced with a diagnosis of terminal illness for their loved one. Because the patient should be in charge of decision making to the greatest extent possible at this difficult time, it is important to ensure that the patient has a "voice" throughout the course of his or her illness. That voice is legally heard via choices made and documented in **advance directives** (**BOXES 17-3** and **17-4**). Patients should legally define their wishes by use of the advance directives accepted in their state of residence.

Since January 1, 2016, advance care planning between physician and patient has been eligible for reimbursement under the Medicare Physician Fee Schedule and Hospital Outpatient Prospective Payment systems. These discussions do *not* lead to the commonly feared "death panels" that were publicized at the time of implementation of the law; they *do* lead to improved patient–physician communication and understanding. Legal forms, whose availability is mandated by the national Patient Self-Determination Act of 1990 (American Cancer Society, 2016) and that is accepted by each state of residence, are available.

Communicating end-of-life wishes is important because these decisions are deeply personal and are based on each person's unique set of values and beliefs. It is essential for the

---

BOX 17-3 Types of Advance Directives

Living will: Specifies the extent of care desired by a patient if diagnosed with a terminal illness.

Durable power of attorney for health care/health care representative (DPOA/ HCR): States the person who is designated by the patient to make healthcare decisions, sign papers, receive information from medical personnel, and admit the patient to healthcare services if the patient is unable to do so.

Durable power of attorney (POA) (for financial/business issues): Names someone to serve as proxy under specific terms; often part of a greater plan for distribution of assets, trust account development, and property management.

Physician order for life-sustaining treatment/physician order for scope of treatment (POLST/POST): A medical order, signed by a physician, that instructs emergency personnel on which actions to take while a patient is still at home, before emergency treatment is given; it contains sections on cardiopulmonary resuscitation (CPR), medical interventions, antibiotics, and artificially administered nutrition. It was developed primarily for seriously ill persons likely to be in the last year of life.

Do not resuscitate (DNR): An order that instructs healthcare providers not to perform CPR if a patient's breathing stops or the heart stops beating; it is used in hospitals.

(continues)

BOX 17-3 Types of Advance Directives   *(continued)*

Out-of-hospital do not resuscitate (OOH-DNR): A medical order that instructs persons not to initiate CPR for a person at home; in a nursing home, hospice, or assisted-living center; or somewhere other than the hospital.

Life-prolonging procedures: States that a person wants to be actively treated and "kept going" for as long as possible, even if treatment is futile; *contraindicated in hospice care.*

Additional documents specific to healthcare wishes are available to complete the full range of documents dealing with end-of-life:

- *Five Wishes:* A clearly written document that enables the person to designate his or her wishes for (1) the person I want to make decisions for me when I can't, (2) the kind of medical treatment I want or don't want, (3) how comfortable I want to be, (4) how I want people to treat me, and (5) what I want my loved ones to know. This document is accepted in many states and can be an adjunct to a living will in the others.
- *Allow natural death (AND):* Used in some hospitals and large treatment centers as a "kinder, gentler" statement than DNR, which implies taking something away. AND simply states to allow death to come naturally in due time.
- *Organ/body donation:* Some states allow this as an attachment to other advance directives. A specific form is completed, provided by the research agency to whom the body is to be donated. This form should be completed prior to death.
- *Psychiatric advance directives (PAD):* Documents prepared by a currently competent person who lives with a mental illness; they allow that person to be prepared if a mental health crisis prevents them from being able to make decisions. A PAD describes treatment preferences and names a proxy to make decisions if the patient is unable to do so.

BOX 17-4 Advance Directive Resources

General information about advance directives: https://www.cancer.org/treatment/finding-and-paying-for-treatment/understanding-financial-and-legal-matters/advance-directives/types-of-advance-health-care-directives.html

To find advance directives for individual states: National Hospice and Palliative Care Organization, www.nhpco.org or caringinfo@nhpco.org

Information about Five Wishes: https://www.agingwithdignity.org/

Information about the POLST (physician order for life-sustaining treatment): http://polst.org/

---

patient to consider and communicate what is important, because it is impossible to foresee every type of circumstance or illness. Conversations with loved ones that focus on wishes and beliefs will relieve loved ones and healthcare providers of the need to guess what one would want, and to avoid making decisions against their will. Preplanning is very helpful to families of those patients who are dealing with terminal illness.

When considering the myriad of issues at end-of-life, a patient and family may not think first of legal documents. However, that is a place to start long before the need presents itself—so that it is *not* the first thing to think about when the patient and family are in a state of chaos or confusion at the time of diagnosis. The person designated as healthcare representative/power of attorney (POA)/ POA for health care should be someone who is trustworthy and will follow the patient's stated wishes. That person is usually, but not always, a family member.

The documents should be shared with anyone who might be involved in decision making for the patient, including all physicians, agencies involved in care, and family members; these are not documents to hide away for safekeeping.

A person may change his or her mind about the documents by creating a new document that states the current wishes. The subsequent new date on the document will designate the accepted form. A revocation becomes effective when the doctor is notified with the new advance directive document. The nurse is often an important resource in explaining these protocols to patients and families and should be familiar with the basics for his or her state of service.

▶ Referral Process

The referral process for hospice care can be initiated by the patient and family, or by the physician's office that has been treating the patient and determines that additional curative treatments are not helpful. This conversation with the patient and family can be difficult but can be eased if the physician says something other than "There is nothing more I can do for you." A patient and family would likely rather hear, "We can refer you to a specialized program that is in place to help you and your family or caregivers through the next phase of your life." Contact with a hospice provider agency for this referral is helpful to families if it is made sooner rather than later in the patient's illness progression.

Hospice agencies are aware of the criteria for admission to hospice under many different diagnoses. There are national protocols to help agencies with consistency in identifying the patients who are eligible and appropriate for hospice care (Centers for Medicare and Medicaid Services [CMS], 2019). If a patient does not meet the specific criteria, acceptance as a palliative care patient may be offered or the physician or nurse might refer a patient to a nearby palliative care program (**TABLE 17-1**).

TABLE 17-1 Comparison of Palliative Care and Hospice

	Palliative Care	**Hospice Care**
Focus of care	■ May be used along with certain curative treatments ■ Appropriate for both terminal and nonterminal diagnoses ■ May be initiated at any stage of the illness	■ Comfort care for the terminally ill ■ Provided in the last six months of life ■ Provides comfort and quality for remaining life ■ Curative treatments are no longer appropriate or desired
Eligibility	■ Referral must come from a physician	■ Person must be certified as terminally ill by two physicians (patient's physician and hospice medical director)
Care location	■ Provided in a setting associated with palliative care (e.g., hospital or clinic) or home	■ Provided in any setting that is "home" to the patient
Payment sources	■ Medicare Part B ■ State Medicaid ■ Private insurance	■ Medicare Hospice Benefit ■ State Medicaid ■ Private insurance

Payment for hospice services is covered for Medicare beneficiaries by the Hospice Medicare Benefit, a national program. States also cover hospice through their Medicaid programs, and nearly all medical insurance companies have some form of hospice coverage. Some hospices have donated or endowment funds to cover services for those patients with no other ability to pay for care.

In 2016, 1.43 million Medicare beneficiaries were enrolled in hospice care. Of all Medicare decedents, 48% received hospice care. The average length of service for Medicare patients was 71 days; the median length of service was 24 days. Nearly half (44.6%) of the deaths occurred in a home, and almost one-third occurred in nursing facilities. Approximately 98% of days of care billed to Medicare were at the routine home care level; general inpatient level of care made up 1.5% of days of care; and inpatient respite care and continuous home care each accounted for 0.2% to 0.3% of care days (NHPCO, 2017).

▶ Hospice Admission Criteria

The hospice industry has developed standardized criteria for admission, covering a great variety of diagnoses. Primarily, a person must have a life expectancy of six months or less if the disease runs its normal course. This prognosis must be certified by two physicians—usually the patient's own physician as well as the hospice medical director. However, a person is not limited to only six months of hospice care. A patient in the final phase of life may receive hospice care for as long as necessary when a physician certifies that he or she continues to meet eligibility requirements.

For a number of years, cancer, as a more predictable illness, was the primary diagnosis for hospice care. However, in 2015, nearly 72% of patients receiving hospice care had a noncancer diagnosis (NHPCO, 2017). Patients with end-stage diagnoses including, but not limited to, heart disease, stroke, coma, Alzheimer's and other dementias, renal disease, pulmonary disease, and neurologic diseases such as amyotrophic lateral sclerosis (ALS), Parkinson's disease, muscular dystrophy, and multiple sclerosis were all served by hospice care. Additional information about specific criteria for hospice diagnoses is available in CMS's disease-specific guidelines (Hospice by the Bay, 2014).

If the condition of a patient should, at some point in his or her hospice journey, stabilize such that the person no longer meets the eligibility criteria for hospice care, that person could be discharged and return to traditional Medicare or insurance coverage until such time as the disease is again deemed terminal and again meets the hospice admission criteria. A patient is also able to revoke the hospice coverage, if he or she wishes to return to active treatment at any point in the hospice benefit period.

Hospice does nothing to speed up or slow down the dying process. Just as a midwife might lend support during the birth process, the hospice caregiver provides a presence and specialized knowledge and support during the dying process. Hospice care provides medications related to the terminal illness, as well as durable medical equipment and medical supplies as appropriate to the patient's needs.

▶ The Hospice Team

Hospice care is provided by a team of professionals mandated by the certification requirements. The patient and family/caregivers are considered to be the unit of care, and hospice care is **patient driven** according to a jointly developed plan of care.

■ The hospice physician oversees care provided by the team, and the physician or a nurse practitioner may visit for recertification assessments.

- A registered nurse (RN) is assigned to provide regular visits and establish the individualized care plan. The nurse is the case manager for the team.
- A social worker is assigned to assist the family with emotional adjustments to the changes they are facing, and to help set up arrangements for additional resources, caregiving resources, equipment, and other needs.
- Home health aides assist with personal care on a scheduled basis.
- A spiritual caregiver/chaplain may contact the patient's own spiritual person as requested, or may offer spiritual care, prayer, and discussion to promote spiritual reconciliation.
- Therapists (physical/occupational/speech therapy) and a dietitian may be assigned for assessment and intervention related to comfort and safety.
- Volunteers are available to provide scheduled brief respites for caregivers. Some hospices have vigil volunteers who will stay with the family as the patient is actively dying.
- Grief counselors offer bereavement services, providing psychosocial and emotional support both prior to and following the patient's death for at least one year. They assist with issues related to grief, loss, and adjustment.

The team meets to review the care plan at least every two weeks (per Medicare rules) and more often as needed. At times, family/caregivers and/or the patient's spiritual care provider may join the team discussion or may request a conference in the patient's home setting. Hospice staff visit during regularly scheduled times, but are available to consult on a 24/7 basis, with additional visits made as appropriate. Hospices do not provide 24/7 care; caregiving is usually provided by family members, friends, or paid caregivers, depending on the location of the "home" where services are provided. Home is wherever the patient lives—whether a family home, an extended-care facility, an assisted-living facility, a veteran's care facility, or even a prison.

▶ The Patient and Family Journey

When a patient has a terminal medical condition and is facing end-of-life, the family and caregivers are also profoundly affected by the changes experienced by the patient. Nurses are often front-line medical staff who interact with patients during this transition: They must be aware of the issues that the patients and caregivers face, as they in turn care for the patient. Hospice nurses become the teachers for the patients and caregivers assigned to their team.

As noted earlier, the "patient and family" are the unit of care in hospice. The "family" is defined by the patient, and may consist of family of origin, extended family (spouses, in-laws, children), significant others, friends, and sometimes paid caregivers. The configuration may vary, depending on the circumstances. However, the patient *always* makes the distinction as to who is considered family, and medical personnel should honor those choices.

Families are often in a state of confusion, perhaps denial, and general disarray when they are faced with a diagnosis of terminal illness for their loved one. It is important to honor the patient's choice, and his or her voice should be heard even when the ability to speak is gone—specifically, through the patient's advanced directives.

When a person makes the choice for hospice care, the family and caregivers continue their journey alongside the patient. They are often surprised by the changing roles they encounter along the way. The patient should maintain as much participation in life and decision making as possible, recognizing that this ability will diminish over time. The primary patient role is to "experience the process." Elizabeth Kubler-Ross famously identified that a patient experiences a variety of feelings that vary and move back and forth on a continuum of adjustments. These five stages of terminality, which begin at the time of diagnosis, can reappear at each phase of the terminal process: denial, anger, bargaining, depression, and acceptance (Kubler-Ross, 1997). This is useful information for a hospice team to consider, but it is not the team's prerogative to assign these labels to their patients.

Role of the Caregiver

Family/caregivers perform a complex array of support tasks that extend across the physical, psychological, spiritual, and emotional domains. As the patient's condition declines, their role may change to include decision maker, advocate, communicator, hands-on-care provider, and active symptom manager in addition to the expected social support (**BOX 17-5**). The primary caregiver is the main connection with the case manager/nurse when the patient is no longer able to self-advocate. The primary caregiver may also be the direct care provider, using skills that the hospice nurse has taught relative to the patient's medications and personal care. The nurse often acts as a cheerleader/coach, instilling confidence in a caregiver who is less than comfortable with the new roles. Caregivers may find that this is the most meaningful job they never wanted, and experience emotions they never expected.

Stress and Grief

Patients and caregivers undergo a wide range of grief responses over the course of a life-ending illness. Anticipatory grief begins at the time of diagnosis. Even as adjustments are made along the way, both the patient and caregivers may experience a back-and-forth, changeable, unpredictable range and sequence of emotions, including sadness, anger, despair, frustration, anxiety, depression, fatigue, and somatic health issues for the caregiver. The physical and emotional demands of providing care tend to peak as the disease progresses to the final stages.

Hospice team members are available to assist patients and their caregivers in navigating these stressful situations. Studies have shown that appropriate, well-rounded support systems are very helpful in promoting increased patient/family satisfaction and caregiver well-being.

BOX 17-5   Roles of the Family/Caregiver in Hospice

- Participate in planning care and setting goals; you know what is most important to the patient.
- Ask questions about your loved one's condition. Ask if all providers are communicating with each other; request family meetings when you need to clarify goals and improve coordination.
- Inform the care team about any change in symptoms.
- As the nurse taught you, provide direct patient care. Not everyone is willing or able to do so, but for many, it is an important way of caring.
- Talk to your loved one, even if he or she seems unresponsive. Reinforce dignity and express affection. Include your loved one in conversations about day-to-day events.
- Engage in activities that your loved one has enjoyed. Reminisce, pray, sing.
- Touch! Hug, hold hands, massage.

Arenella, C. (n.d.). Roles of the family and health care professionals in the care of the seriously ill patient. Retrieved from https://americanhospice.org /caregiving/roles-of-the-family-and-health-professionals-in-the-care-of-the-seriously-ill-patient/

Patients and families/caregivers are encouraged to ask questions, to actively participate in care planning, to request that all care providers have good communication, to request family meetings when goals need clarification, and to notify the team of any changes in symptoms.

It is important to recognize that cultural and spiritual differences may lead to differing modes of communication or interaction by patients and families, which then require differentiated interventions by hospice team members. National hospice resources, such as the National Hospice and Palliative Care Organization and the National Hospice Foundation, as well as local hospice programs can be resources for additional cultural information.

Recognizing Changes at End-of-Life

It can be helpful for caregivers to recognize that in the last year of life, a patient's decline in physical and mental condition rather mirrors the first progressive year in the life of an infant. Physical abilities regress and diminish over time; sleep may increase as the illness progresses; food and fluid intake may become less important and lessen in amounts; cognitive abilities may decrease; speech may become less frequent and less intelligible. These changes are not purposeful acts by the patient but rather an expected direct result of the life-ending illness and approaching death. When aware of this process, caregivers are less frustrated that their "good care" is not keeping the patient going. Instead, they perceive that their good care allows the patient to rest more, to have fewer demands on waning energy, and to have the dignity of experiencing physical decline without placement of fault or undue concern (Krieger-Blake & Warring, 2017).

Caregivers also should be aware that the patient may, in frustration with increasing debilitation, "act out" against the persons in their circle who provide the most care. Caregivers often wonder why the patient seems angriest with them, yet remains pleasant to other visitors, helpers, and hospice staff. This is not necessarily purposeful on the patient's part; that is, in releasing their frustration, they choose the safest persons—the ones who will not abandon them. An adult child may find herself in the "parent" role, especially if dementia is involved, or as mental clarity declines.

Caregivers often feel physical and emotionally drained by the care they provide. It is important that they develop good coping strategies that work for them. The hospice staff can help with these family/caregiver adjustments as well.

Psychosocial, Emotional, and Spiritual Issues at End-of-Life

Fear of the unknown is a major cause of the anxiety expressed by patients and caregivers alike. The hospice team, including the nurse, social worker, chaplain, and other team members, are trained to help allay these fears (Tracy, 2017). Education is a very important aspect in reducing fear: The old adage "Knowledge is power!" is key, and the nurse is able to provide much knowledge about what to expect to patients and caregivers.

We frequently attempt to distinguish among psychosocial, emotional, and spiritual issues. The reality is that the range and depth of being human make it nearly impossible to recognize where one aspect of our being ends and another begins. It has been suggested to address these issues as a continuum, treating them as "opportunities for growth" rather than "problems."

> For those caring for the terminally ill, psychosocial and spiritual issues that might have been problems in the past can, with information and compassion, become opportunities— that will allow each of us to live fully

until we say goodbye. (McKinnon & Miller, 2002, p. 273)

Some psychosocial and spiritual opportunities for growth near end-of-life might include the following (Byock, 1997):

- Reframe society's view of dying, from "grow old and die" to "grow up and grow on"
- Expand the definition of quality of life
- Focus on the individual, not the disease
- Address as a whole physical pain, psychosocial issues, and spiritual concerns
- Move through fear to peace
- Move through confusion to meaning
- Move through despair to hope
- Move from isolation to community
- Come to terms with the physical body
- Move from loss to closure
- Adjust to new roles
- Get affairs in order

Among issues might be a change in roles, wherein a patient may want to maintain independence beyond his or her capacity to function. Sometimes a younger caregiver may not want to take over, seeing such a move as diminishing the parent's dignity. There may be an increase in financial concerns, as caregivers have more responsibilities, and may need to take a leave from their jobs. The cost of additional caregiver support, which is not covered by Medicare or hospice, may be of concern.

A person's stage in the life cycle affects his or her reaction to end-of-life. Elderly people often look back on their life and reflect on their experiences, seeing death as inevitable. Younger people may contemplate all that they will miss. There is an attempt to emotionally integrate all aspects of one's life, including determination of its meaning and acceptance of its uniqueness.

Emotional concerns include anticipatory grief—a powerful influence on end-of-life patients and families. It is seen in nearly every phase of illness, beginning at the time of diagnosis. Patients and caregivers alike are affected emotionally by the patient's anticipated loss

of everything important to him or her. Many caregivers feel that they grew closer to their patient, despite the inevitable tensions and some awkward experiences. But they were often able to concentrate on what mattered most and let go of the trivialities of life.

▶ The Changing Focus of Hope

When people choose hospice care, they sometimes feel as though they are giving up hope altogether. That is, in fact, what some physicians imply when they say, "There is nothing more I can do for you." People may find comfort and assistance with adjusting to their declining condition by recognizing a changing focus of hope. When a person is confronted with the possibility of a life-ending illness, the first response is often a hope that it is nothing serious, or that it can be easily treated without much disruption to the patient's life. As treatment becomes unsuccessful and as the illness progresses, the person might hope that he or she and the family will have the opportunity to get things done, to have closure, to witness a graduation, to see a child get married, or to meet a new grandchild. It is possible for a patient to hear a terminal diagnosis and still have hopes for the type of life remaining.

Hospice personnel believe that patients' hope can continue, that the changing focus of hope moves from that of getting better to new goals (Krieger-Blake & Warring, 2017):

- Hope for the appropriate help for themselves and their families through the transitions that end-of-life brings
- Hope that they will be provided with guidance and emotional comfort through their journey
- Hope that their care will be provided with respect for their dignity through the dying process
- Hope that their passing will be comfortable and pain free

- Hope that their family members will receive the appropriate support before and after their death
- Hope to be treated holistically—as an individual with unique needs, wishes, and desires

Dr. Ira Byock (1997), a leading proponent of excellence in end-of-life care, in his book *Dying Well: Peace and Possibilities at the End of Life* discusses personal tasks that may need to be addressed as someone approaches death: (1) ask for forgiveness; (2) offer forgiveness; (3) offer heartfelt thanks; (4) offer sentiments of love; and (5) say goodbye. These powerful statements provide a clear path to emotional wellness throughout a lifetime. They also provide a format for resolution of some personal, emotional, and/or spiritual issues at the end-of-life.

▶ Components of Peaceful Dying

In search of a **good death**, patients and families make many emotional, psychosocial, and spiritual adjustments through the course of the patient's illness. A good death is "one that is free from avoidable distress and suffering, for patients, family, and caregivers; in general accord with the patients' and families' wishes; and reasonably consistent with clinical, cultural, and ethical standards" (Field & Cassel, 1997, p. 24). The literature suggests a variety of perspectives from which a good death can be defined. All agree that the patient's perspective or definition of good death is the one most important to the dying experience (**BOX 17-6**). Patients often report religiosity/spirituality as being among their top themes, which also includes concepts such as pain-free status, emotional well-being, life completion, dignity, family presence, and retention of control. Additional components of peaceful dying include instilling good memories; uniting as a team between caregivers and medical staff; maintaining alertness, control, privacy, and dignity; spiritual preparedness; saying goodbye; and a peaceful and quiet death. A good death can and ought to mean different things to different people. In hospice care, the patient defines what a good death might mean to him or her. It might mean having his or her affairs in order, controlling pain and discomfort, having few emotional regrets, and receiving mindful care and support (Repa, 2018).

A good death is possible. Family members and caregivers are comforted by the knowledge that they provided the care needed along the continuum and that their loved one was peaceful at the time of death. Because family members and caregivers live on remembering how the patient died, it is important for all medical professionals who interact with them to strive to provide competent, caring, honest, and appropriate care throughout the terminal illness, promoting peace and comfort for the patient at

---

BOX 17-6 References for Personal Reflections on Dying Well

Albom, M. (1997). *Tuesdays with Morrie: An old man, a young man, and life's greatest lesson.* New York, NY: Doubleday.

Byock, I. (1997). *Dying well: The prospect for growth at the end of life.* London, England: Penguin Books/Penguin & Putnam.

Frankl, V. E. (1984). *Man's search for meaning: An introduction to logotherapy.* New York, NY: Simon & Schuster.

Jobs, S. (2005). Commencement address at Stanford University, June 14, 2005. Retrieved from https://news.stanford.edu/2005/06/14/jobs-061505/

Pausch, R., & Zaslow, J. (2008). *The last lecture.* New York, NY: Hyperion.

all times. Success in these endeavors will allow a family to look back on the hospice experience as a journey that was accompanied by people who cared, and who were willing and able to share the difficult journey with their loved one. Remembering the quality of care markedly helps those who remain to grieve the loss of their loved one, long after the actual death experience (Krieger-Blake & Warring, 2017).

▶ Nursing as Ministry at End-of-Life: The Hospice Nurse

As nurses in many settings are there for persons and families at the most intimate and essential life moments, from birth to death, they are in a unique position for divine appointments to occur. Providing spiritually and culturally competent care for a person at the end-of-life may be one of the most spiritual moments in nursing as ministry. Although much of the care provided to a person during this period is physical, the spiritual and psychosocial aspects of care cannot be overlooked. Comprehensive assessment and interventions for each phase of the dying process are essential. While a detailed description of the interventions undertaken by nurses at end-of-life, about which volumes have been written, is beyond the scope of this chapter, **TABLE 17-2** provides goals of care for the dying phase. The reader is referred to specific resources at the end of this chapter for a more thorough discussion of the scope of practice of the hospice and/or palliative care nurse. In addition, **TABLE 17-3** summarizes aspects of

TABLE 17-2 Major Goal Areas for the Dying Patient	
Comfort measures	Consider medication use and discontinue those not necessary; consider best route for medications and discontinuing all but the most essential interventions for comfort.
Psychological issues	Can the person communicate or is a translator needed? Is the person aware of his/her condition?
Spiritual support	Assess and address the patient's spiritual needs.
Communication	How will information about the patient be conveyed to family or other significant others? How is the patient's primary care provider informed of the patient's condition?
Communication with primary healthcare team	General practitioner is aware of the patient's condition.
Plan of care	The plan of care is discussed with the patient and family. The patient, family, and interprofessional team state understanding of the plan of care.

Data from Ellershaw, J., & Ward, C. (2003). Care of the dying patient: The last hours or days of life. *BMJ (Clinical Research Ed.)*, *326*(7379), 30–44.

major cultures and religions to help nurses be better informed about preferences at death and afterward. Although nurses across settings may be present with patients during end-of-life, those called to this ministry often work in hospice and palliative care, so nursing in this specialty provides an exemplar for this chapter.

TABLE 17-3 Cultural and Religious Practices at End-of-Life

Religion	During Sickness	Dying and Death	After Dying
Buddhism	Important to die in a positive state of mind; organ donation permitted.	Help die peacefully by encouraging forgiveness; position on right side, left hand on left thigh, legs stretched out; no special body preparations.	Leave body alone as long as possible to avoid disturbing the consciousness during transition from death to new life.
Hinduism	Family does daily care; father/oldest son makes health decisions; same-sex caregiver due to modesty.	With terminal diagnosis, dying information given to the family, not the patient; the family decides how much information to share with the patient.	Body washed, usually by eldest son, then cremated.
Islam	Prayer five times per day; clean the area of any body waste, including the person and sheets; can use a pitcher and basin provided; use a clean sheet to cover the patient during prayer. Best efforts provided to maintain life; hardship is a test from Allah; can remove life support; natural death will allow person to accept the will of Allah.	Body on its side, facing Mecca; friends and loved ones pray for mercy, forgiveness, and blessings of Allah.	Person of same gender prepares body for burial; same day as death if possible; cremation forbidden.
Jehovah's Witness	No blood transfusions; organ transplants per individual conscience.	Respectful care for dying person and family; respond to their individual needs.	Generally follow traditional state mandates for burial or cremation.

(continues)

TABLE 17-3 Cultural and Religious Practices at End-of-Life			*(continued)*
Religion	**During Sickness**	**Dying and Death**	**After Dying**
Judaism	In serious illness, patient is not to be left alone—to be attended by family; doctor's duty is to prolong life unless death is imminent and certain; cannot hasten death.	Autopsy not permitted unless required by law; organ donation only after the person is declared dead (not at all by Orthodox Jews).	Cremation forbidden; focus on deceased and funeral; mourning occurs in the home for 7 days after the funeral. Orthodox: Extend arms along the body, fingers outstretched; tubing, body fluids, and sheets/blankets with blood are buried with the body; a designated Orthodox Jew should clean the body. Someone stays with body, praying until the body enters the ground.
Christianity (general)	Respect and dignity for body; organ donation and autopsy allowed; if treatment is of no benefit or unreasonable burden, may forgo and allow natural death; decision up to patient/family.	Open to pastoral care; some have a rite of anointing by the priest; some have service of commendation of the dying.	Practices may vary by denomination, but commonly include a gathering with family and friends after the funeral or memorial service.
Orthodox Christianity	Fasting on certain days = no meat, milk, fish, or eggs; no eating before communion; can use drugs to reduce pain/suffering; removing life support done after prayer and discussion with family members, medical professional, and spiritual director; organ donation acceptable.	Family encouraged to be at the bedside; invite the priest; Anointing of the Sick (Holy Unction).	Body buried in the ground, with a coffin, grave liner, and monument with image of the cross; cremation is not allowed.
Roman Catholicism	If possible, fast one hour before receiving Eucharist; moral obligation to use ordinary or proportionate means of preserving life (in judgment of the patient).	Sacrament of Anointing of the Sick before surgery, for elderly in a weakened condition, by a priest.	May be cremated; remains may be brought to funeral mass.

Data from Toole, M. M. (2006). *Handbook for chaplains: Comfort my people.* New York, NY: Paulist Press. Copyright © 2006 by Mary M. Toole/Paulist Press. Retrieved from www.paulistpress.com

BOX 17-7 Outstanding Nurse Leader: Cicely Saunders (1918–2005)

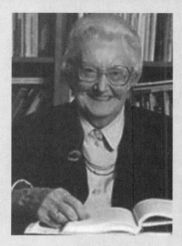

Dame Cecily Saunders

Dame Cicely Mary Strode Saunders. Used with permission from St. Christopher's Hospice. Retrieved from https://www.thelancet.com/action/showPdf?pii=S0140-6736%2805%2967127-9

Dame Cicely Saunders, the founder of the modern hospice movement, started St. Christopher's Hospice in London in 1967, seeking to provide comfort care and dignity to terminally ill patients. She was first a nurse who cared for dying patients as early as the 1940s. Saunders became a social worker, and then a physician in 1957. She was the medical director of St. Christopher's for nearly 20 years. In this role, she advocated for the principle of dying with dignity, and maintained that death is a natural process that could be eased with sensitive nursing and good symptom control. Her philosophy of care was brought to the United States during a seminar she gave at Yale University, which was attended by doctors, nurses, social workers, and chaplains. As a result of her outreach, hospice came to the United States in 1974. Saunders was made a Dame by Queen Elizabeth II in 1980, acknowledging her pioneering work, her research, and her philosophy of dignified care for the dying.

While a hospice team is composed of a variety of members to address the many issues that might pave the way for a good death, the hospice nurse is the case manager of the team, and one of the team members who may visit with the most frequency. Many hospice nurses have said that one of the most enjoyable facets of their work is getting to know the patients and families on a more personal level by visiting in their homes, meeting with extended family, and developing relationships over an extended period of time whenever possible. As the nurse develops these relationships, he or she gains the trust of the patient and caregivers who depend on the nurse to help with symptoms and comfort measures (see **BOX 17-7**).

Often during these somewhat intimate visits, the patient may confide other concerns to the nurse—such as spiritual and emotional concerns. The faith-based nurse generally has a higher degree of comfort with patient/family conversations about spiritual issues and beliefs. It is very important that even at these precious times, the patient remains in charge of the conversations. It is not the nurse's duty to try to proselytize the patient who is nearing death. However, if a patient so requests, a nurse who is comfortable with prayer or intimate spiritual conversations should follow the patient's lead during these conversations, and perhaps choose to share personal beliefs about God, heaven, and the afterlife.

Families frequently comment on the consoling presence demonstrated by their hospice staff. This skill helps a hospice nurse feel comfortable in meeting the needs of the imminently dying patient (see also **BOX 17-8** later in this chapter). This presence enables the nurse to better assess the patient's existential needs and can assist the nurse in meeting some of these needs, in addition to the patient's clergy or the hospice chaplain. Spiritual needs may occur at any time and may not wait for the visit of the "assigned"

BOX 17-8 Evidence-Based Practice Focus

A qualitative study was conducted in which hospice nurses were interviewed individually, with data analysis then being performed using phenomenological hermeneutical methods. The key spiritual and existential themes identified included sensing existential and spiritual distress; tuning in and opening up; sensing the atmosphere in the room; being moved and touched; and consoling through silence, conversation, and religious consolation.

Three additional themes emerged through the discussion: compassionate silence, uncovering the wound, and wounded healers. Results showed that "being there" for the patients and their relatives was at the heart of the nurses' practice. Being there was about conveying consolation through silent presence, companionship, deep existential and religious conversations, and supporting the patients' expressions of faith and rituals.

Willingness to "just be there" for patients—seeing and listening to the patient—demanded personal courage from the nurse, especially if the patient was desolate or despairing. Patients' suffering could sometimes open old wounds for the nurses, triggering feelings of helplessness, vulnerability, and uncertainty. The nurses found that giving and receiving peer support and debriefing were vital to endure the emotional pressures of being with the dying. The authors concluded that:

> Consoling existential and spiritual distress is a deeply personal and relational practice, involving a high degree of sensitivity and the courage to just be there as wounded healers, willing and ready to share the fear of death and the finitude of life with patients and their loved ones. . . . Through the power of consoling presence, nurses have a potential to alleviate existential and spiritual suffering. By connecting deeply with patients and their families, nurses have the possibility to affirm the patients' strength and facilitate their courage to live a meaningful life and die a dignified death. (p. 25)

Tornoe, K., Danbolt, L., Kvigne, K., & Sorlie, V. (2014). The power of consoling presence—Hospice nurses' lived experience with spiritual and existential care for the dying. *BMC Nursing, 13*(1), 25.

professional. A faith-based nurse is usually comfortable providing this comforting presence in the meantime. However, even though whole-person care indicates religious, spiritual, and existential care is to be provided in ways that benefit the patient, hospice teams also need to hear existential pain when it is not voiced in religious language. Training for dealing with these situations is becoming more readily available from agencies such as the National Hospice and Palliative Care Organization (Cheatham, 2017).

Hospice nurses who weather the pressures and find hospice work to be their niche, or heart's mission, and who remain in the hospice profession for extended periods of time seem to have some common characteristics. These include belief in the team concept of care, utilizing all members of the hospice team in their appropriate roles. A nurse soon learns that it is not possible to "be all" to the hospice patient and family and finds a sense of relief in being able to depend on other team members for additional interactions and support to the patient/family unit of care. Those nurses who do not easily find this truth are destined for burnout in a relatively short period of time.

Hospice nurses must have a comfortable concept of death as a fact of life. This concept does not require being brutally honest with a patient in denial but does mean that sensitivity to the dying process and a gentle education of the patient regarding what to expect can be most helpful. A nurse with awareness of the dying process can educate families as death nears, so that relatives can come in from afar, or so that the last goals of the patient can be met with as much comfort and symptom management as possible. The nurse educates the patient and family about the imminence of death, helping family members recognize "the signs" to ensure their awareness and preparation.

Vitas Hospice (2018) has identified several characteristics that make hospice nurses "great":

- They are their patient's advocates as part of the team.
- They are thorough in using the various team members as needed and in taking the time needed by each patient and family they visit.
- They are joyful in the face of death— affirming their patients' lives and living.
- They are compassionate—confident and calm when others are afraid, and capable of sadness and humility as they stand in quiet understanding when death has occurred.
- They are dedicated to their patients/ families and caregivers—providing the education, support, and caring needed at such a sensitive time in life.

▶ Rewards and Challenges in Providing Care at End-of-Life

Challenges found in hospice care as described by hospice nurses include the fact that the nurse is constantly working with dying patients. A sense of attachment can occur when the nurse spends a great deal of time caring for a patient prior to his or her death. Burnout is experienced when job expectations and working conditions are inconsistent over time. High

workloads can be a part of this dissatisfaction. Professional compassion fatigue describes the weariness experienced by healthcare workers who are repeatedly exposed to seriously ill, traumatized, suffering, and dying patients (Melvin, 2015).

Studies have identified some key determinants for these risks, such as trauma, anxiety, life demands, and excessive empathy leading to blurred professional boundaries. Knowledge of these variables can help organizations identify nurses at risk, and then provide interventions and preventions to maintain optimal nursing care (Abendroth & Flannery, 2006). Some agencies provide rituals and healing care practices for their staff members, which provide an outlet for hospice workers to express their grief and reflect on their work in an accepting environment; in turn, this provides for personal closure and decreases the risk of burnout and compassion fatigue.

Rewards are strong when the nurse recognizes the opportunity to really make a meaningful difference in the life of someone who is dying; this is especially true for the families and loved ones who remain behind. The nurse helps the family reduce their distress about the patient's level of comfort, so they can put their energies into the passing of the person they love. The nurse's role is as much about education as it is about caring, providing people with a better understanding about what is happening to their loved one (**CASE STUDY 17-1**). The nurse is a true advocate for each patient at a difficult and important time of life (Box 17-8).

In this author's experience, most nurses who successfully work in hospice over a long period of time have embraced a personal level of faith. They identify rewards of their hospice care as "helping to the nth degree," being able to shepherd patients and families through a very important, trying, and scary period of life. They identify getting to know the patient and family as a highlight, as well as providing education and reassurance through the

🔍 CASE STUDY 17-1

Mary has advanced cancer and came to the hospice center directly from a local hospital with a brief prognosis—perhaps of only a few days. Mary is 67 years old, the mother of an adult daughter, Jane, who is in her mid-30s and from whom Mary has been estranged for nearly 12 years. Jane has come to make peace before her mother dies. She indicates that Mary has had a "hard life," with a history of alcohol and some drug misuse. Jane describes that Mary was not a particularly good mother and is proud that she has overcome some of her childhood issues to become successful and a "better" mother to her own daughter, who is now 13.

Although Mary has been distanced from her congregation for many years, she is visited by her "old pastor" of a conservative religion, arranged by her daughter, who is trying to provide not just personal reconciliation but also a spiritual reconciliation prior to Mary's death. Jane is not present at the time of the visit. The pastor is welcomed on the hospice unit, as spiritual care is an integral part of end-of-life hospice care. The pastor leaves without further consultation with the staff after an approximately 20-minute private visit.

When the nurse enters Mary's room, she observes that Mary is agitated, restless, crying, and indicating increased physical pain. The nurse talks with Mary to assess the causes of her increased multiple symptoms in a short period of time. Mary tearfully reports that the pastor told her that unless she "speaks in tongues" before she dies, she will not have a place in heaven.

Questions

1. As a faith-based nurse with a strong Christian tradition, what would your next steps be? Of course, you would assess and respond to Mary's physical complaints—but what else would you do?
2. What if the physical/medication responses to agitation, restlessness, and physical pain are not enough to ease Mary's symptoms?
3. Describe the resources of the team—daughter, chaplain, social worker, patient's pastor, counselor, and bereavement specialist for anticipatory grief issues.
4. What if Mary remains afraid of going to sleep and is obviously still agitated and restless over the next few days, even as her ability to converse appropriately lessens?
5. What personal resources as her nurse might you bring, especially in the middle of the midnight shift at the hospice center?

process. For these nurses, hospice is about "being more than just a nurse." They voice the awareness that their own life is enriched by participating in such an enriching way with their patients and their families, helping them to recognize what is most important in life. They value the relationships that they develop on a professional level as members of a team— relationships that are just not possible in many other nursing specialties. Finally, they display "hardiness," a personality construct that has three main elements: control, challenge, and commitment (Hutchings, 1997). When hardiness is blended with key hospice elements of critical competence and compassionate care, hospice nurses say, "This is what nursing is all about!"

▶ Conclusion

You matter to the last moment of your life, and we will do all we can, not only to help you die peacefully, but to live until you die.

—**Dame Cecily Saunders**

▶ Clinical Reasoning Exercises

1. Compare and contrast two or more of the additional resources from **BOX 17-9**. How do you react to some of the differing religious perspectives found there?

BOX 17-9 Additional Resources

Catholic Health Association of the United States: *Teachings of the Catholic Church: Caring for People at the End of Life.* Product Code: 3067. https://www.chausa.org/nursing /nursing-overview/faith-community-nursing
Church Health Reader: Innovative, Inspirational, Knowledgeable, Practical. A magazine whose mission is "to reclaim the Church's biblical commitment to care for our bodies and spirits." https://chreader.org
Evangelical Lutheran Church in America: The Parish Nurse program uses The Conversation Project to help people talk about their wishes for end-of-life care. elpna.org/nurses/resources.php; https:// theconversationproject.org/
Gone from My Sight: The Dying Experience. A booklet for families and caregivers about the actual physical, emotional, and spiritual process of dying. https://bkbooks.com
Morningside Ministries: A series of training videos for many aspects of providing care for caregivers. https://training.mmlearn.org /caregiver-training-videos
National Hospice and Palliative Care Organization. (2015, July 23). Hospice FAQs. Retrieved from https://www.nhpco. org/about-hospice-and-palliative-care/ hospice-faqs
National Hospice and Palliative Care Organization. (2017). What are the pros and cons of hospice nursing? Retrieved from https://nursejournal.org/hospice-nursing /what-are-the-pros-and-cons-of-hospice -nursing/

2. *Gone from My Sight: The Dying Experience* by Barbara Karnes (from Box 17-9) is an inexpensive but very useful resource for nurses, team members, and family members who are facing the end-of-life of their loved one. Obtain a copy, review it, and discuss with a classmate the value *you* find in this pamphlet.

▶ Personal Reflection Exercises

1. Have you ever cared for a person who was dying? If so, what was that experience like for you?
2. If you have never cared for someone who was dying, how do you think you would feel?
3. What strategies do you have in your "toolkit" to bring presence and comfort to those who are dying? To a family that is grieving?
4. Of the various cultures and religions discussed in Table 17-3, which is most familiar to you? Which is least familiar? Did you find any specific practices that were surprising?
5. How is being present with a person as they enter into eternity related to the divine appointments we see when practicing nursing as ministry?

References

Abendroth, M., & Flannery, J. (2006). Predicting the risk of compassion fatigue: A study of hospice nurses. *Journal of Hospice and Palliative Nursing, 8*(6), 346–356.

American Cancer Society. (2016). The Patient Self-Determination Act (PSDA). Retrieved from https://www.cancer.org/treatment/finding-and-paying-for-treatment/understanding-financial-and-legal-matters/advance-directives/patient-self-determination-act.html

Byock, I. (1997). *Dying well: Peace and possibilities at the end of life* (pp. 30–34). New York, NY: Riverhead Books.

Centers for Medicare and Medicaid Services (CMS). (2019). Medicare benefit policy manual. Retrieved from https://www.cms.gov/Regulations-and-Guidance/Guidance/Manuals/Downloads/bp102c09.pdf

Cheatham, C. (2017). *Spiritual care for the non-religious.* Webinar from National Hospice and Palliative Care Organization.

Field, M., & Cassel, C. K. (1997). *Approaching death: Improving care at the end of life.* Washington, DC: National Academy Press.

Hospice by the Bay. (2014). Determining a patient's prognosis: CMS disease specific guidelines. Retrieved from http://hospicebythebay.org/resources/lcd-and-physician-letter-3-15-16.pdf

Hutchings, D. (1997). The hardiness of hospice nurses. *American Journal of Hospice and Palliative Care, 14*(3), 110–113.

Krieger-Blake, L., & Warring, P. (2017). End of life care. In K. Mauk (Ed.), *Gerontological nursing: Competencies for care* (4th ed., pp. 845–886). Burlington, MA: Jones & Bartlett Learning.

Kubler-Ross, E. (1997). *On death and dying: What the dying have to teach doctors, nurses, clergy and their own families.* New York, NY: Scribner.

McKinnon, S., & Miller, B. (2002). *Psychosocial and spiritual concerns.* In B. M. Kinzbrunner, N. J. Weinreb, & J. S. Policzer (Eds.), *Twenty common problems at end-of-life care* (pp. 257–274). New York, NY: McGraw-Hill.

Melvin, C. S. (2015). Historical review in understanding burnout, professional compassion fatigue, and secondary traumatic stress disorder from a hospice and palliative nursing perspective. *Journal of Hospice & Palliative Nursing, 17*(1), 66–72.

National Hospice and Palliative Care Organization (NHPCO). (2000). Preamble and philosophy. Retrieved from https://www.nhpco.org/ethical-and-position-statements/preamble-and-philosophy

National Hospice and Palliative Care Organization (NHPCO). (2017). Facts and figures: Hospice care in America. Retrieved from https://www.nhpco.org/sites/default/files/public/Statistics_Research/2017_Facts_Figures.pdf

National Institute on Aging. (2017). What are palliative care and hospice care? Retrieved from https://www.nia.nih.gov/health/what-are-palliative-care-and-hospice-care

Repa, B. (2018). What is a "good death"? Retrieved from https://www.caring.com/caregivers/end-of-life-care/#how-to-have-a-%E2%80%9Cgood-death%E2%80%9D?

Tracy, A. (2017). Hospice and palliative care: Ministry to the dying. Retrieved from https://www.focusonthefamily.com/pro-life/end-of-life/hospice-and-palliative-care-ministry-to-the-dying

Vitas Hospice. (2018). A day in the life of a hospice nurse. Retrieved from https://www.vitas.com/hospice-and-palliative-care-basics/the-hospice-care-team/a-day-in-the-life-of-a-hospice-nurse/

Recommended Readings

Al-Mahrezi, A., & Al-Mandhari, Z. (2016). Palliative care: Time for action. *Oman Medical Journal, 3,* 161–163.

Arenella, C. (n.d.). Roles of the family and health care professionals in the care of the seriously ill patient. Retrieved from https://americanhospice.org/caregiving/roles-of-the-family-and-health-professionals-in-the-care-of-the-seriously-ill-patient/

Meier, E. A., Gallegos, J., Montross-Thomas, L., Depp, C., Irwin, S., & Jeste, D. (2016). Defining a good death (successful dying): Literature review and a call for research and public dialogue. *American Journal of Geriatric Psychiatry, 24*(4), 261–271. doi:10.1016/j.jagp.2016.01.135

Miller, S. C., Lima, J. C., Intrator, O., Martin, E., Bull, J., & Hanson, L. C. (2016). Palliative care consultations in nursing homes and reductions in acute care use and potentially burdensome end-of-life transitions. *Journal of the American Geriatrics Society, 64*(11), 2280–2287.

Tornoe, K., Danbolt, L., Kvigne, K. & Sorlie, V. (2014). The power of consoling presence—Hospice nurses' lived experience with spiritual and existential care for the dying. *BMC Nursing, 13*(1), 25.

Weakland, M. (2018). The five best things about being a hospice nurse. Retrieved from https://www.midlandcareconnection.com/five-best-things-hospice-nurse/

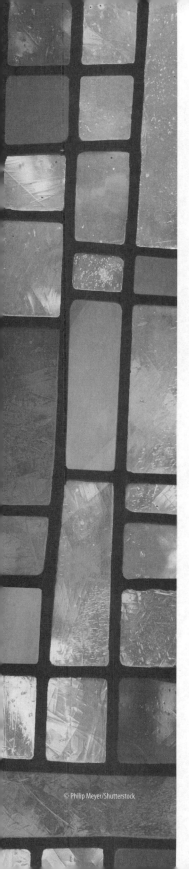

UNIT V

Developing a Personal Commitment to Nursing as Ministry

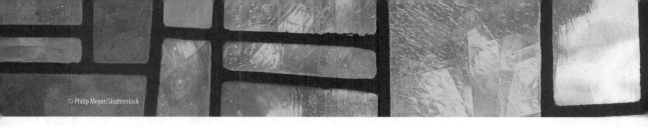

CHAPTER 18

Caring for One's Spiritual Self

David Mulkey, MSN, RN, CCRN

LEARNING OBJECTIVES

At the end of this chapter, the reader will be able to:

1. Recognize the differences between burnout and compassion fatigue.
2. Examine one's spiritual self-care practices.
3. Implement a spiritual self-care plan.
4. Design a method of evaluation of a spiritual self-care plan.
5. Use the ProQOL scale to determine one's professional quality of life.

KEY TERMS

Awareness	Compassion fatigue	Resilience
Burnout	Compassion satisfaction	Secondary traumatic stress
Caring	Empathy	Self-aware
Compassion	Mindfulness	Self-care

▶ Caring for One's Spiritual Self

Casting all your care upon him; for he careth for you. (1 Peter 5:7, King James Version [KJV])

It was four o'clock in the morning, and Kevin stood at the bedside of a 17-year-old patient's hospital bed. Despite spending eight hours performing nonstop life-saving measures, nothing had been good enough to save his life. Kevin had done everything he could, but his efforts did not seem adequate from a life-or-death perspective. The only measures left were to perform postmortem care and to tell the mother and father that their only son had died. They were waiting in the waiting room for the unexpected news. The message was not what they were hoping to receive; they were hoping for good news.

Kevin looked around to his fellow nurse coworkers for support, but they were all too busy caring for other patients to deal with his nonsense emotion. "I have done this before, and I can do it again," he thought to himself (**BOX 18-1**). In fact, he had done it too many times before, three times in the last four weeks. This made number four. How many times could one person do this? Patients were supposed to get better, not die.

Kevin walked to the waiting room and reluctantly stood at the door. The father sat in the corner staring at the ground, while the mother paced back and forth. The glazed look in Kevin's eyes, and his silence, expressed it all. How do you tell a mother and father that their only son has died? "We did everything we could, but your son is dead." Just like that, it was done, no emotion, no **compassion**, just words.

▶ Having Compassion Is Hard

Many people who want to pursue nursing as a career have a passion for helping others. They want to make a difference in people's lives when they are the most vulnerable. In Gallop polls, the profession of nursing was rated the number one most honest and ethical profession for 16 consecutive years (Brenan, 2017). This rating is a testament to nurses and the compassionate care they deliver on a daily basis. Nurses have a professional and moral

obligation to provide compassion, **empathy**, and respect for patients and families (Fowler, 2015). But in addition to caring for others, nurses have a professional and moral obligation to care for themselves. The ANA Code of Ethics Provision 5.1: Duties to Self and Others states:

> Moral respect accords moral worth and dignity to all human beings regardless of their personal attributes or life situation. Such respect extends to oneself as well: the same duties that we owe to others we owe to ourselves. Self-regarding duties primarily concern oneself and include promotion of health and safety, preservation of wholeness of character and integrity, maintenance of competence, and continuation of personal and professional growth. (ANA, 2015, p. 19)

Nurses should care for themselves on the same level that they care for patients and families. Why would the ANA write a provision statement specifically mandating that nurses care for themselves? The answer: Because having compassion for others is hard if you do not have compassion for yourself. Nurses who extend compassion to patients and families without first caring for themselves are at risk for developing **compassion fatigue** and **burnout**.

Compassion Fatigue

The terms *compassion fatigue* and *burnout* are often used interchangeably, but they actually refer to dramatically different phenomena. The differences between compassion fatigue and burnout are clarified in **TABLE 18-1**. Mahatma Gandhi said, "Compassion is a muscle that gets stronger with use"—but as with any muscle, overuse leads to fatigue (Pennington, 2016). Charles Figley (1995) coined the phrase *compassion fatigue* to describe the direct product of **caring** too much for a person. Compassion fatigue is the act of an individual caring so much that he or she

---

BOX 18-1 Kevin's Story: Unfolding Case Study Questions

1. Should Kevin have interrupted his coworkers to help him break the news to this family? Include a rationale for your answer.
2. What actions should Kevin have taken before this incident to cope with the prior deaths?

TABLE 18-1 Compassion Fatigue Versus Burnout	
Compassion Fatigue	**Burnout**
Consistent exposure to emotionally straining situations that affect a person's physical, mental, emotional, and spiritual state and eventually decrease one's compassion over time. Individuals at risk for compassion fatigue are those who care for people, whether it is a job, an assigned position, a divine calling, or a good deed.	Emotional exhaustion to the point that an individual becomes desensitized, or numb, to emotion. Burnout is inherent in the nature of the job and can affect anyone regardless if their primary responsibility is to care for others or not.

suffers physical, mental, emotional, professional, and spiritual side effects because of taking on the burdens of someone else as if they were the individual's own (Compassion Fatigue Awareness Project, 2017; Figley, 1995; Harris & Griffin, 2015; Todaro-Franceschi, 2013).

Burnout

In great contrast, burnout is the result of a situation and can occur independently of compassion fatigue (Lanier, 2017). Although most individuals suffer compassion fatigue first and then proceed to burnout, burnout can also stand independently. Individuals at the greatest risk for developing burnout are often described as those who are the most dedicated and committed to the job (Bridgeman, Bridgeman, & Barone, 2018).

There is a clear distinction between compassion fatigue and burnout. Compassion fatigue is due to caring for a person, whereas burnout is related to the nature of the job. Burnout is not directly related to a person.

▶ Suffering in Silence

Kevin had to stay past the end of his shift, charting everything he did for that young patient. It took him a lot longer than usual to chart his assessments and interventions because he just

> **BOX 18-2** Kevin's Story: Unfolding Case Study Questions
>
> 1. Is Kevin suffering from compassion fatigue?
> 2. Is Kevin suffering from burnout?
> 3. How does compassion fatigue lead to burnout?

could not focus. He kept thinking back to the parents. Kevin got home from work late that morning. His wife called out, "I was starting to worry about you." Kevin responded, "What does it matter?" He walked by his wife, went into the bedroom, and slammed the door. He was angry—so angry he could not seem to control his emotions. Kevin's wife followed him into the room and asked, "What's wrong?" Kevin yelled, "Leave me alone!" If he did not have to talk about it, it would go away, right?

He would feel better after sleeping. Kevin laid down, but the problem was that he could not sleep. He tossed back and forth. He was tired and exhausted, but he was unable to clear his mind. He laid there awake all day until his alarm rang. It was time to get ready for work again. He could not go into work without sleep. He did not want to go to work. Kevin called his supervisor to say that he was sick. He knew he had lied, but he did not care (**BOXES 18-2** and **18-3**).

Risk Factors

Compassion fatigue and burnout can happen to anyone, but newly graduated nurses and oncology nurses have an increased risk of developing compassion fatigue (Mattioli, Walters, & Cannon, 2018; Mendes, 2017; Wu, Singh-Carlson, Odell, Reynolds, & Su, 2016). In one study, newer, younger nurses (younger than age 40) had an increased risk of developing compassion fatigue as compared to their older, more experienced colleagues (Wu et al., 2016). This greater risk was due to two factors: (1) a sense of inferior self-worth and (2) a **secondary traumatic stress** event. New nurses believe that they need to prove themselves worthy—a belief that manifests as skipping breaks, working extra shifts, or not asking for help. Although newer nurses believe they are building their self-worth, in reality they are increasing their risk for compassion fatigue and burnout by failing to provide self-care.

A secondary traumatic stress event occurs when a nurse, or caregiver, who has strong emotional ties to a person, observes that person experience a traumatic event, whether it be illness, treatment, or death. It is crucial for nurses to exhibit caring, compassion, and empathy with patients, but boundaries must remain in intact. The greatest risk to developing compassion fatigue is breaking professional boundaries (Sheppard, 2016).

Signs and Symptoms

As outlined in **TABLE 18-2**, signs and symptoms of compassion fatigue often present in four categories: (1) behavioral, (2) physical, (3) professional, and (4) spiritual (Harris & Griffin, 2015; Lanier, 2017). Put simply, individuals who are experiencing compassion fatigue are often feeling depressed, stressed, anxious, joyless, and unreliable.

Compassion fatigue is a process that can happen either suddenly or over time (Henson,

---

> **BOX 18-3** Kevin's Story: Unfolding Case Study Questions
>
> 1. Which signs and symptoms of compassion fatigue does Kevin exhibit?
> 2. Should Kevin seek support from his wife? How does the Health Insurance Portability and Accountability Act (HIPAA) play into this decision?

TABLE 18-2 Signs and Symptoms of Compassion Fatigue

Behavioral	Physical	Professional	Spiritual
■ Depression	■ Tiredness	■ Calling in sick	■ Questioning belief in God
■ Anger	■ Exhaustion	■ Unreliable	■ Changing beliefs
■ Irritability	■ Headaches	■ Helplessness	■ Anger toward God
■ Difficulty focusing	■ Gastrointestinal changes	■ Apathy	■ Hopelessness
■ Substance abuse	■ Hypertension	■ Lack of joy	■ Suffering
■ Eating disturbances	■ Muscle tension	■ Medication errors	■ Emptiness
■ Insomnia		■ Poor judgment	■ Abandonment
■ Avoiding			■ Forgotten
■ Anxiety			
■ Stress			

Harris & Griffin, 2015; Lanier, 2017; Todaro-Franceschi, 2013.

2017). Nurses typically ignore the antecedents of compassion fatigue. Indeed, nurses who consistently overextend compassion may not realize that they are experiencing a decrease in spiritual commitment, an increase in emotional investment, and a diminished support system. Nurses often believe the myth that they need to be able to do everything with a smile on their face; in fact, it is okay to ask for help when needed. Otherwise, the antecedents will turn into consequences and defining attributes (Harris & Griffin, 2015). Nurses who do not pay attention to their own **self-care** and suffer from compassion fatigue or burnout have a greater risk of leaving the profession of nursing. If compassion fatigue is caught in its earliest phase, it can be prevented.

▶ A Perfect Biblical Example

Humanly speaking, having compassion is hard. Because compassion is something that takes effort, the Bible encourages self-care. **TABLE 18-3** identifies several key verses that mandate Christians to take time to care for themselves.

God wants us to rely on Him for our strength. Our human nature often grows physically, emotionally, and spiritually tired and weary. God illustrated this firsthand through His son, Jesus Christ. Jesus modeled the perfect example of how to embrace suffering. In the book of Mark, Jesus had compassion on many people and healed them from their diseases. Nevertheless, Jesus, who was entirely God and entirely man, emulated self-care to prevent himself from getting compassion fatigue. Mark 1:35 (New International Version [NIV]) states that after Jesus had finished this miracle, "Very early in the morning, while it was still dark, Jesus got up, left the house and went off to a solitary

TABLE 18-3 Caring for Yourself: A Biblical Mandate

Theme	Reference
Your body is a temple used to glorify God.	Psalms 139:13–14 Proverbs 11:17 Isaiah 58:11 1 Corinthians 3:16–17 1 Corinthians 6:19–20 Ephesians 2:10 Philippians 4:6–7 Galatians 5:14 1 Peter 3:4
Stay healthy.	Proverbs 17:22 1 Corinthians 10:31 1 Timothy 4:8 3 John 1:2
Glorify God with all that you do.	Psalms 23: 1–6 Romans 12:1–2 1 Peter 5:7–9
Love others as you love yourself.	Matthew 22:39 Mark 12:31 Romans 13:9
Pray and dwell in God.	Jeremiah 17:7–8 Mark 6:31–32 Mark 1:35 Luke 5:16
Renew your body, mind, and spirit.	Matthew 11:28 Romans 12:2
Rest	Genesis 2:1–3 Matthew 11:26–30

place, where he prayed." This is one example of Jesus performing self-care. **TABLE 18-4** highlights additional verses where Jesus demonstrated self-care.

TABLE 18-4 Jesus Demonstrates Self-Care (New American Standard Bible [NASB])

Matthew 14:13	He withdrew from there in a boat to a secluded place by Himself.
Matthew 14:23	After He had sent the crowds away, He went up on the mountain by Himself to pray; and when it was evening, He was there alone.
Mark 1:35	In the early morning, while it was still dark, Jesus got up, left the house, and went away to a secluded place, and was praying there.
Mark 6:46	After bidding them farewell, He left for the mountain to pray.
Luke 5:16	But Jesus Himself would *often* slip away to the wilderness and pray.

BOX 18-4 Kevin's Story: Unfolding Case Study Questions

1. Even though Kevin's coworkers were not available, was he ever alone?
2. What would have changed Kevin's situation if he spent time alone in prayer after each death he experienced in the last four weeks?
3. Is it professionally acceptable to ask to spend a moment alone after a difficult situation?

Jesus demonstrates two excellent ways of self-care. First, he spent time alone. Second, he prayed. However, his use of these approaches does not mean that Jesus suffered silently. Jesus was never completely alone, because he always had his heavenly Father with him. His alone time was specifically to pray. As Christian nurses, we never suffer alone: We have our heavenly Father. One way for Christian nurses to prevent compassion fatigue and burnout is to spend time alone in prayer with our heavenly Father (**BOX 18-4**). Spiritual self-care leads to improved physical and emotional well-being (Goncalves, Lucchetti, Menezes, & Vallada, 2015). Jesus knew that, embodied as a human, he needed to care for his spiritual self, to be physically and emotionally well to carry

out his purpose. His purpose was not fulfilled yet; he still needed to have compassion for the world on the cross.

▶ The ART of Caring

The signs and symptoms of compassion fatigue can be subtle but dangerous. But is compassion fatigue preventable? Absolutely! An individual must be **self-aware** of his or her feelings and actions to prevent compassion fatigue. Nurses need to be in tune with their spiritual self to prevent compassion fatigue.

The ART model is one method that nurses can use to prevent compassion fatigue (Todaro-Franceschi, 2013). This three-step, cyclic model asks the nurse to Acknowledge, Recognize, and Turn (**FIGURE 18-1**).

Acknowledge

The first step in the ART model is to acknowledge what you are feeling. Are you experiencing anger? Do you feel sad or depressed? Does helping patients bring you joy? This step of the ART model requires you to be self-aware. You may need a mentor to help you discover some of those feelings that you are experiencing. Todaro-Franceschi (2013) suggests paying attention to what irritates you throughout the day. When a patient asks you to do something for him or her, does that bring you joy? Or is it burdensome?

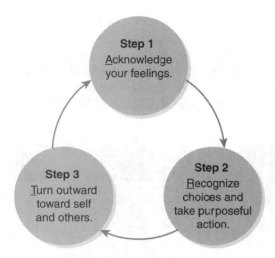

FIGURE 18-1 The ART model: three steps to prevent compassion fatigue.

Recognize

After you acknowledge your feelings, the second step involves recognizing that you are at risk for becoming fatigued. You have a choice to allow yourself to not be self-aware. It takes purposeful action to recognize that you are at risk and that you choose not to be fatigued. One method to accomplish this step is to recognize and choose to spend a few minutes alone in prayer with God.

Turn

The final—and most important—step in the ART model is to turn toward yourself or reflect on what you acknowledged and recognized (Box 18-4). Self-reflection is where the most learning will take place. One method to accomplish this step is, as mentioned earlier, to first reconnect with God, and then reconnect with yourself. The stronger your spiritual relationship with God is, the stronger your physical and emotional connection will be.

Although Turn is the final step of the ART model, this ongoing process is a continuous cycle, something that you will repeat many times in your life.

▶ Achieving Compassion Satisfaction

When applying the ART of Caring model, the goal is for caregivers to be able to achieve **compassion satisfaction**. Compassion satisfaction does not just happen overnight. Instead, nurses must achieve **awareness** and become attuned to their physical, mental, and spiritual needs. Many resources describe this state as **mindfulness**. Achieving compassion satisfaction (**BOX 18-5**) also does not mean that you will never experience traumatic or emotional situations, but rather that you develop **resilience** strategies and techniques to prevent compassion fatigue and burnout (**BOX 18-6**). "For God gave us a spirit not of fear but of power and love and self-control" (2 Timothy 1:7, English Standard Version [ESV]).

BOX 18-5 Research Highlight

In this research study, oncology nurses were surveyed about their experiences of compassion fatigue, burnout, and compassion satisfaction. In 2016, Wu and colleagues conducted a quantitative, descriptive study using a non-experimental design and involving 486 American and 63 Canadian oncology nurses. "All participants were members of the Canadian Association of Nurses in Oncology (CANO) and the Oncology Nursing Society (ONS)" (p. E163). The results were comparable between both the American and Canadian nurses. How nurses perceived team cohesiveness in the workplace positively impacted their reported compassion satisfaction. Nurses aged 40 years or younger showed higher risk of compassion fatigue than older nurses. Further research is warranted to increase generalizability to all areas of nursing practice.

Wu, S., Singh-Carlson, S., Odell, A., Reynolds, G., & Su, Y. (2016). Compassion fatigue, burnout, and compassion satisfaction among oncology nurses in the United States and Canada. *Oncology Nursing Forum, 43*(4), 161–169. Reprinted with permission from the Oncology Nursing Forum. Copyright © 2016. Oncology Nursing Society. All rights reserved.

▶ Conclusion

Compassion fatigue is a devastating complication that affects both Christian nurses and nursing as a profession. Spiritual self-care is the best means to prevent compassion fatigue. The master of compassion, Jesus Christ, demonstrated spiritual self-care for us to model. Remember, as nurses, we extend compassion to others (**BOX 18-7**), but we should also extend compassion to ourselves: "You shall love your neighbor as yourself" (Romans 13:9, ESV).

BOX 18-6 Evidence-Based Practice Focus

This article presents an evidence-based approach to integrate reflective debriefing after a traumatic event in an effort to prevent compassion fatigue and burnout, and to promote compassion satisfaction and resiliency. "Debriefing after adverse outcomes using a structured model has been used in health care as a nonthreatening and relatively low-cost way to discuss unanticipated outcomes, identify opportunities for improvement, and heal as a group" (p. 320). Debriefing in a group setting allows nurses to explore their emotions and develop interventions to be used for future situations. Schmidt and Haglund suggest that debriefing is a way to promote resiliency in environments where compassion fatigue is prevalent. Increasing resilience to secondary traumatic stress events can prevent compassion fatigue and burnout—the key to prevention is to be proactive.

Schmidt, M., & Haglund, K. (2017). Debrief in emergency departments to improve compassion fatigue and promote resiliency. *Journal of Trauma Nursing, 24*(5), 317–322. doi:10.1097/JTN.0000000000000315

BOX 18-7 Outstanding Nurse Leader: Katie Gold, BSN, RN

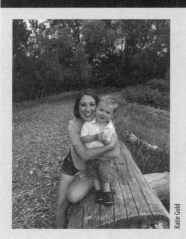

Katie Gold

"Love the Lord your God with all your heart and with all your soul and with all your mind." This is the first and greatest commandment. And the second is like it: "Love your neighbor as yourself." (Matthew 22:37–39, NIV)

A great misconception in the Christian faith is that we miss a key phrase in the second greatest commandment of loving others. Love God first, and love others *as yourself*. We cannot be compassionate and caring nursing professionals if we don't know how to extend that love to ourselves. It is easy to believe that others are worthy of love, but ourselves . . . that is more complicated. Spiritual self-care is not perfection but a constantly evolving journey—a journey that I know all too well. What experiences and lies taught me not to love myself? Why would I not believe God when He tells me that I do not have to hustle for my worthiness, earn my salvation, or prove myself to anyone else?

Death was the beginning of my career as a registered nurse (RN) on the oncology floor, and I was not prepared for it. My first day off orientation, I was assigned three patients, two of whom were receiving hospice care. Both had died by the end of my shift. Completely devastated, I began my struggle to work alongside cancer warriors. Of course, there were plenty of holy moments. Yet, when I found myself holding a sobbing teenager after his mother had died from a brain aneurysm as a complication from leukemia, I could not take it anymore. I called in sick the next shift, sobbing and unintelligibly saying, "I can't do this anymore." I was terrified of cancer and was convinced that everyone I loved would die soon.

My mind immediately flashed back to nursing school. Nurses, staff, and even faculty at my clinical rotations did not display the fulfilled, compassionate, caring professionalism we were supposedly being trained to demonstrate. Unknowingly, I was being introduced to what *not* to do and how *not* to perform self-care. I thought to myself, "I don't want to end up like this!" Things I did during nursing school came in handy as I began down a path of fatigue on the oncology floor: (1) I joined a boxing gym, (2) I created an encouragement journal full of scripture to read when I was feeling anxious, (3) I was intentional in where I studied (in the light, near a garden, outside), (4) I surrounded myself with beauty, (5) I made friends with positive people who were not obsessive about grades and assignments, and (6) I did my best to have fun with fellow classmates.

After doing all of these things, something was different inside me. It made me realize that sometimes self-care is buying yourself flowers, or knowing when enough is enough, or being brave enough to change RN jobs despite intense loyalty to your colleagues. The truth is that self-care takes courage, bravery, confidence, grace, and—most of all—practice.

The Bible does not shy away from showing us that life is hard, but God always shows up to offer grace. God uses imperfect people to perform ordinary tasks that shape the world. When we open the book of Psalms, we are opening the heart of what it means to be human. Psalms explains the range of emotional and spiritual experiences that shape our relationship with God (Psalms 6, 22, 95, and 113). The good news is that God is not intimidated by our complexity. I had to allow myself to thaw and feel my feelings. Hiding and pretending led nowhere. I am a human who is designed to eat, sleep, breathe, worship, and work. Work is a part of who I am, but it does not define me. As my pastor says, "We are not active participants in the gospel but rather passive recipients of grace."

Jesus demonstrated great Biblical boundaries and self-care throughout his life. Jesus spent time alone (Luke 4:1, 4:42, and 5:16). My introverted heart says AMEN. Jesus took time to pray to his Father (Mark 1:35, 6:45–46, and Luke 6:12). He did not do it all. He did not heal everyone. He was not best friends with everyone. Jesus did not allow himself to be manipulated into meeting the expectations of others. He relied on who God sent him, and his purpose was clear. I want to live my life with that peace and confidence provided by Jesus's example.

My advice for a nursing student, a new nurse, or even an experienced nurse comes from my mother: "You cannot give what you do not have." You cannot be an excellent nurse who is caring and compassionate if you do not know how to extend care and compassion to yourself. So take five minutes for yourself, even if it is five minutes of peace in the supply closet with a Graham cracker. Self-care does not need to be extreme, such as a monthly massage or a weekend getaway. It can be as simple as breathing slow and deep, using the restroom when needed, eating when you are hungry, resting when you are tired, starting a spiritual self-care journal, talking with other nurses to remind yourself that you are not alone in the chaos, paying attention to how you are feeling (physically, mentally, emotionally, and spiritually), creating boundaries for yourself, and learning how to say "no" without guilt.

As you enter this journey, you will learn about disease processes, pharmacology, and skills such as how to start an intravenous line, but you will also begin exposure therapy. That is, difficult circumstances will reveal who you are, what you believe, and how you cope with hard things. Know thyself. Ask yourself questions and pay attention to your responses. Are your responses grounded in truth? God declares you to be His lovingly redeemed child. When you believe the truth about who you are in Christ, there is a sigh of relief. No more hustle. No more striving. No more comparison or self-degrading thoughts. Instead, there is peace and great hope when we live out the truth that we are enough because of Jesus Christ. Through this truth, we can be the light of the world, and be the excellent, compassionate, caring nurses that we all long to be.

▶ Clinical Reasoning Exercises

Dr. Beth Hudnall Stamm originally developed the Professional Quality of Life (ProQOL) scale to assess how caring for others affects a professional caregiver's perceived quality of life (Center for Victims of Torture, 2019). ProQOL measures the extent to which a professional caregiver is experiencing compassion satisfaction, burnout, or secondary traumatic stress because of caring for others. The Center for Victims of Torture (2019) suggests that nurses use the ProQOL scale to determine their level of compassion fatigue or burnout. Caregivers can use the ProQOL scale on one occasion; however, an ongoing assessment is best to catch compassion fatigue in its earliest stages.

1. Complete the ProQOL scale found at https://proqol.org/uploads/ProQOL _5_English_Self-Score.pdf.
2. Score your responses according to the instructions.
3. Discuss your findings with a mentor.
4. Answer these questions based on your findings:
    a. How do the findings apply to your spiritual life?
    b. How do the findings apply to your professional life?
    c. Regardless of your score (low, average, or high), list five interventions that you will implement over the next month to achieve compassion satisfaction.

▶ Personal Reflection Exercises

This exercise is intended to help you assess your overall spiritual well-being and develop a plan of action to enhance your perception of spiritual well-being. The Spiritual Well-Being Scale (Paloutzian & Ellison, 1982) is a self-perceived scale assessing your overall spiritual life in relation to God. Reflect on your past clinical or caregiving experiences. You have educated yourself on compassion fatigue, burnout, and the ART of Caring model. You understand the importance of spiritual self-care. To go a step further, do the following:

1. Complete the Spiritual Well-Being Scale that can be ordered from https://www.lifeadvance.com /products.html. It should take 10 minutes or less to complete.
2. Use the scoring instructions to determine your spiritual well-being.
3. Use the concepts of the nursing process to complete a Spiritual Self-Care Plan based on your Spiritual Well-Being Scale score.
4. Implement your interventions to achieve your goals.
5. Evaluate your progress toward your spiritual self-care goals.
6. Continue to reevaluate your progress each day until you have achieved your goals.
7. Repeat this personal reflection as needed.

References

Brenan, M. (2017). Nurses keep healthy lead as most honest, ethical profession. Retrieved from https://news.gallup.com/poll/224639/nurses-keep-healthy-lead-honest-ethical-profession .aspx?g_source=CATEGORY_SOCIAL_POLICY_IS-SUES&g_medium=topic&g_campaign=tiles

Bridgeman, P., Bridgeman, M., & Barone, J. (2018). Burnout syndrome among healthcare professionals. *American Journal of Health-System Pharmacy, 75*(3), 147–152. doi:10.2146/ajhp170460

Center for Victims of Torture. (2019). The ProQOL measure in English and non-English translations. Retrieved from https://proqol.org/ProQol_Test.html

Compassion Fatigue Awareness Project. (2017). What is compassion fatigue? Retrieved from http://compassionfatigue.org/pages/compassionfatigue.html

Figley, C. R. (Ed.). (1995). *Compassion fatigue: Coping with secondary traumatic stress disorder in those who treat the traumatized.* New York, NY: Brunner/Mazel.

Fowler, M. D. M. (2015). *Guide to the code of ethics for nurses with interpretive statements: Development, interpretation, and application* (2nd ed.). Silver Spring, MD: American Nurses Association.

Goncalves, J. P., Lucchetti, G., Menezes, P. R., & Vallada, H. (2015). Religious and spiritual interventions in mental health care: A systematic review and meta-analysis of randomized controlled clinical trials. *Psychological Medicine, 45*(14), 2937–2949. doi:10.1017/S0033291715001166

Harris, C., & Griffin, M. T. Q. (2015). Nursing on empty: Compassion fatigue signs, symptoms, and system interventions. *Journal of Christian Nursing, 32*(2), 80–87. doi:10.1097/CNJ.0000000000000155

Henson, J. (2017). When compassion is lost. *Medsurg Nursing, 26*(2), 139–142.

Lanier, J. (2017). *Running on empty: Compassion fatigue in nurses and non-professional caregivers.* Columbus, OH: Ohio Nurses Association.

Mattioli, D., Walters, L., & Cannon, E. (2018). Focusing on the caregiver: Compassion fatigue awareness and understanding. *Medsurg Nursing, 27*(5), 232–327.

Mendes, A. (2017). How to address compassion fatigue in the community nurse. *British Journal of Community Nursing, 22*(9), 2041–2050. doi:10.1111/jan.12686

Paloutzian, R., & Ellison, C. (1982). Loneliness, spiritual well-being and the quality of life. In L. A. Peplau & D. Perlman (Eds.), *Loneliness: A sourcebook of current theory, research and therapy* (pp. 224–237). New York, NY: Wiley.

Pennington, A. (2016). Compassion is like a muscle: It gets stronger with practice. *HuffPost.* Retrieved from https://www.huffpost.com/entry/compassion-is-like-a-muscle-it-gets-stronger-with_b_576559e7e4b0ed0729a1b196

Sheppard, K. (2016). Compassion fatigue: Are you at risk? *American Nurse Today, 11*(1), 53–55.

Todaro-Franceschi, V. (Ed.). (2013). *Compassion fatigue and burnout in nursing: Enhancing quality of life.* New York, NY: Springer.

Wu, S., Singh-Carlson, S., Odell, A., Reynolds, G., & Su, Y. (2016). Compassion fatigue, burnout, and compassion satisfaction among oncology nurses in the United States and Canada. *Oncology Nursing Forum, 43*(4), 161–169. doi:10.1188/16.ONF.E161-E169

Recommended Readings

Gentry, E. (2018). Fighting compassion fatigue and burnout by building emotional resilience. *Journal of Oncology Navigation and Survivorship, 9*(12), 532–535.

Harris, R. (2008). *The happiness trap: How to stop struggling and start living.* Boulder, CO: Trumpeter.

Khamisa, N., Oldenburg, B., Peltzer, K., & Ilic, D. (2015). Work related stress, burnout, job satisfaction and general health of nurses. *International Journal of Environmental Research and Public Health, 12*(1), 652–666. doi:10.3390/ ijerph120100652

McMillan, K. (2016). Employee spiritual care: Supporting those who care for others. *Journal of Christian Nursing 33*(2), 98–101. doi:10.1097/CNJ.0000000000000258

Murphy, L. S., & Walker, M. S. (2013). Spirit-guided care: Christian nursing for the whole person. *Journal of Christian Nursing, 30*(3), 144–152. doi:10.1097/CNJ.0b013e318294c289

O'Brien, M. E. (2011). *Servant leadership in nursing: Spirituality and practice in contemporary healthcare.* Sudbury, MA: Jones and Bartlett.

O'Brien, M. E. (2014). *Spirituality in nursing: Standing on holy ground* (5th ed.). Sudbury, MA: Jones and Bartlett.

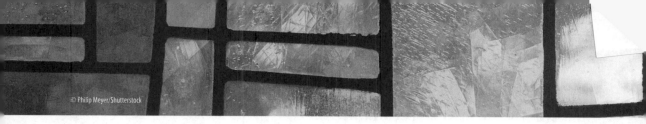

CHAPTER 19

Caring for One Another with Christ's Light

Mary E. Hobus, PhD, MSN, RN

LEARNING OBJECTIVES

At the end of this chapter, the reader will be able to:

1. Appraise Christian characteristics that promote civility among colleagues in the profession of nursing.
2. Understand the importance of maintaining and sustaining civility as nurses across all practice and academic settings.
3. Demonstrate civility among colleagues in the healthcare system and the educational learning environment.
4. Analyze the importance of shining Christ's light on one another.
5. Value the importance of encouraging, honoring, and caring for one another.
6. Reflect on one's own experiences with incivility.

KEY TERMS

Bullying	Compassion	Incivility
Called to care	Forgiveness	Lateral (horizontal)
Christian nursing	Grace	violence
Civility		

▶ Introduction

As does author Barbara White in the *Divine Appointment: Fulfilling Your Call* chapter of this text, the author of this chapter shares her personal stories about caring for other nurses as a leader and administrator. The topic of incivility is a sensitive but timely one and is best discussed through this author's personal experiences. Throughout this chapter, readers will have an opportunity to reflect on their own attitudes, beliefs, and experiences.

Christian nurses must be strong and courageous when caring for one another with Christ's light shining bright. It is through Christ's light that we can care for one another in our daily work by demonstrating civility toward one another. Joshua 1:9 states, "Have I not commanded you? Be strong and courageous. Do not be frightened, and do not be dismayed, for the Lord your God is with you wherever you go" (English Standard Version [ESV]). Another Bible passage on strength and courage is in Isaiah 41:10: "Fear not, for I am with you; be not dismayed, for I am your God; I will strengthen you, I will help you, I will uphold you with my righteous right hand."

It was a journey of trust with Christ to ensure that my nursing practice was of high quality, providing healing and safety in Jesus. Along this journey, to my surprise, I found that the stress of work and the demands of perfection could be extremely overwhelming for a nurse. At times, incivility became part of nursing practice in a number of environments and in varying experiences. This chapter seeks to use the author's personal and professional nursing experiences as a lens through which to view Christian caring for one another as essential to the profession of nursing. After completing this chapter, nurses should have an increased awareness of the importance of Christian nurses as they practice attributes of Christ's forgiveness, love, and care to promote civility in the healthcare practice environment and the educational learning environment. All Christian nurses should shine Christ's light and love among their colleagues, just as they do with all their patients. Encouraging, honoring, and caring for each nurse is an important role of nursing as ministry.

▶ Personal Nursing Experience: A Walk with Jesus and the Holy Spirit

My **Christian nursing** journey as a practicing registered nurse (RN) has been directed by Jesus and the Holy Spirit. I grew up believing that Jesus died for me and saved me from all my sins. I also believed that I was a *called* servant of God, expected to practice nursing with lovingkindness and care toward all of God's children. I was *called* to learn and practice with a caring consciousness toward others: patients, students, nurses, colleagues, administrators, friends, family, and acquaintances. This caring consciousness was important to me and essential to everyday Christian living and life. I wanted to be a shining light of Jesus for my patients and others when they were experiencing a birth of a child, life-changing events with or without hope, suffering, pain, or even death. When I entered into a patient's room, I knew I was standing on holy ground in the presence of God to assist His children in recovery, if that was His will. I can remember standing in a patient's room on several occasions asking for God's presence at the bedside and God's words to be said in a kind and gracious manner.

As an RN with a servant's heart toward your patients and their families, it becomes a privilege to be there to listen and care for those in need. These caring moments between patients, families, and nurses remind you that you are on holy ground in the presence of God, which can bring hope, love, and peace at a moment that is often filled with desperation, discouragement, and a loss of hope. O'Brien (2018) stated the following:

> When the nurse clinician, nurse educator, nurse administrator, or nurse researcher stands before a patient, a student, a staff member, or a study participant, God is also present, and the ground on which the nurse is standing is holy. For it is here, in the act of serving a brother or sister in need, that the nurse truly encounters God. God is present in the nurse's practice of caring just as surely as He was present in the blessed meeting with Moses so many centuries ago. (p. 1)

The story of Moses and the burning bush can be found in the book of Exodus, Chapter 3.

I have loved nursing since the first day I started nursing school. I have been passionate about practicing nursing safely and providing high-quality care. I have read the Bible often as a Christian nurse to find forgiveness, grace, peace, comfort, and understanding, which has provided me with the strength and courage to continue to practice nursing in a profession that I love dearly. As a beginning nursing student at St. John's College in Winfield, Kansas, I often prayed in a little chapel in the basement in our dormitory building. I would go there and quietly kneel before the altar, behind a closed door, asking for God's forgiveness, grace, peace, comfort, and strength to understand nursing and to always provide safe nursing care to everyone whom God created. When we had classes, the nursing students would walk from the nursing building to the chapel for services about three blocks away. I remember walking through snow, rain, and hot weather to listen to God's Word, seek His wisdom, and ask for strength to be a successful nurse and to pass all my examinations. When I was a student, it was not unusual for nursing students to leave nursing school throughout the program due to failing grades or poor judgment in clinical practice. Several of my favorite passages that gave me comfort daily at

that time, and even today help me find strength and courage, are the following:

- Philippians 4:13: "I can do all things through him who strengthens me."
- Philippians 4:4–7: "Rejoice in the Lord always; again I will say, Rejoice. Let your reasonableness be known to everyone. The Lord is at hand; do not be anxious about anything, but in everything by prayer and supplication with thanksgiving let your requests be made known to God. And the peace of God, which surpasses all understanding, will guard your hearts and your minds in Christ Jesus."
- Galatians 5:22–25: "But the fruit of the Spirit is love, joy, peace, patience, kindness, goodness, faithfulness, gentleness, self-control; against such things there is no law. And those who belong to Christ Jesus have crucified the flesh with its passions and desires. If we live by the Spirit, let us also walk by the Spirit. Let us not become conceited, provoking one another, envying one another."

After earning my first degree, I knew I wanted to experience and work in different areas of nursing so as to be a nursing educator and work with students in a faith-based university, which I believe would enable me to share my love of Jesus with others. I recognized during this time in my early years of nursing this was a *calling from God* to work with His children and serve Him daily in my nursing practice. Following this path meant returning to school for a bachelor of science in nursing (BSN), a master of science in nursing (MSN), and a doctoral degree (PhD). So my journey began with the Holy Spirit and with a sincere trust in Jesus that I could do this because of my calling to serve God and His children. By the power of the Holy Spirit, I continued my practice in nursing in many various areas of practice, always learning new knowledge, attitudes, and skills. With the strength and courage from Jesus and constantly trusting him, I was able to raise three children; be a wife; care for a home; slowly obtain a BSN, MSN, and PhD; and work at several faith-based universities and healthcare systems. God was my strength, and God provided the courage I needed to accomplish this calling. Nursing as ministry was always the priority when providing care to others. This journey was not always easy, especially during my nursing practice when incivility would cause deep pain, sorrow, and anxiety.

Even though this journey was difficult at times, I believed that as Christian nurses we are the light of Christ in each aspect of our nursing calling. Therefore, during my nursing practice, I primarily focused on nursing care and ways to improve that care as I worked. Christian nursing care focuses on the holistic care of each individual. As O'Brien (2018) explained:

> Overall, holistic nursing is supported by and alternately supports the intimate connection of body, mind, and spirit. Nursing of the whole person requires attention to the individuality and uniqueness of each dimension, as well as to the interrelatedness of the three. (p. 8)

As we care for our patients, families, and communities, we must walk with Jesus and the Holy Spirit because our patients and families have deep pain, sorrow, and anxiety. As humans, we do cast a shadow, but with Christ there is no shadow because he is the light that shines so brightly in our hearts, minds, and souls. 1 John 1:5 states that "God is light; in him is no darkness at all"; John 8:12 explains, "Again Jesus spoke to them, saying, 'I am the light of the world. Whoever follows me will not walk in darkness, but will have the light of life.'" So even when we are in darkness, we need to remember that God is always with us to be our source of light.

During my nursing practice, I would pray in the car on the way to work, I would pray in the elevator before reaching the nursing unit, and I would pray with patients when they requested a prayer. As I reflect on the past

36 years as an RN, I often went to work with Jesus and focused just on nursing and caring for my patients to the best of my abilities. If I knew a nurse was complaining, unhappy, or causing trouble for other healthcare providers, I stayed away from that individual to avoid falling into a tangled web of negativity. Consequently, throughout my early practice as an RN, I did not always reach out to other RNs to develop professional trusting relationships. If a nurse was caring and compassionate, worked hard to provide high-quality care, and followed the institutional policies, then a professional trusting relationship usually began. Even today, a few of us from that period in my life are still nursing colleagues. During my early practice as an RN, from a professional perspective, I did observe an increase in subtle incivility among colleagues within the healthcare system.

As a young nurse in the 1980s, I was not aware of incivility in the professional world of nursing in either the healthcare system or the educational learning environment. I did not want to believe such behavior existed or even address the possibility of pain from actions of other nurses being uncivil toward others or myself. I did not believe that nurses would intentionally be disrespectful toward others, be insubordinate, or persistently intimidate other nurses in an effort to harm another RN. However, in time I did experience both civility and incivility within the healthcare system and the educational learning environment. I would often defend the profession of nursing to my colleagues and deny the fact that other nurses would demonstrate incivility toward me and attempt to prevent me from achieving goals of continuing my nursing education. Unfortunately, the reality is that incivility does occur in many environments.

Nursing was my chosen profession, and one where I envisioned providers would always be caring and loving. As I have grown in knowledge and wisdom, however, I have had to admit that there is a subtle darkness to the practice of nursing. I call it a subtle darkness because of my experiences with incivility in nursing education as a professor and as an administrator. These experiences of incivility have demonstrated specifically to me that incivility does exist and it can destroy you as a person, as well as your love and passion for the profession and the practice of nursing. As noted by Phillips, MacKusick, and Whichello (2018), "incivility in the nursing workplace is important because a patient's quality of care may be adversely affected, directly or indirectly" (p. E7). According to Oja (2017), "being subjected to uncivil behaviors affects the individual nurse, patients and organizational outcomes" (p. 345). Furthermore, it can be just as harmful in the nursing educational learning setting between faculty members and students.

My hope was always to be an instrument of God, and to be joy-filled and caring toward all of God's creation. Romans 15:13 says, "May the God of hope fill you with all joy and peace in believing, so that by the power of the Holy Spirit you may abound in hope." I prayed and worked hard to keep focused on the positive aspects of professionalism and ignore the negativity of incivility. As a Christian nurse, I was **called to care**, to be civil to others, and to be respectful.

▶ Definitions of Incivility

A plethora of scholarly writing and research focuses on incivility among nurses in the healthcare and educational systems. The list of scholarly journal references that speak directly to incivility, found at the end of this chapter, is intended to foster a deeper understanding of what incivility is and how it affects nurses in their workplace. These journal articles demonstrate the painful reality that nursing incivility is truly a profound concern and can be present in many nurses' everyday work experience.

Several definitions of **incivility** are reviewed here to increase understanding of this negative behavior. According to

Merriam-Webster Dictionary, incivility is "the quality or state of being uncivil" or "a rude or discourteous act" ("Incivility," 2005). Phillips et al. (2018) stated "uncivil behaviors are characteristically rude and discourteous, revealing a lack of regard for others. Incivility begins with rude behavior and branches into negative aggressions called **horizontal or lateral violence**, **bullying**, sexual harassment, or work place violence" (p. E7).

In my own career, a faculty member once became confrontational toward me when the upper administrators from the university were meeting with me and the other faculty members. I had left the room, and on my return, this faculty member spoke forcefully toward me about an issue; the bullying was observed by the other people present. In the past, when confronted with a problem, I would think of a solution and reply in a professional manner or provide information to the faculty member in a timely manner. This faculty member kept trying to add information and raising her voice about the significance of the problem. She kept moving forward toward my personal space, which made me feel uncomfortable. I continued to remain calm and attentive to her needs. I agreed with her, provided a solution, and continued my meeting with administration and other faculty members. This person often gossiped about issues that did not always go her way, and it often angered her when things did not go her way. She was an excellent teacher, and I often complimented her on her excellent teaching methods, positive student outcomes, and positive relationships with students—but her incivility continued.

As I personally experienced workplace incivility, I sought out God's guidance, strength, and courage to stop this behavior from occurring to others and myself. As time continued, I felt powerless, as I received no support from the administrative staff to assist me in dealing with problem faculty members. I knew that I needed to be a Christian nurse leader who told the truth, followed God's commandments, and followed the law. Most importantly, I was to be forgiving and caring toward all involved. Matthew 22:37–39 says, "You shall love the Lord your God with all your heart and with all your soul and with all your mind. This is the great and first commandment. And a second is like it: You shall love your neighbor as yourself." As a nursing administrator, it was important for all members of the faculty to respect one another, including their colleagues' differing beliefs and values. Indeed, Andersson and Pearson (1999) described incivility as a social interaction: "The instigator(s), the target(s), the observers(s), and the social context all contribute to and are affected by an uncivil encounter" (p. 457).

Working with faculty can often be complex and challenging. Sometimes, certain faculty members might not support students attending chapel at a faith-based university. These faculty members would continue class and ignore the requests of students who wanted to attend chapel; they disregarded the requests of the nursing administration to allow students and faculty members time to attend chapel. At other times, faculty members would allow students to go to chapel, yet continue with class or nursing skills lab and teach important information or work with students on their nursing skills while those students were absent. This created great tension between the faculty members, the nursing students, and the nursing administration. I prayed for God's guidance, will, strength, and courage to be a Christian leader, to know how to speak the loving words of Jesus, be forgiving, and be filled with the peace of the Holy Spirit so as to move forward with God's plan. But God had a different plan for me—a plan that I had to accept and move forward with. I had learned that incivility was so very harmful to who I was and what I believed in Jesus. During this very hurtful time, I prayed and prayed not to be bitter, but instead to be a Christian leader who was forgiving and caring toward others and still shining Christ's light for others to see and experience.

A number of organizations have made notable efforts to discuss the topics of bullying, violence, and incivility in the workplace; some of these appear as resources at the end of the chapter. They have sought to examine incivility to identify its causes, host environments, and impacts; identify appropriate interventions; and address actions of administrators and productivity in nursing practice environments.

For example, the American Nurses Association (ANA), in its *Guide to the Code of Ethics for Nurses with Interpretive Statements*, Provision 1, confirms the importance of "Affirming Health through Relationships of Dignity and Respect" (Fowler, 2015, p. 1). Provision 1.5 further describes the importance of "Relationships with Colleagues and Others" (p. 18). "Lateral violence or bullying (or mobbing)" is addressed in Provision 1.5, and its presence is denounced in the nursing work environment (p. 18). "The nurse practices with compassion and respect for the inherent dignity, worth, and unique attributes of every person" (p. 1). Provision 1 "is meant to be applied to everyone, not only patients" (p. 18). It is clear that the interpretative statement includes the whole team of healthcare providers: those nurses who are present at the bedside, those who may have other roles in nursing that are not at the bedside providing direct patient care, and other members of the healthcare team. "The hallmark of these relationships are respect, caring, fairness, transparency, integrity, civility, kindness, dignity, respect, and collaboration. This is a relational environment in which all might thrive and flourish" (p. 18). With positive relationships in place among nurses and other interprofessional team members, safe, effective, and high-quality patient care can be achieved. Indeed, Provision 2.3 notes that "high-quality patient care cannot exist without welcoming and embracing both interdisciplinary and intradisciplinary collaboration in today's healthcare system" (p. 35).

ANA's Provision 6 discusses "The Moral Milieu," which is also mentioned in Provision

1.5. "The nurse, through individual and collective effort, establishes, maintains, and improves the ethical environment of the work setting and conditions of employment that are conducive to safe, quality health care" (p. 95). Provision 6 is divided into three important considerations in nursing practice. Provision 6.1, "The Environment and Moral Virtue," describes normative ethics such as "right and wrong, good and evil" (p. 102). Provision 6.2, "The Environment and Ethical Obligations," highlights that "nurses in all roles must create a culture of excellence and maintain practice environments that support nurses and others in the fulfillment of their ethical obligations" (p. 105). Provision 6.3, "Responsibility for the Healthcare Environment," is an important undertaking for all leaders and nurses. It emphasizes the importance of constructing and building this environment with intentionality. Nurses should work both individually and collectively to develop an ethical environment to enhance patient healthcare outcomes (**BOX 19-1**). According to Hoglund (2013), "the *Code of Ethics for Nurses* gives a professional obligation to practice in a compassionate and respectful way that is unaffected by the attributes of the patient" (p. 228).

BOX 19-1 Reflection Exercises

1. Describe your perceptions of the behaviors of incivility.
2. How would you develop or maintain a culture of civility as a staff nurse on your nursing unit?
3. What are the detrimental effects of incivility on the nursing profession?
4. After reading the ANA's *Guide to the Code of Ethics for Nurses with Interpretive Statements,* analyze the importance of using this information to empower the RN. How can it be used to foster safe, high-quality care?

▶ Definitions of Civility

Another stream of literature deals with the opposite of incivility—that is, **civility**. Thus, the literature is beginning to focus on civility, recognizing that fostering a culture of civility is important in both academic and practice settings. The list of references at the end of this chapter highlights additional scholarly journal articles that can enhance your knowledge of civility.

Porath's (2018) research, conducted over many years, revealed that persons who are continually exposed to negativity in the workplace underperform and tend to make more mistakes than those who engage with a positive work environment. This relationship applies to healthcare workers as well, including physicians. As Porath (2018) noted in her recent TED Talk, businesses could actually save large amounts of money if management created happy employees by implementing small kindnesses such as smiling, "thank you" notes, positive talking, and giving credit for a job well done.

When Clark and Carnosso (2008) performed a concept analysis of civility, they used the following operational definition: "Civility is characterized by an authentic respect for others when expressing disagreement, disparity, or controversy. It involves time, presence, a willingness to engage in genuine discourse, and a sincere intention to seek common ground" (p. 13). Clark and Springer (2010) later stated that "academic incivility is disruptive behavior that substantially or repeatedly interferes with teaching and learning. . . . Academic nurse leaders play a critical role in preventing and addressing academic incivility because these behaviors can negatively affect learning and harm faculty–student relationships" (p. 319). Even though a growing body of nursing research continues to focus on the development of a culture of civility in nursing education, additional studies are needed to find ways that nurses can best support and care for one another. Indeed, Clark and Carnosso (2008) have confirmed the need for additional nursing research to focus on civility. In today's nursing curriculum, it is critical to address the importance of creating a culture of civility and understanding the implications of incivility across all healthcare settings. If these topics are not addressed in the academic learning environment, patients' health care may be negatively affected in real-world settings (**BOX 19-2**).

Even though the professional nursing literature is expanding the depth of knowledge and research about preventive strategies for stopping incivility among nurses and other healthcare providers, more work is needed to elucidate the relationships between nurses. To date, there has been a dearth of research on nurse-to-nurse caring and relationships (**CASE STUDY 19-1**). The ANA's (2015) position statement on incivility, bullying, and workplace violence asserts, "Evidence-based best practices

must be implemented to prevent and mitigate incivility, bullying, and workplace violence; to promote the health, safety, and wellness of RNs; and to ensure optimal outcomes across the

---

BOX 19-2   Reflection Exercises

1. Describe your perceptions of civility.
2. Define the attributes of the concept of civility.
3. How would you develop or maintain a culture of civility as an RN, a faculty member, or a nursing student?
4. Why do nurses not care for one another with the same passion that they have for the patient(s) whom they are assigned to care for?

🔎 CASE STUDY 19-1

Susan is a professional registered nurse and the unit manager on the medical–surgical nursing floor in a faith-based hospital. She has been a nurse for 35 years and the unit manager for 8 years. Susan just completed morning rounds with all the nurses and their patient assignments and has returned to her office to complete a report due at the end of the week. A non-nursing staff member, considered an unlicensed assistive personnel (UAP), comes into her office and begins to yell at Susan concerning a comment made by another non-nursing staff member. The UAP is not making sense and continues to use words that she normally does not use. Susan tries to be supportive of the staff member who is yelling at her, not making sense, and is clearly emotionally and physically upset. Susan does not really find out what the issue is, but the yelling continues. Others outside of the office begin to hear the non-nursing member yelling at Susan. No one enters the office. Finally, the UAP leaves the office, and the other nurses gather around this non-nursing member to calm her down and take her blood pressure.

Susan looks for this UAP staff member; she deeply cares for her and wants her to be okay. Susan has trusted this staff member for many years and believes that she has a strong positive work ethic. The UAP yells, "Get out of here." Susan leaves and is distressed from all the yelling. The other nurses gather around the UAP and begin talking about the incident. Susan tries to call security and no one answers the phone. Susan also calls the human resources (HR) department; again, no one answers the phone. Susan tries to call the person to whom she reports, and yet again no one answers the phone. What can Susan do at this time? She sits in her office and feels very discouraged and hurt about the hostile behaviors and harmful verbal attacks that just occurred.

Several days later, Susan finds out that the nursing staff working during the incident all went to the HR department and complained about Susan, the nursing manager, and how she was supposedly yelling at the UAP member, which was untrue.

Questions

1. As a Christian nurse leader, what would you have done to stop this situation?
2. As a Christian nurse leader, ask yourself, "What have I done to contribute to this conflict?"
3. As a Christian nurse leader, how would you pray for your nurses and staff members after finding out that they reported you to the HR department?
4. What can you as the Christian nurse leader do to provide reconciliation for all members in the nursing unit?
5. How do you restore the professional relationships and forgive one another?
6. What scriptures would you share with others?

health care continuum." Evidence-based best practices are necessary to:

- Bring an awareness of our uncivil actions toward one another as nurses
- Strengthen our consciousness that nurses need to care for one another in a caring and civil Christian manner in our working environments
- Promote caring relationships by utilizing positive caring strategies with one another to advocate for civility

▶ Being Christ's Light Among Other Nurses

It is vitally important for all of us to share Christ's light with one another and be that light for other nurses, especially for new graduates and those who are experiencing burnout in nursing or suffering from compassion fatigue (see the *Caring for One's Spiritual Self* chapter). Nursing as ministry should also emphasize the importance of caring for one another as we care for our patients, families, and communities. Nurses most always make a difference in patient care—but as nurses we also need to learn how to care for one another daily in our stressful work environments. Nursing practice will always be stressful because of the demand for high-quality care and the life-and-death situations that we encounter on a daily basis.

Nursing as ministry can assist those of us who want to serve one another and shine

Christ's light on each of us in nursing practice. We can demonstrate and encourage civility within our nursing practice toward one another, just as we do with our assigned patients. The attributes of shining Christ's light should include a caring presence, lovingkindness, faithfulness, forgiveness, humility, courage, relationships, and compassionate care. These Christ-like attributes can promote civility both in the healthcare practice environment and in academic settings. As Shelly and Miller (2006) stated, "the uniqueness of Christ inspired nursing lies in its emphasis on caring for the whole person as embodied, respecting each person as created in the image of God. It is both a science and an art, but primarily it is a response to God's grace and a reflection of his character" (p. 53). In Galatians 5:22–26, the Apostle Paul writes:

> But the fruit of the Spirit is love, joy, peace, patience, kindness, goodness, faithfulness, gentleness, self-control; against such things there is no law. And those who belong to Christ Jesus have crucified the flesh with its passion and desires. If we live by the Spirit, let us walk by the Spirit. Let us not become conceited, provoking one another, envying one another.

Shelly and Miller (2006) go on to say, "Caring is an act of faith, for it involves the risk of opening ourselves to another who may not want to care or be cared for. But unless we take that risk, we cannot claim to be truly nursing"

(p. 250). As a nurse providing compassionate care to others, we must remember to care for ourselves and other nurses. To care for our patients well, we as nurses must be well, too.

▶ Caring for Self

Newbanks, Rieg, and Schaefer (2018) define a Christian as "one who professes belief in the teachings of Jesus Christ." Christians believe caring originates from God. I believe this as well. My deep love and passion for nursing care came from God, who provided me with all the necessary skills, attitudes, and critical thinking to practice nursing safely and to provide high-quality care. I grew up believing that you must take care of everyone around you, such as your neighbor. For most of my life, this is how I functioned: No matter how tired and exhausted I was, I continued serving others before myself. Shelly and Miller (2006) assert that "Christian caring is not just an emotional tug, an intellectual concept or a metaphysical event. It is hands-on, patient-centered, physical, psychosocial and spiritual intervention to meet the needs of a patient regardless of how the nurse feels" (p. 250). This is how I would describe my nursing as ministry—as compassionate caring for all patients, nurses, and others. Kim and Patterson (2016) state, "A better understanding of the self enhances one's growth and enables the nurse to establish a caring relationship with patients in an honest, genuine, and respectful manner" (p. E25).

But as I became older, I realized that I had not taken care of myself. According to Moorman (2015), "to grow in the art of nursing, nurses must be willing to address the broken areas of their lives" (p. E2). Caring for self is honoring God because we are made in His image. He created me, and why would I not care for me, as God cares for all. Matthew 6:26 says, "Look at the birds of the air: they neither sow nor reap nor gather into barns, and yet your heavenly Father feeds them." As we work as servant leaders in our nursing ministry, we need to be cognizant of the importance of who we are and how we care for ourselves. We must remember to think positively about ourselves and to care for ourselves as we care for others by resting our bodies, resting our minds, exercising, enjoying the activities we love, eating healthy balanced meals, respecting ourselves, and belonging to a community either at church or with family for a sense of belonging and well-being. Remember that we cannot fill up the cup of another if our own cup is empty. Nurses need to learn how to manage the calendar for realistic expectations of what they can accomplish and what is essential to accomplish immediately. Matthew 6:34 reminds us: "Therefore do not be anxious about tomorrow, for tomorrow will be anxious for itself. Sufficient for the day is its own trouble."

▶ Caring for Other Nurses

I met wonderful nurses along my path of growth as an RN who helped me understand the role of the RN and the importance of caring and being present with my patients. They demonstrated how to be a compassionate servant leader while being a nurse either at the bedside or in the educational learning environment. I learned not only to look at my perspectives, experiences, and knowledge, but also to reflect on the other nurse's perspectives, experiences, and knowledge to try to be that role model of a servant leader. By reading God's Word, I found strength each and every day to work with whatever came my way. God provided the strength, courage, humility, knowledge, **compassion**, and competence that was needed to be a strong Christian woman and a nurse servant leader. As a nurse servant leader who was responsible for caring for many individuals and families, it was an honor and privilege to provide Christ's light among them through my attitude, presence, and skills. In 1 John 4:19, the Bible states, "We love because he [God] first loved us." As nurses, we provide high-quality care to our patients—yet all too often, we do not recognize this need among the fellow RNs on our nursing team. The following section suggests ways to initiate caring for your fellow nurses, professors, and students to promote civility in the diverse learning and practice healthcare environments.

Show Lovingkindness

Showing lovingkindness through a caring consciousness and presence helps nurses understand and define how they practice nursing at the bedside. During my initial education, I remember how important it was to be present at the bedside and work with the patient and family. I wanted to be aware of the needs of my patients and how I could best serve them as their nurse. I wanted to be that caring nurse and provide calmness and peace at the bedside in all my care to alleviate fear, discomfort, and pain. After all, I was a Christian nurse who wanted to be a servant leader for all the needs of all my assigned patients. Reality hit hard when I began to understand that the organizations and systems were not necessarily interested in that special touch, care, presence, or ministry. Even so, the desire to enter each room while being conscious of the care needed for the patient and the status of this person as a child of God was still ignited inside me.

By being calm, poised, and in self-control, you can provide high-quality care to each of your patients. Sometimes real-world demands may affect your work, to the point that they can be overwhelming. Although we should be practicing lovingkindness toward all patients at all time, doing so can be a challenge when we are feeling exhausted, overworked, or unsupported. We need to ask our Heavenly Father for assistance so that we can provide high-quality care for each patient and family, just as Jesus cares for us daily and meets all of our needs. Matthew 7:7 affirms: "Ask, and it

will be given to you; seek, and you will find; knock, and it will be opened to you." As nurses, we should ask to share God's lovingkindness and to care deeply for our patients, who are often strangers to us.

When working on your busy assignments, did you stop to think about what your nursing colleagues were experiencing, what their patient assignment for the day looked like, and what might be distracting their thinking? Did you demonstrate to them any lovingkindness with a caring consciousness and presence during morning report, during a break, or during the evening report? Did you express any words of lovingkindness or comfort to lighten their burdens? During the shift, if you noticed that other nurses were extremely busy with their patients and new admissions, did you take time to assist them to accomplish and complete their work? Matthew 11:28–30 states, "Come to me, all who labor and are heavy laden, and I will give you rest. Take my yoke upon you, and learn from me, for I am gentle and lowly in heart, and you will find rest for your souls. For my yoke is easy, and my burden is light." Why not assist your fellow nursing colleague to lighten their burden (**BOX 19-3**)?

As a nursing professor, I found that being caring and loving toward students often assisted students who were often experiencing high levels of stress and discomfort. I had to learn to think of the student's perspectives and needs as well. Providing safe patient care was certainly essential, but as I practiced with students, I also learned how important it was for professors to be nurturing toward students. I found that developing a calm environment in which to practice nursing was enormously beneficial to students. This peaceful atmosphere allowed students to think for themselves, to succeed in answering questions, and to accomplish high-quality care. Some students may be juggling full-time coursework, a family, and full- or part-time employment, and a calm environment may help focus on the immediate nursing issue at hand.

BOX 19-3 Reflection Exercises

1. How can you, as a Christian nurse, care for the fellow nurses with whom you work on either a daily or weekly basis with lovingkindness and a caring consciousness?
2. For nurses, what are barriers to being present for one another and developing professional relationships to empower and value one another?
3. If we do practice lovingkindness with a caring consciousness for our fellow nurses, then why has nursing as a profession not focused on the importance of this practice?
4. What stops nurses from developing those caring relationships with other nurses? Are you afraid?
5. If we do create lovingkindness with a caring consciousness with fellow nurses, then why does incivility develop on our nursing units?

In my own experience, being compassionate and demonstrating lovingkindness toward the nursing students in any environment, such as the classroom, clinical lab, simulation lab, or clinical learning setting, often brought a sense of relief to these students and created a safe place for them to be who they were. New students learning the art and science of nursing may not realize how challenging and demanding nursing school is. Therefore, it is essential to practice lovingkindness and care within the context of a caring consciousness of their needs.

Seeking to promote professional, legal, and ethical caring can be difficult at times. Seek God's guidance in these situations, because conflict and negativity have the potential to emerge in some of the conversations (for example, between nursing professor and student). Providing lovingkindness and a peaceful and calm environment often assists in decreasing the uncivil behavior of a student or a faculty member involved in such a situation.

When struggling with discouragement in a difficult situation or workplace environment, find comfort in God's Word such as Psalm 23 or words from the New Testament. In Psalm 23:1–6, David affirms:

> The Lord is my Shepherd; I shall not want.
> He makes me lie down in green pastures.
> He leads me beside still waters.
> He restores my soul.
> He leads me in paths of righteousness for his name's sake,
> Even though I walk through the valley of the shadow of death,
> I will fear no evil, for you are with me; your rod and your staff, they comfort me.
> You prepare a table before me in the presence of my enemies;
> you anoint my head with oil; my cup overflows.
> Surely goodness and mercy shall follow me all the days of my life,
> and I shall dwell in the house of the Lord forever.

Clark (2017a) inspires us in her article that "presents an evidence-based approach to integrate concepts of civility, professionalism and ethical practice into the nursing curricula to prepare students to foster healthy work environments and ensure safe patient care" (p. 120). How these terms—civility, incivility, professionalism, and ethical practice—are defined helps to increase understanding and provide a common language around the issue. Clark further explains that students need to comprehend the "vision, mission and shared values statements with an intentional focus on civility, professionalism, and ethical conduct" (p. 121). Many universities have students read and sign a Civility Pledge "to foster an ethical, respectful, professional academic work and learning environment" (Clark, 2017a, p. 122). The civil behaviors outlined in this pledge

1. Identify the causes of incivility in the classroom, the procedural simulation lab, or the simulation center learning environments.
2. Identify the causes of incivility in the clinical learning environment.
3. How can professors show grace and forgiveness toward students when incivility has occurred in any of the previously mentioned learning settings?
4. What strategies can be utilized to advance students' learning while fostering healthy work environments and ensuring patient safety (Clark, 2017a)?

should be maintained in the learning and healthcare practice environments both as students and later as professional RNs (**BOX 19-4**).

Sometimes, a student may not adhere to the Civility Pledge. On such an occasion, the professor will need to address this behavior and, depending on the severity of the action, a professional learning contract may be issued to the student or the student may be dismissed from the nursing program. The nursing professor should be a positive role model and set the tone for this learning experience. The instructor should acknowledge the importance of listening to the student, trying to understand the situation from both the professor's and the student's perspectives, and providing the correct consequence for their behavior. **Grace** and **forgiveness** are often necessary in these circumstances, along with the student taking responsibility for his or her actions and behaviors. By providing guidance to the students on how to correct their uncivil behaviors and actions, professors promote a strategic learning plan for developing civility, professionalism, and ethical practice for the future.

As a nursing administrator, I discovered that developing lovingkindness and caring was vital to the nursing department and the organization. Faculty members and staff often experienced similar anxieties and conflicts in their everyday life experiences, and providing them with a safe place to talk and share their fears or concerns was important. As an administrator, I was greatly appreciative of all members of the faculty and staff, whose work enabled the nursing department to be successful and to promote successful student outcomes. These faculty members often worked hard and additional hours in the evening or on the weekends to complete their grading or prepare for classes. Likewise, the staff kept things running smoothly during the week and often helped faculty members and students who needed additional support.

Unfortunately, there will always be some people who create an environment that is uncivil toward others or who disagree with leadership. Academic discourse is generally healthy—but sometimes the development of uncivil behavior occurs in such a subtle manner that no one sees it except for the targeted person (who could be a staff member, nursing faculty member, or even another administrator). Identify this behavior, and ask about it in a nonconfrontational, private manner. Then, seek out God daily in prayer, attend Bible study, take time to reflect and relax, recite Psalm 23, and attend church; all of these steps are valid ways to find the strength and courage to face these challenges. One must seek the Holy Spirit for his strength and wisdom to be the light among others. Perhaps walking, bicycling, running on the beach, hiking in the mountains, or just enjoying God's presence or Word will enable you to discover the sense of peace and calmness that your Heavenly Father provides you. Even Jesus needed to rest: "he withdrew from there in a boat to a desolate place by himself" (Matthew 14:13).

Honor One Another

As a child, I was raised by Christian parents who believed that everyone was created by

God, in the image of God; therefore, you regarded each individual, family, and member of the community with respect, honor, and kindness in all circumstances. As I grew up, I realized that this was a most important lesson that I learned from my parents, and one that I have used throughout my nursing practice. Our Heavenly Father instructs us to love our neighbor. He also requires us not to be judgmental of others. Matthew 7:1–3 says, "Judge not, that you be not judged. For with the judgment you pronounce you will be judged, and with the measure you use it will be measured to you. Why do you seek the speck that is in your brother's eye, but you do not notice the log that is in your eye?"

Many years ago, when I was a young nurse, an elderly African American woman coded during my shift. I called the code and began cardiopulmonary resuscitation (CPR). I remember looking at the young African American medical resident attending the code and noticing how shocked he was that I was giving mouth-to-mouth resuscitation to this patient. This patient was a child of God and an assigned patient in my care; I didn't see color or even think about it. She was simply a child of God in my care at that moment.

Being faithfully present for your patient is a necessity to provide high-quality care, but it is also honoring the patient as a person and a child of God. It is through conversations and active listening that a nurse finds meaning in his or her practice and extends warmth and caring to another individual who may be experiencing pain, stress, grief, trauma, or some type of loss. If you are faithfully present with kind words during your conversations, and actively listening well, a caring professional relationship of trust can develop so that patients may confide their innermost thoughts and feelings. You must always respect the patient's beliefs, even if they are different from yours. You must be open to others and how they believe and choose to live.

Nursing entails much more than running around and completing required tasks; the profession of nursing is exciting and fulfilling as we honor and assist others in developing a professional trusting relationship by being faithfully present at the bedside. I have known a few female nursing instructors and administrators who wanted to release other nursing instructors from their contracts because they allegedly did not fit in with others on the nursing team. Their gifts, talents, and skills were often different; some of the Christians who were nice to everyone on the nursing team taught differently from them. But the truth of the matter is that these instructors were responsible, were accountable, and completed their work well—yet these faithful and dedicated nurses continued to experience the subtle darkness of uncivil behavior and unkindness toward them as a member of the team.

Sometimes nursing staff may be upset because the nursing instructors' schedules do not match their expectations; they may not understand the culture and responsibilities of the university system and what it takes to manage a classroom, prepare for a four-hour lecture, and prepare for a procedural simulation lab, simulation experience, or even a clinical practicum. Even nursing instructors have experienced unjust and unprofessional attitudes and behaviors targeting them by others who felt they were not present enough. In some cases, only a few instructors or staff members were able to empower, sustain, and honor the faith, hope, values, and beliefs of others to maintain a civil environment.

If you are experiencing incivility in the workplace, seek the Word of God, and rely on support from other Christians—those with more experience in wisdom, courage, and strength in managing collegial relationships. Doing so will help you to develop the professional, legal, ethical, and trusting professional relationships (**BOX 19-5**) needed to be faithfully present during all communication, and to listen to both verbal and nonverbal communication. All nurses have different gifts, and we should honor them because these gifts come

1. How can nurses be effective in developing a professional trusting relationship if they are faithfully present at the bedside but not with each other as nurses?
2. Why do you think that only a few instructors were able to empower, sustain, and honor the faith, hope, values, and beliefs of others?
3. Reflect on the different gifts that you have received from your Heavenly Father.

from God. Romans 12:6–8 states, "having gifts that differ according to the grace given to us, let us use them: if prophecy, in proportion to our faith; if service, in our serving; the one who teaches, in his teaching; the one who exhorts, in his exhortation; the one who contributes, in generosity; the one who leads, with zeal; the one who does acts of mercy, with cheerfulness."

Forgive One Another

Not all nurses have had the privilege to grow up in a Christian home where life is centered on God, the community, and the church. Passion and compassion for nurses and nursing are a gift from God. I learned how to be that caring, forgiving person over the many years of working as a nurse, professor, and administrator.

Ask yourself these questions: What would Jesus do? How should I act as a Christian nurse? It was through my Heavenly Father that I grew in mindfulness of God's Word and in forgiveness toward others. I had to learn how to forgive others as our Heavenly Father forgives us of all of our sins. It was through continuous reflection and listening to trustful colleagues that I learned the importance of forgiveness toward others, no matter what the circumstances were. As nurses, we try to practice perfection, but we are humans and we make mistakes. Sometimes

in nursing, the hardest thing to do is to forgive yourself when an error has occurred. At other moments, we need to forgive our colleagues.

Incivility may take the form of harmful gossip, verbal abuse, acting on incorrect assumptions, bullying (cyber or other), pushing, hitting, or being held against your will. Clark (2017b) reports:

> According to 2016 data from the Workplace Bulling Institute, 27 percent of Americans have suffered abusive conduct or incivility at work; 30 percent of bullied employees will leave and 20 percent of those who witness bullying will leave; 40 percent of bullied individuals do not report the problem; and 45 percent of bullying targets suffer stress-related health problems. (pp. 56–57)

As Christian nurses whose ministry is nursing, we need to address these kinds of uncivil actions with compassionate care, honesty, truthfulness, and clear communication of forgiveness. We do not know what is going on in the other person's thoughts or what that person has been told. Meet and discuss these situations, so that each of you can forgive the other and move forward in Christ's love. Incivility is complicated and involves one or more unpleasant occurrences. Not every person is able to speak truthfully and forgive another person. But as 1 John 1:9 promises, "If we confess our sins, he [God] is faithful and just to forgive us our sins and to cleanse us from all unrighteousness." Furthermore, Ephesians 4:31–32 tells us, "Let all bitterness and wrath and anger and clamor and slander be put away from you, along with all malice. Be kind to one another, tenderhearted, forgiving one another, as God in Christ has forgave you." Shelly and Miller (2006) explain, "Caring is an act of faith, for it involves the risk of opening ourselves to another who may not want to care or be cared for" (p. 250).

Your responses to these uncivil actions define your character as a Christian nurse.

Such uncivil actions can destroy your colleagues, poison the work environment, and affect patient care outcomes when you cannot forgive those who have done wrong against you. We must seek reconciliation to these occurrences for healing of all involved members of the team. Clark (2017b, pp. 57–59) suggests the following strategies for promoting civility:

1. Take an accurate inventory of your own behaviors and interactions and consider the impact they may have on others.
2. Institute measures to define desired behavior and discourage incivility from occurring.
3. Determine the consequences of the problem behavior.
4. Address the problem.
5. Attend to your physical, emotional, and spiritual health.
6. Stay civil.

By forgiving one another and implementing these strategies, nurses can begin to foster civility in learning and healthcare environments. When we are civil toward one another (**BOX 19-6**), we respect each other, empower each other in our professional nursing practice, and create safe environments for patients and nurses alike.

Be Sensitive to Others

By trusting in God and being in His Word, we learn to be caring just as Jesus was caring to so many others, His children. I remember caring for a woman with cancer located in her jaw; the cancer was eating away the muscle, bone, and flesh from her face. Her jaw was held in place with an abdominal bandage and tape. I was required to change that dressing every 4 hours, flush the side of her mouth and jaw with medication and normal saline, and replace the dressing. I stood in front of that closed door focusing on prayer that God would give me the strength and courage to love this woman—that no facial expression,

---

BOX 19-6 Key Civil Behaviors

- Trusting in God
- Respectfulness toward all
- Loving others in a professional manner by accepting them and their thoughts, even though you might not agree with them
- Being open to their perspectives, values, beliefs, concerns, worries, or anxieties
- Being present and actively listening to others
- Displaying caring attitudes and appropriate therapeutic touch
- Forgiving others, as God has forgiven you in misunderstandings or failed actions
- Being gracious toward others, because we all have sinned and need God's grace and forgiveness

---

bone, or muscle in my body would display a negative response to such an odorous wound. I wanted to enter that room with a sense of peace and calmness, demonstrating caring and compassion for this woman and her family. I needed to show her that I was an instrument from God to care for her and be sensitive to her needs. She was dying. I looked into her eyes and tried to tell her that God was near and would help her through this situation with His comfort and peace.

God gives us the strength to do the impossible when we need it the most. Mark 9:23 states, "And Jesus said to him, 'If you can! All things are possible for one who believes.'" Our Heavenly Father provides the light, the words, and the approaches we need to embrace others in Jesus's love and to understand their sensitivities in the current situation. When nurses care for patients in a compassionate way, they must also think about their fellow colleagues and how they can care for them in a compassionate way. Our colleague may be experiencing the death of a child or spouse, a loss of their home from a natural disaster, or even personal illness such as cancer; during these times we need to demonstrate our love, compassion, and care for them as well.

Another memorable experience for me was in pediatrics as a nursing instructor. A young boy was admitted to the hospital because his legs were weak; eventually, he could not walk. His father stood by me in the treatment room while a spinal tap was being completed. I remember the father crying and saying to me, "How can this be? Yesterday he was running, walking, and playing, and now today he is not able to move his legs." As the nursing student assisted in the procedure, I stood with this patient's father and was caring as I actively listened to his story and was very sensitive to his needs at that moment of helplessness. I looked to God for the correct words to say and to provide God's love and hope. I know that active listening is preferred over false hope. The words were few, but I know they came from my Heavenly Father that day. A week later, this young boy was up walking with a walker. This moment was a moment filled with joy and excitement as I saw this young boy learning to walk with the support of the walker, his physical therapist, and his father.

I have seen miracles as a nurse. These miracles are a true gift from our Heavenly Father: He does answer our prayers. But even our nursing colleagues may need someone to actively listen to them and pray for them. Prayers can be said together privately in a conference room or in a hospital's chapel. These moments of caring for others can bring Christ's light to our fellow nurses and comfort that allows them to focus their care for others.

All nurses who want to care and be sensitive to others can grow both personally and professionally during their nursing practice (Box 19-6). Rely on God every day for His strength and courage to meet the daily challenges as a nurse by being sensitive and caring toward others. To have the courage and strength to work with God's miracles in

life-and-death situations, one must seek guidance from Jesus to continue to be sensitive to the needs of others and ourselves. A prayer that I enjoy saying is the following from *Luther's Small Catechism* (Luther, 2017):

> I thank You, my Heavenly Father through Jesus Christ, Your dear Son, that You have kept me this night from all harm and danger; and I pray that You would keep me this day also from sin and every evil, that all my doings and life may please You. For into Your hands I commend myself, my body and soul, and all things. Let Your holy angel be with me, that the evil foe may have no power over me. Amen. (p. 30)

Foster Therapeutic Professional Relationships

Therapeutic professional relationships with patients, families, communities, and other healthcare providers are essential in the care of patients. But in nursing school, do we discuss the significance of our relationships with other nurses and how to respect other nurses' thinking, practice, and knowledge? Do we talk about the care of self, which enables us to truly be present for the development and the sustainment of a therapeutic professional relationship to help and trust our fellow nurses?

As a Christian nurse leader, I placed a lot of pressure on myself to practice with perfection. It took me a long time to realize that I am human and that I make mistakes—that being kind to self and others was key, but to forgive yourself was equally as important for my career. I was always developing therapeutic professional relationships with nurses on the team whom I knew I could trust to do a good job with my assigned patients or their assigned patients. Thinking back, I wish I had reached out more to nurses on my team to build better helping, trusting, and therapeutic professional relationships. I was always concerned for my patients and their outcomes. When the nurses did have time to talk with each other, I can remember meaningful conversations, laughing, and enjoying these new professional relationships develop.

It seemed much easier to develop helping–trusting professional relationships with fellow nurses in the faculty role. Nursing professors often worked in groups on projects for nursing courses, curriculum, and assessment. Administrators, deans, or directors in the nursing department also promoted and supported the development of helping, trusting, and professional therapeutic relationships with one another.

In academic nursing leadership, it can be difficult at times to develop these kinds of helping, trusting, and professional therapeutic relationships among nursing professors. Understanding the relational aspects of interpersonal, social, personal, and interactive attributes within a diverse faculty pool could be challenging.

However, seeking God's guidance, strength, and courage allowed me to build positive helping, trusting, and therapeutic professional relationships with some of the nursing professors and other administrators. In the following words, Jesus explains to us the important attributes of Christian nurses and what we should do in our practice of nursing with other nurses. Colossians 3:12–17 states:

> Put on then, as God's chosen ones, holy and beloved, compassionate hearts, kindness, humility, meekness, and patience, bearing with one another and, if one has a complaint against another, forgiving each other; as the Lord has forgiven you, so you also must forgive. And above all these put on love, which binds everything together in perfect harmony. And let the peace of Christ rule in your hearts, to which indeed you were called in one body. And be thankful. Let the word of Christ dwell in you richly, teaching and admonishing one another in all wisdom, singing psalms and hymns and spiritual songs, with thankfulness in your hearts to God. And whatever you do, in word or deed, do everything in the name of the Lord Jesus, giving thanks to God the Father through him.

▶ Conclusion

Nursing as ministry has been my focus throughout this journey. I was so very grateful that I was called to be a nurse to serve God and His children. It has always been an honor and privilege to be standing on holy ground at the bedside of assigned patients or in the community serving God's people. Likewise, it has been an honor and privilege to work with many nursing students, nursing professors and instructors, pastors, and administrators. God has continuously provided the courage and strength to care for His children. Caring for one another with Christ's light and through God's strength brings brightness and joy to the nursing profession. As nurses, we must care for one another as we care for our patients. Being civil toward each nurse and neighbor is essential to the profession of nursing (**BOX 19-7**). By demonstrating these key behaviors toward their nursing colleagues, nurses can create safer learning and healthcare practice environments (**BOXES 19-8** and **19-9**).

"Christian nurses are aware of science, research, and advanced technology for better health outcomes, while acknowledging it is God who grants these revelations" (Moorman, 2015, p. E6). Believe and trust that Christ's light will shine on us and through us as we provide high-quality, safe care to our patients. It is through this trust from our Heavenly Father that we continue on our journey as *called* servants. Shelly and Miller (2006) remind us

BOX 19-7 Outstanding Nurse Leader: Kathleen Kennedy, PhD, RN, PHN

According to Dr. Kathleen Kennedy, her "passion is to encourage and support the next generation of nurses to be excellent in practice, inspirational in nursing education, and exemplary in nursing research." Her research interest focuses on the importance of exclusive breastfeeding to public health locally and globally, and how nurses can make a difference. Kennedy recently graduated from Azusa Pacific University, where she received her PhD in nursing. Her dissertation topic was "examining the influences on mothers' commitment to maintain exclusive breastfeeding within the 48 hours after birth." She earned an MSN from California State University, Fullerton, in 2011. There, her research thesis topic was "influences of knowledge, attitudes, and beliefs on student nurses' intention to promote breastfeeding." In addition to receiving a post-master's certificate in instructional design and technology, Kennedy earned a BSN and public health certificate from Azusa Pacific University in 2006 and her ADN from Cerritos College in Norwalk, California, in 1974.

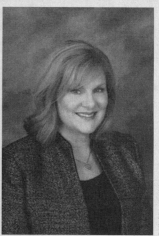

Dr. Kathleen Kennedy

Kennedy has received the following honors:

- MSN Graduate Assistance in Areas of National Need (GAANN) Fellow (grant), 2008–2011
- Jonas Nurse Leader Scholar Award ($20,000 grant), 2016–2018
- Member: Sigma Theta Tau Nursing Honor Society, 2006–present

Currently, Kennedy serves as an assistant professor of nursing at Concordia University Irvine (CUI) in California. Her past work experience in the acute healthcare setting includes medical–surgical, maternal–newborn, neonatal intensive care unit (NICU), and newborn nursery experiences in Southern California and working as a school readiness nurse at the Orange County Children and Families Commission.

An outstanding nurse leader, Kennedy is both a compassionate person and a devoted RN. She loves to develop positive, strong relationships with colleagues and her nursing students. Her passion to assist students and fellow colleagues goes beyond her calling as a Christian nurse. She demonstrates a commitment to Christ daily and in her nursing care through her dedication to students, colleagues, and administrators in her work environment. She has a deep passion for working with students and assisting them to see the larger global lens used in nursing. A lifelong learner, she shares her knowledge so as to enhance the knowledge of her students and colleagues, thereby making nursing practice more effective and ensuring high-quality care.

Kennedy has been married for 45 years, with four children and nine grandchildren. She enjoys Bible studies and attending church; has traveled to South Africa for graduate school; and has lived in Japan while supporting her husband's ministry. Her mission as a Christian has been a true calling from God and she has utilized her spiritual gifts to serve others.

that "the common theme in all these aspects of Christian nursing is the glory of God. Nurses, committed to Jesus Christ, holistically caring for the sick, the poor and the needy, demonstrate the character of God to the world. They bring the light of Christ into dark situations with humility, love, passion and power" (p. 256). May the comfort of God's light, love, grace, and forgiveness fill you with hope and peace as you care for each other as nurses.

BOX 19-8 Evidence-Based Practice Focus

This article presents an evidence-based approach to integrate civility, professionalism, and ethical practice in nursing academics. Nursing educators have a unique role in changing nursing curricula and practice to incorporate the important concepts of civility, professionalism, and ethical practice. When students learn in and practice developing healthy work environments, the result is safe patient care. This evidence-based approach allows nursing educators to integrate pertinent concepts by providing strategies for faculty to address the issue of incivility in the classroom and the clinical practicum. The author suggests that changes to new-student orientation, strategies for laying the foundation for success on the first day of class, white coat ceremonies, and faculty serving as positive role models, among other steps, can enhance the learning of civility.

Modified from Clark, C. M. (2017a). An evidence-based approach to integrate civility, professionalism, and ethical practice into nursing curricula. *Nurse Educator, 42*(3), 120–125. doi: 10.1097/NNE.0000000000000331

BOX 19-9 Research Highlight

In this research study, nurses from intensive care units (ICUs) were surveyed about their perceptions of incivility and professional comportment. A survey was conducted to understand nurse-to-nurse incivility and how this behavior could be decreased within these settings. A quantitative, cross-sectional, descriptive survey was completed in 14 ICUs within three healthcare systems. According to the author, when nurses were aware of the importance of professional comportment along with professional education, improvements in behavior occurred. A decrease in nurse-to-nurse incivility was associated with better conflict management, shared processes, improved professionals, and better communication and collaboration. Thus, ensuring that nursing education incorporates the concept of professional comportment holds out the hope of developing a more civil nursing culture with improved patient safety outcomes.

Modified from Oja, K. J. (2017). Incivility and professional comportment in critical care nurses. *AACN Advanced Critical Care, 28*(4), 345–350. doi: 10.4037/aacnacc2017106

▶ Clinical Reasoning Exercises

1. Why is it important to consider how you might have contributed to an uncivil occurrence?
2. Nursing is considered a relational profession between many individuals. How do you plan to remain a positive professional RN during a conflict or while being a victim of incivility?
3. Do you think you would be able to identify what caused an incivility to occur? If you can, how would you address the issue with your colleague?
4. Would you consider getting help from a counselor if you were unable to resolve the conflict with incivility that is toward you?
5. Can you forgive a colleague who has caused you great harm and pain? How would you do this?
6. What Bible passages would support you during this difficult time?

▶ Personal Reflection Exercises

Being respectful to all nursing colleagues and nursing students is essential in the practice and clinical learning environment for one's growth in the profession of nursing, to promote safe, high-quality patient care, and to demonstrate moral and ethical behavior toward one another in developing positive relationships during our work. Take an hour to reflect on the significance of "caring for one another as nurses." Then answer each question.

1. What does it mean to care for one another as nurses?
2. How would Jesus want us to care for our fellow nurses and the nursing students with whom we work?
3. What attributes of a Christian nurse would you use when caring for another nurse who has been uncivil toward you at work?
4. How would you care for another nurse with whom you work and who has caused you to be distracted by incivility?
5. As Christian nurses, why do we need to care for other nurses on our healthcare team?
6. Will caring for other nurses on my team impact the care for our patients?
7. As a registered nurse, reflect on a time that you may have been uncivil to a colleague—perhaps when you were stressed during your second 12-hour shift? What triggered you to lose your temper at the nursing station with another colleague with whom you enjoy working? Did you realize that you were being uncivil toward a fellow colleague? What did you do after realizing that you lost your temper and you were feeling guilty of your behavior? Did you apologize for losing your temper and ask for forgiveness? If not, why not?
8. Read the research article by Oja (2017). Do you think that understanding the meaning of civility and professional comportment would assist you in preventing incivility at work with fellow colleagues? Do you see a need for nurses to care for one another? To forgive one another? To be respectful toward one another? Should we provide compassionate care to each other if we are having a stress-filled day?

9. What will you try to do to bring civility to your nursing unit and improve patient safety outcomes?

References

American Nurses Association (ANA). (2015). ANA position statement on incivility, bullying, and workplace violence. Retrieved from https://www.nursingworld.org/practice-policy/nursing-excellence/official-position-statements/id/incivility-bullying-and-workplace-violence/

Andersson, L. M., & Pearson, C. M. (1999). Tit for tat? The spiraling effect of incivility in the workplace. *Academy of Management Review, 24*(3), 452–471.

Clark, C. M. (2016). Principled leadership and the imperative for workplace civility. *American Nurse Today, 11*(11), 32–33.

Clark, C. M. (2017a). An evidence-based approach to integrate civility, professionalism, and ethical practice into nursing curricula. *Nurse Educator, 42*(3), 120–125. doi:10.1097/NNE.0000000000000331

Clark, C. (2017b). Seeking civility among faculty: A nursing professor could see the damaging effects of incivility and bullying in academe. So she's delving into how faculty can treat each other better. *ASHA Leader, 22*(12), 54–59.

Clark, C. M., & Carnosso, J. (2008). Civility: A concept analysis. *Journal of Theory Construction Testing, 12*(1), 11–15.

Clark, C. M., & Springer, P. J. (2010). Academic nurse leaders' role in fostering a culture of civility in nursing education. *Journal of Nursing Education, 49*(6), 319–325. doi:10.3928/01484834-20100224-01

Fowler, M. D. M. (2015). *Guide to the code of ethics for nurses with interpretive statements: Development, interpretation, and application* (2nd ed.). Silver Spring, MD: American Nurses Association.

Hoglund, B. A. (2013). Practicing the code of ethics, finding the image of God. *Journal of Christian Nursing, 30*(4), 228–233.

Incivility. (2005). In *Merriam Webster Dictionary*. Retrieved from https://www.merriam-webster.com/dictionary/incivility

Kim, M. S., & Patterson, K. T. (2016). Teaching and practicing caring in the classroom: Students' responses to a self-awareness intervention in psychiatric–mental health nursing. *Journal of Christian Nursing, 33*(2), E23–E26.

Luther, M. (2017). *Luther's Small Catechism with explanation*. St. Louis, MO: Concordia Publishing House.

Moorman, S. (2015). Nursing from a Christian world view: Being transformed to care. *Journal of Christian Nursing, 31*(1), E1–E7.

Newbanks, S. R., Rieg, L. S., & Schaefer, B. (2018). What is caring in nursing? Sorting out humanistic and Christian perspectives. *Journal of Christian Nursing, 35*(3), 160–167. doi:10.1097/CNJ.0000000000000441

O'Brien, M., E. (2018). *Spirituality in nursing: Standing on holy ground* (6th ed.). Burlington, MA: Jones & Bartlett Learning.

Oja, K. J. (2017). Incivility and professional comportment in critical care nurses. *AACN Advanced Critical Care, 28*(4), 345–350. doi:10.4037/aacnacc2017106

Phillips, G., MacKusick, C. I., & Whichello, R. (2018). Workplace incivility in nursing: A literature review though the lens of ethics and spirituality. *Journal of Christian Nursing, 35*(1), E7–E12.

Porath, C. (2018). Why being respectful to your co-workers is good for business. Retrieved from https://www.ted.com/talks/christine_porath_why_being_nice_to_your_coworkers_is_good_for_business/transcript?language=en

Shelly, J. A., & Miller, A. B. (2006). *Called to care: A Christian worldview for nursing*. Downers Grove, IL: InterVarsity Press.

The Lutheran study Bible, English standard version (ESV). (2009). St. Louis, MO: Concordia Publishing House.

Recommended Readings

Alexander, S. (2017). Promoting civility in education and practice: One nurse's experience. *Clinical Nurse Specialist, 31*(2), 79–81. doi:10.1097/NUR.0000000000000274

Clark, C. M. (2010). From incivility to civility: Transforming the culture. *Reflections on Nursing Leadership, 36*(3).

Clark, C. M. (2010). The sweet spot of civility: My story. *Reflections on Nursing Leadership, 36*(1). Retrieved from https://www.reflectionsonnursingleadership.org/features/more-features/Vol36_1_the-sweet-spot-of-civility-my-story

Clark, C. M. (2010). Why civility matters. *Reflections on Nursing Leadership*. Retrieved from https://www.reflectionsonnursingleadership.org/features/more-features/Vol36_1_why-civility-matters

Clark, C. M. (2014). Seeking civility. *American Nurse Today, 9*(7), 18, 20–21, 46.

Clark, C. M. (2017). *Creating and sustaining civility in nursing education* (2nd ed.). Indianapolis, IN: Sigma Theta Tau International.

Clark, C. M., & Cardoni C. (2010). What students can do to promote civility. *Reflections on Nursing Leadership, 36*(2). Retrieved from https://www.reflectionsonnursingleadership.org/features/more-features/Vol36_2_what-students-can-do-to-promote-civility

Clark, C. M., & Kenski, D. (2017). Promoting civility in the OR: An ethical imperative. *AORN Journal, 105*(1), 60–66. doi:10.1016/j.aorn.2016.10.019

Clark, C. M., Landrum, R. E., & Nguyen, D. T. (2013). Development and description of the Organizational Civility Scale (OCS). *Journal of Theory Construction Testing, 17*(1), 11–17.

Clark, C. M., Olender, L., Cardoni, C., & Kenski, D. (2011). Fostering civility in nursing education and practice nurse leader perspectives. *Journal of Nursing Administration, 41*(7/8), 324–330. doi:10.3928/01484834-20100224-01

Clark, C. M., & Springer, P. J. (2017). Academic nurse leaders' role in fostering a culture of civility in nursing education. *Journal of Nursing Education, 49*(6), 319–325.

Jenkins, S. D., Kerber, C. S., & Woith, W. M. (2013). An intervention to promote civility among nursing students. *Nursing Education Perspectives, 34*(2), 95–100.

Kile, D., Skarbeck, A., & Thruby-Hay, L. (2018). Bullying and lateral incivility: Have you and your patients been affected? Retrieved from https://www.nursingald.com/articles/22069-bullying-and-lateral-incivility-have-you-and-your-patients-been-affected

Lachman, V. D., O'Connor Swanson, E., & Winland-Brown, J. (2015). The new "Code of Ethics for Nurses with Interpretive Statements" (2015): Practical clinical application, part 2. *Medsurg Nursing, 24*(5), 363–368.

Laschinger, H. K. S., Finegan, J., & Wilk, P. (2009). New graduate burnout: The impact of professional practice environment, workplace civility, and empowerment. *Nursing Economic$, 27*(6), 377–383.

Pfeiffer, J. (2018). Strategies Christian nurses use to create a healing environment. *Religions, 9*. doi:103390/rel9110352

Pinckney, M. Y. (2015). Increasing civility in the workplace. *Journal of Chi Eta Phi Sorority*. Retrieved from https://sigma.nursingrepository.org/bitstream/handle/10755/560732/MichelleYPinckneyDNPProject.pdf?sequence=2&isAllowed=y

Shanta, L. L., & Eliason, A. R. M. (2014). Application of an empowerment model to improve civility in nursing education. *Nurse Education in Practice, 14*, 82–86. doi:10.1016/j.nepr.2013.06.009

Smith, G. T. (2011). *Courage and calling: Embracing your God-given potential* (2nd ed.). Downers Grove, IL: InterVarsity Press.

Smith, J. G. (2018). Establishing norms of respect: Strategies for nurses and managers. *American Nurse Today, 13*(6), 44–45.

Winland-Brown, J., Lachman, V. D., & O'Connor Swanson, E. (2015). The new "Code of Ethics for Nurses with Interpretive Statements" (2015): Practical clinical application, part 1. *Medsurg Nursing, 24*(4), 268–271.

Additional References on Incivility

Bambi, S., Becattini, G., Giusti, G. D., Mezzetti, A., Guazzini, A., & Lumini, E. (2014). Lateral hostilities among nurses employed in intensive care units, emergency departments, operating rooms, and emergency medical services: A national survey in Italy. *Dimensions of*

Critical Care Nursing, 33(6), 347–354. doi:10.1097/DCC.0000000000000077

Blake, N. (2016). Building respect and reducing incivility in the workplace: Professional standards and recommendations to improve the work environment for nurses. *AACN Advanced Critical Care, 27*(4), 368–371. doi:10.4037/aacnacc2016291

Blevins, S. (2015). Impact of incivility in nursing. *Medsurg Nursing, 24*(6), 379–380.

Clark, C. M. (2008). Faculty and student assessment of experience with incivility in nursing education. *Journal of Nursing Education, 47*(10), 458–465.

Clark, C. M. (2008). Student voices on faculty incivility in nursing education: A conceptual model. *Nursing Education Perspectives, 29*(5), 284–289.

Clark, C. M., Barbosa-Leiker, C., Gill, L. M., & Nguyen, D. (2015). Revision and psychometric testing of the Incivility in Nursing Education (INE) survey: Introducing the INE-R. *Journal of Nursing Education, 54*(6), 306–315. doi:10.3928/01484834-20150515-01

Clark, C. M., Farnsworth, J., & Landrum, E. (2009). Development and description of the Incivility in Nursing Education (INE) survey. *Journal of Theory Construction Testing, 13*(1), 7–15.

Clark, C. M., Juan, C. M., Allerton, B. W., Otterness, N. S., Jun, W. Y., & Wei, F. (2012). Faculty and student perceptions of academic incivility in the People's Republic of China. *Journal of Cultural Diversity, 19*(3), 85–93.

Clark, C. M., Olender, L., Kenski, D., & Cardoni, C. (2013). Exploring and addressing faculty-to-faculty incivility: A national perspective and literature review. *Journal of Nursing Education, 52*(4), 211–218. doi:10.3928/01484834-20130319-01

Clark, C. M., & Springer, P. J. (2007). Incivility in nursing education: A descriptive study of definitions and prevalence. *Journal of Nursing Education, 46*(1), 7–14.

Clark, C. M., & Springer, P. J. (2007). Thoughts on incivility: Student and faculty perceptions of uncivil behavior in nursing education. *Nursing Education Perspectives, 28*(2), 93–97.

Clark, K. R. (2017). Managing the higher education classroom. *Radiologic Technology, 89*(2), 210–213.

Elmblad, R., Kodjebacheva, G., & Lebeck, L. (2014). Workplace incivility affecting CRNAs: A study of prevalence, severity, and consequences with proposed interventions. *AANA Journal, 82*(6), 437–445.

Evans, D. (2017). Categorizing the magnitude and frequency of exposure to uncivil behaviors: A new approach for more meaningful interventions. *Journal of Nursing Scholarship, 49*(2), 214–222. doi:10.1111/jnu.12275

Glasper, A. (2018). Protecting health care staff from abuse: Tackling workplace incivility in nursing. *British Journal of Nursing, 27*(22), 1336–1337. doi:10.12968/bjon.2018.27.22.1336

Guidroz, A., Burnfield-Geimer, J. L., Clark, O., Schwetschenau, H. M., & Jex, S. M. (2010). The Nursing Incivility Scale: Development and validation of an occupation-specific measure. *Journal of Nursing Measurement, 18*(3), 176–200.

Kolanko, K. M., Clark, C., Heinrich, D. O. Serembus, J. F., & Sifford, K. S. (2006). Academic dishonesty, bullying, incivility, and violence: Difficult challenges facing nurse educators. *Nursing Education Perspectives, 27*(1), 34–43.

Lachman, V. D. (2014). Ethical issues in the disruptive behaviors of incivility, bullying, and horizontal/lateral violence. *Medsurg Nursing, 23*(1), 56–60.

Lachman, V. D. (2015). Ethical issues in the disruptive behaviors of incivility, bullying, and horizontal/lateral violence. *Urologic Nursing, 35*(1), 39–42.

Leiper, J. (2005). Nurse against nurse: How to stop horizontal violence. *Nursing, 35*(3), 44–45.

Moreland, J. J., & Apker, J. (2016). Conflict and stress in hospital nursing: Improving communicative responses to enduring professional challenges. *Health Communication, 31*(7), 815–823. doi:10.1080/10410236.2015.1007548

Rainford, W. C., Wood, S., McMullen, P. C., & Philipsen, N. D. (2015). The disruptive force of lateral violence in the health care setting. *Journal of Nurse Practitioners, 11*(2), 157–164.

Spiri, C., Brantley, M., & McGuire, J. (2017). Incivility in the workplace: A study of nursing staff in the military health system. *Journal of Nursing Education and Practice, 7*(3), 40–46. doi:10.5430/jnep.vn3p40

Torkelson, E., Holm, K., Backstrom, M., & Schad, E. (2016). Factors contributing to the perpetration of workplace incivility: The importance of organizational aspects and experiencing incivility from others. *Work and Stress, 30*(2), 115–131. doi:10.1080/02678373.2016.1175524

Townsend, T. (2016) Not just "eating our young": Workplace bullying strikes experienced nurses, too. *American Nurse Today.* Retrieved from https://www.americannursetoday.com/just-eating-young-workplace-bullying-strikes-experienced-nurses/

Ward-Smith, P., Hawks, J. H., Quallich, S. A., & Provance, J. (2018). Workplace incivility: Perceptions of urologic nurses. *Urologic Nursing, 38*(1), 20–26. doi:10.7257/1053-816X2018.38.1.20

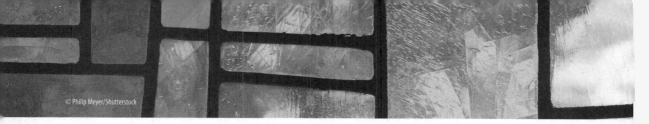

CHAPTER 20

Mentoring in the Example of Christ

Cheryl King, MSN, RN, CNS

LEARNING OBJECTIVES

At the end of this chapter, the reader will be able to:

1. Describe how mentoring can transform lives to be more like Christ.
2. Integrate the concepts of servant, shepherd, steward, and scholar into the role of mentor.
3. Analyze the mentoring process.
4. Examine the mentoring process across different generations.
5. Create a mentoring program for someone you know.

KEY TERMS

Eschatology
Mentee
Mentor

Nursing as ministry
Scholar
Servant

Shepherd
Steward

▶ Mentoring

A **mentor** is a trusted guide, tutor, or coach. Mentoring is helping someone grow stronger in his or her faith and pursue God. It could be said that to be Christ-like is to be a mentor to those whom we encounter. To be a mentor in the same manner as Christ is to be a **servant**, **shepherd**, **scholar**, and **steward**, sharing humbly what we know with God in the lead. This certainly holds true for **nursing as ministry**.

Jesus was the ultimate mentor. God sent His Son to live among us and teach us more about the ways of God. Jesus mentored his 12 disciples while here on earth and challenged them to do the same to others.

> Therefore go and make disciples of all nations, baptizing them in the name of the Father and of the Son and of the Holy Spirit, and teaching them to obey everything I have commanded you. And surely I am with you always, to the very end of the age. (Matthew 28:19–20, New International Version [NIV])

▶ Exploration of Biblical Mentoring

Mentoring can be seen as a Biblical concept. Numerous examples of mentoring relationships appear in the Bible, although the word *mentor* is not actually used. In fact, the principles of mentoring are found throughout scripture. These relationships occurred either in group settings or, as is most experienced today, on a one-on-one basis; on occasion, individuals were involved in multiple mentoring events at the same time. For example, Jesus mentored his 12 disciples as a collective, sometimes two or three at a time, and on rare occasions on a one-on-one basis. His intent was to have the groups be small enough to interact with, have active listening occur, answer the questions posed, and examine personal perspectives. This is how it went: First Jesus mentored the 12 apostles, and then the apostles mentored hundreds of other leaders, including Paul. Paul mentored Titus, Timothy, and many others. Timothy mentored the faithful men of his time, such as Epaphras. Epaphras and the other faithful men mentored others as well, which led to a chain reaction that resulted in dozens of new churches in Asia. Ultimately, this specific mentoring chain is the beginning point of our churches today.

So Christ himself gave the apostles, the prophets, the evangelists, the pastors and teachers, to equip his people for works of service, so that the body of Christ may be built up until we all reach unity in the faith and in the knowledge of the Son of God and become mature, attaining to the whole measure of the fullness of Christ. Then we will no longer be infants, tossed back and forth by the waves, and blown here and there by every wind of teaching and by the cunning and craftiness of people in their deceitful scheming. Instead, speaking the truth in love, we will grow to become in every respect the mature body of him who is the head, that is, Christ. From him the whole body, joined and held together by every supporting ligament, grows and builds itself up in love, as each part does its work. (Ephesians 4:11–16)

Like a ripple spreading across a pond, by acting as mentors we can influence many nurses to be the hands and feet of Christ today in the care of patients who trust in us. Those Christian nurses can spread the word of God through the interactions, role modeling, and caring behaviors exhibited to patients and families across the healthcare system (see **BOXES 20-1** and **20-2**).

BOX 20-1 Reflective Questions

1. How is mentoring a Biblical concept?
2. Consider the many mentoring relationships in the Bible. Describe what went well and what did not go well in each relationship.
3. Why might God want us to assume the role of mentor or mentee?
4. What can be learned from being a mentor? From being a mentee?

BOX 20-2 Reflective Questions: Time to Ponder

1. How is Jesus the ultimate mentor?
2. Utilize the terms *servant*, *shepherd*, *steward*, and *scholar* in mentoring for nursing as ministry.
3. Consider how mentors help the mentee find their calling.

Here are some more examples of mentoring from the Old Testament:

- Jethro mentored Moses; Moses mentored Joshua and the elders of Israel; and Joshua mentored the other remaining leaders of his army.
- Eli mentored Samuel; Samuel mentored Saul and David. Ahithophel and Nathan the prophet also mentored David. David, who became Israel's greatest king, mentored his army commanders and government officials to establish the united nation of Israel. David also mentored Solomon. Solomon mentored the Queen of Sheba, who returned to her people with his wisdom in the form of Proverbs that applied God's laws.
- Elijah mentored Elisha; Elisha mentored King Jehoash and others.
- Daniel mentored Nebuchadnezzar, who humbled himself before God.
- Mordecai mentored Esther; Esther mentored King Artaxerxes, which led to the liberation of God's people.

One might ask, "Why should we mentor?" The answer goes back to the definition of mentoring: It is a close personal relationship with another. Mentoring provides us with an opportunity to share, guide, support, and help grow another person in our area of expertise and to help that individual be transformed through spiritual, personal, and professional growth. It is about being in relationship with another, with both parties ultimately benefiting as the relationship grows. When we seek a closer personal relationship with God, we are enlightened, transformed, and engaged more deeply in that relationship as we learn more about the will of God. Mentoring relationships can be similar, yet different from our relationship with God.

▶ The Mentoring Process

For the mentoring relationship to be most effective, the first step is to seek the wisdom of God to know ourselves and to be directed as to how we can be effective to the mentee for the Kingdom of God. Through this exploration, God draws us closer to Him. We pray and seek His wisdom, insight, and discernment to follow His direction in the mentoring process (Ephesians 4:11–16). Just as we seek to walk in relationship with God, so it should be with the **mentee**, the person being mentored. We need to know ourselves and know what we can offer the mentee; we can achieve those goals through thoughtful reflection and prayer, seeking God's Word. We then can assist the mentee by determining how best to interact, direct, and provide the information needed to help the mentee grow spiritually, personally, and professionally to serve God.

It is also important to recognize that the mentoring relationship will change over time. The first step in the relationship is to identify the needs of the mentee. As Christian nurses, we need to establish a therapeutic relationship with our patients; the same is true for the mentor–mentee relationship. Mentors need to learn from their mentees:

- Are they aware of the need to learn? To change?
- What are their needs at this time?
- What do they want to learn? To change?
- What is their relationship with God?
- What are their expectations of the mentor?
- Is there a willingness to change?

- Do they have courage to do the work of self-reflection?
- Do they have the ability to listen?

Initially, the mentee will be dependent on the mentor for direction and guidance. This type of relationship can be time-consuming and overwhelming for the mentor. Remember to seek God's guidance in challenging times in the mentor relationship. Timing is very important in the relationship, and the mentor needs to be astute in determining when to push and when to back off. The expectations of both parties need to be clear and frequently revisited.

The mentor may need to help the mentee gain courage to attempt the steps suggested and provide words of encouragement as the mentee learns new knowledge and skills. Mentees will need specific steps to guide their path and help them gain confidence in themselves and their abilities. Some modification of the steps and refinement of the process may be necessary to increase the chance for success and for the mentee to gain confidence. The mentor will need patience and the ability to change steps quickly for the mentee as the mentee embraces new skills and abilities. The mentee can be expected to have struggles along the way—sometimes there needs to be "a breakdown before there is a breakthrough." Indeed, those struggles can be the most powerful learning moments.

The mentor will need to adjust and remain flexible as the relationship changes over time. As the mentee becomes more successful and confident, a shift in the relationship will occur as the mentee becomes more autonomous and independent. There may be less frequent interactions. Instead of directing the process for the mentee, the mentor's role will change to one of an advisor and facilitator, validating that the mentee is on the right path. Growing independence for the mentee is an essential component that indicates a successful mentor–mentee relationship is evolving to the next level. At various points along the way, both parties are advised to stop and evaluate the process, celebrate the successes, and plan for the future of the relationship.

▶ The Successful Mentoring Relationship

Anthony K. Tjan (2017) published an article in the *Harvard Business Review* online entitled "What the Best Mentors Do." In that article he states, "The best leaders practice a form of leadership that is less about creating followers and more about creating other leaders" (para. 2). Tjan recommends five points for mentors to consider: (1) put the relationship before the mentorship, (2) focus on character rather than competency, (3) shout loudly with your optimism, (4) keep quiet with your cynicism, and (5) be more loyal to your mentee than you are to your company. Moreover, he notes that "the best mentors avoid overriding the dreams of their mentees" (para. 3). Mentors help their mentees find their calling by guiding, supporting, and nurturing their dreams and aspirations.

▶ Principles of Great Mentoring

When we mentor, we also grow in our own faith as we teach, role model, and pray for insight and wisdom to assist our mentee (see **CASE STUDY 20-1**). On the website *Pursue God* (Dwyer, 2016b), three pertinent "Mentoring Principles for Biblical Discipleship" are delineated.

- *Principle 1: Mentor a few.* Start influencing by mentoring a few, just as Jesus did—and look at how he impacted the world! The key idea is that a mentoring relationship eventually leads

🔍 CASE STUDY 20-1

The following scenario is based on a true story of a mentoring relationship. Judy was about to begin nursing school. She was excited, but also scared, because she had heard that it was hard and would take up most of her time. Judy admitted to being a Christian but had not been in a close relationship with the Lord for several years. She wanted to be a critical care nurse when she completed her education.

On the first day of class, Judy met Karen, a critical care nurse and Christian nurse, who was going to teach the health assessment course. Judy was quickly drawn to Karen, mostly because of her critical care experience. Judy grew to admire Karen for her abilities as a nurse. When the class ended, Judy approached Karen for some advice—and that is how the mentoring relationship began.

During their first meeting, it became apparent to Karen that Judy wanted and needed a mentor. Karen learned that Judy wanted to become a critical care nurse, and Karen agreed to coach her as she went through the nursing program. Karen encouraged Judy to look at each clinical experience as an opportunity to explore different areas as a Christian nurse. Judy was adamant that she wanted to be a critical care nurse. She stated that she was not really interested in any other areas but knew that she had to do them to complete the program.

As the relationship continued, Karen could see that Judy was struggling in her walk with God and decided to broach the subject during one of their encounters. At first, Judy was not willing to talk about her relationship with God, and Karen realized that she needed to back off but not give up. Karen prayed to God for insight, wisdom, and discernment on how to mentor Judy as a Christian.

Over the course of time, God provided opportunities for Karen to talk to Judy about God. With gentle persuasion, Judy began to open up to Karen. Karen and Judy did devotions together during their meetings, and Judy began to read the Bible again and ask Karen questions about what she had read. Judy graduated from the nursing program, passed the National Council Licensure Examination (NCLEX), and went to work in the oncology unit at a local hospital. Although she still wants to become a critical care nurse at some point, Judy knows that at this moment in time God has placed her in the oncology unit so that she can connect with patients in an emotional and spiritual way while providing physical care.

Questions

As the Mentor:

1. Was Karen the best mentor for Judy? Explain.
2. What was effective in Karen's approach to Judy?
3. What did Karen do well to develop the mentoring relationship?
4. What could Karen have improved upon in the mentoring relationship?
5. How effective was their communication over time? How could it be improved?
6. How effective was Karen in facilitating Judy's growth as a Christian nurse? Explain.
7. What else could Karen have done to enhance Judy's growth as a Christian nurse?
8. Other thoughts?

As the Mentee:

1. Was Judy's choice of mentor the best choice for her? Explain.
2. Was Judy's initial investment in the mentoring relationship made for the right reason? Explain.
3. From Judy's perspective, did the relationship change over time? How? Why?
4. How effective was the mentor–mentee communication over time? How could it be improved?

(continues)

5. Was Karen's approach of backing off when Judy did not want to talk about her relationship with God effective? What else could she have tried?
6. What was the trigger for Judy to open up to Karen?
7. How did Judy's first nursing position as an oncology nurse reflect her path as a Christian nurse?
8. Other thoughts?

the mentee to become a mentor; then that mentee becomes a mentor; and so on. Over a period of time, the original relationship can blossom and expand to the multitudes—that was God's plan for Jesus and God's plan for discipleship (2 Timothy 2:2).

- *Principle 2: Speak truth in love.* As mentors, we must know, as guided through prayer, when to bring up topics for our mentees so that they can hear what must be said—both the good and the bad. Following God's lead in this relationship is a very powerful way to share God's truth, insight, and wisdom with the mentee. Our goal is transformation of the mentees, speaking truth through love to help them discover a new Biblical worldview (Ephesians 4:15).

- *Principle 3: Keep moving forward.* Mentors have been transformed through God's Word, discovered Biblical truth, and are willing to share what they have learned. This is a process for the mentors that will evolve as they continue the journey walking with God. There is no true endpoint; instead, these life-changing events, when shared, spread like ripples in a pond to help the next mentee become a mentor to help others. As a result, discipleship happens as Jesus intended it to happen (Luke 14:27).

To mentor is to create opportunities for both parties to intentionally examine well-being, self-care practices, opportunities for personal discovery, professional discovery, and the vision of caring as a Christian and a nurse. Mentoring has also been called the process of making disciples to go among the masses and be like Christ.

▶ Development of Disciples

The website *Pursue God* (Dwyer, 2016a) identifies three phases of mentoring:

1. *Inviting:* In this phase, a relationship is started with another. This may begin with a simple conversation, finding out about the other person. Practical solutions to what the person needs in the mentoring relationship should be addressed.

2. *Investing:* In this second phase, the mentor helps the mentee to honor God through a trusting relationship with Christ. The mentor invests time with the mentee and discusses what matters in his or her life.

3. *Empowering:* In this last phase, the mentee is able to apply what he or she has learned, and eventually may become a mentor as well, inviting another mentee into the process and allowing the process to begin again (**BOX 20-3**).

Mentoring is a form of discipleship. Meryl Herr (2017a) stated, "I define vocational

BOX 20-3 Reflective Questions: Time to Ponder

1. How can each principle of mentoring described in this section be applied in society today to instill Christ-like behavior and a Biblical worldview?
2. Defend how mentoring can lead to discipleship for God.

BOX 20-4 Research Highlight

Meryl Herr (2017a) saw a need to develop a pedagogical tool and conduct a qualitative research study to test her hypothesis that Christians could change their future. The purpose of her research was to explore the 4D-R method as a means to develop vocational discipleship. In the study, participants gain a new perspective on work, vocational discernment, and an intention to live and act differently as a result of the experience. In addition, their journaling indicated learning in four areas: themselves, God, their relationship with God, and a new-to-them theological perspective on their work. In the area of vocational discipleship, Herr noted the following goals among participants (p. 416):

- To seek out more information and resources to be better equipped to live out their calling
- To be courageous
- To live in congruence with God's call
- To take small, easy steps toward their imagined futures

Herr concluded that the 4D-R method did offer a way of imagining the future for individuals to develop skills, reflect on, and perform vocational discipleship.

discipleship similarly—as equipping Christians to discover and live out their callings; it is the training and development of Christians to connect their belief with practice in their various spheres of influence" (p. 406). Spheres of influence can be both personal and professional. Herr (2017a) saw a need to develop a pedagogical tool and conduct a qualitative research study to test her hypothesis that Christians could change their "future shaped by an eschatological vision" (p. 406). *Merriam-Webster Dictionary* defines **eschatology** as the branch of theology concerned with the final events in the history of the world or of humankind and a belief concerning death, the end of the world, or the ultimate destiny of humankind ("Eschatology," n.d.).

Herr developed the 4D-R method, a pedagogical tool designed to help Christians imagine themselves in a personal future shaped by an eschatological vision. In a qualitative study, she explored the role that the 4D-R method might play in vocational discipleship. To understand the impact of the 4D-R method on vocational discipleship, embedded in this tool was a reflective journal, called the Imagine the Future Journal (IFJ). Adult evangelical Christians were invited to use the IFJ and then share about their experiences. This study was guided by the following research questions (Herr, 2017a, p. 409):

1. How do adult evangelical Christians describe the IFJ as a discipleship tool?

2. How do adult evangelical Christians describe their experience of using the IFJ?

3. How do adult evangelical Christians describe what they learn as a result of using the IFJ?

Findings from the study included that study participants gained a new perspective on work, vocational discernment, and an intention to live and act differently as a result of the experience. Herr (2017b) concluded that the 4D-R method did offer a way of imagining the future for individuals to develop skills, reflect on, and perform vocational discipleship (**BOX 20-4** and **FIGURE 20-1**).

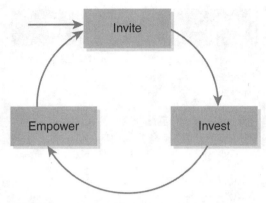

FIGURE 20-1 Phases of discipleship (mentoring).

▶ Types of Mentoring Relationships

Many types of nurses need mentoring and would benefit from learning from a more experienced Christian nurse. Here are some examples:

- Faculty mentoring new faculty, lab/simulation faculty, and clinical faculty
- Faculty mentoring students and students mentoring students (peer mentoring)
- Clinical nurses mentoring new graduate nurses or new hires
- Clinical managers mentoring staff
- Senior nursing management mentoring middle management nurses

▶ Generational Differences

Understanding the difference between generations may help the mentor in a relationship. The generalizations made here are meant to aid in understanding; they are not intended to represent stereotypes (**TABLES 20-1** and **20-2**). Certainly, it is the mentor's responsibility to get to know the mentee personally enough to discover his or her unique gifts, talents, and needs.

Traditionalists

Traditionalists were born between approximately 1922 and 1945. They have been called the veterans, as well as the Silent Generation. Growing up during the Great Depression, they became generally conservative in all aspects of their lives. They came back into the workforce when the economy declined several years ago, and typically place a high emotional value on work because of their life experiences when growing up. They believe in conformity, rules, logic, and a sense of right and wrong. The Silent Generation exhibits some degree of resistance to technology and frequently asks for help from the younger generations. They are dependable, show great loyalty, and follow the chain of authority. "Traditionalists invented the 'box' that every other generation is trying to get out of" (Tokar, 2013, p. 42).

Baby Boomers

The term *Baby Boom* is used to identify the massive increase in births following World War II, between 1946 and 1964. The first Baby Boomers reached the traditional retirement age of 65 in 2011 and represent approximately 28% of the U.S. population. "These Baby Boomers were blessed to have been born at the height of America's international prestige, military power and economic strength" (Tokar, 2013, p. 42). They wanted to change the status quo, were anti-establishment, and burst out of the "box" created by the traditionalists. As they gained more experience in the workplace, they discovered that the competition for jobs was intense and began to work 60 or more hours per week to feel secure in their jobs. Baby Boomers tend to be hard workers and vigilant due to the competition for jobs and success. For some, work became the focus of their lives. Boomers are goal oriented, work well in teams, and value individual choice. Because they did not grow up with technology but experienced the exponential growth in technology and have the latest cellular devices, they still prefer holding meetings, watching presentations, and printing out documents to review (Tokar, 2013).

TABLE 20-1 Generational Mentoring			
Generation Name	**Characteristics**	**Values**	**Mentoring Needs**
Traditionalist = Silent Generation (1922–1945)	Grew up in Great Depression era, places high emotional value on work, believes in rules, dependable; knows the value of money since did not have it growing up, created the "box" in the workplace	Conservative, strong sense of right and wrong, loyalty, hard workers	Technology, thinking out of the box, finding balance in life
Baby Boomers (1946–1964)	Born at the height of U.S. international prestige, military power, and economic strength; obsessed with climbing the steps of the corporate ladder; goal oriented; work well in teams	Anti-establishment, out of the box, work-focused life, face-to-face meetings, printing documents to read, embracing technology	Technology, finding balance in life, distant communication styles
Generation X = Latchkey Generation, Xers (1965–1979)	Lack of adult/parental supervision, increased divorce rates, mothers working outside home, childcare providers, do not want to be micromanaged, innovators and entrepreneurs, embrace technology	Not loyal to company, relationships with coworkers, growth opportunities in workplace, autonomy, creativity	Expand creativity, how to be entrepreneurs, growth opportunities, technological advances
Generation Y = Next Gen, millennials (1980–1994)	More racially and ethnically diverse; technological advances increased exponentially; creative, very bright, highly flexible, and confident; want to contribute to the bottom line	Instant information and communication, internet, working hard, being involved in purchases/decision making, want to impact the world based on technology, driven to make a difference in the world, collaboration	Make a difference in the workplace and world, technological advances, achievement of high expectations of self, goals and dreams

(continues)

TABLE 20-1 Generational Mentoring (continued)

Generation Name	Characteristics	Values	Mentoring Needs
Generation Z = Gen Z, Instant Generation (1995–2012)	Grew up with cellular devices in their hands; able to run multiple apps at the same time, get instant answers from the internet, and multi-task because they can quickly shift; cost-conscious; disengaged from political participation; motivated by a desire to help and please others; willing to take personal risks if they will gain more	Instant, clear, and concise communication; texting; speed more than accuracy; change; peer group; being entrepreneurial; loyal to peer group; career-minded; "we-centric"; collaboration	Practical real-life experience and worldview, desire to help and make a difference, want something to believe in

TABLE 20-2 Where to Start to Be Inclusive of All Generations

Where to Start	An Opportunity	Challenges
Make a commitment	Create a place that is multigenerational friendly, all-inclusive	Breaking old habits, changing culture
Take an organizational pulse	Determine the organization's generational exposure	There will probably be disparities of the generations in place
Train your leadership	Senior and middle management/leadership will need generational training and exposure	Management may not be open to learning about the differences between the generational groups
Develop your strategy	Put together groups that can develop strategies for changing to a multigenerational-friendly environment, include members from all levels of the organization	Getting commitment from all levels of organization to form groups to develop the strategies
Test drive your strategy and tweak	Define a period in the planning process for a trial period prior to implementation, determine where it will be trialed, include an evaluation process and steps along the trial, review the results of the trial and tweak the strategy based on lessons learned	Resistance to the trial by certain parties, potentially saboteurs of the trial

Where to Start	An Opportunity	Challenges
Implement your revised strategy	Put the revised strategic plan into place within the organization	Lack of engagement by members of the organization that may stall or impede the implementation
Seek feedback regularly	The organization will need feedback regarding the implementation process, and what is going well and what is not; include evaluation from participants; make modifications to the strategic plan as identified	Feedback may not be well received

Data from Tokar, P. (2013). GEN busting. *Economic Development Journal, 12*(1), 41–46.

Generation X

Born between 1965 and approximately 1979, and also referred to as the Latchkey Generation, the Slackers, or the GenXers, Generation X accounts for approximately 34% of the U.S. population (David, Gelfeld, & Rangel, 2017). Because the Baby Boomers were working a lot, Xers may have experienced a relative lack of adult supervision compared to previous generations. This generation also experienced increased divorce rates, maternal participation in the workforce, and availability of childcare options outside the home. As a result of seeing their parents experience work layoffs, they do not have the loyalty to a company that prior generations did. They are hard workers with strong interpersonal skills and opt to stay at a company because of their relationships with their coworkers rather than out of any loyalty to the company. Xers are open and always looking for new and growth opportunities in the workplace. They want autonomy to exhibit creativity in a project or job and do not want to be micromanaged. Having a flexible job and time off to enjoy leisure activities is often an important value for them. Xers see themselves as innovators and entrepreneurs, even when they are working for someone else. They embrace technology and are willing to spend the time to learn how to use it effectively.

Generation Y/Millennials

Born between approximately 1980 and 1994, and also referred to as the Next Generation, millennials, or Gen Next, this group represents approximately 12% of the U.S. population (Hernandez, Poole, & Grys, 2018; Sherman, 2015). In terms of sheer numbers, the millennials are the largest birth cohort since the Baby Boomers. Gen Y members are much more racially and ethnically diverse. They are also much more segmented as an audience owing to technological advances such as the expansion of cable TV channels, satellite radio, the internet, e-zines, and more. Gen Yers are less brand-loyal, and the speed of the internet has led this group to be extremely flexible.

The millennials are creative, hard-working, and very bright. It has been said that they are the most "child-centric generation in history" (Tokar, 2013, p. 45). Many were raised in dual-income or single-parent families and have been more involved in family purchases—everything from groceries to new cars. Their parents took a great deal of interest in their children academically, emotionally, and personally; as a result, this generation tends to be confident in all that they do. They are driven by technology and want to impact the world from that standpoint; they have high expectations of themselves and the companies for which they work. They want to contribute to the bottom line and make a difference. Moving between jobs and locations is common for members of this generation.

Generation Z

Born between 1995 and 2012, also often called the Instant Generation, Generation Z represents the next generation to enter colleges and the workforce. This is the most tech-savvy group, as these individuals have grown up with the small screen of the cell phone with multiple apps running at the same time. As a result, they want instant answers and search the internet for those answers—in their opinion, Google and Alexa know all. They value speed more than accuracy and can multitask. It has been said that they think in hyperlinks (Desai & Lele, 2017). "Generation Z is named after the name 'zappers,' characterized by quick shifts. They will be ready for sudden change if they don't like something such as 'workplace,' they live in a faster rhythm than the earlier generations" (Desai & Lele, 2017, p. 7). This generation engages more with Twitter, Instagram, and Snapchat than with Facebook. They want clear and succinct communication, especially through e-mail, but prefer texting. They describe themselves are being influential, thoughtful, loyal, compassionate, open-minded, and responsible. They are also career oriented.

Gen Z typically prefers one-on-one communication with face-to-face interactions. Members of this generation express interest in social issues and want to make the world a better place. They value input from their peer group more than from their parents or other role models when compared to other generations. In the education arena, Gen Z wants practical, real-life experiences and is concerned about the cost of education. These individuals often see themselves working for themselves at some point and being entrepreneurial (Loveland, 2017).

Mentoring Younger Generations

Even though mentoring of individuals from all generations is of value, it is the younger generations (Generations Y and Z) who are in most need of mentoring. As nursing's future, they need insight, guidance, and wisdom about respecting the past, engaging in the present, and creating a vision for the future as Christian nurses, ensuring nursing as ministry. The following steps, developed by Charles Eaton (2017) and adapted from "Mentoring the Next Generation of Technologists," are worth considering when mentoring members of Generations Y and Z:

1. Develop a strategic plan of action to work with them and get them involved in the process.
2. Understand that they have a passion for solving problems especially if it involves their community.
3. Construct contextual meaning to help them learn new things all the time and helping others is very important part of their future.
4. Encourage human contact by working in collaborative groups and emphasizing respect, cooperation, and collaboration are key points to help them make a difference for the good of humanity.
5. Act as a role model to have further influence beyond their current capabilities.
6. Work together in a collaborative approach in which the mentor role-models mentality more than method to help them visualize what the future holds.
7. Help them find their passion and love for specific work that has meaning for them.

▸ Developing a Mentoring Program

Phases of the Mentoring Relationship

Kathy E. Kram's landmark article, published in the *Academy of Management Journal* in 1983, remains applicable today when discussing the phases of a mentor relationship. Kram (1983) defined four phases of a mentor relationship: initiation, cultivation, separation, and redefinition. The initiation phase spans the first six months to a year and is the period in which the mentor and the mentee begin to develop the relationship and understand its significance. The cultivation phase is characterized by an expansion of the psychosocial function and development of career potential that comes to fruition; this phase ranges from two to five years in duration. The next phase is separation, which features a significant change in roles between mentor and mentee, as the mentee becomes more independent and less reliant on the mentor. This phase generally lasts from six months to two years. In redefinition, the mentoring relationship either ends or changes significantly to become more of a peer-like friendship. Kram (1983) also described the major "turning points" (p. 622) in each of the four phases of her model (**FIGURE 20-2**).

As the mentor and the mentee develop their relationship, an understanding of these phases will help each adapt to the changes that occur as the relationship evolves. In the center of this relationship is God; the relationship will flourish when both parties use God as the pillar of all. As part of the relationship, both mentor and mentee should discuss goals, expectations, and logistics of meeting after prayerful time with God. Also, they should take into consideration any generational differences (discussed earlier) that might exist in

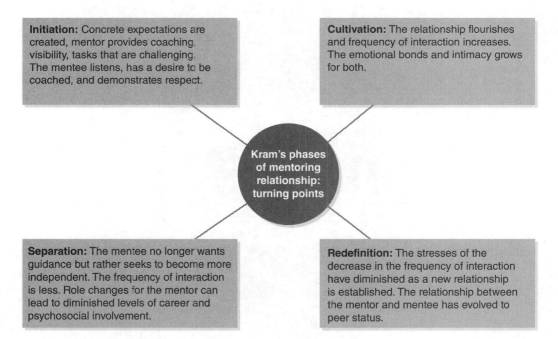

FIGURE 20-2 Kram's phases of the mentoring relationship: turning points.

Data from Kram, K. E. (1983). Phases of the mentor relationship. *Academy of Management Journal (pre-1986), 26*(4), 608–625.

the relationship. Both should recognize that entering into such a relationship is a large responsibility for all involved, and God is in the center of it all. This relationship will become an integral part of the mentor's and the mentee's lives. There needs to be time to celebrate successes in God's Holy Name, as well as time to come together in the presence of God when conflict or disagreement arises. God is pivotal in the faith-based mentor–mentee relationship.

Formalizing a Mentor Program

Creating a formal mentor program is a demanding, yet valuable, task for any entity, whether it be a school of nursing, a full-time or part-time faculty development program, a new-graduate program, or a clinical agency. The goal of any formalized mentor program is to increase the competency of the nurse mentee, promote professional development, and support the growth of the mentee. The goal of such a program for the mentor is to share expertise, insight, and wisdom to the mentee, further enhancing the professional growth of the mentor.

A distinction is made between formalized mentoring and natural mentoring. Formalized mentoring is assigned; there is a structured, definitive plan for both the mentor and the mentee to accomplish (**BOX 20-5**). Natural mentoring, by comparison, is informal and more spontaneous, with its own internal structure in which the mentee and the mentor are not assigned to each other. Instead, this type of

---

BOX 20-5 Evidence-Based Practice Focus

The following steps can be used in developing a formalized mentor program (adapted from Humberd & Rouse, 2016):

1. Pray to God for guidance.
2. Create a mission statement that is Christ centered.
3. Form a steering committee of believers.
4. Establish a definition of mentoring from a Christian perspective.
5. Establish a purpose based on Biblical principles.
6. Consider the financial aspects of the program.
7. Recruit mentors who will fulfill the mission.
8. Provide education to the mentor from a Biblical worldview.
9. Provide some structured guidelines to support mentor and mentee:
   a. Initial period: Plan for introductions, a getting-acquainted period, and time to establish goals and expectations. "The program includes face-to-face meetings, forums on topics relevant to ethnically diverse students, projects to help the student become familiar with their income and study habits, and other activities as deemed appropriate" (Crooks, 2013, p. 48).
   b. Growth period: Communication expands, the frequency of interactions increases, opportunities for teaching and learning arise, feedback and structured assignments are provided, some goal attainment occurs, goals may be modified and restricted, and new goals are developed.
   c. Transition period: Let go of the old ways of doing things; emphasize growth and movement toward independence; communication patterns change and the relationship is reestablished.
10. Recruit and assign mentees—based on education, diversity of the population, and matching of mentee with mentor.
11. Provide for evaluation points along the way.

relationship emerges over time and is mutually agreed upon by both parties (**BOX 20-6**). Summarizing a research study by McKinsey (2016) on faculty's mentoring of undergraduate students, the author stated:

> Based on the research literature and student and faculty testimony from a residential liberal arts college, this article shows that unplanned "natural" mentoring can be crucial to student learning and development and illustrates some best practices. It advances understanding of faculty mentoring by differentiating it from teaching, characterizing several functional types of mentoring, and identifying the phases through which a mentoring relationship develops. Arguing that benefits to students, faculty, and institutions outweigh the risks and costs of mentoring, it is written for faculty who want to be better mentors and provides evidence that administrators should value and reward mentoring. (p. 1)

BOX 20-6 Outstanding Nurse Leader: Linda Richards

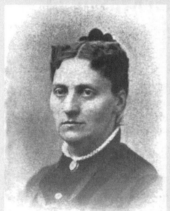

From Mary Adelaide Nutting, Lavinia L. Dock. (1907). *A History of Nursing: The Evolution of Nursing Systems from the Earliest Times to the Foundation of the First English and American Training Schools for Nurses, Vol. 2.* New York, NY: G.P. Putnam's Sons.

Linda Richards (1841–1930) was both a mentor and a mentee. Richards was the first nurse to graduate from a U.S. nursing program. She became discouraged with the status of nursing, working 16-hour shifts, having no written (only verbal) physician orders, and the lack of patient charts. Later in her career, she was mentored by Florence Nightingale, the mother of all nursing, with whom she did an intensive study for seven months. Although she did not meet Nightingale until the late 1870s in Great Britain, Richards pioneered many innovations in nursing on her own, including written patient charts.

One of her most significant accomplishments in nursing was not at the bedside. Ms. Richards was the founder of the first U.S. medical records system.

Richards' analytical mind, an essential element for every great nurse, helped reinvent the records division at hospitals all across the nation, then to the United Kingdom. This administrative revolution created a system where diseases, allergies, and past procedures could be tracked, and doctors were able to see a long view of their patients' histories. (Concordia University Portland, 2017, para. 10)

Richards was also an educator: She established the first nursing school in Japan. Some of her work was as a missionary nurse.

After returning to the U.S. and establishing a training school at Boston City Hospital, Richards traveled to Kyoto, Japan, at the behest of the American Board of Foreign Missions. She spent four years in Japan, working as a missionary and establishing that nation's first nurse training school. The Japanese later remembered her as the nurse who stayed up all night to wash the eyes of a young child afflicted with ophthalmia neonatorum. (Hanink, 2019, para. 10)

Richards is considered one of the pioneers of nursing both in the United States and internationally. She provides a fitting example of the process of mentoring as both a mentee and a mentor, passing along her wisdom and nursing knowledge to others.

▶ Conclusion

It is an honor to be a Christian nurse, and while on the earth, to be the hands and feet of God. We are called to serve God and others through nursing as ministry. God encourages and challenges us to become a mentor like Christ, sharing our insight, wisdom, and discernment in a compassionate way under God's direction. The ultimate guide to becoming a mentor is to follow in Jesus's footsteps (**FIGURE 20-3**): His life was to serve. Jesus was sent by the Father to live among men and to teach the ways of God. The challenge is to follow God's lead and mentor another into discipleship. The late Billy Graham (2016) once said, "A disciple is simply someone who believes in Jesus and seeks to follow him in his or her daily life. Originally, of course, a disciple was someone who literally knew Jesus in the flesh and followed him—but after he was taken up into heaven, anyone who was committed to Jesus was called a disciple.

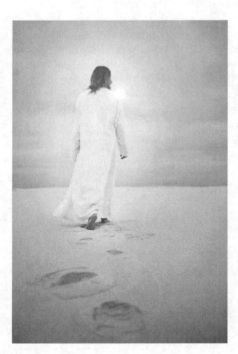

FIGURE 20-3 Follow me!
© Cecilie Arcurs/iStock/Getty Images

And that's what you are, now that you have come to Christ and are seeking to follow him."

> Therefore go and make disciples of all nations, baptizing them in the name of the Father and of the Son and of the Holy Spirit, and teaching them to obey everything I have commanded you. And surely I am with you always, to the very end of the age. (Matthew 28:19–20)

> Whoever serves me must follow me; and where I am, my servant also will be. My Father will honor the one who serves me. (John 12:26)

▶ Clinical Reasoning Exercises

1. Look at Figure 20-1. Discuss the various phases of the mentoring relationship according to the 4D-R method.
2. Examine Figure 20-2 and then explain it from the viewpoint of a new mentor and a new mentee.
3. Imagine that you are a consultant to a hospital who wants to implement a robust mentoring program for new RNs to increase their retention and job satisfaction. Assuming there is no program currently in place at this facility, where would you begin? Outline your plan for a successful mentoring program.

▶ Personal Reflection Exercises

1. Have you ever been mentored by another person? Who was it? What do

you recall from that relationship? How did it start? How did it end?

2. Have you ever been a mentor to another nurse? If so, what was that experience like for you? If not, do you have a desire to do this? Why or why not?

3. What phase of the mentoring relationship seems the most difficult to you? Give a rationale for your answer.

4. Which generation do you come from? Do you believe the description given in this chapter is accurate for you? For members of other generations with whom you have worked? Why or why not?

References

Concordia University. (2017). National nurses's week: Four nursing role models that changed nursing forever. Retrieved from https://acceleratednursing.cu-portland.edu/blog/national-nurses-week-four-nursing-role-models-changed-nursing-forever/

Crooks, N. (2013). Mentoring as the key to minority success in nursing education. *ABNF Journal, 24*(2), 47–50.

David, P., Gelfeld, V., & Rangel, A. (2017). Generation X and its evolving experience with the American dream. *Generations, 41*(3), 77. Retrieved from https://www.aarp.org/content/dam/aarp/research/surveys_statistics/life-leisure/2018/genx-american-dream.pdf

Desai, S. P., & Lele, V. (2017). Correlating internet, social networks and workplace: A case of generation Z students. *Journal of Commerce & Management Thought, 8*(4), 802–815. doi:10.5958/0976-478X.2017.00050.7

Dwyer, B. (2016a). What is mentoring and who should do it? Retrieved from https://www.pursuegod.org/what-is-mentoring-and-who-should-do-it/

Dwyer, B. (2016b). What is PursueGOD mentoring all about? Retrieved from https://www.pursuegod.org/what-is-pursuegod-mentoring-all-about/

Eaton, C. (2017). Mentoring the next generation of technologists. *Professional Development*, 27–29. Retrieved from https://www.itspmagazine.com/from-the-news room/how-to-mentor-the-next-generation-of-technologists

Eschatology. (n.d.). In *Merriam Webster Online*. Retrieved from https://www.merriam-webster.com/dictionary/eschatology

Graham, B. (2016). Billy Graham: What does it mean to be a disciple of Jesus? *Tribune MediaServices*. Retrieved from https://www.kansascity.com/living/liv-columns-blogs/billy-graham/article77272832.html

Hanink, E. (2019). Profiles in nursing: Linda Richards. Retrieved from https://www.workingnurse.com/articles/Linda-Richards-1841-1930-and-Nursing-Education

Hernandez, J. S., Poole, K. G. Jr., & Grys, T. E. (2018). Discussion: Mentoring millennials for future leadership. *Physician Leadership Journal, 5*(3), 41.

Herr, M. (2017a). The 4D-R method of imagining the future, part 1: Implications for vocational discipleship. *Christian Education Journal, 14*(2), 405–420. https://doi.org/10.1177/073989131701400212

Herr, M. A. C. (2017b). The 4D-R method of imagining the future, part 2: Considerations on design, development, and use 2. *Christian Education Journal, 14*(2), 421–436. doi:10.1177/073989131701400213

Humberd, B. K., & Rouse, E.D. (2016). Seeing you in me and me in you: Personal identification in the phases of mentoring relationships. *Academy of Management Review, 41*(3), 435–455. http://dx.doi.org/10.5465/amr.2013.0203

Kram, K. E. (1983). Phases of the mentor relationship. *Academy of Management Journal (pre-1986), 26*(4), 608–625.

Loveland, E. (2017). Instant generation. *Journal of College Admission*, 34–38. Retrieved from https://files.eric.ed.gov/fulltext/EJ1142068.pdf

McKinsey, E. (2016). Faculty mentoring undergraduates: The nature, development, and benefits of mentoring relationships. *Teaching & Learning Inquiry, 4*(1). http://dx.doi.org/10.20343/teachlearninqu.4.1.5

Sherman, R. O. (2015). Recruiting and retaining generation Y perioperative nurses. *AORN Journal, 101*(1), 138–143.

Tjan, A. K. (2017). What the best mentors do. *Harvard Business Review Digital Articles*, 2–4. Retrieved from https://hbr.org/2017/02/what-the-best-mentors-do

Tokar, P. (2013). GEN busting. *Economic Development Journal, 12*(1), 41–46.

Recommended Readings

Aragon, S. (2016). Washington Center for Nursing's Diversity Mentoring Program aims to support nurses from underrepresented communities, promote a culture of health. *Washington Nurse, 46*(2), 34–35.

Ayu, S., K, Ayu Kartika, S., & Pande Putu, J. (2018). Achieving ideal mentoring: Working patterns among clinical instructors, nurses, and nursing students. *Public Health and Preventive Medicine Archives, 6*(1), 1–5. doi:10.15562/pphma.v6i1.9

"Be a lamp, a lifeboat or a ladder . . .": Be a nursing mentor. (2013). *Nursing News, 37*(2), 4–5.

Brannagan, K. B., & Oriol, M. (2014). A model for orientation and mentoring of online adjunct faculty in nursing. *Nursing Education Perspectives, 35*(2), 128–130.

Casey, D., Clark, L., & Gould, K. (2018). Developing a digital learning version of a mentorship training programme. *British Journal of Nursing, 27*(2), 82–86. doi:10.12968/bjon.2018.27.2.82

Chatmon, B. (2018). A call to action: Mentoring as a tool to increase diversity in the nursing profession. *Pelican News, 74*(2), 5.

dos Santos, L., Monteiro, D., da Silva, C. M., & da Silva, P. S. (2015). The undergraduate degree in nursing and the meanings derived from the mentoring. *Revista De Pesquisa: Cuidado E Fundamental, 7*(1), 1783–1795. doi:10.9789/2175-5361.2015.v7i1.1783-1795

Eliades, A. B. (2017). Mentoring practice and mentoring benefit 6: Equipping for leadership and leadership readiness: An overview and application to practice using mentoring activities. *Pediatric Nursing, 43*(1), 40–42.

Fleming, K. (2017). Peer mentoring: A grass roots approach to high-quality care. *Nursing Management, 48*(1), 12–14.

Ford, Y. (2015). Development of nurse self-concept in nursing students: The effects of a peer-mentoring experience. *Journal of Nursing Education, 54,* S107–S111. doi:10.3928/01484834-20150814-20

Green, J. L. (2018). Peer support systems and professional identity of student nurses undertaking a UK learning disability nursing programme. *Nurse Education in Practice, 30,* 56. doi:10.1016/j.nepr.2017.11.009

Hulton, L. J., Sawin, E. M., Trimm, D., Graham, A., & Powell, N. (2016). An evidence-based nursing faculty mentoring program. *International Journal of Nursing Education, 8*(1), 41–46. doi:10.5958/0974-9357.2016.00008.8

Jakubik, L. D. (2016). Leadership series: "How to" for mentoring. Part 1: An overview of mentoring practices and mentoring benefits. *Pediatric Nursing, 42*(1), 37–38.

Jakubik, L. D. (2017). Leadership series: "How to" for mentoring. Mentoring in the career continuum of a nurse: Clarifying purpose and timing. *Pediatric Nursing, 43*(3), 149–152.

Joubert, A., & de Villiers, J. (2015). The learning experiences of mentees and mentors in a nursing school's mentoring programme. *Curationis, 38*(1), E1–E7. doi:10.4102/curationis.v38i1.1145

Kramer, D., Hillman, S. M., & Zavala, M. (2018). Developing a culture of caring and support through a peer mentorship program. *Journal of Nursing Education, 57*(7), 430–435. doi:10.3928/01484834-20180618-09

Merrill, A. S. (2017). Helping educators become teachers through mentoring. *Reflections on Nursing Leadership, 43*(3), 1–6.

Milner, K. A., Foito, K., & Watson, S. (2016), Strategies for providing spiritual care and support to nursing student. *Journal of Christian Nursing, 33*(4), 238–243. doi:10.1097/CNJ.0000000000000309

Nick, J. M., Delahoyde, T. M., Prato, D. D., Mitchell, C., Ortiz, J., Ottley, C., . . . Siktberg, L. (2012). Best practices in academic mentoring: A model for excellence. *Nursing Research & Practice,* 1–9. doi:10.1155/2012/937906

Hosseinabadi, R., Gholami, M., Biranvand, S., Tarverdian, A., & Anbari, K. (2015). Effect of multi mentoring educational method on clinical competence of nursing students. *Journal of Medical Education and Development, 10*(2), 119–128.

Rosser, E. (2017). Developing our future leaders: The role of a global mentoring programme. *British Journal of Nursing, 26*(18), 1045. doi:10.12968/bjon.2017.26.18.1045

Rylance, R., Barrett, J., Sixsmith, P., & Ward, D. (2017). Student nurse mentoring: An evaluative study of the mentor's perspective. *British Journal of Nursing, 26*(7), 405–409.

Schleisman, A., & Gruber-Page, M. (2016). Response to "the value of mentoring in nursing: An honor and a gift." *Oncology Nursing Forum, 43*(6), 677. doi:10.1188/16.ONF.677

Walker, D., & Verklan, T. (2016). Peer mentoring during practicum to reduce anxiety in first-semester nursing students. *Journal of Nursing Education, 55*(11), 651–654. doi:10.3928/01484834-20161011-08

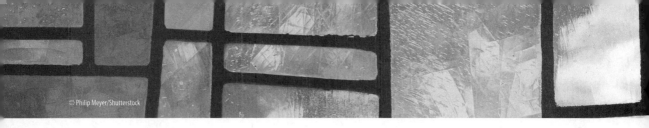

CHAPTER 21

Christian-Based Leadership in Nursing

Karen Hessler, PhD, RN, FNP-BC

LEARNING OBJECTIVES

At the end of this chapter, the reader will be able to:

1. Describe leadership and followership in the nursing profession.
2. Compare the different leadership styles and their impact on leaders and followers.
3. Acknowledge the calling of Christian-based leaders within the framework of servant as leader.
4. Discuss Biblical application within the process of building character and skills as a nurse leader.
5. Explore the nurse as leader using an ecological framework.

KEY TERMS

Attributes
Christian-based leader
Ecological framework

Follower
Leader
Leadership style

Servant as leader (servant leadership)
Team player

I n this chapter, the role, definition, and impact of great nursing leadership are examined in depth. In addition, the chapter explores leadership styles and the unique approach of the **Christian-based leader**. To that end, God's word is intertwined with guidance and wisdom in learning about the leadership journey. One cannot discuss Christian-based leadership without taking a deep dive into the world of servant leadership and considering how it can change both **leader** and **follower** in the most amazing and productive manner. Due to the many layers of leadership that can be found in different contexts, nursing leadership is also examined through the lens of the **ecological framework** in this chapter. Finally, the chapter explores how nurse leaders are developed and refreshed to do the good work that the Lord has prepared them to do.

▶ The Concept and Definition of Leadership

Leadership and nursing go hand in hand. It is difficult to take on one role without automatically adopting the other. Nurses may hesitate to assume the role of leader for many reasons. But if these same nurses would stop to examine the work that they do every day, they would readily see that leadership is an innate characteristic of one's calling to the profession. As a result, there lies within each nurse a leadership instinct. When that instinct is nurtured properly, it can be used to do the good work that each nurse is called to perform under the direction of the Heavenly Father. When calling someone to become a nurse, God sets each one of us upon a particular path. As Christian men and women, we are called to something much more than a job: We are called to be the hands and feet of Jesus. Nurses are in a perfect position to walk in this path. With specialty information about how we are created and how God has developed each body to work and fight disease and illness, we are equipped with life-saving skills and abilities.

When our fellow man or woman is in pain, whether it be physically or spiritually, nurses are in a unique position to be able to help. Indeed, that role is part of the job description. What higher calling or responsibility could there be than to care for the lost and hurting, much like Jesus did during his ministry on earth? As nurses learn how God would choose to use them, it becomes clear that leadership is a part of that master plan. Leaders provide direction, guidance, inspiration, and hope to those around them. Part of this leadership includes a call to do the good work of nursing and care for our fellow humans. God wants to prepare us ahead of time for the work He has planned for each specific nurse's career. As Paul teaches in Ephesians 2:10, "For we are His workmanship, created in Christ Jesus for good works, which God prepared beforehand, that we should walk in them" (English Standard Version [ESV]).

Defining a word such as *leader* can be challenging. To see this difficulty, just think of all the different contexts in which the word could be used. For example, U.S. children often play a game called "Follow the Leader." In this game, one child is chosen or demands to be the "leader," and the rest of children must follow the leader and do exactly what the leader does. Some organizations may perceive leadership as working in this manner. Another context for the word *leader* arises when thinking about the structure of a government. Several leaders exist in this type of context, with each defined leader having a leader of his or her own. Still another context would be in a church setting, where the word *leader* is used to describe people who are in charge of specific aspects of a church service. For example, the worship leader is the individual who directs the worship music for a service, but that person is rarely the pastor or the leader of the entire organization.

Given all of the preceding context-based examples, and the endless additional possible contexts one might consider, what does it really mean to be a leader in health care? In other words, how can nurses provide a definition of a "leader" that is specific to their profession? The real answer is that one definition may not fit all nursing scenarios. The practical outcome of this discussion would be to consider which traits and qualities a leader might need to be a person whom others choose to follow. While recognizing that one definition does not always encompass the importance and brilliance of a leader, the following definition provides a starting point for further elaboration and discussion: A "leader" in nursing is someone who is able to use experience and available evidence to guide and inspire fellow nurses toward the collective goal of providing best nursing practice for optimal patient and family outcomes. A leader must have the skills, attitudes, and abilities to manage each patient, family, and staffing situation with grace, strength, knowledge, and wisdom. Based on this description, a leader could be a nurse who has been out of school for two months and who orchestrates a Code call for the first time. Perhaps this nurse might not have extensive experience with this particular scenario, but as a leader, he or she would be able to put the right people and tools in place to ensure the best patient outcome possible.

All nurses continually develop their leader skills and abilities with each experience that God brings to their lives. For example, the inexperienced nurse running a Code for the first time has begun a journey on the road to leadership development. God molds and shapes each nurse for a specific purpose and work on earth to be the hands and feet of Jesus to patients and families. Providing experiences that are married with knowledge of Biblical principles can produce the most fruitful and productive leaders in the nursing profession. God teaches each individual nurse that He has created how to be a leader through this experiential and iterative process. In other words, nurses are continually challenged with new experiences that assist them in developing their unique and blessed leadership qualities. Each experience brings not only knowledge but also a new appreciation for the work that the Father can do through each individual. As part of this paradigm, nurses are continually shaped and molded as God prepares each individual for the work He will bring to that person in the future. Similarly, the development of the nurse as leader is never finished. When the Father is working within and through a Christian nurse, the nurse's influence cannot be understated or underappreciated. As Christian nurses, we bring a fresh perspective to patients, families, and coworkers as we do our best to be the hands and feet of Jesus, our ultimate leadership mentor.

In nursing, as in many other professions, it is often assumed that the most seasoned nurse is the best leader. In reality, a leader is more than just the most experienced nurse or the nurse that has been in the job for the longest period of time. Although the seasoned nurse may be the best nurse at the bedside, that definition does not always translate to being the best nurse in the boardroom. In short, the collective abilities of a nurse leader are complex and numerous.

Who Are the Leaders in Nursing?

Given the many different ways that a nurse can show leadership abilities, one might ask who the leaders are in nursing. As previously discussed, all nurses are called to be leaders at different times in their career (see **BOXES 21-1** and **21-2**). Some would describe leaders in nursing as those who step out of the status quo and offer options for improvement that often involve change. Speaking out for change or improvement, particularly if the nurse is less developed in his or her career, can be scary

---

BOX 21-1 Research Highlight

Research by Dr. Jennifer Manning aimed to evaluate the influence of nurse manager leadership styles on staff nurse work engagement levels. Using a descriptive, correlational design, 441 staff nurses from three different hospitals were surveyed. Transactional and transformational leadership styles used by nurse managers were positively correlated with increased staff nurse work engagement, which was hypothesized to have the potential to improve organizational outcomes.

Modified from Manning, J. (2016). The influence of nurse manager leadership style on staff nurse work engagement. *Journal of Nursing Administration, 46*(9), 438–443.

BOX 21-2 Evidence-Based Practice Focus

Adopting evidence-based practice (EBP) into the clinical setting can be easier to talk about than to actually implement. This study assessed the beliefs of nurse leaders and registered nurse clinicians about the use of EBP, their perceptions of organizational readiness for EBP, and the frequency of implementing EBP before and after interventions to achieve and maintain Magnet status designation. Between the pre- and post-survey time periods, registered nurses' self-reports of positive attitude and organizational readiness perceptions improved. Although the nurse leader scores were originally high for positive attitude and perception of organizational readiness, these scores did not increase after the preparations for Magnet status. The authors had some ideas about why scores for registered nurses versus nurse leaders differed in the study. First, they hypothesized that registered nurses' attitudes and perceptions may have been more affected by the Magnet preparation, whereas the nurse leaders had higher scores on these items originally and, therefore, experienced little change in the post-study survey results. A second hypothesis was that nurse managers could be more proactive in their role in implementing EBP initiatives in the organization. Realistic expectations for EBP implementation, accessible resources, and clarifying expectations for the process of EBP in the facility are important aspects of incorporating the EBP process in organizational settings.

Modified from Warren, J. I., Montgomery, K. L., & Friedmann, E. (2016). Three-year pre-post analysis of EBP integration in a magnet-designated community hospital. *Worldviews on Evidence-Based Nursing, 13*(1), 50–58. doi: 10.1111/wvn.12148

and intimidating. However, true nurse leaders recognize that their actions can improve outcomes for their patients and charge forward despite the intimidation. In this sense, the nurse leader can be described as an advocate.

The American Nurses Association (ANA) suggests that advocacy is both the pillar of nursing and a multifaceted concept (ANA, 2018). Nurses can advocate for safe and high-quality health care for their patients and communities in direct patient care, or they can assume a more indirect role when advocating in politics and within policy realms. In short, being a leader in nursing is more than having a certain title or holding an administrative position as the official person in charge.

Every time nurses use their skills and abilities to provide better patient care, they are exuding leadership qualities. When nurses implement evidence-based practice with the goal of improving patient and organizational outcomes, they are working as advocates. Although students may not recognize themselves as leaders, they are also exhibiting leadership every day as they learn the ways of professional nursing. The many hours of studying, clinical work, classwork, and paper writing culminate in each nursing student learning how to care for patients and families in a safe and evidence-based manner. Why do nursing students do all of this work? One could argue that it is not for the paycheck, but rather as part of a higher calling to care for their fellow man and woman. This is God's ultimate call for a nurse.

As all nurses are called to be leaders in their current roles, they must recognize their important role as leaders in the profession. Learning what it means to be an effective and productive leader will bring each nurse to a higher level of ability and advocacy in the profession of nursing.

▶ Leadership Styles

Not all leaders do the work of leadership in the same manner. Although each leader brings a unique perspective and set of skills to the role, researchers have delineated a set of well-known leadership styles over the years. A **leadership style** is a general description of how a person in a leadership position completes his or her daily tasks. One definition of leadership style, offered by Cherry (2018), is a leader's characteristic behaviors when directing, motivating, managing, and guiding a group of people. As Cherry notes, leaders go about the work they do in very different ways.

In the 1930s, Kurt Lewin and a group of psychologists began research aimed at identifying and classifying styles of leadership. From this research came three major leadership styles: authoritarian, democratic, and laissez-faire (Cherry, 2018). Since then, many more researchers have further developed Lewin's work, and other theories and leadership styles have emerged from this original work. Although Lewin's research was conducted using children who were being led to do an arts and crafts project, the conclusion was a fairly broad one: Human behaviors change depending on the type of leader to whom individuals are exposed.

In the remainder of this section, the three main types of leadership styles are described, followed by additional leadership styles that have been thoroughly researched. Although some of the styles may seem to overlap, they also have nuances that distinguish them from one another. As you read, consider which types of leaders you have encountered and how their leadership style may have changed the way you went about your work as a follower.

Autocratic Leaders

Autocratic leaders provide clear expectations for their followers regarding what needs to be done, when it needs to be done, and how it needs to be done (Cherry, 2018). Such leaders often assume control of all the decisions, requesting and accepting little or no input from others in an organization ("Definition of 'autocratic leadership,'" 2018). There exists a clear division between leader and follower that is fostered by a command (of the leader) and control (of those following) system. It is not uncommon for an authoritarian leader to make decisions completely independently and announce

them without discussion or advice. This type of leadership is akin to the "Follow the Leader" game discussed earlier in this chapter. When autocratic leadership is applied in an abusive manner, followers may experience a dictatorship, with bossing and controlling being part of the everyday leadership tactics (Cherry, 2018).

Sometimes the autocratic approach is beneficial—particularly if a certain situation demands a rapid decision. Over time, however, this approach has the potential to create a dysfunctional or hostile environment in which the followers are pitted against a domineering leader (Cherry, 2018).

Democratic Leaders

In contrast to autocratic leadership, the democratic or participatory leadership style offers guidance to followers, who are encouraged to participate in the organization's decision making. As such, team members can feel more invested in the organization, and therefore more engaged in the day-to-day work that needs to be completed toward organizational goals. The leader typically takes input and suggestions from the team, but often retains the final decision-making role. Team members can be more creative and motivated when sharing ideas and solutions to corporate dilemmas. When assuming this more active role, the members of a team often feel that they have an important part in the work done by the organization, which can also foster commitment to the collective goals of both the group and the organization at large (Cherry, 2018).

Delegative (Laissez-Faire) Leaders

The third type of leadership discussed in Lewin's early work is a delegative leadership style, also known as laissez-faire (Cherry, 2018). The delegative leader provides little or no guidance and leaves the ultimate decision making for the organization or unit up to the group members. As one might imagine, this hands-off approach means that team members have no true direction and may face the challenge of competing ideas and directions on a project. Even in situations in which the team members are highly qualified to do the work and make the decisions appropriately, the delegative leadership style is often unproductive. It is not uncommon for the team members to be frustrated, making demands to the leader and showing little cooperation due to the lack of direction provided by the leader. Unfortunately, team members also often turn against one another, blaming one another for mistakes or poor decisions. Without a clear goal or direction for the team members to strive for, those team members lack personal responsibility and motivation and fail to make progress on work to be completed.

Those individuals assuming a laissez-faire leadership style may feel uncomfortable making decisions and accepting their role as leader of the team. They may prefer an environment in which they can be liked or be a friend of each employee or team member. Allowing free reign to the team and attempting to give everyone what they want, when they want it, can initially give followers a positive view of their leader. Over time, however, the leader may learn that the leadership role does not include the same social interactions experienced as a follower or team member.

Laissez-faire leaders do provide the tools and resources necessary for their team to do the work at hand. In addition, they allow for a great deal of creativity, as the lack of direction from the leader leaves open the road for innovative ideas and solutions. Some team members may value this independence to work as they see fit. Particularly when the team members are highly motivated and have a great deal of expertise necessary to complete the work, the laissez-faire style may be beneficial. Having the right people on the team is essential to the success of a laissez-faire leader. Otherwise, the laissez-faire leadership style is likely to yield poor involvement and motivation of the team,

low accountability, lack of role awareness and direction, and frustrated team members. At its worst, the laissez-faire leader can be passive or totally avoid the leadership role. In these cases, no motivation, direction, encouragement, or feedback is provided to the team. Eventually the members of a team with this type of leader will seek someone with more expertise and inspiration as their next leader (Cherry, 2018).

Transformational Leaders

Falling within the larger category of the democratic or participatory leadership style established by Lewin's work, the transformational leadership style provides the opportunity for each team member or follower to provide input and share in a collective organizational vision. Transformational leaders are known for inspiring staff by creating an environment of intellectual stimulation and effective communication. Characteristics of such a leader include charisma, inspiration, self-confidence, self-direction, and intellectual stimulation (Atkinson, 2011). These leaders are experts at motivating followers under their leadership but do so in a sensitive and determined manner that keeps the organization's vision and mission at the forefront of the team's efforts.

Inspiring followers in the profession of nursing requires the use of evidence-based practice (Box 21-2). Moreover, effective communication and the ability to foster teamwork are essential traits of the transformational leader. However, great ideas and vision are only one part of this leadership equation: A transformational leader must also direct the positive outcomes of the inspired work. To do this, the leader must be optimistic, respectful, passionate, and honest. Self-reflection is a regular habit of the transformational leader, and these types of leaders encourage those persons under their leadership to be self-reflective as well (Atkinson, 2011).

When developing the Multifactor Leadership Questionnaire (MLQ), Bass and Avolio (1995) listed five factors associated with the transformational leadership style. The first two of these factors have been labeled *idealized influence* and associated with a more specific set of behaviors and **attributes**. Idealized influence behaviors are described as the trust and confidence a leader builds with his or her followers through behaviors and personal associations. Similarly, idealized influence attributes comprise the way a leader builds a collective sense of mission and values with the followers. A third factor, *inspirational motivation*, has been described as how the transformational leader disseminates a clear vision to the followers, whereas *intellectual stimulation* is the way the leader promotes innovation and creativity among and within the group. Finally, *individual consideration* is the empowerment that the leader disseminates and supports in the followers (Bass & Avolio, 1995).

Although quite abstract, each of these factors contributes to the collective idea that a transformational leader is a person who does not dictate, but rather inspires. By capitalizing on the internal motivation of each follower, the transformational leader can move a group forward toward a collective goal. Within this general movement, each follower can find his or her own passion and innovation within the shared goal. When done well, transformational leadership can be inspirational to followers, providing a sense of personal satisfaction, empowerment, and connection to one's work (Garcia-Sierra & Fernandez-Castro, 2018).

Given the wonderful skills associated with this leadership style, one might ask why everyone does not strive to be a transformational leader. In fact, many leaders may aspire to be transformational leaders but are on a journey rather than at the final destination. Some critics of this type of leadership believe transformational leaders are too abstract and therefore have unrealistic expectations within their role. There is a risk of creating an environment that is full of ideas and inspiration, but in which the necessary work is not completed owing to a lack of planning and directed, goal-oriented outcomes. This type of leadership may need to be balanced by followers who are more detail focused and goal oriented.

Transactional Leaders

Group organization and establishment of a clear chain of command are the focus of transactional leaders. As the term *transactional* indicates, this kind of leader uses a carrot-and-stick approach, in which followers are rewarded for good performance and punished for poor performance (Willis, Clarke, & O'Connor, 2017). In regard to Lewin's early work on leadership styles, transactional leadership is akin to autocratic leadership but adds more details about how the leader most often motivates the team. Notably, this leadership style allows the leader to have more control and direct action in the management of the organization, much like described in an autocratic leadership style. In transactional leadership, goals of positive performance are typically established by the leader, creating a "top-down" direction of leadership that dictates expectations to followers. While this can be a clear and, in many cases, productive way to lead, it may not allow for any individual goal setting by followers in the organization. Workers are not likely to meet their own professional goals if those goals are not directly linked to the organizational goals already set by the leader. In addition, this leadership style seldom allows for creativity among members of the organization, which is likely to stifle innovative and potentially productive ideas and outcomes.

The main attributes of transactional leadership style are *contingent reward*, *management by exception (active)*, and *management by exception (passive)* (Manning, 2016). The idea of contingent reward revolves around an exchange of, and expected performance of an employee based on, a reward from the leader. Management by exception is an attribute of transactional leaders that includes negative feedback, negative reinforcement, and corrective criticism of the leader directed toward an employee or follower. It can be either active or passive. A transactional leader using active management by exception is likely to provide negative reinforcement and corrective criticism, waiting for employees to make a mistake and then correcting them accordingly (Manning, 2016). While this approach to leadership may sound negative, it is highly effective and appropriate in some contexts. Willis et al. (2017) have suggested that in work environments where safety is critical, such as nursing, transactional leadership is preferred. High attention to details and tracking of employee performance errors can be beneficial for prevention of similar errors in the future. In their research, Willis et al. (2017) found that the higher the followers perceived the possibility of making errors to be, the more accepting they were of active management by exception in their leaders.

Situational Leaders

Some leaders can adjust their leadership style to the situation or team at hand. Situational theories of leadership focus on how the environment, situation, and members on the team affect the way leaders choose to do their work (Cherry, 2018). They suggest that no single leadership style is best; instead, the situation and team should dictate the kind of leadership style that is used. In this view, the most effective leader is one who can adapt the leadership style to the current situation after assessing certain cues and clues about each job at hand. Situational leadership theory is also referred to as the Hersy–Blanchard situational leadership theory after its developers (Cherry, 2018).

▸ The Servant as Leader

The **servant as leader** concept was first introduced and described by Robert Greenleaf in 1970. Greenleaf (2018) defined servant leadership as "a philosophy and set of practices that enriches the lives of individuals, builds better

organizations and ultimately creates a more just and caring world" (para. 1). The premise of servant leadership builds upon the natural (or unconscious) feeling one may have to want to serve others. This natural service to others leads one to a more conscious choice to aspire to lead. In Greenleaf's opinion, this is very different from the motivation experienced by the person who wants to lead first due to a natural affinity to be in power or acquire status or material possessions (Robert K. Greenleaf Center for Servant Leadership, n.d.). The servant leader focuses primarily on the well-being of the people and communities being served. As such, the servant leader does not aspire to be at the top of some invisible leadership pyramid, but instead wishes to help others develop and perform at their highest level possible.

Greenleaf was a Quaker with years of leadership experience, but he was inspired to write about the concept of servant as leader after reading a short novel, *Journey to the East* (Greenleaf & Spears, 1998). The story concerned a group of people on a journey who were nurtured by a servant in their midst. As the story goes, the servant disappeared, and the group of people became lost without their servant there to help them along. Eventually, the journey was abandoned. After many years of searching, the narrator of the story found the missing servant and was taken to his religious order. The narrator learned that the servant was not a servant in this environment, but rather the head of the order, the leader. Greenleaf recognized the importance of the story and became inspired by the idea that the best leader is a servant first. The servant has a deep desire and primary motivation to help others. From this framework of humility, a true leader can emerge (Greenleaf & Spears, 1998).

Although many writings after Greenleaf's original work have played with the wording a bit, Greenleaf believed that the phonetics of the model were very important. He wanted those reading his work to understand that the servant came first, and so used the term *servant as leader* rather than *servant leadership* or *servant leader* (Greenleaf & Spears, 1998). To stay true to Greenleaf's legacy, the title of this section and the remainder of the chapter use the term *servant as leader*. Elsewhere, the terms are considered interchangeable, with servant leader and servant leadership representing the same set of ideals and characteristics (**CASE STUDY 21-1**).

A great deal of literature deals with the servant as leader concept, and each nurse is encouraged to learn more. Within the pages of this chapter, the main characteristics of servant as leader are very briefly described. Larry Spears (Greenleaf & Spears, 1998) provided his perspective on the key aspects of Greenleaf's work and offers a set of 10 characteristics of the servant as leader style of leadership:

1. *Listening.* The servant leader has a deep commitment to listening and hearing what others have to say. Listening is a key component of great communication and decision-making skills. Listening to oneself and being self-reflective are as important as the ability to listen to others and find a collective voice. These are all aspects of a servant as leader but are ongoing and continual as the leader continues to develop and grow.

2. *Empathy.* Understanding and empathizing with others can lead to acceptance and recognition of each individual's talents and spirits. Even when the leader finds it necessary to correct behavior or performance in the workplace, the servant as leader does not reject anyone. "The most successful servant-leaders are those who have become skilled empathetic listeners" (Greenleaf & Spears, 1998, p. 22).

🔍 *CASE STUDY 21-1*

Read the following case study and answer the subsequent questions based on your understanding of servant leadership.

Judy has been a nurse in the intensive care unit (ICU) for 17 years. She is considered an expert nurse, and other nurses on the unit go to her with questions about patient care, medications, and procedures on a regular basis. The director of nursing in the ICU is retiring and the upper management is attempting to find her replacement. The current director has regular meetings with each staff member and helps them prepare goals during the evaluative process. She has been an expert at maintaining a safe environment for nurses, patients, and families.

The search for a new director has been going on for two months with no qualified applicants. Judy is seen by her colleagues as the most qualified for the director position due to her expert abilities as an ICU nurse over the past 17 years.

Questions

1. Assume that hospital management wants a servant leader in the director position for the ICU. You are on the search committee and need to prepare a list of interview questions for the position. What kinds of interview questions could they ask to determine if an applicant has the attributes of a servant leader?
2. Assume that Judy is being interviewed for the job. As part of the team who is interviewing Judy, which responses to the interview questions you developed in question 1 would lead you to believe that Judy is a servant leader?
3. Do you believe that Judy is qualified to take the director role at this point in her career? Why or why not? Support your answer with a sound rationale and evidence.

3. *Healing.* It might be odd to see the word "healing" in a list of leadership attributes. However, healing of relationships can be a very necessary and often-used characteristic of a successful leader. Included in this attribute is healing of oneself and one's relationship with others. The people with whom we work will come from all walks of life, and some have had experiences that left them emotionally scarred and currently scared or feeling apprehensive when asked to trust others. The servant as leader recognizes this human trait and realizes that there is an opportunity to "help make whole" (Greenleaf & Spears, 1998, p. 22) those persons. Quite unique to a leadership model or style, Greenleaf believed that the servant as leader could recognize the innate human condition of searching for wholeness.

4. *Awareness.* The servant as leader has general awareness and self-awareness that strengthens his or her ability as a leader. Being aware can bring to bear ethics, values, and an ability to view situations holistically. To exercise this kind of awareness, the leader cannot be a seeker of solace, but rather pursues inner serenity.

5. *Persuasion.* The servant as leader does not depend on authority to influence followers, but instead relies on persuasion. This type of leader works to convince others, rather than dictate or coerce them into compliance. A servant as leader is skilled at building consensus among group members. The emphasis on persuasion over coercion may have come from Greenleaf's religious roots.

6. *Conceptualization.* As a visionary, the servant as leader has the ability to dream big and look toward the future to solve current and upcoming problems. In doing so, the servant as leader is called to find a balance between conceptual and practical foci. As Spears noted, "Trustees need to be mostly conceptual in their perspective; staff need to be mostly operational in their perspective; and, the most effective CEOs and managers probably need to develop both perspectives" (Greenleaf & Spears, 1998, p. 23).

7. *Foresight.* The servant as leader has the ability to understand and learn from past experiences, then apply those lessons to the present and future. Applying an intuitive mind can provide foresight, or the ability to foresee a likely outcome of a situation.

8. *Stewardship.* The servant as leader assumes first and foremost a commitment to serving the needs of others and holding in trust the greater good of society. Preservation of a company, organization, legacy, or profession for those to come afterward represents one aspect of stewardship.

9. *Commitment to the growth of people.* An especially beautiful quality of a servant as leader is the belief that people in an organization have intrinsic value. The servant as leader is, therefore, deeply committed to the growth of each and every person in the organization. The leader seeks to nurture and mentor each person who has chosen to follow him or her. As such, "the

servant-leader recognizes the tremendous responsibility to do everything within his or her power to nurture the personal, professional, and spiritual growth of employees" (Greenleaf & Spears, 1998, p. 23).

10. *Building community.* The servant as leader believes that true community can be created among those whom work together. Developing a working environment that fosters caring by the leader can create a specific community-related group. When part of a community, workers are more likely to invest and build, care for one another as the leader has cared for them, and instill servant-like qualities toward one another on a regular basis without conscious effort.

This list of the qualities of the servant as leader paints a beautiful picture of harmony within the work environment. Ultimately, that harmony must begin with the leader. As a leadership style, the servant as leader can allow for self-growth and self-worth of each employee or follower. As one might imagine, it takes time to develop as a servant leader. Creating an environment of caring like that described here can be overwhelming and emotionally taxing for a leader depending on the team in place. Although the leader may be extremely attuned to the process of servant as leader, it may take some time for the followers to begin to understand this approach. The leader may feel taken advantage of when fulfilling the caring and servant role. He or she may also feel a lack of respect or authority in some instances. Over time, studying and practicing the art of servant as leader should help further the development of this style of leadership. Although it is not perfect, it most aligns with the philosophy of most nurses and Christians alike.

Servant Leaders for Nurses to Follow

Reflecting on the 10 characteristics of Greenleaf's servant as leader (Greenleaf & Spears, 1998), one cannot deny the obvious connections to the Bible and Jesus Christ as an example of a servant as leader. God sent Jesus to earth to serve His people, to provide the ultimate sacrifice of service by laying down his life for his friends on the cross (John 15:13, 10:11). The Bible also has many examples of how Jesus served the people and taught service to all of his followers before he went to the cross. Perhaps the most beautiful of these moments can be found during the account of the Last Supper in John 13. Jesus washed the feet of each of his disciples in an act of humility and servitude. In John 13:12–17 (New American Standard [NAS]), Jesus teaches his disciples (and us) the significance of his actions:

> So when He had washed their feet, and taken His garments, and sat down again, He said unto them, [12]"Do you know what I have done to you? [13]You call me Teacher, and Lord: and you say well: for so I am. [14]If I then, the Lord and the Teacher, have washed your feet, you also ought to wash one another's feet. [15]For I have given you an example that you also should do as I have done to you. [16]Verily, verily, I say unto you, A servant is not greater than he that sent him. [17]If you know these things, blessed are you if you do them."

It is noteworthy that Jesus did not just talk about what to do; that is, he showed his disciples in his own actions what they should do.

The Bible includes many examples of Jesus wanting to serve first, rather than wanting to be in power. Recall that this is the ideal attribute of a servant leader. Although the people were really hoping for a dominant king, what they needed was a leader who would come to serve them. What an amazing example Jesus gives all of us who aspire to be servant leaders.

Jesus: A Servant Leader

A full discussion of how Jesus demonstrated the 10 attributes of servant as leader described earlier in the chapter would be too lengthy to fit within these pages. Therefore, a few examples of how Jesus exuded the servant as leader characteristics will have to suffice.

Jesus was an excellent listener. He would listen intently to what was being verbalized but could also read spiritual and nonverbal communication. Jesus had the ability to listen to the heart and one's intention of the spoken word, which allowed him to understand in a supernatural way. The best example of this might be in Mark, Chapter 2, when Jesus not only forgave the sins of the paralytic who was lowered through the roof top by his friends but also healed his physical deformity so that he could take up his bed and walk. In Mark 2:8, Jesus knew that some in the crowd were doubting him in their hearts; he did not have to hear them say the words. In Mark 2:10–12, Jesus revealed through the healing that he had the authority on earth to forgive sins.

Jesus was also an expert communicator, speaking in parables and stories that his followers could understand and find relatable to their current situations. In this manner, his communications became relevant and applicable to those whom he was teaching. The crowds were amazed by Jesus's ability to teach others in this tangible and meaningful way. The Bible provides several instances in which Jesus used parables, or stories, to teach the people the Word of God. He had a unique way of knowing how to reach those around him.

Nurses are called to be excellent communicators, teachers, and listeners, just like Jesus. When nurse leaders want to serve first, they will naturally gravitate toward listening to be able to fully understand what is necessary for service to take place. Tuning into each follower, nurse leaders can "read" their followers, watching for nonverbal cues and behaviors as well as monitoring verbal expressions. When nurse leaders really listen, they also hear and comprehend each follower's needs so as to tailor the service necessary to lead.

Each time Jesus performed a miracle, one could argue that he first had compassion, which requires empathy. He loved his followers and felt the pain or struggle that they were feeling, which compelled him to serve them through each miracle he performed. The nurse leader who is empathetic like Jesus is not fearful of assessing followers' fears and doubts. Understanding through listening and then committing oneself to be empathetic can be risky. However, the nurse leader who strives to be a servant leader might consider the love of Jesus for his followers, and the love of God for each of us as He sent Jesus to earth for our benefit.

Jesus was the ultimate healer. So many biblical examples of the healing power of Jesus might be cited that it seems unfair to mention only one. Each physical healing of Jesus was powerful and undeniable by those who witnessed and later wrote about the incidents in the text of the Bible. Indeed, John 21:25 states that Jesus did so many miraculous things that "if every one of them were written down, the whole world would not have enough room for the books that would be written." Although the New Testament writers provide substantial proof of Jesus's healing power, it is quite humbling to think about all of the additional, miraculous things Jesus was able to do for those he served during his time of ministry.

As nurse leaders, we also need to consider each day to be a miraculous beginning from which we can be the hands and feet of Jesus. Being in tune with Jesus through reading scripture and engaging in quiet prayer time each day can allow us to listen to the will of God for ourselves and those we are leading. James 1:5 states, "If any of you lacks wisdom, you should ask God, who gives generously to all without finding fault, and it will be given to you." One of the great promises that Jesus makes in John 14:16–17 is to send the spirit of truth to be our advocate. All we need to do is ask God for guidance and wisdom, then take the time to listen for the solutions and actions to each issue or problem we face as leaders.

Nightingale: A Servant Leader

Another excellent example of a servant leader who must be mentioned in the history and profession of nursing is Florence Nightingale. Known for her efforts to establish nursing as a profession built on statistical evidence, Nightingale has become the epitome of nursing's promise. Nightingale's work in nursing began with a personal calling by God to care for others (Nightingale & Barnum, 1992). In fact, she believed that "the highest honor is to be God's servant and fellow worker" (p. 4). Nightingale's personal calling to help others in their suffering and her use of the word "servant" in her writings fit the description of servant as leader. Nightingale did not aspire to be a leader; instead, she aspired to serve her fellow human. She was driven throughout her life by an intense commitment to help humanity.

Nightingale was born on May 12, 1820, and grew up in England (Nightingale & Barnum, 1992). During this era, it was highly unusual for a woman to be as educated as Nightingale was, and even more unusual for a woman to pass up marriage and social status in exchange for nursing and serving others. Educated primarily by her father, Nightingale was a brilliant statistician: She applied statistical concepts to demonstrate the need for improvement in health care and sanitation in many different instances. Perhaps the most well-known example involves Nightingale's work in the Crimean War, where she was responsible for significantly decreasing the mortality rate in the army hospital and improving the sanitation and care practices.

Like Jesus, Nightingale was an incredible communicator. She was not only an expert at the spoken word but also used written letters and her statistical analyses to describe the current conditions and relay the need for improvements in care to decrease mortality and morbidity rates among those she served. She used awareness and persuasion to educate those in power to listen to her ideas for improvement of patient care. Nightingale was a visionary, with the ability to conceptualize how things could be and should be, rather than how they were. In her service, she built stronger and healthier communities, and left the legacy of the Nightingale School of Nursing to teach others how to serve in the same ways. When reviewing her wonderful accomplishments in the profession of nursing, however, we must not forget that she was motivated by empathy, compassion, and a desire to serve. Nightingale is an exquisite example of servant as leader in the nursing profession. Each nurse is encouraged to read her *Notes on Nursing* and contemplate the accomplishments of Florence Nightingale in context of the time period and culture in which she lived (Nightingale & Barnum, 1992).

Being a servant as leader is a high calling, and one that should not be taken lightly. To fully fit the description of servant as leader, one must have an innate passion to serve others. There is an iterative process in developing as a servant leader, a process that takes time and commitment as well as patience and diligence. The servant as leader model is a wonderful reflection of the attributes of our Lord and Savior as well as the historical foundations of nursing.

▶ The Roles of Leader and Manager

You might think that being a leader means being a manager, or vice versa. However, there are differences and similarities between the role of leader and manager. Management involves a set of processes and tasks such as planning shifts and staffing, making schedules, measuring professional performance, and solving problems (Garcia-Sierra & Fernandez-Castro, 2018). Leadership, by contrast, focuses on taking an organization into the future, finding and exploiting new opportunities for improvement for an organization, and finding and promoting a vision to those who work within the organization (Garcia-Sierra & Fernandez-Castro, 2018). A successful leader is able to provide a vision and empower followers to assimilate with that vision for improvement of the organization and movement toward future goals. Can a nurse be both a leader and a manager? The answer is yes, if the nurse is multitalented and well developed in both roles. Even so, many nurse leaders are not great managers, and some great nurse managers are not good leaders.

▶ The Follower

A follower, in the nursing context, is a person who is under leadership of the nurse leader. If the nurse leader is the chief nursing executive, then all of the nurses who work in that particular facility would be considered followers.

The idea of being a follower might not seem very glamorous or exciting, but being a follower is an important part of the leadership dynamic. A leader may be very skilled and have excellent abilities, but if he or she has no followers, the role is useless. Followers and leaders who work together and support, motivate, and believe in one another have the most success (Raso, 2017). No leader works alone to accomplish organizational goals. Instead, a team, with the leader providing the motivation and direction, is needed to get the work at hand done in an effective and timely manner.

What makes a good follower? Becoming a good follower entails more than blindly being led by another who is in a position of power. The best followers are loyal, but also think for themselves and feel comfortable with well-informed and productive questioning geared toward achieving the goal of understanding their role and how they fit into the organizational goals (Raso, 2017). "Following" may not be the best word to describe how each person becomes a part of the functioning team—"active following" might be a more descriptive term. The active follower is engaged and competent, truthful and productive, motivated and energetic. It is the nurse on the team who is constantly thinking about how to improve patient care outcomes, make everyone's job easier, and make the organization's systems work well and be effective. As previously mentioned in the chapter, nurses take part in providing leadership in each position that they hold in nursing. Active followers show their own leadership skills by working with the leadership to improve the goals and plans to make their organization the best it can be. Another term that might be used to describe this type of follower is **team player**: A team player is known for selfless work or giving up his or her own glory to achieve the best outcome for the team as a whole.

Perhaps the best perspective on followership can be found in the Bible in 1 Corinthians 12:12–27 (American Standard Version [ASV]). Paul reminds us in this set of verses that we are all working together, much like the parts of the human body:

> [12]There is but one body, but it has many parts. But all its many parts make up one body. It is the same with Christ. [13]We were all baptized by one Holy Spirit. And so we are formed into one body. It didn't matter whether we were Jews or Gentiles, slaves or free people. We were all given the same Spirit to drink. [14]So the body is not made up of just one part. It has many parts. [15]Suppose the foot says, "I am not a hand, So I don't belong to the body." By

saying this, it cannot stop being part of the body. [16]And suppose the ear says, I am not an eye. So I don't belong to the body. By saying this, it cannot stop being part of the body. [17]If the whole body were an eye, how could it hear? If the whole body were an ear, how could it smell? [18]God has placed each part in the body just as he wanted it to be. [19]If all the parts are the same, how could there be a body? [20]As it is, there are many parts, But there is only one body.

In this amazing piece of scripture, Paul teaches that each person is a part of the greater whole. In the same way, each nurse has a specific role that is essential in helping the entire organization function and carry out the goals of its existence. Being an active follower is about taking an energetic and engaged approach to your work in your current role. It is also about understanding a collective goal and doing your part to reach that goal.

▶ Nursing Leadership Principles Within an Ecological Framework

As previously discussed, nurses take on different leadership roles at different times in their lives. At any given time, nurses may also have the opportunity to convey leadership qualities within different contexts on a daily basis. For this discussion, an ecological framework will be employed as a method to categorize these contexts. This ecological framework was first described by Urie Bronfenbrenner (1977) as a framework for child development but has since been used in numerous contexts and in countless research studies as a framework to understand the layers of influence within our society. Bronfenbrenner theorized that a child exists in, and therefore is influenced by, different ecosystems in which he or she is enmeshed (**FIGURE 21-1**). Thus, the child is "nested" within the different ecosystems, which all affect the

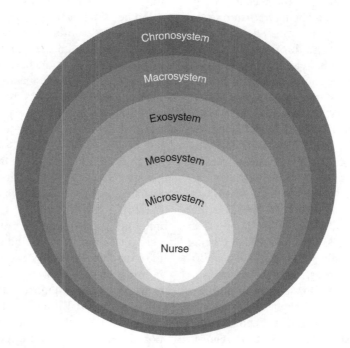

FIGURE 21-1 Ecological systems model.

outcome of human development. Although Bronfenbrenner's theory was first used for the conceptualization of human development, it can be a helpful framework for considering how each individual exists within and interacts with different ecosystems.

As seen in Figure 21-1, each nurse is first influenced by the microsystem. The microsystem comprises the home environment—how the nurse was raised, and the experiences and the ways the nurse engages with the home environment. As examples, consider a nurse who is 25 years of age, is single, and lives alone in an apartment versus a 45-year-old nurse who is married, has three children, and lives in the suburbs in a large house. No matter what the microsystem, each nurse has the opportunity to be a leader in his or her own personal world. We can show leadership qualities in our own health, our home, and our habits.

One very important aspect of leadership on a personal level is taking control of one's own health. Each nurse has specialized knowledge about how to be healthy, what nutrition his or her body needs, and the need for engaging in daily exercise and being free from stress. Too many nurses become stressed and in danger of being unhealthy during their careers. We must consider the "care of the caregiver" lessons that we teach to patients' families, which essentially state that we cannot take care of anyone if we are ourselves unhealthy. If we want to be the best nurses we can be, our work starts with keeping ourselves healthy. For many nurses or aspiring nurses, this might seem like a selfish suggestion. How can servants put themselves before those whom they wish to serve? But consider the problems that arise when the unhealthy nurse attempts to do service work. When we envision being healthy, we typically think about the physical body—but we must also pay attention to our spiritual health. Our leadership and service, much like that of Nightingale, may be most successful when they are connected to our Heavenly Father. Spending time spent in prayer, reading the Bible, and seeking spiritual

growth through Bible studies are some ways nurses can foster their spiritual connection and maintain spiritual health.

While nurses are affected by their environment and those persons in their microsystem, they also have a direct influence on those individuals in their microsystem. Using their nursing knowledge and ability to serve those within their microsystem, nurses can show leadership qualities by being a good example in their own lives. Using the characteristics of a servant leader, nurses can choose to serve those with whom they are in direct contact at home first. The microsystem is where nurse leaders can practice and hone their skills in leadership, so that they can later apply them in the greater ecosystems to which they will be exposed.

The next system in the ecological framework is the mesosystem. This is where nurses experience their different microsystems interacting a little more with the world around them. School, work, peer groups, and church are some examples. A nurse can work on many leadership characteristics in these types of settings. Perhaps a nurse is working hard to develop her skills as a new graduate, and she is feeling more confident in her abilities. She volunteers to be on the quality improvement committee to work on her followership and leadership skills simultaneously. She may experience positive feedback from peers or superiors for her work, but it may also create more stress for her as she attempts to continue assimilating into her role as a bedside nurse while she works on the committee tasks. Ultimately, her leadership on the committee might lead to a change in the way patients are admitted to the unit, improving the workflow within the unit and improving nurse satisfaction among her peers. She might also find that her work on the committee provides her with much needed information about how to do her job and improves her work as a nurse at the bedside.

The exosystem includes institutional and organizational factors such as policies, regulations, and informal operating procedures within the larger institution ("Ecological Models,"

2018). For example, the nurse described previously may be affected by hospital policies that regulate the work of the quality improvement committee. In this case, the nurse may need to use communication, much like Nightingale, to speak about the changes needed on a unit, and how they would lead to improved working conditions or better patient care outcomes. Nurses who will be interacting with higher management in a large institution need to be very well prepared with evidence when bringing ideas and requests forward. Leadership is necessary in these types of instances.

The macrosystem extends even further from the individual nurse and includes cultural patterns and values as well as political and economic systems within the community. Nurses can provide leadership in the form of advocacy for their patients and their fellow nurses by becoming and staying politically active. Such political activity can occur at the local, state, and national levels. Many nurses may find politics intimidating but informing oneself about the policies is the beginning of changing the laws and systems that govern our work environments. Nurses possess specialty knowledge about health promotion and disease prevention that can be extremely beneficial to those in political positions and those making the laws. Becoming a member of professional organizations is a good starting point in this leadership endeavor, but really getting involved and understanding the macrosystem one lives in is more beneficial.

The chronosystem is the dimension of time and global environment in which the nurse's life occurs ("Ecological Models," 2018). What happens on a global level can impact an individual's health and environment. Nurses must stay informed about global issues in disease progression and treatments, health promotion, and disease prevention. The chronosystem may not be under our immediate control but being knowledgeable about what is happening in the chronosystem is essential to becoming a leader in nursing care for those whom we serve on a daily basis.

▶ Conclusion

Leadership in nursing is dynamic and ever-changing. It is challenging and exhausting, but it is also rewarding and fruitful. Much as nurses learn from their peers those skills and abilities needed to take care of patients and do their job more efficiently, so nurses must learn from the leaders to whom they are exposed (**BOXES 21-3** and **21-4**). Taking each

---

BOX 21-3 Outstanding Nurse Leader: Susan Wilhelm, PhD, RN

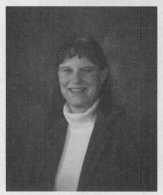

Dr. Susan Wilhelm has been the assistant dean of the Western Division of the University of Nebraska Medical Center College of Nursing for the past 13 years. Prior to assuming this prestigious leadership position, Wilhelm felt an early calling to be a nurse from a very young age. Growing up in a family full of brothers playing war, even her childhood play was focused on taking care of the imaginary wounded. Her original goal in nursing school was to become a pediatric nurse practitioner. Knowing that she would have to perform invasive procedures on pediatric patients who were fearful and upset made her realize that it would be a challenge for her emotions to do this work on a long-term basis. God had other plans for Wilhelm, who continued to hone her nursing skills in the float

(continues)

BOX 21-3 Outstanding Nurse Leader: Susan Wilhelm, PhD, RN *(continued)*

pool, where she was exposed to a variety of patients. She had a desire to serve her patients, and that meant getting to know more about each one. Unfortunately, the fast-paced medical–surgical nursing environment would not allow for this kind of care to take place. Ultimately, Wilhelm found that she enjoyed the challenge of helping patients through the pain and fear of labor on the obstetric floor.

One of Wilhelm's instructors encouraged her to obtain her master in nursing degree and teach. As this path became a goal for Wilhelm, she worked to complete first her master's degree and then her doctoral degree after her husband had finished his degrees to further his pastoral work. Throughout this process, she continued to work as a nurse and teach maternal–child nursing for more than 30 years. Wilhelm has a passion to teach others the art and profession of nursing. She still loves to teach nursing and has been flexible in learning the new technology of simulation to further student experiential learning. For the last seven years, she has been instrumental in implementing and developing a concept-based curriculum at the University of Nebraska Medical Center. She and her colleague are consultants and teach other nursing instructors about concept-based curriculum across the nation.

How did Wilhelm answer the call of God to be a nurse leader? When the assistant dean for the West Nebraska campus retired, she applied for the position. The local community college decided to add an associate degree program, which was in direct competition to her program. Since she had many contacts in nearby states, Wilhelm believed that she could recruit students from that area and keep the bachelor's degree in nursing (BSN) program thriving. Accepting this leadership position meant making a challenging transition, as Wilhelm had been a coworker of those whom she was leading for a number of years. However, she felt a peace about accepting the assistant dean position, one of the confirmatory signs that she was where God would want her for that place in time.

In this new role, Wilhelm practices from a servant as leader perspective, with the goal of giving her followers the benefit of the doubt and working hard to increase their job satisfaction and prevent burnout. In her position, she is accountable for recruitment and retention of qualified students in the traditional BSN and accelerated programs. She is also responsible for the quality of teaching on the campus and adherence to the curriculum and is the ambassador for the dean of the College of Nursing in her area of the state. Wilhelm is a member of the dean's team, the executive council, and the academic program team at the University of Nebraska Medical Center. Her official position is considered to be 50% administration and 50% faculty role.

Wilhelm considers one of her most important leadership positions to be her role as a pastor's wife. God called her husband to attend seminary and become a minister. She struggled with the fact that God did not call her to full-time service; however, she was informed that God called her to follow her husband's calling. When she accepted God's assignment, she was able to not only support her husband but also find her own mission field as a nurse instructor and leader. There are countless students and faculty whom Wilhelm has been able to quietly and humbly serve and minister to along the way. The impact on each and every person she has touched in this way cannot be understated. The caring and serving demeanor of Wilhelm is inspirational to others, who strive to be like her in their own mission fields.

As previously stated, Wilhelm believes in servant leadership. She matches this philosophy with a strong work ethic, which she considers a requirement for a strong leader. The most difficult part of being an effective leader is being able to contend with the problems that occur. Conflict is inevitable in a leadership position, and unresolved conflict never produces an optimal environment for either the leader or the followers. Wilhelm believes that nurses who are able to make tough decisions and not worry about all of the repercussions are likely to be good leaders. Many leaders and many nurses are "fixers," but not everyone wants to change. Wilhelm knows firsthand that waiting too long to deal with a conflict situation does not help solve conflict or help followers adapt to new paradigms. Sometimes a leader needs to make a tough decision, and sometimes not everyone on the team will agree.

Wilhelm's favorite Bible scriptures help her in her daily leadership role:

- 1 Peter 5:7: Casting all your cares upon him because he cares for you.
- Isaiah 26:3: He whose mind is stayed on you will have perfect peace.

In closing, Wilhelm offers the following advice to all nurses:

> God would have us all be servant leaders. Establishing positive working relationships is critical for success as a leader.

BOX 21-4   Outstanding Nurse Leader: Barbara White, EdD, RN, CNS

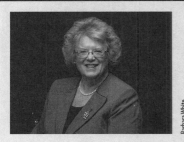
Barbara White

Dr. Barbara White came to Colorado Christian University in August 2007 to start the nursing program and has held the dean position there for more than 11 years. As founding dean, she has had the privilege of overseeing the development of the university's BSN, RN-to-BSN, MSN, and DNP nursing programs. As dean of the School of Nursing and Health Professions, she is responsible for the nursing, health sciences (biology), and healthcare administration programs. Her responsibilities are to provide vision, leadership, and oversight of all school programs and personnel, so as to ensure effective and efficient management of all matters related to academics. In collaboration with faculty members, she is also responsible for creating, directing, and supporting the integration of faith and the university's strategic priorities into the teaching–learning practices of each program. As the dean, White is also responsible for monitoring and maintenance of ongoing national program accreditation, annual program budgets, program curricula, assessment of student learning outcomes, and systematic program evaluation. She delegates, empowers, and promotes faculty and staff in their work for the university as well as serves as a role model for teaching, scholarship, service, professional development, and Christian ministry. In addition to all of these responsibilities, White is to be a leader in health care, with expert knowledge of the changing environment of health care locally, nationally, and globally. Her position requires expertise in professional trends and networks that impact current and future program development. As such, she is responsible for representing the nursing and health professions internally to the university and externally to the community at large.

As shared in her *Divine Appointment: Fulfilling Your Call* chapter in this book, White felt a specific call from God to be a nurse leader. She has held several leadership positions in her lengthy career including administrative director in a hospital-based school of nursing in the 1980s; chair and developer of various programs in the 1990s; chair of the Rocky Mountain Regional Council, Nurses Christian Fellowship (1991–2000); Fulbright Senior Scholar, Yonsei University College of Nursing, Seoul, Korea (2006–2007); president of the Nurses Christian Fellowship International (2008–2016); and chair of the board of directors of the Nurses Christian Fellowship International (2016 to the present).

(continues)

BOX 21-4   Outstanding Nurse Leader: Barbara White, EdD, RN, CNS   *(continued)*

White believes that all nurses have the potential to become great leaders. A nurse may lead from any position, as a person does not have to be in an official leadership role to have influence. But others will clearly see leadership traits in the person who is interested in becoming a leader. White shared four important characteristics that she believes make a leader effective in the profession of nursing:

- Vison: A clear picture of how things can be different and better in the future.
- Integrity: Being honest and trustworthy as a leader.
- Humility: Considering the needs of others before your own, a key aspect of servant as leader.
- Wisdom: Seeing things from God's perspective.
  When asked about the scripture that she refers to often in relationship to leadership, White chose the following:

- Mark 10:42–44, NIV: Jesus called them together and said, "You know that those who are regarded as rulers of the Gentiles lord it over them, and their high officials exercise authority over them. [43]Not so with you. Instead, whoever wants to become great among you must be your servant, [44]and whoever wants to be first must be slave of all."
- Esther 4:14, NIV: And who knows but that you have come to your royal position for such a time as this?
- Jeremiah 29:11, NIV: [11]"For I know the plans I have for you," declares the Lord, "plans to prosper you and not to harm you, plans to give you hope and a future."
- Proverbs 3:5–6, NIV: Trust in the Lord with all your heart and lean not on your own understanding; [6]in all your ways submit to him, and he will make your paths straight. [Some versions say "direct your paths."]
- Ephesians 2:10, NIV: For we are God's handiwork, created in Christ Jesus to do good works, which God prepared in advance for us to do.

In closing, White shared her belief that being a Christian leader is being a leader like Jesus, a servant to others. Robert Greenleaf, in his book *The Servant as Leader*, describes it best in contemporary language: The servant leader is servant first. Becoming a servant leader begins with the natural feeling that one wants to serve first. Then a conscious choice brings one to aspire to lead. The best test is this: Do those served grow as persons? Do they, while being served, become healthier, wiser, freer, more autonomous, more likely themselves to become servants? White would like those who aspire to be nurse leaders to know that God's timing is always perfect. He is a God of economy and He uses everything in our lives to prepare us for what He has in store for us next. Everything in our lives is filtered through the hands of God.

---

skill that is positive and remembering the negative aspects of these leaders can help each individual nurse form his or her own leadership style. The question is not whether a nurse aspires to be a leader, but rather how he or she will choose to lead others as the nurse's career develops. Keeping spiritually and physically healthy and remembering the characteristics of a servant as leader, we can all aspire to be leaders in nursing.

▶ Clinical Reasoning Exercises

Karie has been working successfully as a nurse in the same institution for the last 15 years. She is a great nurse, is always on time, is responsible, and cares for her patients and fellow coworkers. She is a work colleague of yours, and you have grown to respect her and the work she does each day. Karie took a leadership role as charge nurse for the last year but found that it took her away from the nursing work at the bedside that she loved far too often. She mentioned to you that she is better at caring for patients then "staffing and putting out fires." You heard that Karie decided to step down from the charge nurse position in favor of resuming her staff nurse position. She was up for a big pay raise at work, as she has met the years in service criteria. She also shared with you that she has received 5 out of 5 on all of her evaluation goals by the nurse manager.

You go to work one morning to find the staff nurse talking quietly during report about what has happened to Karie. When you ask, they tell you that Karie was not given her raise and is being reprimanded by the current charge nurse for things that she did not do. It is a well-known fact that Karie is an excellent nurse and coworker, so there are many questions about how the manager is treating her and what the staff should do about it.

Later in the same week, you find out that Karie asked to be transferred to the surgical unit, where she would be in charge of the patient and family education. The job would have been a step up in the career ladder for Karie, and she would have also received a large pay increase. The current nurse manager called the manager of the surgical unit and prevented Karie from getting the position, even though she was the only person who applied and she was highly favored by the surgical unit staff and management.

1. From this scenario, what has occurred that you are concerned about, if anything?
2. Do you believe that anyone has behaved in an unprofessional or unethical manner? Why or why not?
3. When the leader in your institution is not behaving ethically and you have evidence of this fact, what should you do?
4. What aspects of leadership would you be showing by the actions you have described?

5. Have you experienced any unethical or questionable practices by leadership in your work or personal experiences? If so, please share with the group and discuss your actions or inactions.

▶ Personal Reflection Exercises

Consider a nurse leader to whom you have had exposure through your nursing career or nursing education experiences and answer the following questions:

1. What type of leadership style did this leader have? What are some of the leader's actions that made you choose this leadership style?
2. What did you appreciate about this leader?
3. What things did this leader not do well? How could the leader have improved his or her leadership?
4. Describe how you followed this leader. How were you successful and not so successful in your following?
5. How will you use the information you've reflected on in this section as you approach leadership in nursing in your own career? What type of leader would you strive to be and why?

References

American Nurses Association. (2018). ANA leadership competency model. Retrieved from https://www.nursingworld.org/~4a0a2e/globalassets/docs/ce/177626-ana-leadership-booklet-new-final.pdf

Atkinson, S. M. (2011). Are you a transformational leader? *Nursing Management, 42*(9), 44–40.

Bass, B., & Avolio, B. (1995). *Multifactor leadership questionnaire (MLQ)* (2nd ed.). Redwood City, CA: Mindgarden.

Bronfenbrenner, U. (1977). Toward and experimental ecology of human development. *American Psychologist, 32*(7), 513–531.

Cherry, K. (2018). Leadership styles and frameworks you should know. Retrieved from https://www.verywell mind.com/leadership-styles-2795312

Ecological models. (2018). *Rural Health Information Hub*. Definition of "autocratic leadership." (2018). *The Economic Times*. Retrieved from https://economictimes .indiatimes.com/definition/autocratic-leadership

Ecological models. (2018). *Rural Health Information Hub*. Retrieved from https://www.ruralhealthinfo.org/tool kits/health-promotion/2/theories-and-models /ecological

Garcia-Sierra, R., & Fernandez-Castro, J. (2018). Relationships between leadership, structural empowerment, and engagement in nurses. *Journal of Advanced Nursing, 74*, 2809–2819.

Greenleaf, R. K., & Spears, L. C. (1998). *The power of servant leadership*. San Francisco, CA: Berrett-Koehler.

Manning, J. (2016). The influence of nurse manager leadership style on staff nurse work engagement. *Journal of Nursing Administration, 46*(9), 438–443.

Nightingale, F., & Barnum, B. S. (1992). *Notes on nursing: What it is and what it is not* (commemorative ed.). Philadelphia, PA: Lippincott Williams and Wilkins.

Raso, R. (2017). In favor of followership. *Nursing Management, 48*(10), 6.

Robert K. Greenleaf Center for Servant Leadership. (n.d.). Homepage. Retrieved from https://www.greenleaf.org/

Willis, S., Clarke, S., & O'Connor, E. (2017). Contextualizing leadership: Transformational leadership and management-by-exception-active in safety-critical contexts. *Journal of Occupational and Organizational Psychology, 90*, 281–305.

Coeling, H. V., Chiang-Hanisko, L., & Thompson, M. (2011). Living out our values: The legacy of Christian academic nursing leadership. *Journal of Christian Nursing, 28*(1), 24–30. doi:10.1097/CNJ .0b013e3181fe3288

Fahlberg, B., & Toomey, R. (2016). Servant leadership: A model for emerging nurse leaders. *Nursing, 46*(10), 49–52. doi:10.1097/01.NURSE.0000494644.77680.2a

Hughes, V. (2018). Authentic leadership: Practices to promote integrity. *Journal of Christian Nursing, 35*(2), E28–E31. doi:10.1097/CNJ.0000000000000491

Jeffs, L. (2018). Moving beyond the quality and safety quagmire: Collective wisdom from nurse leaders. *Nursing Leadership, 31*(4), 32–39C.

Murray, M., Sundin, D., & Cope, V. (2017). The nexus of nursing leadership and a culture of safer patient care. *Journal of Clinical Nursing, 27*, 1287–1293.

Olvera, L., Hunt, K., Johnson, K., & Li, S. Y. (2018). The APRN as servant leader. *Journal of Christian Nursing, 35*(1), 13. doi:10.1097CNJ.0000000000000457

Parris, D. L., & Peachey, J. W. (2013). A systematic literature review of servant leadership theory in organizational context. *Journal of Business Ethics, 113*(3), 377–393. doi:10.1007/s10551-012-1322-6

Robinson, F. P. (2018). Leading from the heart: It's okay to want to be liked. *Nurse Leader, 16*(6), 414–417.

Shaughnessy, M. K., Quinn Griffin, M. T., Bhattacharya, A., & Fitzpatrick, J. J. (2018). Transformational leadership practices and work engagement among nurse leaders. *Journal of Nursing Administration, 18*(11), 574–579. doi:10.1097/NNA.0000000000000682

Recommended Readings

Akerjordet, K., Furunes, T., & Haver, A. (2018). Health-promoting leadership: An integrative review and future research agenda. *Journal of Advanced Nursing, 74*, 1505–1516.

Glossary

A

ADPIE A model that includes five steps: assess, diagnose, plan, implement, and evaluate.

Advance care planning A conversation with patient and family members that seeks to understand their values and goals regarding end-of-life care and medical interventions, and that is documented to be prepared for the time when the patient can no longer communicate.

Advance directives Spoken and written instructions about future medical care and treatment; legal documents outlining a person's wishes for medical treatments to be (or not to be) provided at some point in the future, at a time the individual is not able to verbalize or make his or her wishes known.

Agape God's self-sacrificial love.

Agape Model A tool that describes the development and the character of a nurse who is dedicated to Christ.

Alcohol use disorder (AUD) A severe problem with drinking alcohol, characterized by excessive alcohol use, lack of control over drinking habits, and negativity when not using alcohol.

Assistive technology A mechanical aid that can support or improve a physical or mental impairment.

Attributes Qualities, character, or characteristics ascribed to someone or something.

Awareness Perception of a situation.

B

Bibliotherapy The use of literature or spiritual readings to support mental or spiritual health.

Bullying Unwanted actions that cause harm and distress to another person; can include degrading remarks, hostility, verbal attacks, threats, and intimidation.

Burnout Emotional exhaustion to the point that an individual becomes desensitized, or numb, to emotion. Burnout is inherent in the nature of the nursing job and can affect anyone, regardless of whether his or her primary responsibility is to care for others.

C

Called to care The assertion that nursing is a vocation, giving nurses a framework for understanding their mission and living out their calling service to God through caring for others.

Calling The life focus to which God calls a believer in ministry or vocation.

Cannabidiol (CBD) A major cannabinoid that indirectly antagonizes cannabinoid receptors, which may attenuate the psychoactive effects of tetrahydrocannabinol.

Cannabinoids Any chemical compound that acts on cannabinoid receptors; includes both endogenous and exogenous cannabinoids.

Cannabis Any raw preparation of the leaves or flowers from the plant genus *Cannabis*; a shorthand term that also includes cannabinoids.

Caring Those values held by an individual, which are influenced by his or her worldview, and are reflected in caring behaviors.

Caritas Christian love; caring.

Christian-based leader A person in a leadership position who uses Biblical principles and a Biblical worldview in his or her daily tasks and activities.

Christian nursing Nursing as ministry from a biblical worldview that aims to promote optimum health and comfort to the whole person.

Christian worldview (of nursing) A nurse's approach to care that is rooted in the characteristics of Christ.

Civility A behavior characterized by sincere respect for others with intent to foster clear communication and discourse.

Compassion The emotional investment in one's situation.

Compassion fatigue Consistent exposure to emotionally straining situations that affect a person's physical, mental, emotional, and spiritual state and eventually decrease the individual's compassion over time. Individuals at risk for compassion fatigue are those who care for people, whether it is a job, an assigned position, a divine calling, or a good deed.

Compassion satisfaction The positive pleasure, sense of fulfillment, or gratification a person receives from helping others.

Correctional forensic nursing A nursing specialty related to care of those in jail, prison, or juvenile detention.

Creation God-made earth, beings, animals, and man; God's handiwork.

Crisis poverty Poverty due to a sudden loss of income or possessions. This loss can be the result of fire, tornado, hurricane, or some other natural disaster, or it can be the result of an accident or injury making it so the individual or family suddenly do not have the resources to cover their food, shelter, and/or medical expenses.

D

Debriefing A careful review of information upon completion of a task or incident.

Delta-9-tetrahydrocannabinol (THC) One of many cannabinoids found in cannabis, which is believed to be responsible for most of the characteristic psychoactive effects of cannabis.

Dementia Progressive neurodegeneration that is irreversible, negatively affecting memory, learning, and mood.

Deployment The action of bringing resources into effective action.

Disaster A sudden event, such as an accident or a natural catastrophe, that causes great damage or loss of life.

Displacement The forced departure of people from their homes, typically because of war, persecution, or natural disaster.

Distributive justice Allocating scarce resources fairly; it involves evaluating situations and using ethical concepts to determine how to divide and allocate scarce resources.

Divine appointment A time when God clearly speaks and moves one toward fulfilling one's calling through otherwise unexplainable circumstances.

Divine monergism The concept that God is sole power and cause.

E

Ecological framework The interaction between, and interdependence of, factors within and across all levels of a health problem. It highlights people's interactions with their physical and sociocultural environments.

Elder abuse A situation in which a caregiver or trusted person causes psychological or physical harm by their intentional or negligent treatment of a person older than age 65.

Empathy A sense of closeness, understanding, and sensitivity toward the emotions of another person.

Environment The complex conglomeration of internal and external factors that influence health.

Eschatology A branch of theology related to the end of the world or of humankind.

Evaluation The stage of the nursing process/care plan defined as examining the effectiveness of the plan of care related to established nursing goals and revising the approach as needed.

F

Florence Nightingale The mother or founder of nursing.

Follower A person who is part of the team and being led by a designated leader.

Forgiveness Not being held accountable for one's sins. Forgiveness comes from our Heavenly Father, who sent His Son to die on the cross for our sins.

Fruit of the Spirit Given by God to believers through the indwelling Holy Spirit. With a transformed life, the believer reflects Christ's character in actions, attitudes, behaviors, and thoughts, as an extension of the love of Christ. Includes love, joy, peace, patience, kindness, goodness, faithfulness, gentleness, and self-control.

G

Generational poverty Poverty that is passed down from parents to children to grandchildren, often as a result of learned behavior as well as a lack of resources to pull out of the cycle of poverty.

God-man The concept that Christ is fully God and fully man in one person.

Good death A death that is free from avoidable distress and suffering, according to patient/family wishes, and consistent with clinical, cultural, and ethical standards.

Grace The saving gift of God through faith and not works; undeserved favor.

Guided imagery A focused relaxation technique that embraces the mind and imagination by thinking of peaceful images as a form of mental escape, creating harmony between the mind and body.

H

Health The person's own perception of his or her state on a wellness–illness continuum.

History Things occurring in the past.

Holy Spirit The third person of the Trinity; Father, Son, and Holy Ghost (Spirit). He guides us, protects us, teaches us, and strengthens us.

Homelessness As defined by the Department of Housing and Urban Development, the lack of a fixed, regular, and adequate nighttime residence.

Hospice care A program to deliver palliative care to individuals in the last stages of a terminal illness; it also provides personal support and care to the patient, support to the patient's family/caregivers while the patient is dying, and offers bereavement support after the patient's death.

I

Image of Christ The righteousness and life of Christ in and through the Christian.

Imago Dei Created in the image and likeness of God.

Incarcerated The state of detained in a facility for crimes committed.

Incivility Being rude, discourteous, disrespectful, or uncivil.

J

Jails Short-term detention facilities, usually run by the county or local authorities.

L

Lateral (horizontal) violence Negative, hostile, or aggressive behavior by an individual or group towards a member or members of the same larger group (for example: nurse to nurse).

Leader In nursing, a person who is able to use experience and available evidence to guide and inspire fellow nurses toward the collective goal of providing best nursing practice for optimal patient and family outcomes.

Leadership style A general description of how a person in a leadership position completes his or her daily tasks.

M

Malnutrition Insufficient energy intake, resulting in weight loss from a combined loss of muscle mass and fat, leading to weakness and decreased functional capacity.

Marijuana A cultivated cannabis plant, whether for recreational or medicinal use.

Meaning The goal or purpose of life; that which gives life value.

Medical marijuana programs (MMPs) The official jurisdictional resource for the use of cannabis for medical purposes.

Mentee A person who is being mentored; a protégé.

Mentor A trusted counselor or guide; a tutor or coach.

Mindfulness Cognizance of self, surroundings, and situation.

Models A framework or blueprint, although not an entire theory, to guide nursing practice in a specific area, domain, or curriculum; it often appears in the form of a figure or diagram.

N

Neighborhood poverty A state in which a neighborhood consists of several families living in persistent poverty. Homes may become rundown because of insufficient funds to maintain the home or landlords who are unresponsive to calls to maintain the home. Because of psychosocial factors, such neighborhoods can become unsafe.

Nurse A professional who is educated to provide expert care to persons across the lifespan and health continuum.

Nursing as ministry To serve God and others as Jesus did, as He is our example. The unique calling of the Christian nurse is the realization that one is gifted by God for a specific nursing practice to make a significant difference in the world. Nursing as ministry encompasses compassionate care and is directed by the nurse's faith, which shapes the understanding of roles, privileges, and responsibilities within practice and health care.

Nursing process/care plan A process used by nurses to direct the care of patients. It consists of five stages: assessment, diagnosis, planning, implementation, and evaluation. A systematic approach the nurse develops and implements in order to provide focused patient/client-centered care.

O

Objective The way that something is, apart from any person or any bias. Something is objectively the case if it is accurate apart from any personal experience.

Objective gospel The fact that Christ won salvation for all (the good news for all people).

Original (hereditary) sin Spiritual disease residing in the heart of all people that brings sinning and death.

P

Palliative care A concept of medical care designed to promote comfort and holistic management of symptoms at any stage of illness or disease.

Patient/client In some facilities (e.g., hospitals), the term for the person being cared for. In other facilities (e.g., nursing homes, assisted living, home care), this person may be referred to as a client or resident.

Patient driven The patient is at the center of medical decision making; care is based on the patient's preferences as opposed to the clinician's decisions about what is best for the patient.

Person (personhood) The individual, family, group, or population receiving care.

Polypharmacy The use of five or more prescription medications daily.

Post-hospital syndrome (PHS) The increased vulnerability of hospitalized patients to many other adverse health events.

Poverty A matter of perspective, but traditionally thought of as a lack of resources to cover the cost of food, clothing, housing, utilities, health care, and other necessities. Those who grow up with very little may not consider themselves poor if all of their friends and classmates are in the same financial condition.

Prayer Communication with God requesting strength of spirit, guidance, wisdom, knowledge, discernment, boldness, and/or any other petition in line with Biblical teachings. Important elements of prayer include forgiveness, faith, trust, thanksgiving, praise, and requests for spiritual, emotional, and physical needs of self and on behalf of others.

Praying circles Based on the legend of Honi the Circle Maker, a strategy to pray around our biggest dreams and greatest fears to experience God's divine appointments and see His hand in our work.

Presbycusis Progressive hearing loss due to age-related changes, which negatively impacts communication ability, leading to social stress, family frustration, and a decreased perception of quality of life.

Presbyopia An inability of the eyes to focus or accommodate appropriately, causing a heavy negative impact on independence and activities of daily living.

Presence The therapeutic use of self to bring comfort to those who are hurt or grieving, just by being there.

Prioritization The action or process of deciding the relative importance or urgency of a thing or things.

Prison A longer-term detention facility that houses persons convicted of crimes; usually run by the state.

Prisoner An inmate who resides in a prison facility.

Professional nursing The roles and processes that the nurse engages in to promote health, prevent disease, treat illness, encourage rehabilitation, and manage the environment in the person.

Professional spiritual assessment An in-depth assessment of spiritual beliefs, values, and needs that is conducted by a spiritual care provider (preferably a board-certified chaplain) who is trained in dealing with spiritual issues related to death and illness.

R

Resilience The development of strategies and techniques to prevent compassion fatigue and burnout. A nurse's ability to recover from a difficult situation that leads to compassion fatigue or burnout.

S

Saline Process A framework for living as a witness. As is indicated by the name, witnesses are encouraged to be like saline—a specific solution of salt and water that sustains life. This analogy emphasizes how it is important for witnesses to balance God's love and truth in their interactions with others.

Scholar A critical thinker who is intelligent, wise, and profound. Scholars take action based on evidence, reflect on their behavior by seeking feedback from others, and engage others in thoughtful discourse. A scholar renews the mind by thinking on those things that bring peace and harmony to the team.

Secondary traumatic stress Indirect exposure to stressful or traumatic situations that causes physical, behavioral, professional, or spiritual symptoms.

Self-aware Having an unbiased, conscious knowledge of a person's emotional strengths and weaknesses. This includes an understanding of your feelings, motives, desires, character, thoughts, and beliefs in response to a situation.

Self-care A personalized, intentional, and deliberate plan to renew an individual's mind, body, and soul.

Self-neglect A situation in which an elderly person has impairments that cause him or her to be unable to meet basic needs or perform personal care.

Servant A devoted person towards others; a devoted follower.

Servant as leader (servant leadership) A philosophy and set of practices that enrich the lives of individuals, build better organizations, and ultimately create a more just and caring world. One who serves others first, yet inspires others as a leader.

Service Helping others without receiving anything in return.

Shalom God's perfect healing in mind, spirit, and body.

Shepherd A person who nurtures enduring trusting relationships with team members. In the relationship model of shepherd leadership, the shepherd leader is available, committed, and trustworthy, providing direction, correction, mentoring, and safety. Shepherds enable others on the team to act with success and encourage the heart of team members.

SMART Nursing goals for patients that are specific, measurable, achievable, relevant, and timely.

Social justice Advocating that all persons have worth and should be treated fairly. Social justice may require changes in social structures, policies, and laws that marginalize, exclude, and/or exploit vulnerable social groups.

Social poverty A lack of social support and the loss of resources upon whom to call in times of need. The elderly experience social poverty when they become isolated as family members move away and friends die. Young people can experience this phenomenon when they move away from their extended family and friends due to job, college, or a relationship.

Spiritual assessment A collaborative process to assess for the presence of spiritual distress or other spiritual needs or resources. It typically includes the following spiritual care methods or inquiry: spiritual screen, spiritual history, and professional spiritual assessment with different healthcare providers engaged in different methods based on time and spiritual expertise.

Spiritual barriers A condition that gets in the way of someone meeting Jesus.

Spiritual Care Implementation Model An interdisciplinary model for spiritual care that outlines the spiritual assessment process, spiritual care methods of inquiry, and the individuals responsible for obtaining data for each respective method.

Spiritual care methods of inquiry The different ways in which spirituality can be assessed; they include spiritual screening, spiritual history, and professional spiritual assessment.

Spiritual care plan A systematic approach that the nurse develops to help provide care, support, and interventions for the body, soul, mind, and spirit of the patient/client.

Spiritual care provider A person trained in dealing with spiritual issues associated with illness and dying; includes chaplains, religious leaders, spiritual care counselors or directors, pastors, and faith community nurses or providers.

Spiritual distress An approved nursing diagnosis of NANDA International (NANDA-I) related to the impaired ability to find meaning and purpose in life that has the potential to impact the patient's health, healing, and well-being.

Spiritual gifts Individual specialized gifts and abilities given by God through the Holy Spirit to believers in Christ, useful in furthering His Kingdom on earth by serving and equipping others. They include apostleship, prophecy, evangelism, shepherding, teaching, serving, exhortation, giving, giving aid, compassion, healing, working miracles, tongues, interpretation of tongues, wisdom, knowledge, faith, discernment, helps, and administration.

Spiritual history A set of health history questions that are used by healthcare providers as part of a comprehensive hospital history and physical examination or a complete health history during an annual or new patient visit to elicit information related to spiritual values, needs, and preferences that have the potential to impact care and individuals' healthcare decisions.

Spiritual journey The process that occurs over time as someone who does not have a relationship with Jesus moves closer (or further away) from coming into relationship with him.

Spiritual poverty A sense of hopelessness, or a lack of meaning or purpose in life. An individual may not be able to sense love and forgiveness and may become acutely aware of the emptiness that comes with a lack of relationship with God.

Spiritual screen A set of one or two questions aimed at quickly screening the patient for the presence of spiritual distress or immediate needs for which a chaplaincy referral should be made.

Spiritual vitality A measurement of spiritual health indicative of one's connection to God and one's level of empowerment to express God's character.

Steward A person who manages the property, finances, resources, and affairs of an organization. Good stewardship involves wisdom and discernment in allocating and managing the resources provided. Stewards view themselves as change agents and recognize patterns of behavior that become habits.

Subjective The manner in which persons know things about the world. Persons are "subjects" and therefore know things subjectively—that is, from their point of view.

Subjective faith Saving trust in the heart; personal faith.

Substance abuse disorders (SADs) Addiction to drugs or other substances that negatively affect the brain and one's behavior.

Substance use disorder (SUD) A life-affecting problem caused by the use of alcohol, prescription medications, or illicit drugs.

Sustainable relief Methods that empower an individual or a group of individuals to create solutions that are self-efficient.

T

Team player An individual known for selfless work or giving up his or her own glory to ensure the best outcome for the team as a whole.

Theory A framework from which to view practice, which identifies prepositions, assumptions, unique terms defined by the author, and relationships between concepts.

Therapeutic communication A purposeful verbal interaction between a healthcare provider and a patient with a goal of having meaningful dialogue that fosters understanding.

Transitional Care Model (TCM) An evidence-based, nurse-driven model that targets the elderly and seeks to reduce poor outcomes and cost as they move across settings.

Triage The assignment of degrees of urgency to wounds or illnesses to decide the order of treatment of a large number of patients or casualties.

U

Universal atonement Christ shed his blood to cover all sin of all people.

Universal truths Truths of the faith applicable to all people.

V

Vicarious satisfaction Christ as humanity's substitute on the cross.

Vocations Callings and stations in life.

Vulnerable elder An adult age 65 or older with multiple chronic comorbidities, which often interact, and atypical responses, which often slow or confuse the accuracy of health care.

W

Witness (noun) One who communicates (verbally or nonverbally) about a situation based on personal experience.

Working poor Individuals and families who remain as poor even though they have regular employment. The working poor may not be eligible for government aid or charity because their income slightly exceeds the federal poverty guidelines.

Worldview The interpretive matrix through which someone sees the world. Worldviews encompass fundamental beliefs relating to matters of ultimate concern, such as the meaning of life, creation, and morality.

Index

Note: Page numbers followed by *b*, *f*, and *t* denote boxes, figures, and tables.